Repair and Regeneration of Craniofacial Tissues and Organs

Repair and Regeneration of Craniofacial Tissues and Organs

Editor: Doug Hickman

AMERICAN
MEDICAL PUBLISHERS
www.americanmedicalpublishers.com

AMERICAN
MEDICAL PUBLISHERS
www.americanmedicalpublishers.com

Cataloging-in-Publication Data

Repair and regeneration of craniofacial tissues and organs / edited by Doug Hickman.
p. cm.
Includes bibliographical references and index.
ISBN 979-8-88740-432-5
1. Skull--Histology. 2. Facial bones--Histology. 3. Face--Histology. 4. Mouth--Histology. 5. Bone regeneration.
6. Regeneration (Biology). 7. Tissue engineering. I. Hickman, Doug.
RC936 .R47 2023
617.510 757 2--dc23

American Medical Publishers,
41 Flatbush Avenue,
1st Floor, New York,
NY 11217, USA

ISBN 979-8-88740-432-5 (Hardback)

Contents

Preface

The craniofacial complex encases the brain along with other organs for vital functions of the body, such as taste, mastication, vision, smell, breathing, hearing, and balance. The fusion, patterning, outgrowth and shaping tissues with heterogeneous developmental origins are necessary for craniofacial development. Mesenchymal stem cells (MSCs) have the potential to be used in the repair of craniofacial tissues, because these cells are adept at changing into cartilage, tendon, bone, muscle, and fat. Craniofacial bone reconstruction is significant when it comes to craniofacial repairs, because it provides support to nearby soft tissues. Furthermore, it provides anchorage for dental structures which guide facial appearance, as well as structural stability. The regeneration of craniofacial tissue and organs is possible using bio-ink along with various stem cells and biomaterials in 3D bio printers. This book unravels the recent studies on craniofacial tissues and organs. It aims to shed light on the processes of repair and regeneration of these tissues and organs. This book will help new researchers by foregrounding their knowledge in this area of study.

This book unites the global concepts and researches in an organized manner for a comprehensive understanding of the subject. It is a ripe text for all researchers, students, scientists or anyone else who is interested in acquiring a better knowledge of this dynamic field.

I extend my sincere thanks to the contributors for such eloquent research chapters. Finally, I thank my family for being a source of support and help.

Editor

1

Retinoic Acid Excess Impairs Amelogenesis Inducing Enamel Defects

Supawich Morkmued[1,2,3,4,5]***, Virginie Laugel-Haushalter***[1,2,3,4]***, Eric Mathieu***[6]***, Brigitte Schuhbaur***[1,2,3,4]***, Joseph Hemmerlé***[6]***, Pascal Dollé***[1,2,3,4]***, Agnès Bloch-Zupan***[1,2,3,4,7,8,9,10] ***and Karen Niederreither***[1,2,3,4,7]*****

[1] Developmental Biology and Stem Cells Department, Institute of Genetics and Molecular and Cellular Biology (IGBMC), Illkirch, France, [2] Centre National de la Recherche Scientifique, UMR 7104, Illkirch, France, [3] Institut National de la Santé et de la Recherche Médicale, U 964, Illkirch, France, [4] Université de Strasbourg, Illkirch, France, [5] Pediatrics Department, Faculty of Dentistry, Khon Kaen University, Khon Kaen, Thailand, [6] Université de Strasbourg, INSERM UMR_1121, Biomaterials and Bioengineering, Strasbourg, France, [7] Faculté de Chirurgie Dentaire, Université de Strasbourg, Strasbourg, France, [8] Faculté de Médecine, Fédération de Médecine Translationnelle de Strasbourg, Université de Strasbourg, Strasbourg, France, [9] Hôpitaux Universitaires de Strasbourg, Pôle de Médecine et Chirurgie Bucco-Dentaires, Centre de Référence des Manifestations Odontologiques des Maladies Rares, CRMR, Strasbourg, France, [10] Eastman Dental Institute, University College London, London, UK

***Correspondence:**
Karen Niederreither
niederre@igbmc.fr

Abnormalities of enamel matrix proteins deposition, mineralization, or degradation during tooth development are responsible for a spectrum of either genetic diseases termed *Amelogenesis imperfecta* or acquired enamel defects. To assess if environmental/nutritional factors can exacerbate enamel defects, we investigated the role of the active form of vitamin A, retinoic acid (RA). Robust expression of RA-degrading enzymes *Cyp26b1* and *Cyp26c1* in developing murine teeth suggested RA excess would reduce tooth hard tissue mineralization, adversely affecting enamel. We employed a protocol where RA was supplied to pregnant mice as a food supplement, at a concentration estimated to result in moderate elevations in serum RA levels. This supplementation led to severe enamel defects in adult mice born from pregnant dams, with most severe alterations observed for treatments from embryonic day (E)12.5 to E16.5. We identified the enamel matrix proteins *enamelin* (*Enam*), *ameloblastin* (*Ambn*), and *odontogenic ameloblast-associated protein* (*Odam*) as target genes affected by excess RA, exhibiting mRNA reductions of over 20-fold in lower incisors at E16.5. RA treatments also affected bone formation, reducing mineralization. Accordingly, craniofacial ossification was drastically reduced after 2 days of treatment (E14.5). Massive RNA-sequencing (RNA-seq) was performed on E14.5 and E16.5 lower incisors. Reductions in *Runx2* (a key transcriptional regulator of bone and enamel differentiation) and its targets were observed at E14.5 in RA-exposed embryos. RNA-seq analysis further indicated that bone growth factors, extracellular matrix, and calcium homeostasis were perturbed. Genes mutated in human AI (*ENAM, AMBN, AMELX, AMTN, KLK4*) were reduced in expression at E16.5. Our observations support a model in which elevated RA signaling at fetal stages affects dental cell lineages. Thereafter enamel protein production is impaired, leading to permanent enamel alterations.

Keywords: retinoids, tooth, enamel, RNA-seq, mouse models, *enamelin*

INTRODUCTION

Enamel formation is a unique biomineralization process involving a highly organized matrix protein scaffold deposition and degradation, leading to hydroxyapatite crystal nucleation generating a dense and tightly aligned network of hydroxyapatite crystals. Mature enamel is the body's hardest tissue. Ameloblasts are cells of ectodermal origin responsible for enamel development. These cells secrete enamel proteins, which are required for correct mineralization and structural maturation. Enamel proteins self-assemble and provide a matrix organization that aligns the thin ribbons of calcium phosphate deposited during enamel appositional growth. Enamel formation is characterized by inductive, secretory, and maturation stages. During the inductive stage, the inner enamel epithelium begins to differentiate. Then at the secretory stage, polarized differentiated ameloblasts release enamel proteins, contributing to the enamel matrix (Bei, 2009). Finally at the maturation stage, ameloblasts absorb water and organic matrix. This dehydration allows dense crystal deposition. Mature enamel is thus extremely strong, because of the density and fine organization of its crystal layers (Bei, 2009; Simmer et al., 2010).

Amelogenesis imperfecta (AI) refers to a group of rare genetic diseases presenting with defects in enamel formation either as isolated trait, or in association with other symptoms. Patient cases of AI are classified into hypoplastic, hypomineralized, or hypomaturation categories based on enamel quantitative or qualitative defects, i.e., thickness, hardness, and/or color. To date, mutations in over 30 genes are associated with non-syndromic or syndromic AI (Bloch-Zupan et al., 2012). These diseases can be recapitulated in several mouse models. For example, hypoplastic or aplastic enamel deficiencies are produced by *amelogenin (Amel)*, *ameloblastin* (*Ambn*), and *enamelin* (*Enam*) mutations, recapitulating defects in patients (Gibson et al., 2001; Fukumoto et al., 2004; Masuya et al., 2005; Hu et al., 2008, 2014). Studies in mouse models have contributed to understanding how defective ameloblast protein secretion contributes to these diseases. For a given genetic defect, interfamilial, intrafamilial, and individual intraoral variations in phenotype severity are often seen, suggesting that environmental factors come into play. Indeed, ameloblasts are highly sensitive to their environment (Simmer et al., 2010). Body stressors including high fever (Ryynänen et al., 2014), excess fluoride (Yang et al., 2015), and endocrine disrupters such as bisphenol A disrupt ameloblast function (Jedeon et al., 2014). It is likely that a variety of factors contribute to clinical heterogeneity found in AI and to acquired enamel defects such as molar incisor hypomineralization (MIH) or hypomineralized second primary molars (HSPM; Alaluusua, 2010; Jeremias et al., 2013). Our objective is to discover novel factors initiating and influencing enamel regulatory networks, with the aim of designing new strategies to alleviate dental defects. To further characterize nutritional and environmental factors regulating enamel formation, we have focused on the role of retinoic acid (RA), the main active form of vitamin A that plays key roles during vertebrate development (Niederreither and Dollé, 2008). RA is the ligand for nuclear receptors (RARα, β, and γ), which bind as heterodimers with RXRs to DNA regulatory elements termed RA-response elements (RAREs, Rochette-Egly and Germain, 2009). Through this mechanism, RA regulates expression of various target genes (Balmer and Blomhoff, 2002). RA distribution within embryonic tissues is tightly controlled through an interplay between enzymes involved in its synthesis (mainly retinol dehydrogenase 10 and retinaldehyde dehydrogenases [Raldh]1, 2, and 3) and catabolism (Cyp26A1, B1, and C1). As both RA deficiency and excess results in diverse developmental defects, the distribution of active retinoid signaling requires tight regulation to limit potent adverse effects (Rhinn and Dollé, 2012).

Expression of RA receptors, synthesizing, and catabolizing enzymes has been detected in the developing teeth (Bloch-Zupan et al., 1994; Berkovitz et al., 2001; Cammas et al., 2007). Severe dietary vitamin A deficiency in rats leads to hypoplastic enamel, enamel organ metaplasia, dentine dysplasia, and delayed tooth eruption (Mellanby, 1941; Punyasingh et al., 1984; McDowell et al., 1987). Hypervitaminosis A during rodent pregnancy induces exencephaly and craniofacial malformations, along with tooth fusions and supernumerary incisors (Knudsen, 1967 and references therein). These effects may reveal an evolutionary role of RA signaling in the posterior pharyngeal region controlling tooth number (Seritrakul et al., 2012). In culture, RA excess can retard molar growth (Mark et al., 1992), reduce ameloblast differentiation (Kronmiller et al., 1992), and diminish tooth alkaline phosphatase production (Jones et al., 2008). Retinoids may also regulate incisor cervical loop maturation, increasing mitosis and laminin gene expression (Bloch-Zupan et al., 1994).

In vivo models to substantiate RA actions in tooth development are lacking. Interestingly, though, *Cyp26b1* knockout mice show a defect in maxillary bone compaction around upper incisors (Maclean et al., 2009). Observing that the fetal tooth has robust expression of *Cyp26b1* and *Cyp26c1* RA-degrading enzymes, we hypothesized that *in vivo*, conditions of RA excess may have adverse effects on osteoblast and ameloblast growth regulatory networks. We report that mice born from dams exposed to RA during mid-late pregnancy using a food-based supplementation suffer adult-stage enamel hypoplasia. Effects were strongest when treatments began at the tooth dental lamina-placode stage (E12.5), and continued until early bell developmental stages. Reductions of *Enam*, *Ambn*, and *Odam* mRNA expression in E16.5 lower incisors were observed. High throughput RNA sequencing (RNA-seq) analysis of lower incisors revealed that RA excess perturbs neural crest lineage determinants and pro-ossification growth factor and transcription networks. Combinatorial changes in collagen, extracellular matrix, and calcium homeostasis genes occur at E14.5, followed by a decrease at E16.5 of transcripts encoding pre-ameloblast secretory-stage proteins. These alterations in gene expression are observed several days before the ameloblast lineage begins to differentiate. Retinoid excess targets fetal odontoblasts, along with a range of epithelial enamel protein targets. Our data provides potential avenues through which environmental and nutritional changes may alter the penetrance and expressivity of human enamel defects such as AI or MIH.

MATERIALS AND METHODS

Ethics Statement

All animals were maintained and manipulated under animal protocols in agreement with the French Ministry of Agriculture guidelines for use of laboratory animals (IGBMC protocol 2012–097) and with NIH guidelines, provided in the Guide for the Care and Use of Laboratory Animals. CD1 mice were purchased from Charles River, France. All-*trans*-RA (Sigma) suspended in ethanol (5 mg/mL) was mixed into 50 mL water and 50 g powdered food to a final concentration of 0.4 mg/g food. The RA-containing food mixture (protected from light) was left in the cage for the mice to feed *ad libitum* and changed every day. Control groups consisted of CD1 mice given a matching food treatment, but with no added RA. Equal numbers of RA-treated samples vs. controls were randomly assigned to treatment or control groups.

In situ Hybridization, Beta-Galactosidase (X-gal) Staining, and Skeletal Analysis

In situ hybridization was performed using digoxigenin-labeled RNA probes on 200 μM vibratome sections of paraformaldehyde-fixed embryos, which were processed using an Intavis InSituPro robot, as described in detail on the website http://empress.har.mrc.ac.uk/browser/ (Gene Expression section). To analyze patterns of RA-response, we used the *RARE-hsp68-lacZ* reporter transgenic line (Rossant et al., 1991). At least 20 randomized fetal samples from control and matching RA-treated samples were used to test each probe. All expression studies were confirmed in at least 3 independent experiments. X-gal assays were performed on 200 μm vibratome sections. Whole-mount fetal alizarin red/alcian blue staining was carried out as described in http://empress.har.mrc.ac.uk/browser/ (Bone, Cartilage, Arthritis, Osteoporosis section).

Real-Time Quantitative RT-PCR

RT-PCR assays were performed in duplicate on 3 RNA samples for control or RA-treated incisors dissected at E14.5 and E16.5. Total RNA (1 μg) was subjected to real-time RT-PCR using SYBR Green Reagents (Qiagen). RNA was extracted using the RNeasy Micro-kit. Oligo-dT primed cDNAs were generated using the Superscript II kit (Invitrogen). The incorporation of SYBR Green into the PCR products was monitored in real-time with a Roche 480 LightCycler. Sequences of primers are given in supplemental Table S1. Target genes were normalized relative to the glyceraldehyde-3-phosphate dehydrogenase (*Gapdh*) housekeeping gene.

X-Ray Microtomography

Seven week-old mice were analyzed by X-ray micro-computed tomography (micro-CT) using a Quantum FX micro-CT *in vivo* Imaging System (Caliper Life Sciences), which operates at 80 kV and 160 μA, with high-resolution at 10–80 μm pixel size, to assay skull and tooth morphology. Data reconstructions were performed with the Analyze software (v 11.0; Biomedical Imaging Resource, Mayo Clinic, Rochester, MN).

Scanning Electron Microscopy

The lower incisors of 7 week-old control and RA-treated mice were dissected out of the alveolar bone, rinsed, dehydrated in a graded series of ethanol, and then transferred in a propylene oxide/epon resin (v/v) solution. After embedding the teeth in Epon 812 (Euromedex, Souffelweyersheim, France), they were sectioned sagittally and polished with diamond pastes (Escil, Chassieu, France). The embedded half incisors were etched with a 20% (m/v) citric acid solution for 2 min, rinsed with distilled water, dehydrated in a graded series of ethanol and dried at room temperature. The samples were then coated with a gold-palladium alloy using a HUMMER JR sputtering device (Technics, CA, USA) before performing scanning electron microscopy with a Quanta 250 ESEM (FEI Company, Eindhoven, The Netherlands) with an accelerating voltage of the electrons of 5 kV.

RNA Sequencing

Total RNA was extracted in quadruplicate from lower incisors at E14.5 and 16.5 (2 days or 4 days after RA treatment) and respective controls. The mRNA-seq libraries were prepared as detailed in the Illumina protocol (supplemental Experimental Procedures). Sequence reads mapped to the mouse reference genome mm10/NCBI37 using Tophat. Only uniquely aligned reads were retained for further analysis. Quantification of gene expression was performed with HTSeq-0.6.1. (see http://www-huber.embl.de/users/anders/HTSeq/doc/overview.html). For each transcript the resulting reads per kilobase of exon model per million mapped reads (RPKM) were converted to raw read counts, which were then added for each gene locus. Data normalization was performed as described (Anders and Huber, 2010) and resolved using the DESeq Bioconductor package. Resulting *p*-values were adjusted for multiple testing, according to Benjamini and Hochberg (1995). Regulated transcripts with an RPKM of >2, an adjusted $p < 0.050$, and a log2 fold change of >0.3 and < −0.3 at E14.5 and >0.5 and < −0.5 at E16.5 were considered.

RESULTS

To analyze RA-dependent tooth alterations, we employed a protocol where RA added to the food supply was administered to pregnant CD1 mice (Niederreither et al., 2002), at a concentration of 0.4 mg/g food beginning at E12.5 or later. The treatment period began after craniofacial neural crest migration into the head was complete (Minoux and Rijli, 2010), avoiding earlier stage lethality due to exencephaly. In another study, HPLC analysis carried out after similar RA treatment at 0.1 mg/g food showed that serum RA levels were moderately increased (∼20%) compared with untreated controls (Mic et al., 2003). Treated dams bore litters with 50% lethality, typically with 5–7 pups. Incisors in both groups erupted at the same age. Once the pups reached adulthood (4–7 weeks-old), we compared 100 randomized control and RA-treated groups macroscopically for dental defects. The labial side of rodent incisor (analog of the crown and covered with enamel) normally has a yellow/orange pigmentation, due to iron present at a net weight of about

0.03% in enamel (Pindborg, 1953). It gives mouse teeth a characteristic color, which is a dark orange in the upper incisors (**Figures 1A,E**). When RA treatments were performed from E12.5 to 16.5, they were found to produce a chalky lightening and length reduction of incisors, changes more pronounced in lower incisors (**Figures 1B,F**). The whiter color and less shiny surface may reflect reduced enamel thickness typical of mouse enamel hypoplasia models (Gibson et al., 2001; Masuya et al., 2005; Hu et al., 2014). Treatments performed at later stages (E13.5–16.5: **Figures 1C,G**, or E14.5–17.5: **Figures 1D,H**) had less severe effects on enamel, suggesting RA has early roles in the oral epithelium starting at the placode stage of tooth initiation.

Samples shown in **Figures 1A,E** (WT) and B,F (RA-treated) were analyzed by X-ray micro-computed tomography (micro-CT). This analysis confirmed lower incisor shortening (**Figures 2A,B**; Figure S1). Optical sections revealed a reduction in enamel mineral density and thickness (molars in **Figures 2C,E**; incisors in **Figures 2D,F**). Alveolar bone at the level of the molars showed greater porosity in the RA-treated animals (boxes in **Figures 2C,E**; Figure S2). Although retinoid gradients shape pharyngeal tooth evolution (Seritrakul et al., 2012), our micro-CT analysis revealed normal molar eruption and cusp morphology (Figure S3), as predicted because RA treatments are initiated at E12.5, after neural crest has completed its migration into the jaw. This analysis also revealed no evident signs of dental attrition from both groups. **Figure 2G** shows scanning electron micrographs (SEM) of enamel prisms of control lower incisor, exhibiting a well-organized decussating pattern. This was disrupted following RA treatment. The most outer enamel was less mineralized when compared with the control tooth, as outer enamel appeared darker in RA-treated animals. Enamel rods of RA-supplemented animals were less densely packed, and as a consequence, areas normally filled with interprismatic enamel seemed empty and showed holes-like pattern (**Figure 2H**), similar to *Enam* haploinsufficent mice (Hu et al., 2014).

Histological analysis of 1-week old mice after hematoxylin-eosin staining confirmed that RA treatments produced a shorter, smaller, and disorganized layer of ameloblasts in both molars (**Figures 3A,B**) and incisors (**Figures 3C–H**). This was clearly seen in the secretory zone, where ameloblasts displayed disrupted epithelial sheet organization (**Figure 3H**). In all treated samples, ameloblast adhesion to enamel was impaired (**Figures 3B,D,G,H**). This was first seen histologically as a detachment of the basement membrane, likely causing preameloblast separation from forming odontoblasts (**Figure 3G**, red arrowhead). Non-cellular

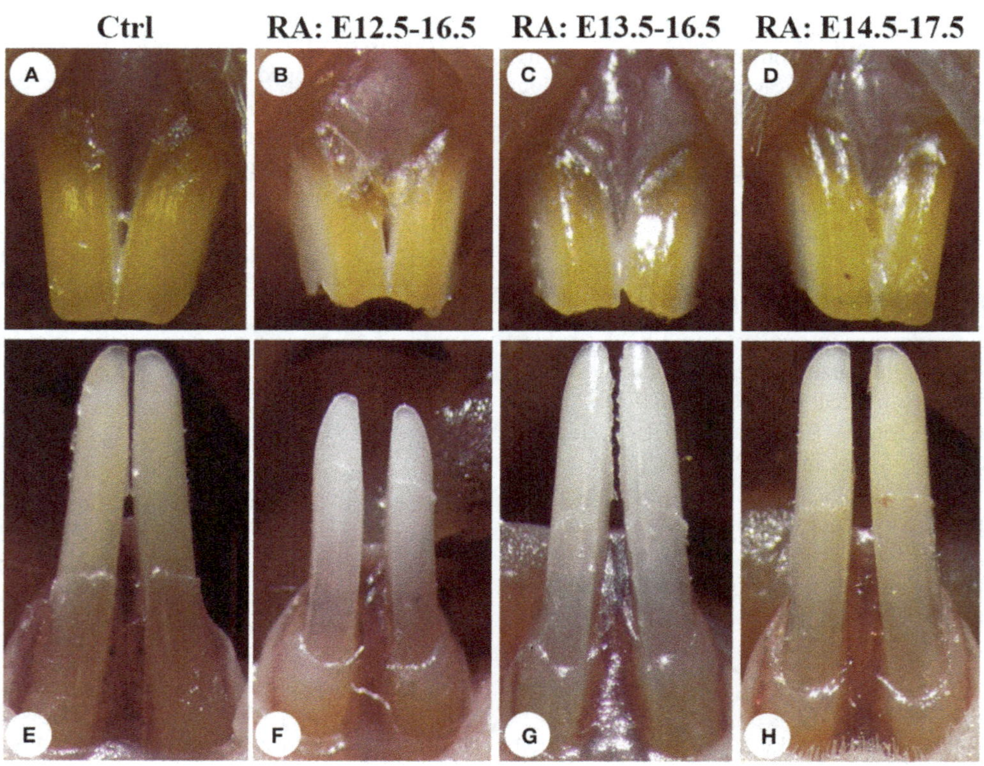

FIGURE 1 | RA excess during pregnancy produces stage-specific whitening and size reductions of mouse incisors. Enamel of the upper **(A)** and lower **(E)** incisors of 7 weeks-old CD1 control (non-RA treated) mice has a characteristic yellow/orange color, which is consistently darker in the upper incisor. Retinoic acid treatment from E12.5 to 16.5 reduces incisor length (by ~20%) and lightens enamel color **(B,F)**, suggesting reduced iron accumulation typical of murine models of hypoplastic enamel formation. When RA treatment begins at E13.5 **(C,G)** or E14.5 **(D,H)**, incisor length reductions and lightening of incisor color are progressively less severe.

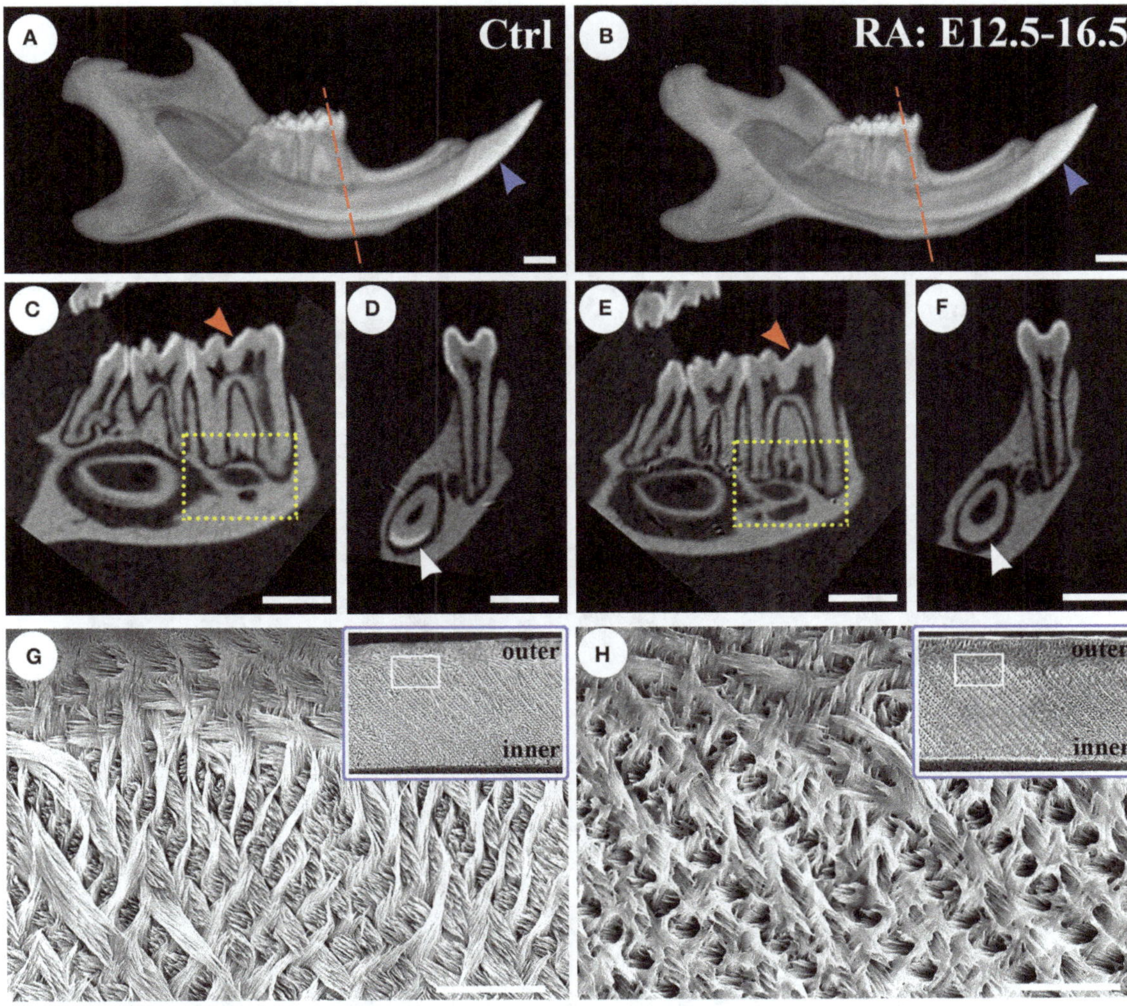

FIGURE 2 | Micro-CT and SEM imaging of 7 weeks-old control (A,C,D,G) and RA-treated **(B,E,F,H)** mice. **(A)** Shows the typical length of a control incisor, which is longer and exhibits an opaque whiter region reflecting high density where enamel is present. Comparing the E12.5–16.5 RA-treated mouse **(B)**, incisor length and enamel density are reduced throughout the tooth. Optical sections in a sagittal plane reveal regions with less surface enamel on lower molars of the treated mouse (arrowheads in **C,E**). Optical cross-sections of the first molar and lower incisor (dotted lines in **A,B**) show reduced density of enamel in the lower incisor (arrowheads in **D,F**). An increased porosity of the alveolar bone is observed below the molars in the RA-treated mouse (compare boxed areas in **C,E**). Scale bars: 1 mm. **(G,H)** Are SEM images from the central longitudinal plane of fully-formed lower incisor enamel from control and RA-treated samples (arrowheads in **A,B**). The enamel of control presented a constant thickness and a clear decussating prism pattern **(G)**. A reduced mineralization and impaired organization (especially in the outer enamel) is observed in RA-treated samples **(H)**. The area from which SEM views are taken is shown in the insert box. Scale bars: 10 μm.

organic material was present between layers (**Figure 3B**, black arrowhead). The lower incisor secretory zone enamel layer was slightly thinner (**Figure 3H**), suggesting RA treatment delayed enamel maturation and/or reduced overall mineralization.

Enamel matrix proteins are secreted by ameloblasts and form a matrix directing enamel mineral deposition. Among these proteins, amelogenin is the most abundant (Eastoe, 1979). Enamel fails to form or is hypoplastic in amelogenin-deficient mice (Gibson et al., 2001), and in *Enam*- or *Ambn*-null mutant mice (Fukumoto et al., 2004; Masuya et al., 2005; Hu et al., 2014). Our real-time RT-PCR analysis of E16.5 lower incisors following E12.5–16.5 RA treatment revealed up to 20-fold reductions in *Enam*, *Ambn*, and *Odam* mRNAs (**Figure 4**). Notably, no RA-induced alterations in *Enam*, *Ambn*, or *Odam* were observed at E14.5 (data not shown).

To assess if reduced enamel protein expression was linked to ectopic activation of RA signaling, we used RARE-hsp68-*lacZ* transgenic mice as a reporter for RA activity (Rossant et al., 1991). No expression was seen in the tooth germ areas at E13.5 (data not shown), although activity was found in the mandible next to the tooth germs at E14.5 (**Figures 5A,B**). This retinoid reporter transgene exhibited low level of expression in both mandible and maxilla adjacent to the growing incisors and molars in E16.5 untreated fetuses (**Figure 5C** and data not shown). In E16.5

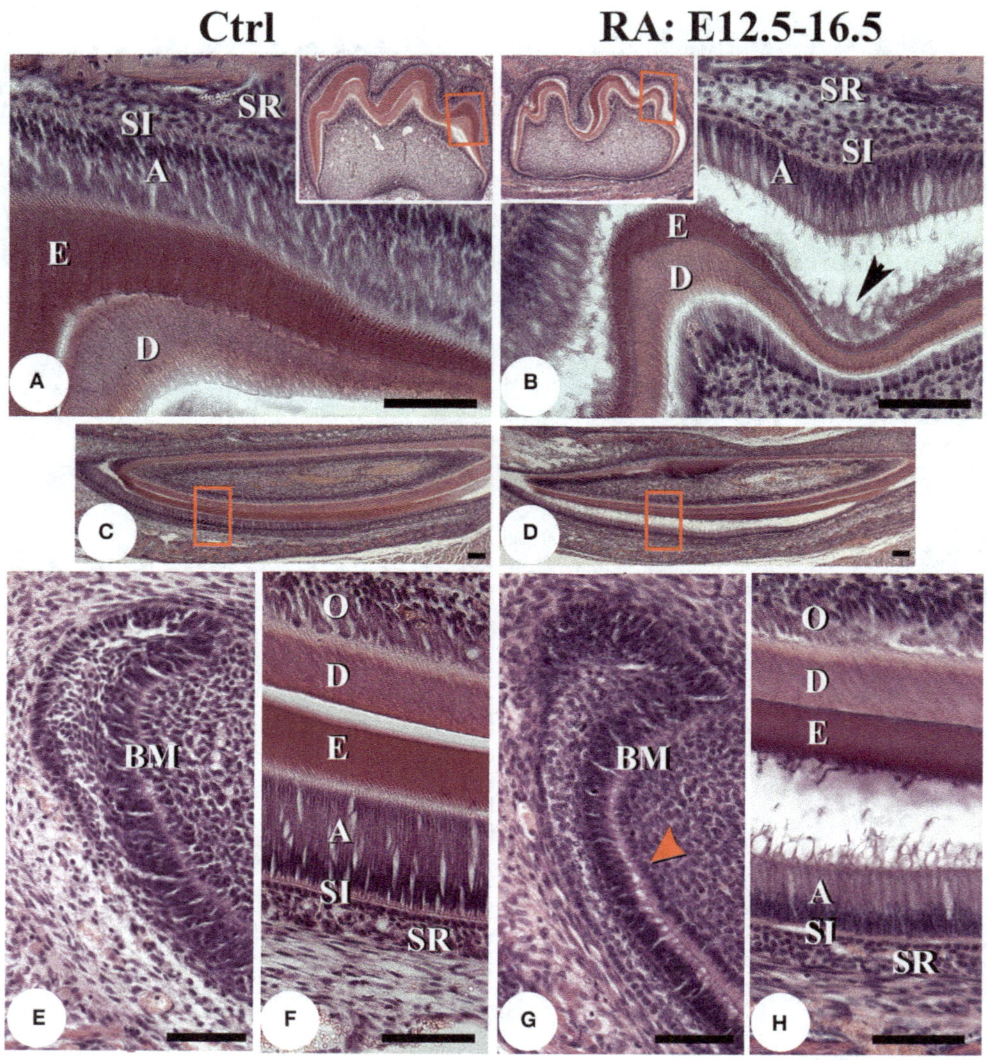

FIGURE 3 | Histological analysis of post-natal day 7 teeth. Hematoxylin and eosin stained sagittal sections of lower first molars of control **(A)** and E12.5–16.5 RA-treated **(B)** mice. The boxed areas in low-magnification insert panels are shown in detail. A black arrowhead in **B** points to cell debris accumulating between separated tissue layers. Lower incisors of untreated **(C,E,F)** and RA-treated **(D,G,H)** mice. **F**, **H** are higher magnification views of the boxed areas in **C,D**. Comparing the cervical loop of untreated **(E)** with RA-treated mice **(G)**, it appears retinoid excess may disrupt the basement membrane (**G**, red arrowhead), potentially leading to ameloblast detachment **(B,D,H)**. The secretory stage ameloblast layer is also slightly thinner and enamel thickness reduced after RA treatment **(B,D,H)**. Scale bars: 100 μm. Abbreviations: A, ameloblasts; BM, basement membrane; D, dentin; E, enamel; O, odontoblasts; SI, stratum intermedium; SR, stellate reticulum.

fetuses following RA treatment from E12.5 to 16.5, domains of RARE-*lacZ* activity broadly extended into alveolar bone and surrounding mesenchyme, but appeared absent from enamel organ and dental ectomesenchyme (**Figure 5D** and data not shown). Note that very low levels of RA signaling may not be detected by such a reporter transgene. Proper control of RA levels is necessary for early neural crest patterning, but RA deficiency does not alter first branchial arch formation (Niederreither et al., 2000). To explore why RA activity was absent from most tissues of the tooth buds, we examined expression of CYP26 family cytochrome P450 enzymes specifically involved in RA catabolism. At E13.5, *Cyp26b1* expression (**Figure 5E**) was found to be prominent in mesenchyme surrounding the forming incisors. At E14.5, *Cyp26c1* (**Figure 5F**) was prominently expressed in the enamel organ, whereas a low amount of *Cyp26a1* transcripts was seen in the dental papilla (**Figure 5F**, insert).

Excesses of vitamin A or RA lead to skeletal fragility by reducing bone formation and by stimulating bone-resorbing osteoclasts (Henning et al., 2015). In the *Cyp26b1* mutant, impaired RA catabolism causes long-bone fusions and induces premature osteoblast differentiation into mineralizing osteocytes, truncating bone development in the craniofacial region (Maclean et al., 2009). Alizarin red/alcian blue staining of E14.5 skulls 2 days into RA regime revealed shortened mandibles, and truncated regions of ossified maxilla and premaxilla in the

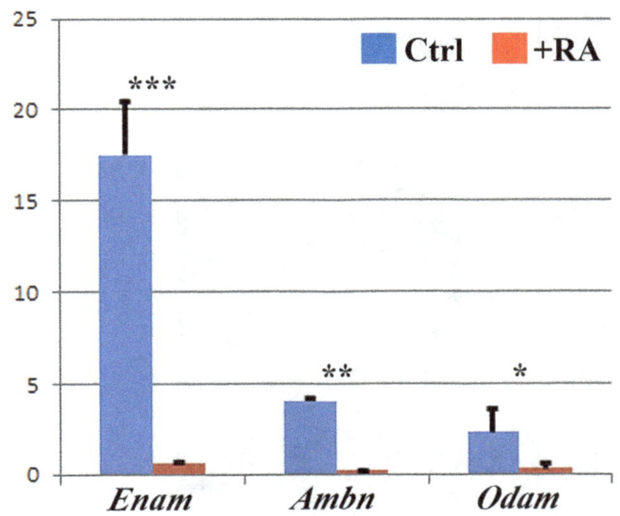

FIGURE 4 | Real-time RT-PCR analysis shows reductions in secretory-stage enamel gene expression. *Enam*, *Ambn*, and *Odam* mRNA levels in lower incisor samples of E16.5 control mice (blue) vs. E12.5–16.5 RA-treated mice. Target genes were normalized relative to *Gapdh*. Mean (*SD*). Student *t*-test: ***$p < 0.001$, **$p < 0.010$, *$p < 0.050$.

RA-treated animals (**Figures 6A,B**). The skull frontal plate was also smaller in treated animals, with less ossification. Malformed Meckel's cartilage and truncated mandibles could lead to incisor shortenings. Skeletal staining performed at E15.5 confirmed RA-reduced mineralization (**Figures 6C,D**). RT-PCR analysis showed reductions in *Runx2* mRNA in both lower incisor and adjacent alveolar bone at E14.5 in RA-treated animals (**Figures 6E,F**). A 3-fold reduction in the expression of this key target might account for reduced bone mineral deposition (Ducy and Karsenty, 1998), and its mesenchymal localization (**Figure 6G**) implies indirect enamel effects. To exclude systemic non-specific RA effects, we cultured isolated lower incisors or lower incisors with adjacent alveolar bone from E13.5 embryos (Figure S4). When 10^{-8} M RA was added to culture medium, *Enam* levels were dramatically reduced in isolated incisor cultures, indicating RA acted directly on tooth.

To compare global gene expression changes in control vs. RA-treated samples, E14.5 and E16.5 lower incisors were analyzed by high throughput RNA sequencing (RNA-seq). Principal component analysis (PCA plot, Figure S5) and scatter plots (Figure S6) revealed the overall changes observed at E14.5 were tightly clustered, statistically significant, yet often seen as net reductions of ~20–50% (**Table 1**). RNA-seq analysis confirmed broad effects of RA treatment affecting mineralization-inducing pathways, extracellular collagens, and calcium networks. Genes reduced in expression at E14.5 included *Runx, Dlx, Bmp*, and *Shh*, all known inducers of inner enamel epithelium differentiation (Bei, 2009). Net reduction in *Runx2* and *Dlx5* (**Table 1**) may act combinatorially to reduce the bone biomarker BGLAP (osteocalcin, (Hassan et al., 2004)), a target reduced by ~2-fold at E16.5 in RA-treated samples (**Table 2**). A novel RA-inhibited target is the matricellular protein Smoc2, whose mutation in human produces oligodontia, microdontia, abnormal root development, dentin dyplasia, and reduced alveolar bone growth (Bloch-Zupan et al., 2011). Retinoids are known to drive uncommitted progenitor cells into neuronal lineages (Maden, 2007). Consistently, DAVID (Database for Annotation, Visualization, and Integrated Discovery) analysis revealed a functional enrichment score of 1.4 E^{-6} for neuronal differentiation pathways. Increased *Neurogenin1* (*Neurog1*), *Neurogenin2* (*Neurog2*), and the notch target *Hes5*, are typical of an RA-induced neuronal differentiation profile (Table S2). At E16.5, *Enam* was the most reduced target (**Table 2**), also markedly reduced by *in situ* hybridization analysis (Figure S7). Reductions in *ameloblastin, X- linked amelogenin, amelotin*, and *kallikrein-related peptidase 4* (*Klk4*), all encoding enamel proteins (Núñez et al., 2015), were observed (**Table 2**). Notably, these reductions at E16.5 occur much earlier than the characterized times of action of the corresponding proteins in inductive, secretory, or maturation stages of rodent enamel development. Odontoblast-originating signals control ameloblast induction (Bei, 2009). Reductions in mineralization targets (*alkaline phosphatase*), odontoblast structural proteins (*dentin matrix protein 1, dentin sialophosphoprotein*), ossification biomarkers (*Bglap1/osteocalcin, Bglap2*), and calcium homeostasis pathways (*calcitonin, vitamin D receptor*) were all observed in E16.5 RA-treated samples. Table S3 summarizes how RA excess at E16.5 increases the expression of genes involved in retinoid signaling (including *Cyp26b1*), Wnt signaling, and neuronal differentiation.

DISCUSSION

RA Excess Affects Enamel Matrix Protein Expression Prior to Ameloblast Differentiation

AI refers to rare, inherited diseases characterized by a defect in enamel formation with clinical heterogeneity even within the same family (Bloch-Zupan et al., 2012). These variations, also observed in acquired enamel defects, have been proposed to be due to environmental excess in fluoride (Yang et al., 2015), or to other nutritional, environmental, or behavioral changes (Li et al., 2013), along with genetic makeup of an individual. Retinoids are regulators of skeletal growth and patterning, known to lead to skeletal fragility when given in excess (Henning et al., 2015). Since reciprocal interactions between enamel organ and ectomesenchyme are necessary for alveolar bone, periodontal, and tooth differentiation, we examined if nutritional RA excess could have additional effects on developing teeth. Prior to this study, little was known about *in vivo* effects of RA on enamel cytodifferentiation. Here we find that RA treatment at a defined window of murine development resulted in permanent defects resembling human AI. Ameloblast differentiation begins at the advanced bell stage (~E18.5 in mouse), when the inner enamel epithelial originating cells express enamel secretory proteins and follow

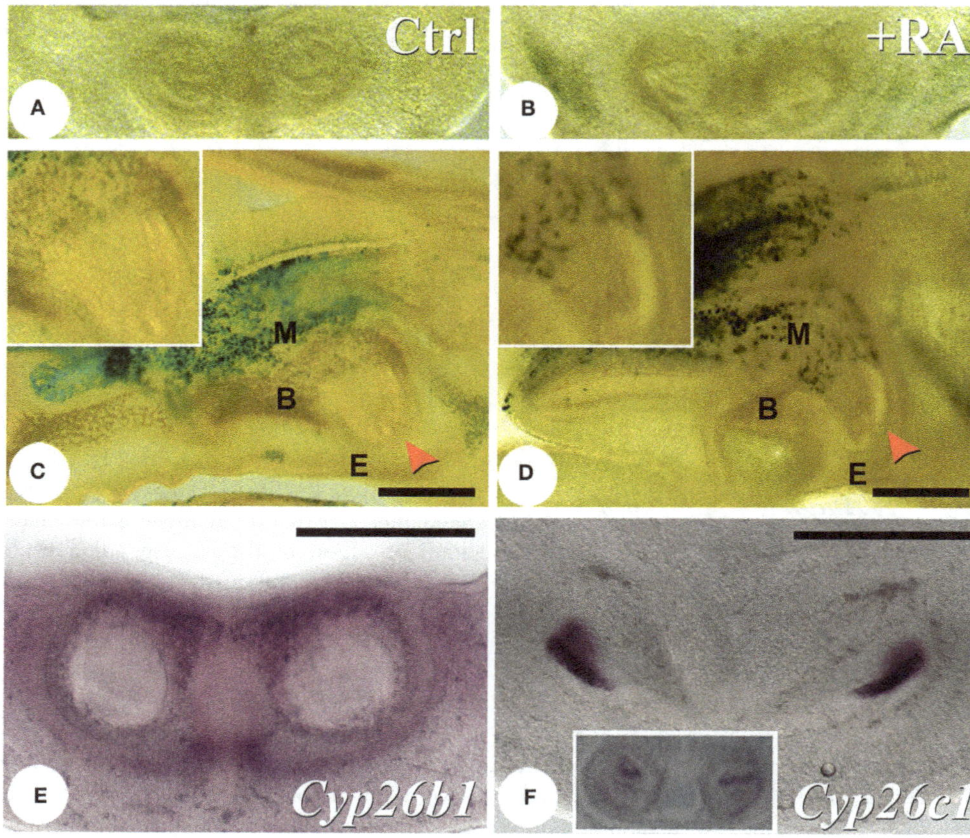

FIGURE 5 | Regions of RA activity and expression of RA-catabolizing enzymes in the developing teeth. X-gal analysis of RARE-hsp68-*lacZ* reporter transgene activation in E14.5 **(A,B)** and E16.5 **(C,D)** untreated and RA-treated (E12.5–16.5) mice. At E14.5 in untreated mice, transgene activity can be observed surrounding the tooth germ, and this activity is increased in treated mice. At E16.5, X-gal activity is detected in alveolar bone adjacent to upper **(C,D)** and lower (data not shown) incisors (arrowhead). After RA treatment, reporter activity is increased in alveolar bone, but is never seen in developing teeth (compare high magnification insert panels in **C,D**). At E13.5, *Cyp26b1* is expressed in mesenchyme surrounding the lower incisors **(E)**. At E14.5 a pronounced expression of *Cyp26c1* is seen in the enamel organ **(F)**, whereas *Cyp26a1* is expressed in the dental papilla epithelium (**F**, insert). Scale bars: 500 μm. Abbreviations: B, bone; E, epithelium; M, mesenchyme.

by processing enzymes (Bei, 2009; Bloch-Zupan et al., 2012). Assuming normal rodent nocturnal feed, in our experimental protocol RA exposure would begin at the bud stage of tooth formation (E13.0). We observed that at E14.5, RA excess impairs expression of *Runx*, *Dlx*, bone morphogenetic proteins, while levels of enamel secretory proteins are not altered in either our RNA-seq analysis or RT-PCR analysis at these same stages (data not shown). RA excess changes likely occur prior to ameloblast differentiation, with molecular alterations indicating effects on pro-mineralization signaling.

Retinoids Have Early Targets in Mineralized Tissue, and Later Effects on Enamel Proteins

Enamel-reducing effects of RA supplementation at E13–14.5 coincide with the initial stages of intramembraneous ossification. An early target is *Runx2*, a master regulator of skeletal mineralization. *Runx2*$^{-/-}$ mouse mutants have a block in endochondral and intramembraneous osteoblast maturation, and site-specific reductions in collagen type I and alkaline phosphatase expression (Ducy and Karsenty, 1998). *Runx2*$^{-/-}$ mutants lack differentiated odontoblast and ameloblast matrices, indicative of late bell-stage defects (D'Souza et al., 1999; Bronckers et al., 2001). We observe RA-dependent *Runx2* reductions at E14.5 bud stage incisors, but not at E16.5, suggesting earlier effects. Cleidocranial dysplasia, an autosomal dominant condition caused by mutations of *RUNX2*, likewise results in insufficient dentin and enamel mineralization (Xuan et al., 2010) and other dental anomalies (Camilleri and McDonald, 2006). Terminal ameloblast differentiation requires odontoblast-originating signals and matrix components (Balic and Thesleff, 2015). Reports of evolutionarily conserved Runx2-binding sites in *Enam, Ambn*, and *Odam* gene promoters Dhamija and Krebsbach, 2001; Lee et al., 2010, suggested a model of RA-inhibitory effects (**Figure 7**). Retinoid excess at E14.5 would induce relatively small, yet combined reductions in *Runx2/3, Dlx3/5*, and *Bmp2/3*, predominantly mesenchymal targets that surround the bud stage tooth (Figure S8). By E16.5 these factors collectively regulate early epithelial (enamel

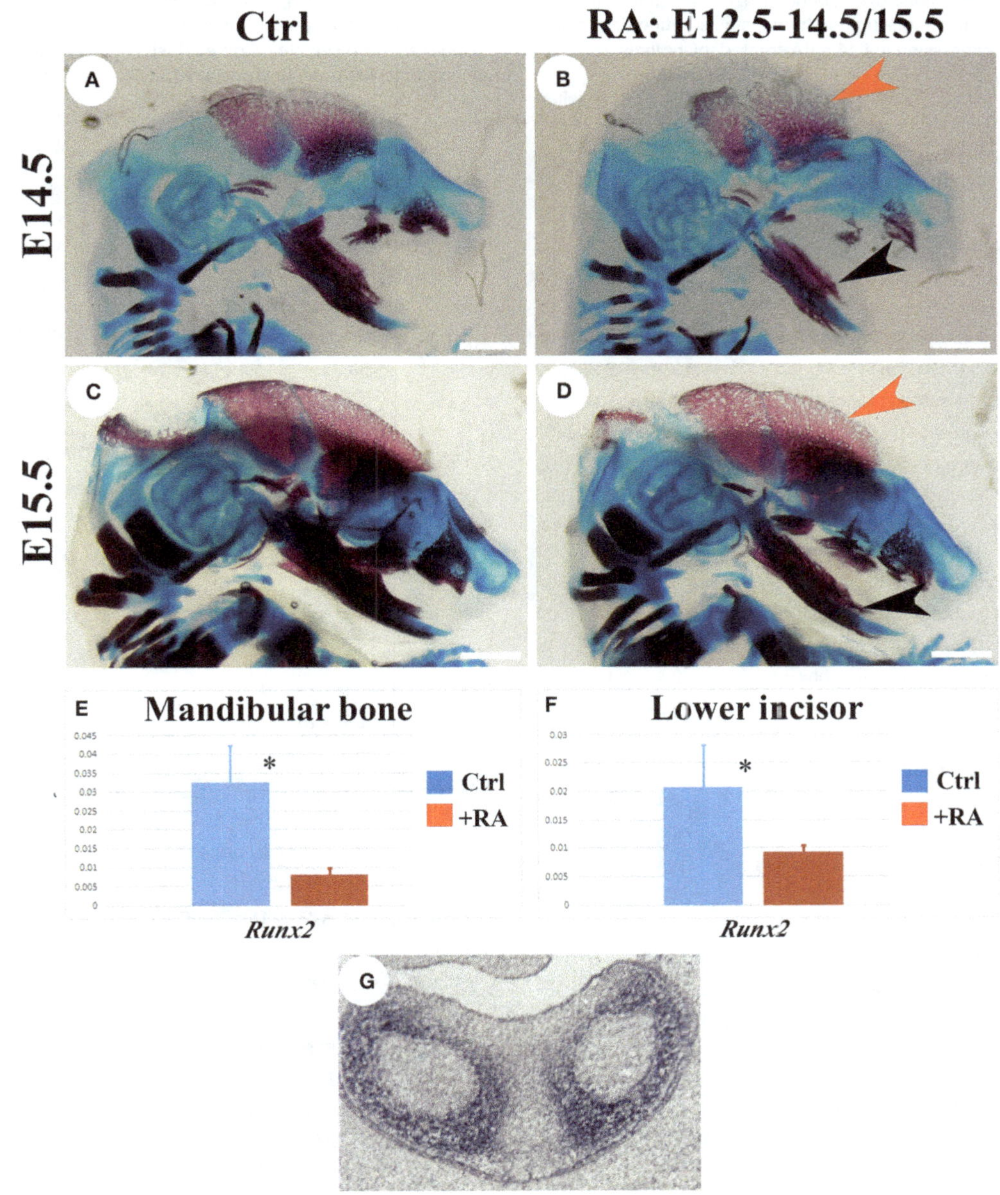

FIGURE 6 | Alizarin red/alcian blue analysis of E14.5 and E15.5 skeleton, RT-PCR and *in situ* hybridization analysis of *Runx2* expression in lower incisors and alveolar bone. Osteoblast mineralization marked by red alizarin staining in untreated E14.5 **(A)** and E15.5 **(C)** heads is reduced in RA-treated **(B,D)** parietal bone (red arrowhead) and mandible (black arrowhead) at equivalent stages. Scale bars: 1 mm. RT-PCR analysis of *Runx2* mRNA at E14.5 shows significant reductions following RA treatments in mandibular bone **(E)** and lower incisor **(F)**. Target genes were normalized relative to *Gapdh*. Mean (*SD*). Student *t*-test: $^*p < 0.05$. **(G)** *In situ* hybridization detection of *Runx2* transcripts in E14.5 lower incisors (in absence of RA treatment).

organ) expression of *Enam*, *Ambn*, and *Amelx*. This is plausible because these enamel targets possess evolutionarily conserved binding site-motifs in their proximal promoters (Loots et al., 2002; Cartharius et al., 2005; **Figure 7C**; Table S4). While the bell stage tooth reacts to the high retinoid environment by up-regulating *Cyp26b1* levels (Table S3), this change is insufficient to offset strong reductions in enamel matrix protein secretion, which then induce ameloblast differentiation defects.

Many Enamel Targets Are in the Secretory Phosphoprotein-Encoding (SCPP) Gene Cluster

Our RNA-seq analysis on the whole lower incisors uncovered many genes significantly reduced at E16.5 that regulate ameloblast differentiation, enamel formation, and dentin/bone development (**Table 2**). Hence combinatorial deficits in enamel secretory protein expression included reductions in X-linked amelogenin (*AMELX*, OMIM: 300391) (Gibson et al., 2001;

TABLE 1 | Genes encoding regulators of bone growth, collagens, and proteins involved in calcium signaling and homeostasis, retinoid, and Shh pathways, reduced in expression in E14.5 RA-treated lower incisors.

Symbol	Name	FC log2	*p*-value
BONE/OSTEOBLAST GROWTH			
Bmp2	Bone morphogenetic protein 2	−0.35	1.08 E-02
Bmp3	Bone morphogenetic protein 3	−0.33	1.93 E-02
Bmp5	Bone morphogenetic protein 5	−0.43	1.72 E-02
Ostn	Osteocrin	−1.30	8,96 E-05
Sp7	Sp7 transcription factor 7	−0.80	2,62 E-05
Smoc2	SPARC modular calcium binding 2	−0.73	1,74 E-08
Runx2	Runt related transcription factor 2	−0.38	2.98 E-02
Runx3	Runt related transcription factor 3	−0.62	7.01 E-06
Dlx5	Distal-less homeobox 5	−0.58	1.64 E-03
Dlx3	Distal-less homeobox 3	−0.53	8.37 E-03
Mef2c	Myocyte enhancer factor 2C	−0.58	6.33 E-05
Ltbp2	Latent transforming growth factor β binding protein 2	−0.86	1.98 E-06
Fgf10	Fibroblast growth factor 10	−0.42	4.17 E-04
Fam20a	Family with sequence similarity 20A	−0.64	2.71 E-04
Tnn	Tenascin N	−1.18	2.01 E-10
Sox6	SRY (sex determining region Y)-box 6	−0.41	1.20 E-02
Tgfb3	Transforming growth factor β 3	−0.31	1.45 E-04
COLLAGEN			
Col1a1	Collagen, type I, α 1	−0.61	6.25 E-03
Col1a2	Collagen, type I, α 2	−0.43	3.62 E-02
Col5a1	Collagen, type V, α 1	−0.37	1,39 E-04
Col6a3	Collagen, type VI, α 3	−0.42	8.34 E-05
Col8a1	Collagen, type VIII, α 1	−0.79	3.74 E-04
Col8a2	Collagen, type VIII, α 2	−0.53	1.25 E-04
Col12a1	Collagen, type XII, α 1	−0.63	1.43 E-04
CALCIUM SIGNALING AND HOMEOSTASIS			
Capn3	Calpain 3	−1.03	1.78 E-03
Otof	Otoferlin	−0.82	3.68 E-03
Kcnma1	Potassium calcium-activated channel Mα 1	−0.54	8.47 E-03
Cacna2d2	Calcium channel, voltage dependent, α2/δ2	−0.48	2.26 E-03
RETINOID SIGNALING			
Aldh1a1	Retinaldehyde dehydrogenase 1	−0.80	1.22 E-02
Aldh1a3	Retinaldehyde dehydrogenase 3	−0.69	2.70 E-03
Rbp2	Retinol binding protein 2	−0.86	4.68 E-02
Cyp26c1	Cytochrome P450 26c1	−0.29	3.77 E-01
SHH SIGNALING			
Ihh	Indian hedgehog	−1.40	1.84 E-06
Hhip	Hedgehog-interacting protein	−0.65	1.64 E-05
Ptch1	Patched 1	−0.42	3.04 E-02

Data are presented as log2 fold changes in RA-treated vs. control samples: for instance, a FC log2 value of −1.00 will correspond to a 50% mRNA level in the RA-treated samples.

TABLE 2 | Summary of genes encoding enamel proteins, extracellular matrix components, proteins involved in bone growth pathways, or calcium and iron signaling/homeostasis, all reduced in expression according to RNA-seq analysis of E16.5 RA-treated lower incisors.

Symbol	Name	FC log2	*p*-value
ENAMEL MATRIX PROTEINS			
Enam	Enamelin	−3.47	4.99 E-013
Amtn	Amelotin	−1.85	1.53 E-004
Amelx	Amelogenin, X-linked	−1.7	1.01 E-004
Ambn	Ameloblastin	−1.42	1.78 E-003
ENAMEL MODIFICATION			
Klk4	Kallikrein peptidase 4	−1.62	1.14 E-003
Ppara	Peroxisome proliferator activated receptor α	−0.74	1.55 E-002
Fam20c	Family with sequence similarity 20, C	−0.66	7.31 E-003
BONE GROWTH FACTOR PATHWAYS			
Bglap	Bone gamma carboxyglutamate protein	−1.67	6.06 E-004
Bglap2	Bone gamma-carboxyglutamate protein 2	−1.15	2.41 E-002
Comp	Cartilage oligomeric matrix protein	−2.89	3.00 E-013
Phex	Phosphate endopeptidase X-linked	−1.01	4.10 E-002
Alpl	Alkaline phosphatase	−0.94	5.79 E-006
Col11a1	Collagen, type XI, α 1	−1.16	4.60 E-006
Col11a2	Collagen, type XI, α 2	−1.4	5.72 E-004
Col13a1	Collagen, type XIII, α 1	−1.34	7.25 E-008
EXTRACELLULAR MATRIX			
Dmp1	Dentin matrix protein 1	−0.94	7.47 E-002
Dspp	Dentin sialophosphoprotein	−0.85	9.79 E-002
Postn	Periostin	−0.56	1.39 E-004
CALCIUM SIGNALING AND HOMEOSTASIS			
Camk2a	Calcium/calmodulin protein kinase II α	−1.31	4.72 E-005
Camk2b	Calcium/calmodulin protein kinase II β	−1.41	1.33 E-005
Smoc2	SPARC related modular calcium binding 2	−0.51	5.02 E-004
Calcr	Calcitonin receptor	−2.91	1.22 E-014
Vdr	Vitamin D receptor	−1.45	6.81 E-008
Slc8a3	Solute carrier family 8 (sodium/calcium exchanger) 3	−1.17	3,80 E-003
Pth1r	Parathyroid hormone 1 receptor	−1.00	3.31 E-006
Ramp1	Receptor (calcitonin) activity modifying protein1	−1.09	1.00 E-006
IRON HOMEOSTASIS			
Hfe2	Hemochromatosis type 2	−1.04	3.70 E-002
Tfr2	Transferrin receptor 2	−0.99	1.34 E-003

Data are presented as log2 fold changes (FC log2) in RA-treated vs control samples: for instance, a FC log2 value of −1.00 will correspond to a 50% mRNA level in the RA-treated samples. Adjusted p-value takes into account a false discovery rate wherein 5% of samples with a p-value of 0.050 will result in false positives.

Barron et al., 2010), *AMBN* (OMIM: 601259) (Fukumoto et al., 2004), *AMTN* (OMIM: 610912) (Nakayama et al., 2015), along with *Odam* (OMIM: 614843). These genes belong to the evolutionarily-related SCPP gene cluster, a linked group of genes also containing members regulating skeletal mineralization (Kawasaki and Weiss, 2008). These SCPP enamel proteins contain structural domains promoting calcium sequestration and regulating crystal adsorption (Addison and McKee, 2010), and their mutations produce hypomineralized enamel phenotypes including altered prism patterning and increased cellular apoptosis in both patients and mouse models (Fukumoto et al., 2004; Bei, 2009; Hu et al., 2014; Núñez et al., 2015). Reductions in the SCPP cluster appeared specific to enamel expression. Other enamel-regulating targets included the kallikrein-related

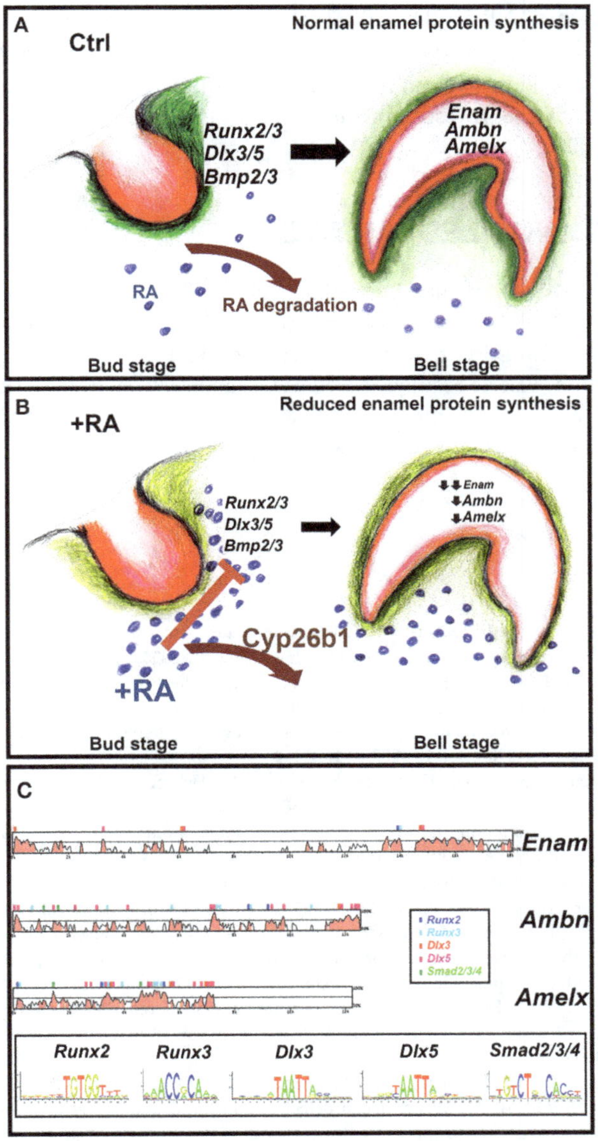

FIGURE 7 | Model of how RA excess impairs enamel formation. Dental mesenchyme (green) and oral epithelium (red) have reciprocal interactions during tooth development (Balic and Thesleff, 2015) **(A,B)**. **(A)** Normally the entire developing tooth is shielded from RA by actions of Cyp26 RA-degrading enzymes. This allows proper expression of *Runx2/3*, *Dlx3/5*, and *Bmp2/3* in the mesenchyme condensing next to the oral epithelium at the bud stage **(B)**. These targets are reduced by excess RA. *Enam*, *Ambn*, and *Amelx* exhibit strong reductions at the late bell stage, impairing enamel crystallization **(C)**. The binding site motifs of *Runx2/3*, *Dlx3/5,* and *Smad2/3/4* were obtained from the JASPAR database (http://jaspar.genereg.net) and used to find potential binding sites in conserved regions using the rVISTA database (http://genome.lbl.gov/vista/index.shtml).

peptidase 4, essential for removing enamel proteins and biomineralization (OMIM: 603767), the peroxisome proliferator-activated receptor (PPAR) alpha, required to achieve normal enamel mineralization (OMIM: 170998) (Sehic et al., 2009), and FAM20C, whose mutation produces severe enamel defects in human and mouse (Wang et al., 2012; Acevedo et al., 2015).

RA Excess Alters the Osteoblast, Odontoblast, and Ameloblast Lineages

Over 80 years ago, severe nutritional vitamin A deficiency was reported to reduce enamel formation (Mellanby, 1941), but since this time no genetic models of RA deficiency have been reported with ameloblast or other primary tooth defects. No defects are observed in mouse mutants for the RA-synthesizing enzymes Raldh2 and Raldh3 (Dupé et al., 2003, our unpublished observations), implicating a more severe RA deficiency is required. More likely vitamin A intake levels are usually quite high, hence cellular RA levels need to be reduced during ossification. Both hypervitaminosis A and very low serum retinol levels produce skeletal fragility, poor bone health, and osteoporosis risk (Henning et al., 2015; Green et al., 2016). During mineralization, site-specific increases in CYP26 enzymes are required for bone formation (Minegishi et al., 2014). $Cyp26b1^{-/-}$ mutants have truncated, under-ossified mandibles, possibly due to RA excess perturbing neural crest migration, or alternatively to defects in osteoblast maturation. Incisor defects, while noted, were not characterized (Maclean et al., 2009). Human mutations (both null and hypomorphic) for this RA-catabolizing enzyme produce calvarial hypoplasia and craniosynostosis (Laue et al., 2011). In our experiments, *Cyp26b1* is potently induced in RA-treated E16.5 incisors (Table S3). Even so, enamel defects are still observed.

The dentino-alveolar bone complex regulates tooth development. We observe rapid *in vivo* effects of RA reducing *Runx2*, and its collagenous and mineralization targets. This rapid rodent response to hypervitaminosis A (Lind et al., 2013) is similar to effects in humans (Henning et al., 2015). These RA excesses target enamel matrix protein production. Phenotypic differences in AI severity have been described between family members with identical mutations (see Prasad et al., 2016, for a recent list). Affected patients could be sensitized to otherwise benign alteration in vitamin consumption, RA catabolism pathways, or defects in the tooth and bone biosynthesis programs. Accumulating mutations might sensitize fetal development to environmental factors, including nutrition, explaining variability in AI morphogenetic phenotypes. Similar models have been proposed for RA interactions with the DiGeorge/chromosome 22q1 deletion syndrome (Maynard et al., 2013). Even physiological RA excesses, in the context of additional genetic alterations (which otherwise would produce benign changes) could have net consequences contributing to clinical variations in oral manifestations of rare diseases.

AUTHOR CONTRIBUTIONS

Study design: SM, AB, and KN. Data collection: SM, VL, EM, BS, and KN. Data analysis: SM, VL, JH, AB, and KN. Drafting manuscript: SM, PD, AB, and KN. Revising manuscript content:

SM, JH, PD, AB, and KN. Approving final version of manuscript: SM, VL, JH, EM, BS, PD, AB, and KN. KN takes responsibility for the integrity of the data analysis.

FUNDING

This work was supported by a grant from the University Hospital of Strasbourg (API, 2009–2012, "Development of the oral cavity: from gene to clinical phenotype in Human"), the EU-funded projects (ERDF) A27 "Oro-dental manifestations of rare diseases" in the framework of the RMT-TMO Offensive Sciences initiative INTERREG IV and INTERREG V No. 1.7 RARENET, the Institut d'Etudes Avancées (Institute of Advanced Studies) de l'Université de Strasbourg (USIAS Fellows 2015), and the grant ANR-10-LABX-0030-INRT managed by the Agence Nationale de la Recherche under the frame program Investissements d'Avenir ANR-10-IDEX-0002-02. Sequencing was performed by the IGBMC Microarray and Sequencing platform, supported by the France Genomics National Infrastructure, funded as part of the Investissements d'Avenir program (ANR-10-INBS-0009).

ACKNOWLEDGMENTS

We wish to thank Amandine Velt, Céline Keime, Bernard Jost, Christelle Thibault-Carpentier, Doulaye Dembelé, Antonio Nanci, Greg Pratt, Rena D'Souza, Sylvain Provot, Dominique Hotton, Valérie Fraulob, Carole Haushalter, Muriel Rhinn, Anna Niewiadomska-Cimicka, and Claire Huber for gift of reagents, technical assistance, and/or knowledgeable insight.

REFERENCES

Acevedo, A. C., Poulter, J. A., Alves, P. G., de Lima, C. L., Castro, L. C., Yamaguti, P. M., et al. (2015). Variability of systemic and oro-dental phenotype in two families with non-lethal Raine syndrome with FAM20C mutations. *BMC Med. Genet.* 16:8. doi: 10.1186/s12881-015-0154-5

Addison, W. N., and McKee, M. D. (2010). ASARM mineralization hypothesis: a bridge to progress. *J. Bone Miner. Res.* 25, 1191–1192. doi: 10.1002/jbmr.110

Alaluusua, S. (2010). Aetiology of molar-incisor hypomineralisation: a systematic review. *Eur. Arch. Paediatr. Dent.* 11, 53–58. doi: 10.1007/BF03262713

Anders, S., and Huber, W. (2010). Differential expression analysis for sequence count data. *Genome Biol.* 11:R106. doi: 10.1186/gb-2010-11-10-r106

Balic, A., and Thesleff, I. (2015). Tissue interactions regulating tooth development and renewal. *Curr. Top. Dev. Biol.* 115, 157–186. doi: 10.1016/bs.ctdb.2015.07.006

Balmer, J. E., and Blomhoff, R. (2002). Gene expression regulation by retinoic acid. *J. Lipid Res.* 43, 1773–1808. doi: 10.1194/jlr.R100015-JLR200

Barron, M. J., Brookes, S. J., Kirkham, J., Shore, R. C., Hunt, C., Mironov, A., et al. (2010). A mutation in the mouse Amelx tri-tyrosyl domain results in impaired secretion of amelogenin and phenocopies human X-linked *Amelogenesis imperfecta*. *Hum. Mol. Genet.* 19, 1230–1247. doi: 10.1093/hmg/ddq001

Bei, M. (2009). Molecular genetics of ameloblast cell lineage. *J. Exp. Zool. Part B Mol. Dev. Evol.* 312B, 437–444. doi: 10.1002/jez.b.21261

Benjamini, Y., and Hochberg, Y. (1995). Controlling the false discovery rate: a practical and powerful approach to multiple testing. *J. R. Stat. Soc. Ser. B. (Methodological)* 57, 289–300.

Berkovitz, B. K., Maden, M., McCaffery, P., and Barrett, A. W. (2001). The distribution of retinaldehyde dehydrogenase-2 in rat and human orodental tissues. *Arch. Oral Biol.* 46, 1099–1104. doi: 10.1016/S0003-9969(01)00081-4

Bloch-Zupan, A., Décimo, D., Loriot, M., Mark, M. P., and Ruch, J. V. (1994). Expression of nuclear retinoic acid receptors during mouse odontogenesis. *Differentiation* 57, 195–203. doi: 10.1046/j.1432-0436.1994.5730195.x

Bloch-Zupan, A., Jamet, X., Etard, C., Laugel, V., Muller, J., Geoffroy, V., et al. (2011). Homozygosity mapping and candidate prioritization identify mutations, missed by whole-exome sequencing, in SMOC2, causing major dental developmental defects. *Am. J. Hum. Genet.* 89, 773–781. doi: 10.1016/j.ajhg.2011.11.002

Bloch-Zupan, A., Sedano, H., and Scully, C. (2012). *Dento/Oro/Craniofacial Anomalies and Genetics*. Amsterdam: Elsevier.

Bronckers, A. L., Engelse, M. A., Cavender, A., Gaikwad, J., and D'Souza, R. N. (2001). Cell-specific patterns of Cbfa1 mRNA and protein expression in postnatal murine dental tissues. *Mech. Dev.* 101, 255–258. doi: 10.1016/S0925-4773(00)00562-1

Camilleri, S., and McDonald, F. (2006). Runx2 and dental development. *Eur. J. Oral Sci.* 114, 361–373. doi: 10.1111/j.1600-0722.2006.00399.x

Cammas, L., Romand, R., Fraulob, V., Mura, C., and Dollé, P. (2007). Expression of the murine retinol dehydrogenase 10 (Rdh10) gene correlates with many sites of retinoid signalling during embryogenesis and organ differentiation. *Dev. Dyn.* 236, 2899–2908. doi: 10.1002/dvdy.21312

Cartharius, K., Frech, K., Grote, K., Klocke, B., Haltmeier, M., Klingenhoff, A., et al. (2005). MatInspector and beyond: promoter analysis based on transcription factor binding sites. *Bioinformatics* 21, 2933–2942. doi: 10.1093/bioinformatics/bti473

Dhamija, S., and Krebsbach, P. H. (2001). Role of Cbfa1 in ameloblastin gene transcription. *J. Biol. Chem.* 276, 35159–35164. doi: 10.1074/jbc.M010719200

D'Souza, R. N., Aberg, T., Gaikwad, J., Cavender, A., Owen, M., Karsenty, G., et al. (1999). Cbfa1 is required for epithelial-mesenchymal interactions regulating tooth development in mice. *Development* 126, 2911–2920.

Ducy, P., and Karsenty, G. (1998). Genetic control of cell differentiation in the skeleton. *Curr. Opin. Cell Biol.* 10, 614–619. doi: 10.1016/S0955-0674(98)80037-9

Dupé, V., Matt, N., Garnier, J. M., Chambon, P., Mark, M., and Ghyselinck, N. B. (2003). A newborn lethal defect due to inactivation of retinaldehyde dehydrogenase type 3 is prevented by maternal retinoic acid treatment. *Proc. Natl. Acad. Sci. U.S.A.* 100, 14036–14041. doi: 10.1073/pnas.2336223100

Eastoe, J. E. (1979). Enamel protein chemistry-past, present and future. *J. Dent. Res.* 58, 753–764. doi: 10.1177/00220345790580022701

Fukumoto, S., Kiba, T., Hall, B., Iehara, N., Nakamura, T., Longenecker, G., et al. (2004). Ameloblastin is a cell adhesion molecule required for maintaining the differentiation state of ameloblasts. *J. Cell Biol.* 167, 973–983. doi: 10.1083/jcb.200409077

Gibson, C. W., Yuan, Z. A., Hall, B., Longenecker, G., Chen, E., Thyagarajan, T., et al. (2001). Amelogenin-deficient mice display an *Amelogenesis imperfecta* phenotype. *J. Biol. Chem.* 276, 31871–31875. doi: 10.1074/jbc.M104624200

Green, A. C., Martin, T. J., and Purton, L. E. (2016). The role of vitamin A and retinoic acid receptor signaling in post-natal maintenance of bone. *J. Steroid Biochem. Mol. Biol.* 155, 135–146. doi: 10.1016/j.jsbmb.2015.09.036

Hassan, M. Q., Javed, A., Morasso, M. I., Karlin, J., Montecino, M., van Wijnen, A. J., et al. (2004). Dlx3 transcriptional regulation of osteoblast differentiation: temporal recruitment of Msx2, Dlx3, and Dlx5 homeodomain proteins to chromatin of the osteocalcin gene. *Mol. Cell. Biol.* 24, 9248–9261. doi: 10.1128/MCB.24.20.9248-9261.2004

Henning, P., Conaway, H. H., and Lerner, U. H. (2015). Retinoid receptors in bone and their role in bone remodeling. *Front. Endocrinol.* 6:31. doi: 10.3389/fendo.2015.00031

Hu, J. C., Hu, Y., Lu, Y., Smith, C. E., Lertlam, R., Wright, J. T., et al. (2014). Enamelin is critical for ameloblast integrity and enamel ultrastructure formation. *PLoS ONE* 9:e89303. doi: 10.1371/journal.pone.0089303

Hu, J. C., Hu, Y., Smith, C. E., McKee, M. D., Wright, J. T., Yamakoshi, Y., et al. (2008). Enamel defects and ameloblast-specific expression in Enam knock-out/lacz knock-in mice. *J. Biol. Chem.* 283, 10858–10871. doi: 10.1074/jbc.M710565200

Jedeon, K., Loiodice, S., Marciano, C., Vinel, A., Canivenc Lavier, M. C., Berdal, A., et al. (2014). Estrogen and bisphenol A affect male rat enamel formation and promote ameloblast proliferation. *Endocrinology* 155, 3365–3375. doi: 10.1210/en.2013-2161

Jeremias, F., Koruyucu, M., Küchler, E. C., Bayram, M., Tuna, E. B., Deeley, K., et al. (2013). Genes expressed in dental enamel development are associated with molar-incisor hypomineralization. *Arch. Oral Biol.* 58, 1434–1442. doi: 10.1016/j.archoralbio.2013.05.005

Jones, D. M., Fabian, B., and Kramer, B. (2008). The effect of retinoic acid on mouse mandibular molar development *in vitro*, using alkaline phosphatase as a molecular indicator of differentiation. *SADJ* 63, 276, 278–280.

Kawasaki, K., and Weiss, K. M. (2008). SCPP gene evolution and the dental mineralization continuum. *J. Dent. Res.* 87, 520–531. doi: 10.1177/154405910808700608

Knudsen, P. A. (1967). Dental malformations in rat embryos with exencephaly induced by hypervitaminosis A. *Acta Odontol. Scand.* 25, 267–287. doi: 10.3109/00016356709104023

Kronmiller, J. E., Upholt, W. B., and Kollar, E. J. (1992). Alteration of murine odontogenic patterning and prolongation of expression of epidermal growth factor mRNA by retinol *in vitro*. *Arch. Oral Biol.* 37, 129–138. doi: 10.1016/0003-9969(92)90008-V

Laue, K., Pogoda, H. M., Daniel, P. B., van Haeringen, A., Alanay, Y., von Ameln, S., et al. (2011). Craniosynostosis and multiple skeletal anomalies in humans and zebrafish result from a defect in the localized degradation of retinoic acid. *Am. J. Hum. Genet.* 89, 595–606. doi: 10.1016/j.ajhg.2011.09.015

Lee, H. K., Lee, D. S., Ryoo, H. M., Park, J. T., Park, S. J., Bae, H. S., et al. (2010). The odontogenic ameloblast-associated protein (ODAM) cooperates with RUNX2 and modulates enamel mineralization via regulation of MMP-20. *J. Cell. Biochem.* 111, 755–767. doi: 10.1002/jcb.22766

Li, Y., Konicki, W. S., Wright, J. T., Suggs, C., Xue, H., Kuehl, M. A., et al. (2013). Mouse genetic background influences the dental phenotype. *Cells Tissues Organs* 198, 448–456. doi: 10.1159/000360157

Lind, T., Sundqvist, A., Hu, L., Pejler, G., Andersson, G., Jacobson, A., et al. (2013). Vitamin a is a negative regulator of osteoblast mineralization. *PLoS ONE* 8:e82388. doi: 10.1371/journal.pone.0082388

Loots, G. G., Ovcharenko, I., Pachter, L., Dubchak, I., and Rubin, E. M. (2002). rVista for comparative sequence-based discovery of functional transcription factor binding sites. *Genome Res.* 12, 832–839. doi: 10.1101/gr.225502. Article published online before print in April 2002

Maclean, G., Dollé, P., and Petkovich, M. (2009). Genetic disruption of CYP26B1 severely affects development of neural crest derived head structures, but does not compromise hindbrain patterning. *Dev. Dyn.* 238, 732–745. doi: 10.1002/dvdy.21878

Maden, M. (2007). Retinoic acid in the development, regeneration and maintenance of the nervous system. *Nat. Rev. Neurosci.* 8, 755–765. doi: 10.1038/nrn2212

Mark, M. P., Bloch-Zupan, A., and Ruch, J. V. (1992). Effects of retinoids on tooth morphogenesis and cytodifferentiations, *in vitro*. *Int. J. Dev. Biol.* 36, 517–526.

Masuya, H., Shimizu, K., Sezutsu, H., Sakuraba, Y., Nagano, J., Shimizu, A., et al. (2005). Enamelin (Enam) is essential for amelogenesis: ENU-induced mouse mutants as models for different clinical subtypes of human *Amelogenesis imperfecta* (AI). *Hum. Mol. Genet.* 14, 575–583. doi: 10.1093/hmg/ddi054

Maynard, T. M., Gopalakrishna, D., Meechan, D. W., Paronett, E. M., Newbern, J. M., and LaMantia, A. S. (2013). 22q11 Gene dosage establishes an adaptive range for sonic hedgehog and retinoic acid signaling during early development. *Hum. Mol. Genet.* 22, 300–312. doi: 10.1093/hmg/dds429

McDowell, E. M., Shores, R. L., Spangler, E. F., Wenk, M. L., and De Luca, L. M. (1987). Anomalous growth of rat incisor teeth during chronic intermittent vitamin A deficiency. *J. Nutr.* 117, 1265–1274.

Mellanby, H. (1941). The effect of maternal dietary deficiency of vitamin A on dental tissues in rats. *J. Dent. Res.* 20, 489–509. doi: 10.1177/00220345410200051401

Mic, F. A., Molotkov, A., Benbrook, D. M., and Duester, G. (2003). Retinoid activation of retinoic acid receptor but not retinoid X receptor is sufficient to rescue lethal defect in retinoic acid synthesis. *Proc. Natl. Acad. Sci. U.S.A.* 100, 7135–7140. doi: 10.1073/pnas.1231422100

Minegishi, Y., Sakai, Y., Yahara, Y., Akiyama, H., Yoshikawa, H., Hosokawa, K., et al. (2014). Cyp26b1 within the growth plate regulates bone growth in juvenile mice. *Biochem. Biophys. Res. Commun.* 454, 12–18. doi: 10.1016/j.bbrc.2014.10.001

Minoux, M., and Rijli, F. M. (2010). Molecular mechanisms of cranial neural crest cell migration and patterning in craniofacial development. *Development* 137, 2605–2621. doi: 10.1242/dev.040048

Nakayama, Y., Holcroft, J., and Ganss, B. (2015). Enamel hypomineralization and structural defects in amelotin-deficient mice. *J. Dent. Res.* 94, 697–705. doi: 10.1177/0022034514565214

Niederreither, K., and Dollé, P. (2008). Retinoic acid in development: towards an integrated view. *Nat. Rev. Genet.* 9, 541–553. doi: 10.1038/nrg2340

Niederreither, K., Vermot, J., Schuhbaur, B., Chambon, P., and Dollé, P. (2000). Retinoic acid synthesis and hindbrain patterning in the mouse embryo. *Development* 127, 75–85.

Niederreither, K., Vermot, J., Schuhbaur, B., Chambon, P., and Dollé, P. (2002). Embryonic retinoic acid synthesis is required for forelimb growth and anteroposterior patterning in the mouse. *Development* 129, 3563–3574.

Núñez, S. M., Chun, Y.-H. P., Ganss, B., Hu, Y., Richardson, A. S., Schmitz, J. E., et al. (2015). Maturation stage enamel malformations in *Amtn* and *Klk4* null mice. *Matrix Biol.* 52–54, 219–233. doi: 10.1016/j.matbio.2015.11.007

Pindborg, J. J. (1953). The pigmentation of the rat incisor as an index of metabolic disturbances. *Oral Surg. Oral Med. Oral Pathol.* 6, 780–789. doi: 10.1016/0030-4220(53)90205-9

Prasad, M. K., Geoffroy, V., Vicaire, S., Jost, B., Dumas, M., Le Gras, S., et al. (2016). A targeted next-generation sequencing assay for the molecular diagnosis of genetic disorders with orodental involvement. *J. Med. Genet.* 53, 98–110. doi: 10.1136/jmedgenet-2015-103302

Punyasingh, J. T., Hoffman, S., Harris, S. S., and Navia, J. M. (1984). Effects of vitamin A deficiency on rat incisor formation. *J. Oral Pathol.* 13, 40–51. doi: 10.1111/j.1600-0714.1984.tb01399.x

Rhinn, M., and Dollé, P. (2012). Retinoic acid signalling during development. *Development* 139, 843–858 doi: 10.1242/dev.065938

Rochette-Egly, C., and Germain, P. (2009). Dynamic and combinatorial control of gene expression by nuclear retinoic acid receptors (RARs). *Nucl. Recept. Signal.* 7:e005. doi: 10.1621/nrs.07005

Rossant, J., Zirngibl, R., Cado, D., Shago, M., and Giguère, V. (1991). Expression of a retinoic acid response element-hsplacZ transgene defines specific domains of transcriptional activity during mouse embryogenesis. *Genes Dev.* 5, 1333–1344. doi: 10.1101/gad.5.8.1333

Ryynänen, H., Sahlberg, C., Lukinmaa, P. L., and Alaluusua, S. (2014). The effect of high temperature on the development of mouse dental enamel *in vitro*. *Arch. Oral Biol.* 59, 400–406. doi: 10.1016/j.archoralbio.2014.01.005

Sehic, A., Khuu, C., Risnes, S., and Osmundsen, H. (2009). Differential gene expression profiling of the molar tooth germ in peroxisome proliferator-activated receptor-alpha (PPAR-alpha) knockout mouse and in wild-type mouse: molar tooth phenotype of PPAR-alpha knockout mouse. *Eur. J. Oral Sci.* 117, 93–104. doi: 10.1111/j.1600-0722.2009.00615.x

Seritrakul, P., Samarut, E., Lama, T. T., Gibert, Y., Laudet, V., and Jackman, W. R. (2012). Retinoic acid expands the evolutionarily reduced dentition of zebrafish. *FASEB J.* 26, 5014–5024. doi: 10.1096/fj.12-209304

Simmer, J. P., Papagerakis, P., Smith, C. E., Fisher, D. C., Rountrey, A. N., Zheng, L., et al. (2010). Regulation of dental enamel shape and hardness. *J. Dent. Res.* 89, 1024–1038. doi: 10.1177/0022034510375829

Wang, X., Wang, S., Lu, Y., Gibson, M. P., Liu, Y., Yuan, B., et al. (2012). FAM20C plays an essential role in the formation of murine teeth. *J. Biol. Chem.* 287, 35934–35942. doi: 10.1074/jbc.M112.386862

Xuan, D., Sun, X., Yan, Y., Xie, B., Xu, P., and Zhang, J. (2010). Effect of cleidocranial dysplasia-related novel mutation of RUNX2 on characteristics of dental pulp cells and tooth development. *J. Cell. Biochem.* 111, 1473–1481. doi: 10.1002/jcb.22875

Yang, T., Zhang, Y., Zheng, D., Hao, Y., Snead, M. L., and Duan, X. (2015). High-fluoride promoted phagocytosis-induced apoptosis in a matured ameloblast-like cell line. *Arch. Oral Biol.* 60, 84–90. doi: 10.1016/j.archoralbio.2014.09.001

2

Site-Specific Variations in Bone Mineral Density under Systemic Conditions Inducing Osteoporosis in Minipigs

Matthias C. Schulz[1], Jan Kowald[2,3], Sven Estenfelder[2,4], Roland Jung[5], Eberhard Kuhlisch[6], Uwe Eckelt[1], Ronald Mai[1], Lorenz C. Hofbauer[7], Christian Stroszczynski[8] and Bernd Stadlinger[9]*

[1] Department of Oral and Maxillofacial Surgery, Medical Faculty "Carl Gustav Carus," Technische Universität Dresden, Dresden, Germany, [2] Department of Radiology, Medical Faculty "Carl Gustav Carus," Technische Universität Dresden, Dresden, Germany, [3] Division of Nephrology, Department of Internal Medicine III, Medical Faculty "Carl Gustav Carus," Technische Universität Dresden, Dresden, Germany, [4] Department of Internal Medicine III, University of Ulm, Ulm, Germany, [5] Experimental Center, Medical Faculty "Carl Gustav Carus," Technische Universität Dresden, Dresden, Germany, [6] Institute for Medical Informatics and Biometry, Medical Faculty "Carl Gustav Carus," Technische Universität Dresden, Dresden, Germany, [7] Division of Endocrinology, Diabetes and Bone Diseases, Department of Medicine III, Medical Faculty "Carl Gustav Carus," Technische Universität Dresden, Dresden, Germany, [8] Department of Radiology, University Hospital Regensburg, Regensburg, Germany, [9] Clinic of Cranio-Maxillofacial and Oral Surgery, University of Zurich, University Hospital Zurich, Zurich, Switzerland

***Correspondence:**
Matthias C. Schulz
Matthias.Schulz@uniklinikum-dresden.de

Osteoporosis is a systemic bone disease with an increasing prevalence in the elderly population. There is conflicting opinion about whether osteoporosis affects the alveolar bone of the jaws and whether it poses a risk to the osseointegration of dental implants. The aim of the present study was to evaluate the effects of systemic glucocorticoid administration on the jaw bone density of minipigs. Thirty-seven adult female minipigs were randomly divided into two groups. Quantitative computed tomography (QCT) was used to assess bone mineral density BMD of the lumbar spine as well as the mandible and maxilla, and blood was drawn. One group of minipigs initially received 1.0 mg prednisolone per kg body weight daily for 2 months. The dose was tapered to 0.5 mg per kg body weight per day thereafter. The animals in the other group served as controls and received placebo. QCT and blood analysis were repeated after 6 and 9 months. BMD was compared between the two groups by measuring Hounsfield units, and serum levels of several bone metabolic markers were also assessed. A decrease in BMD was observed in the jaws from baseline to 9 months. This was more pronounced in the prednisolone group. Statistically significant differences were reached for the mandible ($p < 0.001$) and the maxilla ($p < 0.001$). The administration of glucocorticoids reduced the BMD in the jaws of minipigs. The described model shows promise in the evaluation of osseointegration of dental implants in bone that is compromised by osteoporosis.

Keywords: animal models, bone, bone mineralization, oral cavity, osteoporosis

INTRODUCTION

Osteoporosis is a systemic disease that affects bone mass and architecture, increasing the risk of bone fractures (Rachner et al., 2011). Osteoporosis is prevalent in the United States, Europe, and Japan, causing over 4.5 million fractures annually (WHO Scientific Group on the Assessment of Osteoporosis at Primary Health Care Level, 2004). As consequence of an aging population, an increasing number of people suffer from osteoporosis. The most common form of osteoporosis is post-menopausal osteoporosis in females, due to reduced estrogen levels. Other risk factors for the development of osteoporosis include patient age and long-term systemic exposure to exogenous glucocorticoids. The clinical diagnosis of osteoporosis is usually confirmed radiographically, via dual-energy X-ray absorptiometry (DXA)-based bone densitometry (Felsenberg and Gowin, 1999) and, more recently, with high resolution quantitative computed tomography (hrQCT; Snedeker et al., 2006; Graeff et al., 2013).

The influence of both local and systemic diseases on the osseointegration of dental implants has been a repeated point of discussion. For example, it has been shown that periodontitis in conjunction with smoking (Heitz-Mayfield and Huynh-Ba, 2009), and radiotherapy prior to implant placement (Chambrone et al., 2013), negatively affect implant integration. With regard to osteoporosis, there are contradictory reports on the success rates of dental implants placed in osteoporotic bone. Whereas, some studies describe no influence of osteoporosis on the implant osseointegration (Dvorak et al., 2011a), other authors report higher loss rates of implants in osteoporotic bone (Moy et al., 2005; Alsaadi et al., 2008). It is uncertain whether osteoporosis commonly induces areas of rarefaction in the alveolar processes of the jaws that are of clinical relevance to implant success. While some authors report that osteoporotic skeletal changes are reflected in alveolar bone changes (Jonasson et al., 2006), others have found no correlation between the condition of the general skeletal and alveolar bone structures (Kingsmill and Boyde, 1999).

Such possible correlations can be analyzed in animal models. In osteoporosis research, rodent models have been used for analysis of the integration of biomaterials (Stadlinger et al., 2013). In rodent studies, ovariectomy serves to induce an osteoporotic state. Large animal models more closely resemble human anatomy and human patterns of wound healing, allowing the application of regular-sized surgical instruments and dental implants. However, due to practicalities, it has been uncommon to employ systemically impaired large animal models for the analysis of dental implant integration in bone or soft tissue (Thoma et al., 2012). Sheep, minipigs, and dogs may serve for such studies. The establishment of an osteoporotic state in large animals is possible by various means. Usually osteoporosis is induced by ovariectomy, however this has been reported to have a limited influence on nulliparous pigs (Scholz-Ahrens et al., 1996). Other approaches involve a calcium-deficient diet, the systemic application of glucocorticoids, or a combination of those approaches. Recently, an animal model has been reported, showing mandibular bone loss following a hypothalamic-pituitary disconnection (Oheim et al., 2014).

The application of glucocorticoids in minipigs has been shown to induce reduction of BMD in the lumbar spine as assessed by quantitative computed tomography (QCT; Scholz-Ahrens et al., 2007). QCT enables repeated measurements of the entire skeleton over time and is therefore suitable for large animal studies on bone structure.

In most pre-clinical studies, implant integration is analyzed in pristine bone under unimpaired osseous conditions. The aim of this minipig study was to establish a large animal model with glucocorticoid-induced osteoporosis, for the analysis of implant osseointegration under impaired systemic osseous conditions. To achieve this effect, the experimental animals received systemic glucocorticoid therapy for 9 months. During this period, the animals underwent three QCT assessments. The hypothesis was that glucocorticoid application for 9 months would induce a significant decrease of BMD in both the lumbar spine and the alveolar bone of the jaws.

MATERIALS AND METHODS

Experimental Design

The study protocol was approved by the Commission for Animal Studies at the District Government, Dresden, Germany (file reference: 24-9168.11-1/2008-43). The study was conducted in accordance to the recommendations and guidelines of the Commission for Animal Studies at the District Government, Dresden, Germany.

For the study, 37 adult female miniature pigs (nulliparous, aged 18–20 months, average weight 72.5 $\pm$ 16.7 kg) of the breed Mini-Lewe were used. The animals were randomly divided into two groups: Group I (29 animals) received daily oral prednisolone, 1 mg per kg body weight in the initial phase. After 2 months, the dosage was reduced to 0.5 mg prednisolone per kg body weight per day. Prednisolone administration was performed according to the protocol described by Scholz-Ahrens (Scholz-Ahrens et al., 2007). Group II (eight animals), which received neither prednisolone nor a carrier, served as control. Before the commencement of prednisolone, and at the 6- and 9-month time-points of prednisolone administration, QCT was performed for each animal, and blood samples for laboratory assessment and measurement of biochemical markers of bone turnover were also taken.

Nutrition

Prior to the start of the study, the animals were fed a diet consisting of pollard, wheat bran, and corn silage obtained from a local food producer. The pollard contained 0.57% of calcium and 0.55% of phosphorus. The content of vitamin D3 was 328 international units (IU) per kg. After initiation of the glucocorticoid therapy, the experimental animals were fed a calcium-deficient diet omitting the pollard. The diet contained 58.3% wheat bran and 41.7% corn-based silage. The wheat bran contained 0.07% calcium and 0.05% phosphorus. The content of vitamin D3 was <300 IU per kg. The diet of the control group remained unchanged. Water was available *ad libitum*. The components of the animal nutrition were analyzed prior to the study (LUFA-ITL GmbH, Kiel, Germany).

Sedation

Computed tomography investigations and the collection of the blood samples were performed under sedation, under the surveillance of a veterinarian. The medication for sedation involved a mixture of 1 mg/kg body weight midazolam (Ratiopharm GmbH, Ulm, Germany), 10 mg/kg body weight ketamine (Riemser Arzneimittel AG, Greifswald, Germany), and 0.05 mg/kg body weight atropine (Eifelfango Chem.-Pharm. Werke, Bad Neuenahr-Ahrweiler, Germany), administered intramuscularly.

Quantitative Computed Tomography

The computed tomography scanner was a multislice-CT (SOMATOM 16, Siemens Healthcare, Erlangen, Germany). The minipigs were positioned ventrally due to veterinary aspects of respiration, with mandible and maxilla parallel to the horizontal plane. The images were acquired by applying the spiral technique with a collimation of 16 × 0.75 mm. The data acquisition was performed axial using a slice-thickness of 0.75 mm. The field of view was chosen 265 × 265 mm for the jaw scan and 200 × 200 mm for the scan of the lumbar vertebrae with a matrix of 512 × 512. Thus, a pixel spacing of 0.426 × 0.426 mm for the jaw scan and of 0.445 × 0.445 mm resulted. The optimal set-up conditions for the jaw scan were a tube voltage of 120 kV and 36 mAs. For the vertebra region the same tube voltage was used with 274 mAs.

The data was acquired by a filtered back projection with convolution kernel H60s for the jaw scan and B70s for the vertebra scan. Saving was performed as digital imaging and communication in medicine (DICOM) standard using the Leonardo workstation (LEONARDO VD10B; Syngo VX49B; Siemens Healthcare Diagnostics GmbH, Eschborn, Germany). The analyses and measurements of the CT scans were performed with interactive data language software (IDL 7.0.0, ITT-Visual Information Solutions, Boulder/CO, USA) by two experienced examiners (JK, SE). To calculate the inter- and intra-observer reproducibility, measurements of eight randomly selected animals were repeated twice by each examiner with a time interval of 2 weeks. Calibration was performed using a reference phantom containing a bone-like and a water-like phase (Osteo Phantom, Siemens Healthcare, Erlangen, Germany) placed parallelly to the horizontal plane. A gray scale of Hounsfield units (HU) served for the analysis of the bone mineral density. A threshold was defined in order to ensure that no soft tissue (e.g., fat) or dental structures (e.g., roots) were included in the measurements. In preliminary tests, a mean density of the mandibular and maxillary cortical bone of 1386 HU was assessed (data not shown). Furthermore, the gray values of the soft tissues in the bone marrow were measured to have a peak value below 0 HU. According to the resulting histograms, the thresholds at 0 HU for the minimum and at 1,350 HU for the maximum were defined. As mineralized dental structures show comparable or higher density values than cortical bone they could be precluded from the measurements by the threshold, likewise.

For the radiographic analysis of the jaw region, the radiographs were positioned parallelly to the transversal plane. The vertical position of the transversal cutting plane was determined by the root tips of the three premolar teeth in each jaw. The regions of interest in the mandible and maxilla were defined as follows: The oral and buccal borders were defined by the inner layer of the cortical bone. The distal edge of the canine root served as the anterior border and the mesial root of the third molar as the distal border. The matching of the radiographs of the baseline QCT and of the QCTs after 6 and 9 months was achieved by using constant anatomical structures e.g., pterygoid process, the bony nasal septum and the tuber maxilla in the upper jaw. In the mandible, the profile of the oral and vestibular cortical bone was used for the matching of the images. For the measurement of the BMD in lumbar vertebrae I–III, the radiographs were positioned parallel to the axial plane. The region of interest was defined through the ventral cortical bone and the cortical bone of the spinal canal. The lateral border was defined by a dense trabecula connecting the ventral cortical bone and the spinal canal in dorsomedial direction. The regions of interest are depicted in **Figures 1**, **2** for the jaw region and in **Figure 3** for the vertebral region. For the measurement of the bone density, the gray values of the pixels in the regions of interest were assessed and displayed in Hounsfield Units using the IDL-software. The mean value and standard deviation of each region of interest was calculated. In the upper and lower jaw, the left and right side were measured separately, and were later pooled for the statistical evaluation.

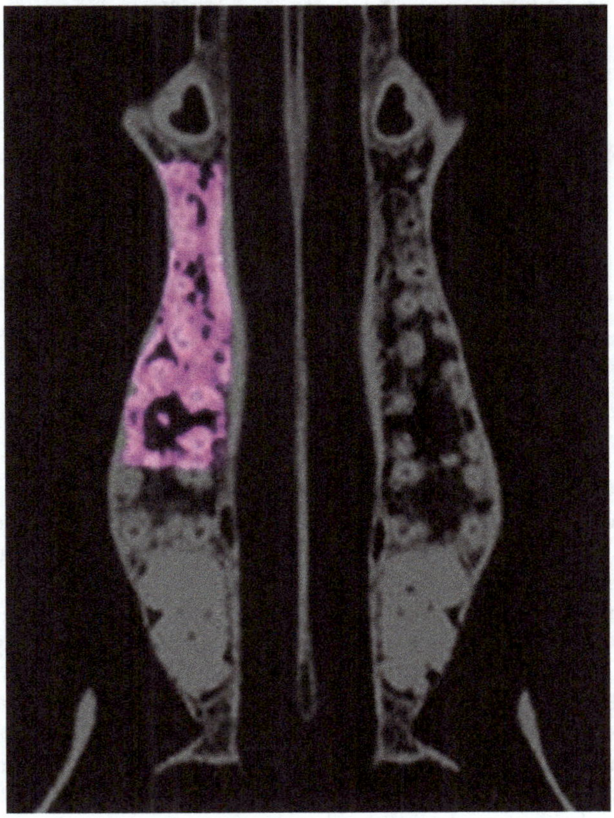

FIGURE 1 | The region of interest for the analysis of the computed tomography scans is depicted in the maxilla. The area is extended between the distal edge of the canine root and the mesial edge of the third molar. Laterally, the cortical bone served as border.

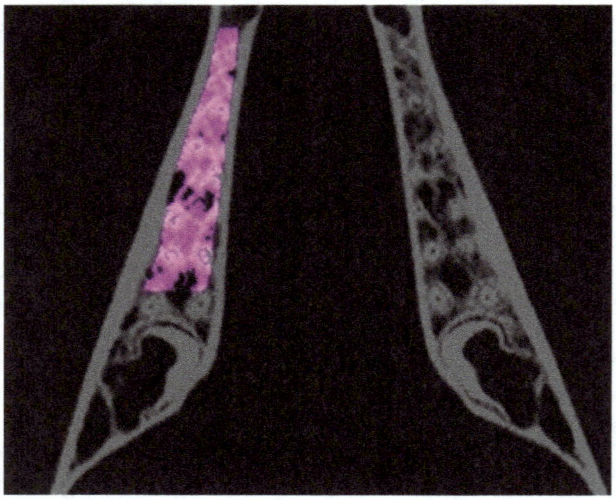

FIGURE 2 | The region of interest for the analysis of the computed tomography scans is depicted in the mandible. The area is extended between the distal edge of the canine root and the mesial edge of the third molar. Laterally, the cortical bone served as border.

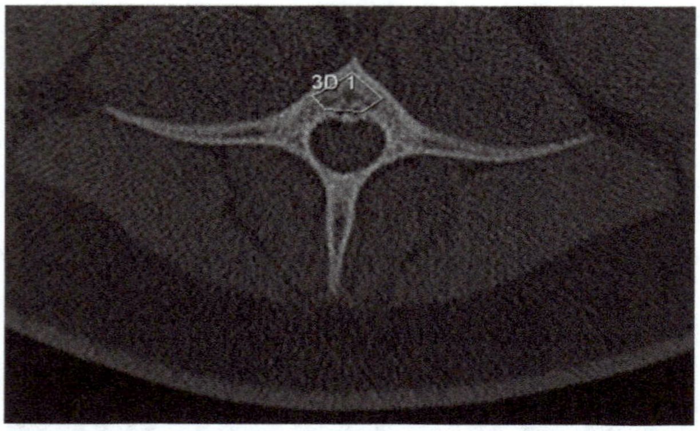

FIGURE 3 | In the vertebrae, the region of interest was defined as a polygon being limited by the ventral and dorsal cortical bone and dorso-laterally by a dense trabecula between the ventral cortical bone and the spinal canal.

Serum Parameters

Blood samples were taken before the commencement of glucocorticoid administration and after 6 and 9 months, respectively. The samples were always obtained from the ear vein at the same time of the day using serum gel monovettes (Sarstedt AG & Co., Nürmbrecht, Germany) and stored at 4°C until centrifugation. Subsequently, the following parameters were analyzed using an automatic test system (cobas c, Roche Diagnostics, Mannheim, Germany). The serum level of ionic calcium and ionic phosphorus were analyzed by photometric test kits (CA2 and PHOS2). The level of total alkaline phosphatase was measured by an extinction test kit (ALP2). For the analysis of the levels of beta crosslaps an immunoassay test kit (ECLIA) was used. All test kits were obtained from Roche Diagnostics, Mannheim, Germany. Bone specific alkaline phosphatase was measured using an immunoassay (MicroVue™ BAP, Quidel Corporation, San Diego, CA, USA). The serum level of 25(OH) Vitamin D was analyzed by a chemiluminescence assay (LIAISON® 25 OH Vitamin D TOTAL Assay). The analysis of the osteocalcin level was performed using a two-site immunoradiometric assay (CA 72-4 IRMA). Both assays were obtained from DiaSorin Inc., Stillwater, MN, USA. Osteoprotegrin (OPG) levels were analyzed by an enzyme-linked immune sorbent assay (Osteoprotegrin ELISA kit, Immundiagnostik AG, Bensheim, Germany). The serum level of $1,25(OH)_2$-Vitamin D was measured using a radioimmunoassay (1,25-Dihydroxy Vitamin D RIA, Immunodiagnostic Systems GmbH, Frankfurt am Main, Germany). All analyses were performed by the Institute for Clinical Chemistry and Laboratory Medicine (Medical Faculty "Carl Gustav Carus," Technische Universität Dresden, Dresden, Germany) using standardized laboratory methods.

Statistical Analysis

The degree of agreement between the two observers and the degree of agreement between the two measurements were assessed by a reliability analysis. The inter- and intra-observer reliability is described by the intraclass correlation coefficient (ICC) taking a two-way random model with absolute agreement definition. The animal experiment was planned and carried out as longitudinal study. Consequentially the analyses were done by ANOVA using linear mixed models. The models included fixed effects associated with treatment, time, and the interaction between treatment and time. The residual covariance matrix was specified as a heterogeneous compound symmetry (CSH), so that the variances differ across the levels of time. Estimated means and their 95%-confidence limits are given. *Post-hoc* tests and confidence limits are alpha-adjusted using the Tukey–Kramer method. The statistical analysis was performed using SPSS 19 (SPSS Inc., Chicago, Illinois, USA) and SAS 9.3 (SAS Institute Inc., Cary, NC, USA).

RESULTS

From the initially 37 minipigs, two animals of the prednisolone group died due to unknown cause and were excluded from the analysis. Thus, 35 animals completed the study period and could be included in the evaluation.

Quantitative Computed Tomography

Intra- and Inter-Observer Control

The intra-observer analysis showed an ICC of 0.992 (95%-confidence interval: 0.987–0.995) for observer I and an ICC of 0.991 (95%-confidence interval: 0.987–0.994) for observer II. The inter-observer analysis showed an ICC of 0.992 (95%-confidence interval: 0.988–0.995) for the first time point and an ICC of 0.990 (95%-confidence interval: 0.984–0.993) for the second time point. A statistically significant difference between both observers could not be found, neither for the first ($p = 0.592$) nor for the second time point ($p = 0.224$).

Control Group—Development of Bone Mass with Aging

With regard to BMD-values, the control group showed a general decrease from baseline to the 6-month examination. This decrease was statistically significant for all regions of interest. From 6 to 9 months, a statistically significant increase of BMD was obvious for all examined regions. When comparing the baseline values to those obtained after 9 months, an overall decrease of BMD was found. However, this decrease was only statistically significant for the maxilla. For vertebrae and mandible no significant changes could be found (vertebrae: $p = 0.988$; mandible: $p = 0.995$).

Effects of Glucocorticoid Exposure on Bone Mass

At the baseline point of the study, the values for BMD in the lumbar vertebrae and the maxilla differed statistically significantly between control and treatment group. For the mandible, no statistically significant difference could be observed ($p = 0.973$). In the computed tomography results after 6 months, the BMD showed a decrease in all evaluated regions. This decrease was statistically significant for both the control and the glucocorticoid group. Between the groups, no statistically significant differences could be found for any region. After 9 months, an increase of BMD in the control group was obvious for all evaluated regions compared to the 6-month values. This increase was statistically significant for all regions. However, the values after 9 months did not reach the baseline level again. Compared to baseline values, the decrease was statistically significant for the maxilla ($p < 0.001$). For the lumbar vertebrae and the mandible, the differences were not statistically significant (lumbar vertebrae: $p = 0.981$; mandible: $p = 0.559$). An example for the rarefied trabecular structure in the jaw bone is given in **Figures 4A,B** for the maxilla and in **Figures 5A,B** for the mandible.

After 9 months, there was an increase in the bone density values in the lumbar vertebrae in the glucocorticoid group compared to the 6-month value. This was statistically significant. In the jaw region, a slight decrease of BMD was observed. However, this decrease did not reach statistical significance when compared to the values after 6 months (maxilla: $p = 0.551$; mandible: $p = 0.559$). Compared to the baseline, the values after 9 months of glucocorticoid administration were lower. For the lumbar vertebrae region, this difference was not statistically significant ($p = 0.981$). In the jaw region, the difference reached statistical significance. When compared to the control group the values for BMD differed statistically significant for all examined regions in the glucocorticoid group. The detailed chronological data and statistical significant differences are shown in **Table 1**.

Serum Parameters

Control Group

In the control group, the level of ionic phosphorus decreased slightly during the period of study while values of ionic calcium, alkaline phosphatase, osteocalcin, and 1,25(OH)2-vitamin D varied. The values of bone specific alkaline phosphatase and beta crosslaps increased. During the study period, an increase could be observed for OPG serum levels. The means and their standard deviations are shown in **Table 2**. Statistical significant differences are depicted in **Figure 6**.

Effects of Glucocorticoid Exposure on Serum Parameters

The serum values for ionic phosphorus showed a decrease over the study period. Ionic calcium values varied over the study period as in the control group. From the baseline to

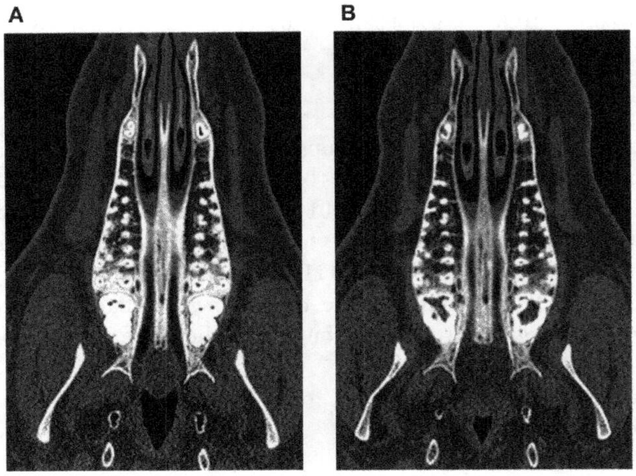

FIGURE 4 | Trabecular rarefication over time shown in the maxilla. Compared to the baseline **(A)** the spongious area in the region of interest appears in darker gray values after 9 months **(B)** indicating a loss of mineralization.

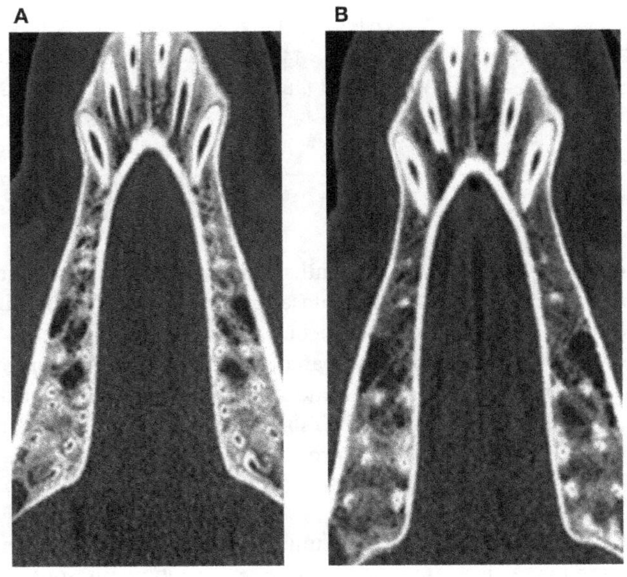

FIGURE 5 | Trabecular rarefication over time shown in the mandible. Compared to the baseline **(A)** the spongious area in the region of interest appears in darker gray values after 9 months **(B)** indicating a loss of mineralization.

TABLE 1 | Values of bone mineral density in Hounsfield Unit (HU).

Region of interest	Baseline (HU)	6 months (HU)	9 months (HU)
Control	**Mean ± SD**	**Mean ± SD**	**Mean ± SD**
Lumbal vertebrae	$464.70^{*1} \pm 46.44$	$382.71^{*+3} \pm 40.90$	$444.67^{+3,10} \pm 43.29$
Maxilla	$569.21^{**\$2,6} \pm 66.24$	$407.25^{**\#4} \pm 72.87$	$474.80^{\#\$4,6,11} \pm 76.36$
Mandible	$613.41^{''} \pm 74.99$	$537.14^{''\wedge 5} \pm 87.46$	$598.83^{\wedge 5,12} \pm 112.85$
GLUCOCORTICOID			
Lumbal vertebrae	$377.80^{1} \pm 51.49$	$339.87^{7} \pm 57.84$	$366.37^{7,10} \pm 71.76$
Maxilla	$421.91^{2,8} \pm 119.20$	323.25 ± 69.74	$315.51^{8,11} \pm 71.23$
Mandible	$541.23^{9} \pm 151.83$	424.40 ± 106.84	$402.89^{9,12} \pm 99.23$

Means and standard deviations (SD) are depicted. The statistical significant differences of the pairwise comparisons are marked (, **, +, $, 2, 3, 6, 8, 9, 11, 12: $p < 0.001$;", #, ^, 1, 4, 5, 7, 10: $p < 0.05$).*

TABLE 2 | The development of serum parameters over the study period.

		CT 1			CT 2			CT 3		
Parameter	**Group**	**Mean**	**SD**	**95% CI**	**Mean**	**SD**	**95% CI**	**Mean**	**SD**	**95% CI**
PO_4^{2-}/mmol*l^{-1}	Control	2.008	0.541	(1.752, 2.263)	1.943	0.188	(1.789, 2.096)	1.950	0.148	(1.712, 2.188)
	Glucocorticoid	2.253	0.285	(2.114, 2.392)	1.716	0.220	(1.633, 1.800)	1.708	0.365	(1.578, 1.838)
Ca^{2+}/mmol*l^{-1}	Control	2.266	0.440	(1.981, 2.552)	2.396	0.086	(2.115, 2.678)	1.368	0.381	(1.095, 1.640)
	Glucocorticoid	2.027	0.385	(1.872, 2.183)	1.993	0.439	(1.840, 2.147)	2.128	0.378	(1.979, 2.276)
AP/μmol*l^{-1}	Control	0.754	0.161	(−0.178, 1.686)	0.776	0.222	(0.459, 1.093)	0.744	0.126	(0.476, 1.012)
	Glucocorticoid	1.678	1.457	(1.171, 2.185)	0.734	0.483	(0.561, 0.907)	0.807	0.415	(0.661, 0.953)
BAP/U*l^{-1}	Control	16.738	4.194	(−24.081, 57.556)	29.588	5.192	(16.734, 42.441)	27.750	2.799	(15.887, 39.613)
	Glucocorticoid	71.830	63.894	(49.611, 94.048)	23.793	19.950	(16.796, 30.789)	25.330	18.523	(18.872, 31.787)
β-Crosslaps/ng*ml^{-1}	Control	0.385	0.099	(0.244, 0.526)	0.736	0.172	(0.426, 1.047)	0.731	0.081	(0.499, 0.963)
	Glucocorticoid	0.838	0.215	(0.761, 0.915)	0.499	0.478	(0.330, 0.668)	0.600	0.361	(0.474, 0.726)
Osteocalcin/ng*ml^{-1}	Control	13.125	3.605	(1.195, 25.055)	34.988	7.618	(21.428, 48.547)	19.763	8.833	(7.210, 32.315)
	Glucocorticoid	121.822	18.591	(115.328, 128.316)	27.563	20.865	(20.182, 34.944)	21.137	19.118	(14.304, 27.970)
OPG/pmol*l^{-1}	Control	0.140	0	(0.042, 0.238)	0.140	0	(−0.257, 0.537)	0.180	0.091	(0.082, 0.278)
	Glucocorticoid	0.286	0.153	(0.233, 0.339)	0.540	0.622	(0.324, 0.756)	0.200	0.146	(0.147, 0.253)
$1,25(OH)_2D_3$/pg*ml^{-1}	Control	141.625	27.184	(118.075, 165.175)	57.463	16.318	(44.053, 70.872)	143.050	51.234	(114.620, 171.480)
	Glucocorticoid	87.433	34.082	(74.614, 100.253)	48.633	19.220	(41.334, 55.932)	101.778	35.721	(86.302, 117.253)
$25(OH)D_3$/ng*ml^{-1}	Control	7.638	2.744	(6.692, 8.583)	4.000	0	(3.975, 4.025)	5.488	1.750	(4.908, 6.067)
	Glucocorticoid	4.315	0.407	(3.800, 4.829)	4.007	0.038	(3.994, 4.021)	4.000	0	(3.684, 4.316)

Means, their 95% confidence intervals (CI) and standard deviations (SD) are depicted.

the measurement after 6 months, alkaline phosphatase and bone specific alkaline phosphatase decreased. After initiating the administration of glucocorticoids, the values for osteocalcin decreased after 6 months compared to the baseline. The serum levels for beta-crosslaps, OPG, and $1,25(OH)_2$-vitamin D varied. The detailed data is depicted in **Table 2** and statistical significant differences are depicted in **Figure 6**.

Inter-Group Comparison

At baseline, the values for all serum parameters differed between the groups. A decrease could be observed for ionic phosphorus in both groups, but was more pronounced in the glucocorticoid group. The decrease differed statistically significant for both time points ($p = 0.008$; $p = 0.009$). When comparing bone-specific alkaline phosphatase, osteocalcin, and 25(OH)-vitamin D, the development in both groups differed significantly (alkaline phosphatase: $p = 0.013$; $p = 0.017$; osteocalcin: $p < 0.001$; 25(OH)-vitamin D: $p < 0.001$). No statistically significant differences were found for the trends of the levels of alkaline phosphatase ($p = 0.076$; $p = 0.111$), OPG ($p = 0.266$; $p = 0.129$). For $1,25(OH)_2$-vitamin D, the development initially differed between the groups ($p = 0.006$) but not for the entire study period ($p = 0.443$).

DISCUSSION

The osseointegration of dental implants is commonly analyzed in animal models prior to clinical application in humans. In treatment clinics however, the situation is often different to ideal pre-clinical laboratory conditions. Many patients suffer

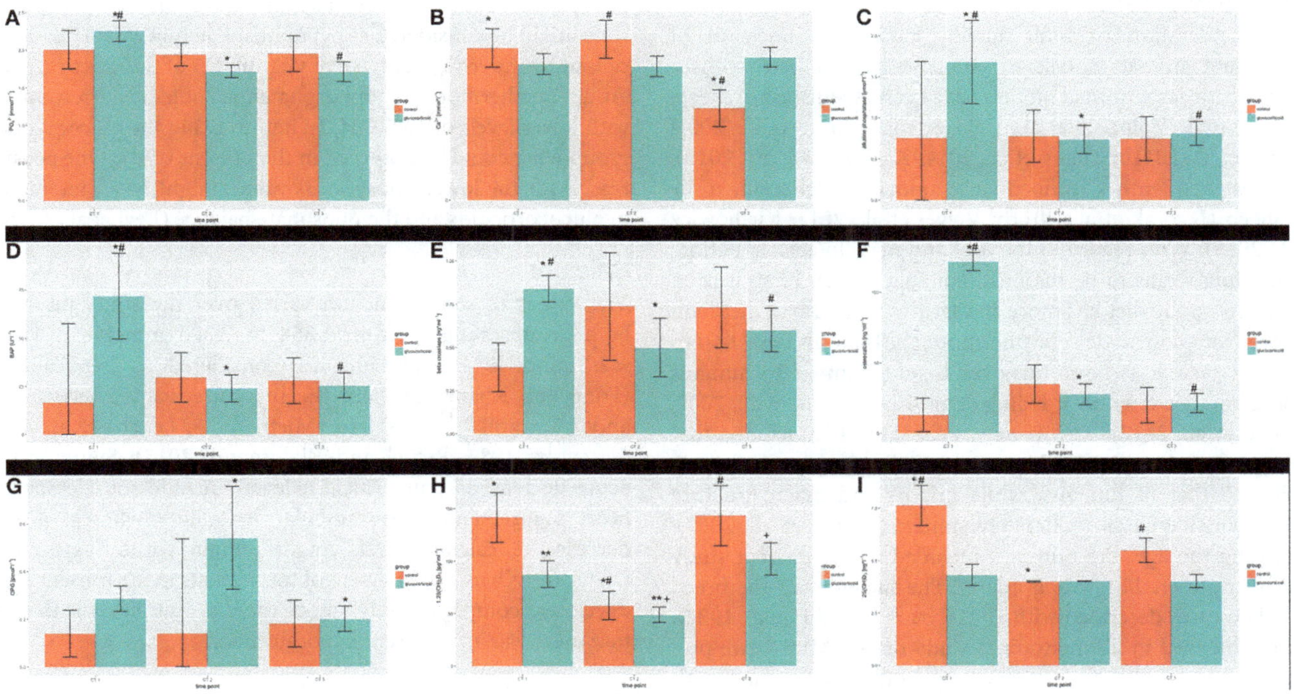

FIGURE 6 | Serum parameters during the study period: **(A)** inorganic phosphorus; **(B)** calcium; **(C)** alkaline phosphatase; **(D)** bone specific alkaline phosphatase (BAP); **(E)** β-crosslaps; **(F)** osteocalcin; **(G)** osteoprotegrin; **(H)** 1,25-dihydroxyvitamin D; **(I)** 25(OH)-hydroxyvitamin D. Statistical significant differences within the groups over the study period are marked (*, **, #, +).

from local bone defects due to bone resorption following tooth extraction or as a consequence of local trauma and require bone augmentation prior to implant therapy. Further, an increasing number of patients suffer from systemic diseases such as diabetes mellitus or osteoporosis, and are receiving medical therapy. These factors might interfere with bone healing, osseointegration of implants, and the health of oral soft tissues (Sachelarie et al., 2016).

Bone Mineral Density

In the present study, BMD was measured using QCT, which is frequently used in animal studies (Scholz-Ahrens et al., 2007; Veigel et al., 2011). The measurements are focused on the trabecular bone mineral density, as glucocorticoid administration seems to have an important effect (Wetzsteon et al., 2009; Paggiosi et al., 2015). Furthermore, the gray values of the cortical bone and the dental structures are in the same range. Thus, cortical bone has usually been excluded from the measurements to avoid a biased analysis through inclusion of dental structures (roots). Scholz-Ahrens et al. found a statistically significant decrease in BMD in lumbar vertebrae after 8 months of glucocorticoid treatment (Scholz-Ahrens et al., 2007). This partially agrees with the results of this current study, which showed a statistically significant decrease in lumbar vertebrae after 6 months with a slight increase of BMD after 9 months. This might be related to an increase of body weight which is described for minipigs after completed adolescence (Richel and Waldmann, 2015). The growing weight might be a stimulus for bone formation in the vertebral region due to an increase of stress. An unexpected finding in the current study were the statistically significant differences considering the baseline values of bone mineral density. One possible reason for the different baseline data might be inter-animal variance. All came from the same herd, however, showed a variance in age and weight. Another reason might be the different group size (8 vs. 27 animals completing the study). If the control group would have had an equal group size to the glucocorticoid group, the differences might have been lower due to the compensation of extremal values.

The results for maxillofacial BMD in animals undergoing the induction of osteoporosis are different to those of lumbar bone. In a study using ovariectomized sheep, a pronounced horizontal and vertical bone loss in the mandible was described after 3 and 12 months (Johnson et al., 1997). However, a metric measurement of bone volume was not performed. Using the same animal model, another study measured BMD 12 months after ovariectomy, and showed no changes in the region of the diastema or the mandibular ramus (Johnson et al., 2002). Bone density in the alveolar regions however was significantly decreased, by 27.8%. This is in accordance with our results, which showed a progressive rarefication of the trabecular structure of the maxilla and the mandible. This rarefication of trabecular bone was found to be more pronounced in mandibular bone. In the experimental group, both a progressive decrease over time and a decrease in comparison to the control group were recorded.

Animal Models

The consideration of bone quality raises the question of appropriate animal models to simulate human osteoporosis. Osteoporotic large animal models have been established in sheep, dog, and pigs (Volozhin et al., 1990; Scholz-Ahrens et al., 2007; Dvorak et al., 2011b; Zhang et al., 2014; Kielbowicz et al., 2015). The most frequently described large animal model seems to be the sheep (Dvorak et al., 2011b; Veigel et al., 2011; Kielbowicz et al., 2015). With regard to the oral and maxillofacial situation, the minipig seems to be the most suitable model. First, it is an omnivore, so the diet has more similarities to a human diet than do sheep and dog models. Furthermore, the bone and oral tissues structure as well as bone turnover is quite similar to humans (Hönig and Merten, 1993; Hönig et al., 1997; Wang et al., 2007; Swindle et al., 2012). In a review, Pearce et al. concluded that both bone composition and bone remodeling in pigs are largely similar to that of humans, while micro- and macrostructure can be considered as moderately similar (Pearce et al., 2007). Regarding the age, the minipigs included in the current study can be considered as young adults. The life span of the breed Mini-Lewe was described with 10–15 years (Leucht et al., 1982). Richel observed in a longitudinal study of 144 Mini-Lewe pigs no further increase in the withers height and crown rump length after an average age of 20 months. Day 600 post-partum was defined as the time point of completed adolescence (Richel and Waldmann, 2015). This is in accordance with the findings of the current study, as no bone growth could be determined when comparing the matched images of the CT scans during the study period. Unlike in humans, in non-primate mammals there is no description of a physiological menopause state in the literature (Finn, 2001). Therefore, the use of young adult minipigs seems to be appropriate as there is no change in estrous cycle expected with increasing age. Additionally, when implant osseointegration is evaluated, the anatomy of the jaw of minipigs allows the application of the same instruments as used for human patients (Stadlinger et al., 2012).

Serum Parameters

Any systemic animal model needs to be validated by systemic parameters. Along with the measurement of bone density, the analysis of serum parameters is of particular interest, providing better understanding of bone metabolism.

Inorganic Phosphorus

The values of the inorganic phosphorus decreased in both groups which was more pronounced in the glucocorticoid group. When comparing the current values to the literature the values of the control group were in the same range (2.38 ± 0.86 to 3.10 ± 0.65 mmol*l^{-1}; Mieth, 1978; Leucht et al., 1982; Gusewski, 1983; Richel and Waldmann, 2015). Increasing age was discussed as a possible reason for this decrease by Gregor et al. but could not be confirmed in other evaluations (Gregor, 1979; Richel and Waldmann, 2015). In a recent study, inorganic phosphorus values between 1.55 and 2.24 mmol*l^{-1} were measured in female Aachen minipigs, a breed descending from the Mini-Lewe strain (Pawlowsky et al., 2017). However, these differences might be due to a different state of growths as the used animals were aged 6 months. When comparing both groups during the study, lower phosphorus levels were obvious in the glucocorticoid group. This state might be considered as hypophosphatemia which possibly is caused by the reduced intake of vitamin D3 of the glucocorticoid group. Furthermore, hypophosphatemia could be corresponding with lower levels of 1,25(OH)2-vitamin D3 in the glucocorticoid group what could be observed in the present study. One possible reason for the lower phosphorus values might be an interaction of glucocorticoids and the phosphate balance (Levi et al., 1995).

Calcium

The values of serum calcium varied over the study period in both groups ranging from 1.368 to 2.396 mmol*l^{-1}. Values <2.1 mmol*l^{-1} in humans are considered as hypocalcemia (Fong and Khan, 2012). In the literature, values between 3.1 and 2.5 mmol*l^{-1} are stated (Mieth, 1978; Leucht et al., 1982; Gusewski, 1983; Richel and Waldmann, 2015). Symptoms of acute decreased serum calcium levels include muscle spasms, heart failure, and neuromuscular irritability whereas a slow decrease of calcium levels might remain without symptoms (Fong and Khan, 2012). As no of the animals in the present study developed comprehensibly any of these symptoms it is unlikely that there was an apparent hypocalcemia.

Alkaline Phosphatase and Bone-Specific Alkaline Phosphatase

The values of total alkaline phosphatase and bone-specific alkaline phosphatase showed a significant decrease after glucocorticoid administration for 6 months. These findings were consistent with those of Ikeda et al., who observed a reduction of bone-specific alkaline phosphatase and osteocalcin values in serum of adolescent miniature pigs under glucocorticoid treatment (Ikeda et al., 2003). This might be explained by decreased bone formation due to supressed osteoblast activity (Lukert et al., 1986; Prummel et al., 1991). Clinically, a statistically significant correlation between bone alkaline phosphatase as well as osteocalcin levels and the age was found in postmenopausal women (Lumachi et al., 2009). However, a correlation between these bone markers and the BMD was not observed.

β-Crosslaps

The C-terminal telopeptide of the type I-collagen is termed as β-Crosslaps. It is considered as bone resorption marker (Okabe et al., 2004). In a clinical study, the changes of β-Crosslaps in serum correlated with the annual changes in BMD in postmenopausal women (Christgau et al., 1998). They are of crucial value to monitor the effect of antiresorptive therapies (Christgau et al., 1998). Furthermore, an increased level of β-Crosslaps and OPG was observed in patients suffering from Wilsons disease and osteoporosis (Hegedus et al., 2002). No such results could be observed in the present study. A reason might be a wide interindividual variety of the serum levels. However, there is little literature describing the levels of β-Crosslaps in pigs.

Osteocalcin

The osteocalcin serum levels in the glucocorticoid group decreased significantly after 6 months of prednisolone administrations. This was not observed in the control group.

In human studies, osteocalcin was described as a sensitive marker for osteoblastic depression under glucocorticoid therapy (Lukert et al., 1986; Ekenstam et al., 1988). The effects were pronounced when doses of glucocorticoids between 5 and 30 mg were administered daily over a period of at least 3 months (Lukert et al., 1986). In our study, a daily average dosage correlating to 35–45 mg prednisolone in human subjects (based on body weight) over a period of more than 4 months was assumed. This implies a comparable effect on the osteocalcin level (Scholz-Ahrens et al., 2007). However, the baseline values of both groups differed significantly, limiting this comparison. One possible reason for low values of osteocalcin might have been the degradation of osteocalcin by proteases of erythrocytes and leukocytes. In cases of difficult blood drawing degradation might have started already before further processing of the blood samples.

OPG

OPG is a glycoprotein that regulates bone density (Yano et al., 1999). A significant correlation was found between OPG serum level and age (Yano et al., 1999; Fahrleitner-Pammer et al., 2003). There was no such finding in the present study. Possibly, the age range of the minipigs was too small for the observation of such an effect. In contrast to our study, where young adult animals were examined the mentioned study evaluated patients with an age ranging from young adults to elderly patients. Furthermore, there is an increased level of OPG in patients suffering from osteoporosis (Yano et al., 1999). In the present study, slightly increased levels of OPG were observed in the glucocorticoid group during the study period. This, however, showed no significant statistical difference when compared to the control group. In a study of ovariectomized rats, a transient increase of OPG was found in the initial stage of osteoporosis, which might correlate with the increase of OPG observed in our study (Miyazaki et al., 2004).

1,25-Dihydroxyvitamin D and 25(OH)-Hydroxyvitamin D

The levels measured for 1,25-dihydroxyvitamin D were variable over the study period in both groups. This is in accordance to the literature, where increases, decreases, and an absence of alterations of the 1,25-dihydroxyvitamin D levels in individuals undergoing glucocorticoid therapy are described (Hodsman et al., 1991; Prummel et al., 1991; van der Veen and Bijlsma, 1992). However, in contrast to our study, higher glucocorticoid doses given intravenously cause a pronounced decrease (van der Veen and Bijlsma, 1992). To minimize extraneous influences, animals were housed in a stable and both groups received an equally vitamin D3 deprived (<300 IU/kg) daily diet. Comparable to other studies, no strong correlation could be found between the changes in bone metabolism and serum levels of 1,25-dihydroxyvitamin D (Seeman et al., 1980).

In summary, the serum parameters in the current study showed a wide range of values. In comparison to the literature, there are concordances but also some discrepancies. One potential reason is the fact, that different breeds of minipigs are being compared. Furthermore, in contrast to humans, there are no standard values for most parameters in minipigs. For some parameters, there were no reference values of pigs available at all. Thus, only a comparison to values obtained from other species was possible. Here, further studies are needed to elucidate potential correlations. Another possible reason might be the use of different analytical methods (Richel and Waldmann, 2015).

Methods of Osteoporosis Induction

The induction of an osteoporotic state in large animal models has been described by means of ovariectomy, calcium-deficient diet, glucocorticoid administration, and combinations of these approaches (Scholz-Ahrens et al., 1996, 2007; Kielbowicz et al., 2015). In comparison to deficient nutrition and glucocorticoid application, ovariectomy carries the disadvantage of a surgical intervention, which is a cause of stress for the animals. Furthermore, the effect of ovariectomy on nulliparous animals has been reported to be limited (Scholz-Ahrens et al., 1996). This would apply to the animals in the current study. Additionally, ovariectomy creates a sudden change in the hormonal balance, which is not entirely comparable to the postmenopausal situation, where the hormone levels change more gradually. In distinction, the administration of glucocorticoids over a period of time might lead to a gradual induction of osteoporosis, more closely mimicking the natural disease condition. However, a longer period of glucocorticoid administration may be required to show measurable effects on bone density. One limitation of this study might be the unequal size of the animal groups. This might cause some bias in the statistical evaluation e.g., statistically significant differences in BMD at the baseline. The reason was to minimize the total number of animals used. This was similar to other studies, where unequal group sizes for treatment and control groups have also been used (Scholz-Ahrens et al., 2007; Kielbowicz et al., 2015).

Compared to intramuscular application of glucocorticoids one limitation of oral administration is the fact that the individual animal dose is not fully calculable, because of the uncertainty about complete ingestion and absorption. Furthermore, glucocorticoids have various metabolic effects not limited to the stimulation of bone resorption and induction of osteoblast apoptosis (Dalle et al., 2001; Spreafico et al., 2008). Regarding the suitability as a model for dental implant research, glucocorticoid administration might lead to delayed wound healing. Morin and Fardet described altered wound healing in a retrospective study in humans, when glucocorticoids were taken for more than 6 months (Morin and Fardet, 2015). Dental implant clinics are seeing an increasing number of patients with progressive osteoporosis secondary to the use of glucocorticoid medications for the treatment of rheumatoid arthritis or following organ transplantation. Thus, despite possible criticisms of the animal model, glucocorticoid-induced osteoporosis might be a fair representation of a common clinical situation.

CONCLUSION

There are advantages and disadvantages of every animal model which involves artificial induction of a compromised metabolic state. However, the induction of an osteopenic state in the minipig by oral administration of glucocorticoids is predictable, and is minimally invasive when compared to surgical ovariectomy. In summary, the induction of osteoporosis in the minipig appears to be a promising model for the evaluation of the osseointegration of dental implants under systemically impaired osseous conditions.

AUTHOR CONTRIBUTIONS

MS was involved in the data acquisition, analysis and interpretation, drafted the manuscript, approved the final version of the manuscript, and agreed to be accountable for integrity and accuracy of the work. JK, SE, and RJ were involved in the data acquisition, drafted the manuscript, approved the final version of the manuscript, and agreed to be accountable for integrity and accuracy of the work. EK and LH were involved in data analysis and interpretation, drafted the manuscript, approved the final version of the manuscript, and agreed to be accountable for integrity and accuracy of the work. RM, UE, and CS were involved in study conception, drafted the manuscript, approved the final version of the manuscript, and agreed to be accountable for integrity and accuracy of the work. BS was involved in the conception of the study, data interpretation, drafted the manuscript, approved the final version of the manuscript, and agreed to be accountable for integrity and accuracy of the work.

ACKNOWLEDGMENTS

The authors are grateful to Mrs. Sylvia Albrecht for the support in acquiring the CT data. Furthermore, the authors thank PD Dr. Volker Hietschold for supporting them with the IDL software. Mrs. Andrea Groß is acknowledged for her technical support. The authors thank Dr. Ian Chambers for the English editing.

REFERENCES

Alsaadi, G., Quirynen, M., Komarek, A., and van Steenberghe, D. (2008). Impact of local and systemic factors on the incidence of late oral implant loss. *Clin. Oral Implants Res.* 19, 670–676. doi: 10.1111/j.1600-0501.2008.01534.x

Chambrone, L., Mandia, J. Jr., Shibli, J. A., Romito, G. A., and Abrahao, M. (2013). Dental implants installed in irradiated jaws: a systematic review. *J. Dent. Res.* 92(12 Suppl.), 119S–130S. doi: 10.1177/0022034513504947

Christgau, S., Rosenquist, C., Alexandersen, P., Bjarnason, N. H., Ravn, P., Fledelius, C., et al. (1998). Clinical evaluation of the Serum CrossLaps One Step ELISA, a new assay measuring the serum concentration of bone-derived degradation products of type I collagen C-telopeptides. *Clin. Chem.* 44, 2290–2300.

Dalle, C. L., Arlot, M. E., Chavassieux, P. M., Roux, J. P., Portero, N. R., and Meunier, P. J. (2001). Comparison of trabecular bone microarchitecture and remodeling in glucocorticoid-induced and postmenopausal osteoporosis. *J. Bone Miner. Res.* 16, 97–103. doi: 10.1359/jbmr.2001.16.1.97

Dvorak, G., Arnhart, C., Heuberer, S., Huber, C. D., Watzek, G., and Gruber, R. (2011a). Peri-implantitis and late implant failures in postmenopausal women: a cross-sectional study. *J. Clin. Periodontol.* 38, 950–955. doi: 10.1111/j.1600-051X.2011.01772.x

Dvorak, G., Reich, K. M., Tangl, S., Goldhahn, J., Haas, R., and Gruber, R. (2011b). Cortical porosity of the mandible in an osteoporotic sheep model. *Clin. Oral Implants Res.* 22, 500–505. doi: 10.1111/j.1600-0501.2010.02031.x

Ekenstam, E., Stalenheim, G., and Hallgren, R. (1988). The acute effect of high dose corticosteroid treatment on serum osteocalcin. *Metabolism* 37, 141–144. doi: 10.1016/S0026-0495(98)90008-7

Fahrleitner-Pammer, A., Dobnig, H., Piswanger-Soelkner, C., Bonelli, C., Dimai, H.-P., Leb, G., et al. (2003). Osteoprotegerin serum levels in women: correlation with age, bone mass, bone turnover and fracture status. *Wien. Klin. Wochenschr.* 115, 291–297. doi: 10.1007/BF03040334

Felsenberg, D., and Gowin, W. (1999). Bone densitometry by dual energy methods. *Radiologe* 39, 186–193. doi: 10.1007/s001170050495

Finn, C. A. (2001). Reproductive ageing and the menopause. *Int. J. Dev. Biol.* 45, 613–617.

Fong, J., and Khan, A. (2012). Hypocalcemia: updates in diagnosis and management for primary care. *Canad. Family Phys.* 58, 158–162.

Graeff, C., Marin, F., Petto, H., Kayser, O., Reisinger, A., Pena, J., et al. (2013). High resolution quantitative computed tomography-based assessment of trabecular microstructure and strength estimates by finite-element analysis of the spine, but not DXA, reflects vertebral fracture status in men with glucocorticoid-induced osteoporosis. *Bone* 52, 568–577. doi: 10.1016/j.bone.2012.10.036

Gregor, G. (1979). Hämatologische und biochemische untersuchungen am miniaturschwein MINILEWE: 2. Mitteilung: elektrolyte und enzyme. *Z. Versuchstierk.* 21, 125–135.

Gusewski, E. (1983). *Klinische und Labordiagnostische Untersuchungen am DDR-Miniaturschwein Mini-Lewe in Einem SPF-Bestand.* Dissertation, Humboldt-Universität, Berlin.

Hegedus, D., Ferencz, V., Lakatos, P. L., Meszaros, S., Lakatos, P., Horvath, C., et al. (2002). Decreased bone density, elevated serum osteoprotegerin, and beta-cross-laps in Wilson disease. *J. Bone Miner. Res.* 17, 1961–1967. doi: 10.1359/jbmr.2002.17.11.1961

Heitz-Mayfield, L. J., and Huynh-Ba, G. (2009). History of treated periodontitis and smoking as risks for implant therapy. *Int. J. Oral Maxillofac. Implants* 24(Suppl.), 39–68.

Hodsman, A. B., Toogood, J. H., Jennings, B., Fraher, L. J., and Baskerville, J. C. (1991). Differential effects of inhaled budesonide and oral prednisolone on serum osteocalcin. *J. Clin. Endocrinol. Metab.* 72, 530–540. doi: 10.1210/jcem-72-3-530

Hönig, J. F. and Merten, H. A. (1993). Das Göttinger Miniaturschwein (GMS) als Versuchstier in der human-medizinischen osteologischen Grundlagenforschung. *Z. Zahnärztl Implantol.* 9, 244–254.

Hönig, J. F., Merten, H. A., Wiltfang, J., and Wiese, K. G. (1997). Der Stellenwert des Göttinger Miniaturschweins in der craniofacialen osteologischen Grundlagenforschung. *Osteologie* 5, 125–133.

Ikeda, S., Morishita, Y., Tsutsumi, H., Ito, M., Shiraishi, A., Arita, S., et al. (2003). Reductions in bone turnover, mineral, and structure associated with mechanical properties of lumbar vertebra and femur in glucocorticoid-treated growing minipigs. *Bone* 33, 779–787. doi: 10.1016/S8756-3282(03)00263-1

Johnson, R. B., Gilbert, J. A., Cooper, R. C., Dai, X., Newton, B. I., Tracy, R. R., et al. (1997). Alveolar bone loss one year following ovariectomy in sheep. *J. Periodontol.* 68, 864–871. doi: 10.1902/jop.1997.68.9.864

Johnson, R. B., Gilbert, J. A., Cooper, R. C., Parsell, D. E., Stewart, B. A., Dai, X., et al. (2002). Effect of estrogen deficiency on skeletal and alveolar bone density in sheep. *J. Periodontol.* 73, 383–391. doi: 10.1902/jop.2002.73.4.383

Jonasson, G., Jonasson, L., and Kiliaridis, S. (2006). Changes in the radiographic characteristics of the mandibular alveolar process in dentate women with varying bone mineral density: a 5-year prospective study. *Bone* 38, 714–721. doi: 10.1016/j.bone.2005.10.008

Kielbowicz, Z., Piatek, A., Biezynski, J., Skrzypczak, P., Kuropka, P., Kuryszko, J., et al. (2015). The experimental osteoporosis in sheep - clinical approach. *Polish J. Vet. Sci.* 18, 645–654. doi: 10.1515/pjvs-2015-0083

Kingsmill, V. J., and Boyde, A. (1999). Mineralization density and apparent density of bone in cranial and postcranial sites in the aging human. *Osteoporos. Int.* 9, 260–268. doi: 10.1007/s001980050146

Leucht, W., Gregor, G., and Stier, H. (1982). "Das miniaturschwein: versuchs- und modelltier in medizin und biologie," in *Einführung in die Versuchstierkunde* (Jena: VEB Gustav Fischer Verlag).

Levi, M., Shayman, J. A., Abe, A., Gross, S. K., McCluer, R. H., Biber, J., et al. (1995). Dexamethasone modulates rat renal brush border membrane phosphate transporter mRNA and protein abundance and glycosphingolipid composition. *J. Clin. Invest.* 96, 207–216. doi: 10.1172/JCI118022

Lukert, B. P., Higgins, J. C., and Stoskopf, M. M. (1986). Serum osteocalcin is increased in patients with hyperthyroidism and decreased in patients receiving glucocorticoids. *J. Clin. Endocrinol. Metab.* 62, 1056–1058. doi: 10.1210/jcem-62-5-1056

Lumachi, F., Ermani, M., Camozzi, V., Tombolan, V., and Luisetto, G. (2009). Changes of bone formation markers osteocalcin and bone-specific alkaline phosphatase in postmenopausal women with osteoporosis. *Ann. N. Y. Acad. Sci.* 1173(Suppl. 1), E60–E63. doi: 10.1111/j.1749-6632.2009.04953.x

Mieth, A. (1978). *Hämatologische und Biochemisch-Klinische Parameter Beim Miniaturschwein MINILEWE.* Berlin: Diplomarbeit.

Miyazaki, T., Matsunaga, T., Miyazaki, S., Hokari, S., and Komoda, T. (2004). Changes in receptor activator of nuclear factor-kappaB, and its ligand, osteoprotegerin, bone-type alkaline phosphatase, and tartrate-resistant acid phosphatase in ovariectomized rats. *J. Cell. Biochem.* 93, 503–512. doi: 10.1002/jcb.20201

Morin, C., and Fardet, L. (2015). Systemic glucocorticoid therapy: risk factors for reported adverse events and beliefs about the drug. A cross-sectional online survey of 820 patients. *Clin. Rheumatol.* 34, 2119–2126. doi: 10.1007/s10067-015-2953-7

Moy, P. K., Medina, D., Shetty, V., and Aghaloo, T. L. (2005). Dental implant failure rates and associated risk factors. *Int. J. Oral Maxillofac. Implants* 20, 569–577.

Oheim, R., Beil, F. T., Krause, M., Bindl, R., Ignatius, A., and Pogoda, P. (2014). Mandibular bone loss in ewe induced by hypothalamic-pituitary disconnection. *Clin. Oral Implants Res.* 25, 1239–1244. doi: 10.1111/clr.12259

Okabe, R., Inaba, M., Nakatsuka, K., Miki, T., Naka, H., Moriguchi, A., et al. (2004). Significance of serum CrossLaps as a predictor of changes in bone mineral density during estrogen replacement therapy; comparison with serum carboxyterminal telopeptide of type I collagen and urinary deoxypyridinoline. *J. Bone Miner. Metab.* 22, 127–131. doi: 10.1007/s00774-003-0460-4

Paggiosi, M. A., Peel, N. F., and Eastell, R. (2015). The impact of glucocorticoid therapy on trabecular bone score in older women. *Osteoporos. Int.* 26, 1773–1780. doi: 10.1007/s00198-015-3078-1

Pawlowsky, K., Ernst, L., Steitz, J., Stopinski, T., Kogel, B., Henger, A., et al. (2017). The aachen minipig: phenotype, genotype, hematological and biochemical characterization, and comparison to the gottingen minipig. *Eur. Surg. Res.* 58, 193–203. doi: 10.1159/000471483

Pearce, A. I., Richards, R. G., Milz, S., Schneider, E., and Pearce, S. G. (2007). Animal models for implant biomaterial research in bone: a review. *Eur. Cells Mater.* 13, 1–10. doi: 10.22203/eCM.v013a01

Prummel, M. F., Wiersinga, W. M., Lips, P., Sanders, G. T., and Sauerwein, H. P. (1991). The course of biochemical parameters of bone turnover during treatment with corticosteroids. *J. Clin. Endocrinol. Metab.* 72, 382–386. doi: 10.1210/jcem-72-2-382

Rachner, T. D., Khosla, S., and Hofbauer, L. C. (2011). Osteoporosis: now and the future. *Lancet* 377, 1276–1287. doi: 10.1016/S0140-6736(10) 62349-5

Richel, N., and Waldmann, K.-H. (2015). *Phänotypische Charakterisierung der Entwicklung von Körpergewicht und -größe, Reproduktionsparametern und Ausgewählten Blutinhaltsstoffen Beim Miniaturschwein der Rasse "Mini-Lewe", Cuvillier; Tierärztl.* Göttingen; Hannover: Hochsch.

Sachelarie, L., Farcas, D. M., Dartu, L., Vasiliu, M., Daraba, O., Nazarie, S., et al. (2016). Comparative study of diseases of the stomatognathic system and specific parameters of osteoporosis. *Osteoporos. Int.* 27, 845–848. doi: 10.1007/s00198-015-3251-6

Scholz-Ahrens, K. E., Delling, G., Jungblut, P. W., Kallweit, E., and Barth, C. A. (1996). Effect of ovariectomy on bone histology and plasma parameters of bone metabolism in nulliparous and multiparous sows. *Z. Ernahrungswissen.* 35, 13–21. doi: 10.1007/BF01612023

Scholz-Ahrens, K. E., Delling, G., Stampa, B., Helfenstein, A., Hahne, H. J., Acil, Y., et al. (2007). Glucocorticosteroid-induced osteoporosis in adult primiparous Gottingen miniature pigs: effects on bone mineral and mineral metabolism. *Am. J. Physiol. Endocrinol. Metab.* 293, E385–E395. doi: 10.1152/ajpendo.00627.2006

Seeman, E., Kumar, R., Hunder, G. G., Scott, M., Heath, H. III., and Riggs, B., L. (1980). Production, degradation, and circulating levels of 1,25-dihydroxyvitamin D in health and in chronic glucocorticoid excess. *J. Clin. Invest.* 66, 664–669.

Snedeker, J. G., Walz, F. H., Muser, M. H., Schroeder, G., Mueller, T. L., and Muller, R. (2006). Microstructural insight into pedestrian pelvic fracture as assessed by high-resolution computed tomography. *J. Biomech.* 39, 2709–2713. doi: 10.1016/j.jbiomech.2005.09.008

Spreafico, A., Frediani, B., Francucci, C. M., Capperucci, C., Chellini, F., and Galeazzi, M. (2008). Role of apoptosis in osteoporosis induced by glucocorticoids. *J. Endocrinol. Invest.* 31(Suppl. 7), 22–27.

Stadlinger, B., Korn, P., Todtmann, N., Eckelt, U., Range, U., Burki, A., et al. (2013). Osseointegration of biochemically modified implants in an osteoporosis rodent model. *Eur. Cells Mater.* 25, 326–40; discussion 339–340. doi: 10.22203/eCM.v025a23

Stadlinger, B., Pourmand, P., Locher, M. C., and Schulz, M. C. (2012). Systematic review of animal models for the study of implant integration, assessing the influence of material, surface and design. *J. Clin. Periodontol.* 39(Suppl. 12), 28–36. doi: 10.1111/j.1600-051X.2011.01835.x

Swindle, M. M., Makin, A., Herron, A. J., Clubb, F. J. Jr., and Frazier, K. S. (2012). Swine as models in biomedical research and toxicology testing. *Vet. Pathol.* 49, 344–356. doi: 10.1177/0300985811402846

Thoma, D. S., Martin, I. S., Muhlemann, S., and Jung, R. E. (2012). Systematic review of pre-clinical models assessing implant integration in locally compromised sites and/or systemically compromised animals. *J. Clin. Periodontol.* 39(Suppl. 12), 37–62. doi: 10.1111/j.1600-051X.2011.01833.x

van der Veen, M. J., and Bijlsma, J. W. (1992). Effects of different regimes of corticosteroid treatment on calcium and bone metabolism in rheumatoid arthritis. *Clin. Rheumatol.* 11, 388–392. doi: 10.1007/BF02207199

Veigel, E., Moore, R. J., Zarrinkalam, M. R., Schulze, D., Sauerbier, S., Schmelzeisen, R., et al. (2011). Osteopenia in the maxillofacial area: a study in sheep. *Osteoporos. Int.* 22, 1115–1121. doi: 10.1007/s00198-010-1289-z

Volozhin, A. I., Stupakov, G. P., and Davydova, N. G. (1990). Changes in the mechanical properties of the femur and jaws in dogs with osteoporosis due to a single acute whole-body irradiation. *Patolog. Fiziolog. Eksp. Terapiia* 4, 44–46.

Wang, S., Liu, Y., Fang, D., and Shi, S. (2007). The miniature pig: a useful large animal model for dental and orofacial research. *Oral Dis.* 13, 530–537. doi: 10.1111/j.1601-0825.2006.01337.x

Wetzsteon, R. J., Shults, J., Zemel, B. S., Gupta, P. U., Burnham, J. M., Herskovitz, R. M., et al. (2009). Divergent effects of glucocorticoids on cortical and trabecular compartment BMD in childhood nephrotic syndrome. *J. Bone Miner. Res.* 24, 503–513. doi: 10.1359/jbmr.081101

WHO Scientific Group on the Assessment of Osteoporosis at Primary Health Care Level (2004). *Summary Meeting Report.* Brussels: WHO.

Yano, K., Tsuda E., Washida, N., Kobayashi, F., Goto, M., Harada, A., et al. (1999). Immunological characterization of circulating osteoprotegerin/osteoclastogenesis inhibitory factor: increased serum concentrations in postmenopausal women with osteoporosis. *J. Bone Miner. Res.* 14, 518–527.

Zhang, Y., Li, Y., Gao, Q., Shao, B., Xiao, J., Zhou, H., et al. (2014). The variation of cancellous bones at lumbar vertebra, femoral neck, mandibular angle and rib in ovariectomized sheep. *Arch. Oral Biol.* 59, 663–669. doi: 10.1016/j.archoralbio.2014.03.013

3

Hoxa2 Inhibits Bone Morphogenetic Protein Signaling during Osteogenic Differentiation of the Palatal Mesenchyme

Paul P. R. Iyyanar* and Adil J. Nazarali†

Laboratory of Molecular Cell Biology, College of Pharmacy and Nutrition and Neuroscience Research Cluster, University of Saskatchewan, Saskatoon, SK, Canada

****Correspondence:***
Paul P. R. Iyyanar
paul.iyyanar@usask.ca

†Deceased.

Cleft palate is one of the most common congenital birth defects worldwide. The homeobox (*Hox*) family of genes are key regulators of embryogenesis, with *Hoxa2* having a direct role in secondary palate development. *Hoxa2*$^{-/-}$ mice exhibit cleft palate; however, the cellular and molecular mechanisms leading to cleft palate in *Hoxa2*$^{-/-}$ mice is largely unknown. Addressing this issue, we found that *Hoxa2* regulates spatial and temporal programs of osteogenic differentiation in the developing palate by inhibiting bone morphogenetic protein (BMP) signaling dependent osteoblast markers. Expression of osteoblast markers, including *Runx2*, *Sp7,* and *Alpl* were increased in *Hoxa2*$^{-/-}$ palatal shelves at embryonic day (E) 13.5 and E15.5. *Hoxa2*$^{-/-}$ mouse embryonic palatal mesenchyme (MEPM) cells exhibited increased bone matrix deposition and mineralization *in vitro*. Moreover, loss of *Hoxa2* resulted in increased osteoprogenitor cell proliferation and osteogenic commitment during early stages of palate development at E13.5. Consistent with upregulation of osteoblast markers, *Hoxa2*$^{-/-}$ palatal shelves displayed higher expression of canonical BMP signaling *in vivo*. Blocking BMP signaling in *Hoxa2*$^{-/-}$ primary MEPM cells using dorsomorphin restored cell proliferation and osteogenic differentiation to wild-type levels. Collectively, these data demonstrate for the first time that *Hoxa2* may regulate palate development by inhibiting osteogenic differentiation of palatal mesenchyme via modulating BMP signaling.

Keywords: Hoxa2, cleft palate, bone morphogenetic protein (BMP), osteoblast, osteoprogenitor, proliferation, RUNX2

INTRODUCTION

Cleft palate is one of the most common structural birth defects in humans with an incidence of 1 in 700–1,000 live births (Dixon et al., 2011). Studies using mouse model which has a high similarity to human palate development helped to identify several key stages and cellular processes during palate formation (Yu et al., 2017). In mice, secondary palate development begins at embryonic day (E)11.5 and is completed with palatal fusion by E15.5 (Ferguson, 1988). During palate development, the

---

Abbreviations: AlpI, alkaline phosphatase I; ARS, Alizarin red S; BMP, bone morphogenetic protein; CNCC, cranial neural crest cells; d, day; E, embryonic day; MEPM, mouse embryonic palatal mesenchyme; pSMAD 1/5/8, phosphorylated SMAD 1/5/8; qRT-PCR, quantitative real-time PCR; Runx2, runt-related transcription factor 2.

vertical palatal shelves grow downward along the sides of the tongue until E13.5 and then elevate above the tongue at E14. The palatal shelves on either side contact each other forming midline epithelial seam at E14.5, which eventually disintegrates leading to palatal fusion by E15.5 (Kaufman, 1992). Impairment in any of these distinct stages during palatogenesis may result in cleft palate. The palate is comprised of the palatal process of the maxilla and the palatal process of the palatine bone derived from the cranial neural crest cells (CNCC) (Iwata et al., 2010), constituting the anterior and posterior part of the hard palate, respectively (Baek et al., 2011). While the structural changes during palate development are well defined, there is a scarcity of knowledge on the molecular mechanisms governing the patterning of the palate.

In murine models, deletion of about 280 genes are known to cause cleft palate (Funato et al., 2015). Among these genes, mutations of 55 genes are associated with cleft palate in humans (Funato et al., 2015). Mutation in the *Hoxa2* gene is associated with cleft palate in humans (Alasti et al., 2008) and mouse models (Gendron-Maguire et al., 1993; Rijli et al., 1993). In *Hoxa2*$^{-/-}$ mice, the cleft palate phenotype was initially attributed to the physical obstruction of the tongue preventing the palatal shelves to elevate and fuse (Barrow and Capecchi, 1999). However, our group has previously demonstrated that *Hoxa2* is expressed in the palatal shelves (Nazarali et al., 2000) and plays an intrinsic role in palatogenesis (Smith et al., 2009). The palatal shelves from *Hoxa2*$^{-/-}$ mouse embryonic maxilla devoid of tongue grown in rolling bottle cultures failed to fuse (Smith et al., 2009). Hence, tongue musculature may not be the principal reason for the cleft palate phenotype in *Hoxa2*$^{-/-}$ mice. *Hoxa2* appears to be a key regulator of palatogenesis, yet the molecular signaling pathways downstream of *Hoxa2* remain largely unknown.

Bone morphogenetic protein (BMP) signaling plays a critical role in palate development regulating cell proliferation (Zhang et al., 2002). *Bmp4* is upstream of *Bmp2* to induce proliferation in the palatal mesenchyme and is able to reverse the reduced cell proliferation and cleft palate phenotype in the *Msx1*$^{-/-}$ mice (Zhang et al., 2002). Defective cell proliferation observed in *Pax9*$^{-/-}$ embryos is consistent with the reduced *Bmp4* expression in the palatal mesenchyme at E13.5 (Zhou et al., 2013). Similarly, reduced expression of *Bmp2* is associated with reduced cell proliferation in the palatal shelves of *Hand2* hypomorphic mice (*Hand2*$^{LoxP/-}$) (Xiong et al., 2009). In addition, growing evidence highlight the importance of osteogenic differentiation in the elevation of palatal shelves and abnormal osteogenic differentiation could lead to cleft palate manifestations (Wu et al., 2008; Fu et al., 2017; Jia et al., 2017a,b). BMP signaling is critical for osteogenic differentiation in the palatal mesenchyme (Wu et al., 2008; Baek et al., 2011; Hill et al., 2014), where it is required for the expression of osteoblast markers such as *Runx2*, *Sp7*, and *AlpI* (Baek et al., 2011). During craniofacial development, *Hoxa2* restricts the bone mineralization in the calvaria (Dobreva et al., 2006). Moreover, *Hoxa2*$^{-/-}$ mice exhibit ectopic *Runx2*-positive osteogenic center in the second pharyngeal arch that results in duplication of tympanic ring (Kanzler et al., 1998).

In this study, we tested the hypothesis that *Hoxa2* inhibits osteogenic differentiation of the palatal mesenchyme *in vivo* and *in vitro* using *Hoxa2*$^{-/-}$ mice. Our findings reveal that *Hoxa2* plays a critical role in the spatial and temporal regulation of osteogenic differentiation via modulating BMP signaling pathway in the developing palate.

MATERIALS AND METHODS

Animals

Wild-type and *Hoxa2*$^{-/-}$ embryos were obtained from timed pregnant *Hoxa2*$^{+/-}$ (heterozygous) mice. Genotype was confirmed using PCR as previously described (Gendron-Maguire et al., 1993). This research was approved by the University of Saskatchewan's Animal Research Ethics Board and adhered to the Canadian Council on Animal Care guidelines for humane animal use.

Primary Mouse Embryonic Palatal Mesenchyme (MEPM) Cell Culture and Osteogenic Induction

Primary MEPM cells were isolated from micro-dissected palatal shelves of wild-type and *Hoxa2*$^{-/-}$ mouse embryos at E13.5. The palatal shelves were treated with 0.25% trypsin-EDTA for 15 min, passed through a 70 μm cell strainer and cultured as monolayer cells (Iwata et al., 2012) in DMEM: Ham's F12 (1:1) media containing 10% FBS, 1% antibiotic-antimycotic solution (Sigma). Osteogenic differentiation was carried out as described previously (Kwong et al., 2008) with minor modifications. Briefly, MEPM cells were seeded on 0.1% gelatin or poly-D-lysine coated plates at a cell density of 5×10^4 cells per well in 24 well plates and cultured until they reached confluence. Osteogenic differentiation was induced with differentiation media (DMEM, 10% FBS, 2 mM L-glutamine and 1% antibiotic-antimycotic solution) supplemented with osteogenic inducing agents, including 50 μg/ml L-ascorbic acid 2-phosphate sesquimagnesium salt (Sigma), 10 mM β-glycerophosphate (Sigma), and 100 nM dexamethasone (Sigma). Cells were differentiated for up to 21 days (d) and samples were collected at d8, d15, or d21. To assess the impact of BMP signaling, MEPM cells were treated with dorsomorphin (5 μM) or DMSO and were harvested at d8 for further experiments.

Alkaline Phosphatase I (ALPI) Staining

ALPI staining in the palatal shelves *in vivo* was carried out as previously described (Baek et al., 2011). Embryonic mouse heads were fixed overnight in freshly prepared 4% paraformaldehyde at 4°C and rehydrated in 30% sucrose at 4°C. Frozen coronal sections (10 μm) were prepared on slides coated with 0.5% gelatin. The sections were air dried for at least 2 h and then rehydrated with TBS with 0.08% tween-20 two times for 10 min each. Subsequently, the sections were treated with alkaline phosphatase buffer (100 mM NaCl, 100 mM Tris-HCl pH 9.5, 50 mM $MgCl_2$, 0.1% Tween-20) for 20 min and stained with alkaline phosphatase buffer containing 4.5 μl/ml of 5-bromo-4-chloro-3-indolyl phosphate (Roche) and 3.5 μl/ml of nitro blue tetrazolium (Roche) for 10 min. The reaction was stopped with PBS containing 20 mM EDTA buffer and counter stained with nuclear fast red. The stained sections were dehydrated in a series of PBS/ethanol, ethanol/xylene and finally mounted in DPX mounting media (Sigma). For osteoblast differentiation in primary MEPM cells, ALPI staining was carried out following the aforementioned protocol after fixing the cells with 4% paraformaldehyde for 15 min.

Alizarin Red S (ARS) Staining and Quantification

ARS staining and quantification was carried out as previously described (Gregory et al., 2004) with minor modifications. Briefly, monolayer MEPM cells were fixed with 4% paraformaldehyde for 15 min and stained with 250 μl of 40 mM ARS (Sigma) solution (pH 4.1) at room temperature for 20 min with gentle shaking. Excess dye was aspirated and washed with deionized water before imaging. ARS quantification was carried using an acid extraction method (Gregory et al., 2004). Standard plot of ARS concentration was constructed by serially diluting the 40 mM ARS in the buffer containing 10% (v/v) acetic acid and 10% (v/v) ammonium hydroxide. The absorbance values of the standard concentrations were used to interpolate the concentrations of the test samples.

Quantitative Real-Time Polymerase Chain Reaction (qRT-PCR)

Total RNA was isolated from the micro-dissected palatal shelves using RNA mini spin column (Bio-Rad) as per the manufacturer's protocol. First strand complementary DNA synthesis (reverse transcription) was performed in 20 μl reactions with 500 ng of total RNA using High-Capacity complementary DNA Reverse Transcription Kit (Invitrogen). qRT-PCR was carried out as described in our previous study (Thangaraj et al., 2017) using SYBR green assay (Applied Biosystems) in 7300-real time PCR system (Applied Biosystems) with primers listed in **Table 1**.

Western Blotting

Western bot analyses were carried out as previously described (Brown and Nazarali, 2010). Briefly, palatal tissues were homogenized in RIPA buffer. Total protein content was quantified using the Bradford assay and proteins were separated in 10% SDS-PAGE. Primary antibodies used were: RUNX2 (1:500; Abcam ab102711), SP7 (1:1500; Abcam ab22552), phosphorylated SMAD 1/5/8 (pSMAD 1/5/8) (1:500; Cell signaling 9511S), SMAD 1/5/8 (1:500; Santa Cruz Biotechnology sc-6031-R), and β-ACTIN (1:2,000; Developmental Studies Hybridoma JLA20). Densitometric analyses were carried out using AlphaView software.

Immunohistochemistry

Embryonic mouse heads were fixed overnight with freshly-prepared 4% paraformaldehyde and rehydrated in 30% sucrose at 4°C. Frozen coronal sections (10 μm) were rehydrated with PBS for 45 min, permeabilized with 0.1% Triton X-100 and blocked with 3% skim milk containing 0.1% Triton X-100 in 1X PBS for 1 h at room temperature. Sections were then incubated overnight with the following primary antibodies: RUNX2 (1:200; Abcam ab23981) or SP7 (1:800; Abcam ab22552) in 1X PBS with 0.1% Triton X-100 at 4°C. Double labeling was carried out by co-incubating: Ki67 (1:100; eBioscience 14569882) and RUNX2 (1:200; Abcam ab23981) overnight at 4°C. Sections were then washed three times and treated with secondary antibodies conjugated with Alexa Fluor® 488 (1:200) or Alexa Fluor® 594 (1:400) in 1X PBS with 0.1% Triton X-100 at room temperature for 1.5 h. Cell counting analyses were carried out manually using ImageJ software platform (NIH).

TABLE 1 | Primer sequences used for the relative quantification of the transcripts by qRT-PCR.

Transcript	Primer sequences	Length (bases)	Amplicon size (bp)
Alkaline phosphatase (*Alpl*)	CCTTGACTGTGGTTACTGCT	20	216
	CCTGGTAGTTGTTGTGAGCG	20	
Bone morphogenic protein 2 (*Bmp2*)	CAGTAGTTTCCAGCACCGAA	20	199
	CACTTCCACCACAAACCCAT	20	
Bone morphogenic protein 4 (*Bmp4*)	AGGAAGGAGTAGATGTGAGAG	21	158
	AGGGACGGAGACCAGATAC	19	
Bone carboxy-glutamic acid containing protein (*Bglap*)	GCAGGAGGGCAATAAGGTAG	20	159
	ATGCGTTTGTAGGCGGTC	18	
CyclinD1 (*Ccnd1*)	ACCCTGACACCAATCTCCTC	20	214
	AAGCGGTCCAGGTAGTTCAT	20	
Sp7 transcription factor (*Sp7*)	CACAAAGAAGCCATACGCTG	20	165
	CCAGGAAATGAGTGAGGGAAG	21	
Runt-related transcription factor 2 (*Runx2*)	TGCCTCCGCTGTTATGAAAA	20	187
	CTGTCTGTGCCTTCTTGGTT	20	

Cell Proliferation Assay

Cell proliferation assay was carried out in MEPM cells using cell-counting kit-8 (Dojindo) as previously described (Iwata et al., 2010). MEPM cells were incubated with CCK-8 reagent for 1 h and the absorbance measured at 450 nm was plotted to calculate the relative cell proliferation rate.

Statistical Analyses

Statistical analyses were carried out using unpaired *t*-test in the case of two groups. One-way ANOVA or two-way ANOVA with Bonferroni multiple comparison test was used for one or two variate analyses, respectively. A *p*-value of <0.05 was considered significant.

RESULTS

Hoxa2$^{-/-}$ Mice Exhibit Increased Expression of Osteoblast Markers during Palate Development *in Vivo*

To investigate the role of *Hoxa2* in osteogenesis of the palatal mesenchyme, we first examined changes in osteogenic differentiation in the embryonic palatal shelves of *Hoxa2*$^{-/-}$ mice at E16.5, a stage when both the prospective palatal process of the maxilla and the palatal process of the palatine bone evidently ossify (Baek et al., 2011). Staining for ALPI, a marker of osteoblast differentiation showed an expansion in ALPI expression domain in the *Hoxa2*$^{-/-}$ palatal mesenchyme compared to wild-type (**Figures 1A–H**). At the anterior region of the hard palate, ALPI staining was restricted to the nasal half in two condensations of the prospective palatal process of the maxilla on either side of the degraded midline epithelial seam in wild-type embryos (**Figures 1A,E**). In contrast, the domain of ALPI positive preosteoblast area was increased and expanded toward the oral side covering oral-nasal axis in *Hoxa2*$^{-/-}$ palatal shelves (**Figures 1B,F**). In the posterior region of the hard palate, ALPI staining was present in the ossifying centers of the palatal process of the palatine bone in wild-type embryos (**Figures 1C,G**), whereas there was an expansion in the expression domain of ALPI positive preosteoblasts toward the oral side in *Hoxa2*$^{-/-}$ embryos (**Figures 1D,H**).

Two well-known regulators of osteogenic differentiation RUNX2 (Komori et al., 1997) and SP7 (previously known as Osterix; Nakashima et al., 2002) have been implicated in the patterning of the palatal bones (Baek et al., 2011).

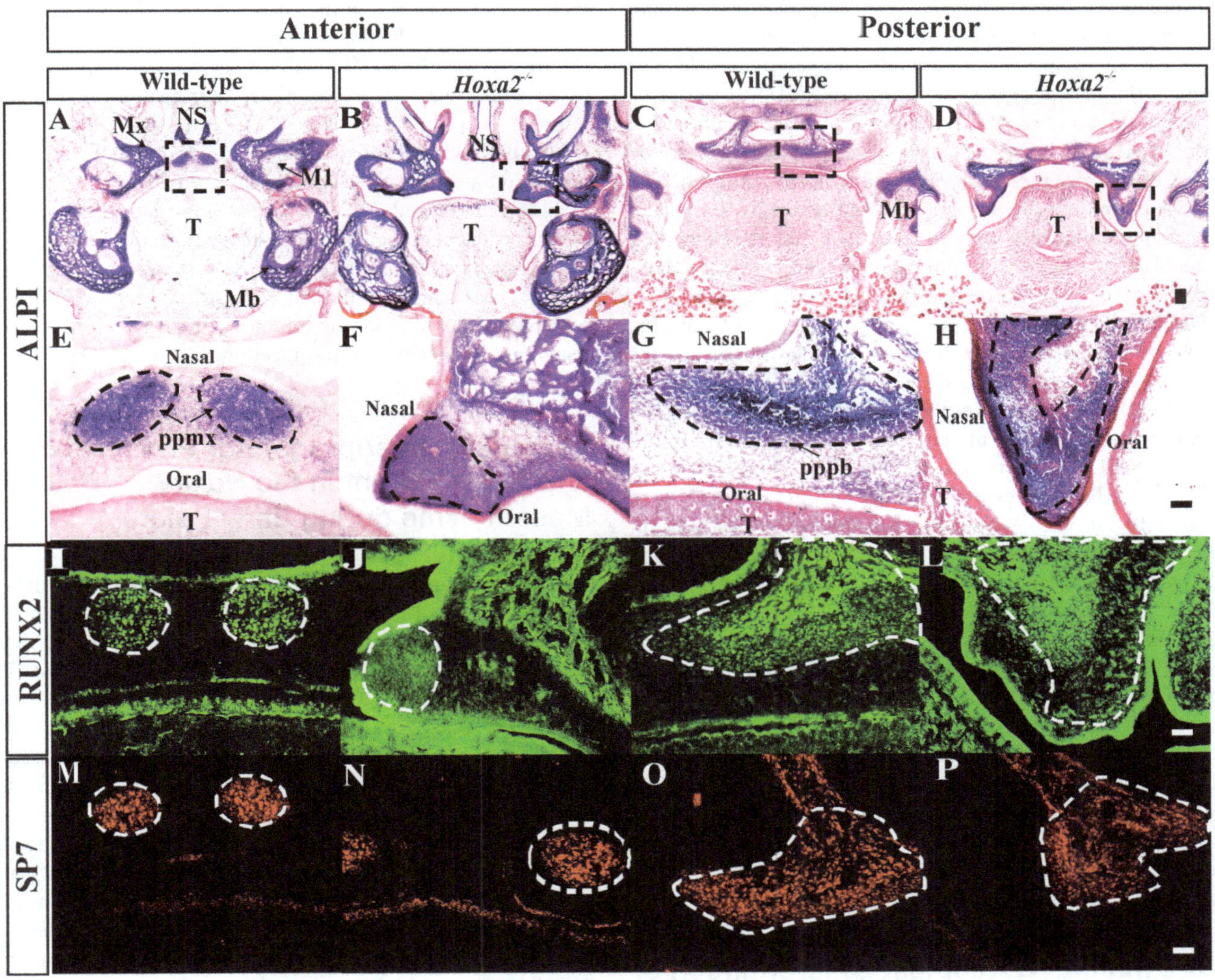

FIGURE 1 | Loss of *Hoxa2* leads to increased osteogenic differentiation of the palatal mesenchyme at E16.5. Position matched coronal sections of wild-type and *Hoxa2*$^{-/-}$ embryos at E16.5 were stained for ALPI **(A–H)**, RUNX2 **(I–L)**, and SP7 **(M–P)**. Sections in the anterior region **(A,B,E,F,I,J,M,N)** were through the middle of the first molar tooth bud to detect osteogenic condensation of the palatal process of the maxilla. Sections in the posterior region **(C,D,G,H,K,L,O,P)** were through the osteogenic centers of the developing palatal process of the palatine bone. **(A–D)** ALPI staining (blue) counterstained with nuclear fast red. Scale bar, 100 μm. Boxed regions in **(A–D)** highlighting the palate are enlarged **(E–H)**. Scale bar, 50 μm. **(E,F)** In the anterior hard palate, ALPI staining in the two condensations of the palatal process of the maxilla (marked in black dotted lines) was evidently increased in the *Hoxa2*$^{-/-}$ embryos **(F)** compared to wild-type **(E)**. **(G,H)** In the posterior hard palate, ALPI stained developing palatal process of the palatine bone (marked in black dotted lines) in the *Hoxa2*$^{-/-}$ embryos **(H)** was increased compared to the wild-type **(G)**, $n = 5$ biological replicates. **(I–P)** Immunohistochemical analyses of RUNX2 (green; **I–L**) and SP7 (red; **M–P**) in wild-type and *Hoxa2*$^{-/-}$ palate at E16.5. RUNX2 was increased in both anterior **(J)** and posterior regions **(L)** of the *Hoxa2* null hard palate, whereas SP7 was increased only in the anterior hard palate **(N)**, $n = 4$ biological replicates. Scale bar, 50 μm. M1, first molar; Mb, mandible; Mx, maxilla; NS, nasal septum; pppb, the palatal process of the palatine bone; ppmx, the palatal process of the maxilla; T, tongue.

To elucidate the spatial mis-regulation of palatal bone formation in *Hoxa2*$^{-/-}$ mice, expression pattern of these two osteoblast-specific transcription factors were assessed at E16.5. Immunohistochemical analyses revealed that RUNX2 (**Figure 1I**) and SP7 (**Figure 1M**) expressions were confined to the condensations of the palatal process of the maxilla at the anterior hard palate in wild-type embryos at E16.5, whereas RUNX2 (**Figure 1J**) and SP7 (**Figure 1N**) expression domains were increased in *Hoxa2*$^{-/-}$ embryos. In the posterior region, along the developing palatal process of the palatine bone, the expression of RUNX2 (**Figure 1L**) was increased in *Hoxa2*$^{-/-}$ embryos compared to wild-type (**Figure 1K**). In this region, the expression of SP7, a downstream target of RUNX2 and a marker of mature osteoblasts, was not evidently increased in the *Hoxa2*$^{-/-}$ palate (**Figure 1P**) compared to wild-type (**Figure 1O**). This suggests that cells toward the oral side of the palatal process of the palatine bone are at immature osteoblast stage and may not have developed bone matrix by E16.5. Collectively, these data indicate that *Hoxa2* could be a potential inhibitor of osteogenic differentiation in the palatal mesenchyme, which may serve to spatially restrict the expression of osteoblast-specific proteins during palate development *in vivo*.

Furthermore, gene expression profiles of osteoblast markers were evaluated during the initiation of ossification of the palatal process of the palatal bone and the palatal process of the maxilla at E13.5 and E15.5, respectively. The loss of *Hoxa2* in the developing palate resulted in an increase in mRNA expression of osteoblast markers such as *Runx2*, *Alpl* and *Sp7* at both E13.5 (**Figures 2A–D**) and E15.5 (**Figures 2E–H**). At E13.5, mRNA expression of *Runx2*, *Alpl* and *Sp7* were increased to ~6.36-, ~9.65-, and ~2.62-fold, respectively, in *Hoxa2*$^{-/-}$ palate compared to wild-type (**Figures 2A–C**). At E13.5, mRNA expression of *Bglap* (previously known as *Ocn*) was not significantly altered (**Figure 2D**). At E15.5, mRNA expression of *Runx2*, *Alpl*, *Sp7*, and *Bglap* were upregulated ~1.86-, ~2.29-, ~1.42-, ~3.27-folds, respectively, in *Hoxa2*$^{-/-}$ palate compared to wild-type (**Figures 2E–H**). Consistent with this, protein expression of RUNX2 was upregulated at E13.5 and E15.5 to ~1.4-fold (**Figures 2I,J**). SP7 protein expression, both long (**Figures 2I,K**) and short isoforms (**Figures 2I,L**) were upregulated at E15.5 to ~1.4-fold. These data reveal that along with regulating the spatial patterning of osteogenic differentiation, *Hoxa2* also regulates the expression of osteogenic markers at the molecular level in the developing palate.

Hoxa2 Inhibits Osteoblast Differentiation of Mouse Embryonic Palatal Mesenchymal (MEPM) Cells *in Vitro*

To evaluate the potential of *Hoxa2* in regulating the temporal pattern of osteogenesis, the primary mesenchyme cells from the wild-type and *Hoxa2*$^{-/-}$ palatal shelves were differentiated *in vitro* for up to 21 days (d). Osteogenesis of mesenchymal cells involves sequential stages of proliferation, osteogenic commitment around day8 (~d8) followed by matrix deposition (~d15) and mineralization (~d21) (Gordon et al., 2010). Differentiating cells were stained for ALPI at d8 and Alizarin Red S (ARS) at d15 and d21. ALPI staining showed an increased osteoblast differentiation at d8 in *Hoxa2*$^{-/-}$ MEPM cells compared to the wild-type MEPM cells (**Figures 3A,B**). In addition, ARS staining followed by quantification of ARS extracted matrix showed that *Hoxa2*$^{-/-}$ MEPM cells exhibited increased extracellular matrix deposition ~2-fold at d15 (**Figures 3C,D,G**) and increased mineralization ~1.5-fold at d21 (**Figures 3E,F,H**) compared to the wild-type MEPM cells.

Next, the gene expression profiles of osteogenic markers were examined in wild-type and *Hoxa2*$^{-/-}$ MEPM cells during osteogenic differentiation *in vitro*. *Runx2* mRNA expression was increased to ~1.9-fold in the *Hoxa2*$^{-/-}$ MEPM cells compared to the wild-type during osteoblast commitment stage at d8 (**Figure 3I**). *Alpl* and *Sp7* mRNA expression were increased ~2.85 and ~3.37-fold, respectively, during matrix deposition stage at d15 in the *Hoxa2*$^{-/-}$ MEPM cells (**Figures 3J,K**). *Bglap* mRNA expression was increased ~6.37-fold during matrix deposition at d15 and ~8.09-fold during matrix mineralization at d21 in the *Hoxa2*$^{-/-}$ MEPM cells (**Figure 3L**). Thus, loss of *Hoxa2* results in upregulation of osteogenic marker expression in a stage-specific manner as early as d8 (osteogenic commitment stage). These data indicate that *Hoxa2* may play a role in early osteoblast differentiation by inhibiting the transcription factors regulating osteogenic fate specification.

Increased Osteoprogenitor Proliferation and Commitment in the *Hoxa2*$^{-/-}$ Palatal Mesenchyme during Early Palate Development

Hoxa2 peaks in its expression in the developing palate at E13.5 (Smith et al., 2009), a stage when the mesenchymal cells simultaneously proliferate and commit to form preosteoblasts of the prospective palatal process of the palatine bone. This suggests that the cleft palate phenotype in *Hoxa2*$^{-/-}$ mice, due to the failure of palatal shelves to elevate and reorient horizontally above the tongue after E13.5 (Barrow and Capecchi, 1999), may be a consequence of abnormal cell proliferation (Smith et al., 2013) and osteogenic differentiation (Wu et al., 2008; Fu et al., 2017; Jia et al., 2017a,b). To gain further insight into the role of *Hoxa2* during this early stage of palate development, the rate of mesenchymal cell proliferation and the commitment of mesenchymal cells to osteoprogenitor fate was investigated *in vivo* at E13.5. Immunohistochemical staining of RUNX2 (**Figures 4A,B**) was used to evaluate osteoprogenitor commitment in the wild-type and *Hoxa2*$^{-/-}$ palatal shelves at E13.5. RUNX2 (**Figure 4A**) expression in the wild-type was restricted to the bend region in the nasal side of the palatal shelves, whereas the expression domain of RUNX2 (**Figure 4B**) was increased spatially toward the medial edge of the palate as well as to the oral side of the palate in the *Hoxa2*$^{-/-}$ mutants. This is similar to the aberrant expression patterns of RUNX2 observed at E16.5 in the *Hoxa2*$^{-/-}$ palatal shelves. In addition, the number of RUNX2-positive osteoprogenitor cells on the nasal side of the palatal shelves were significantly higher in

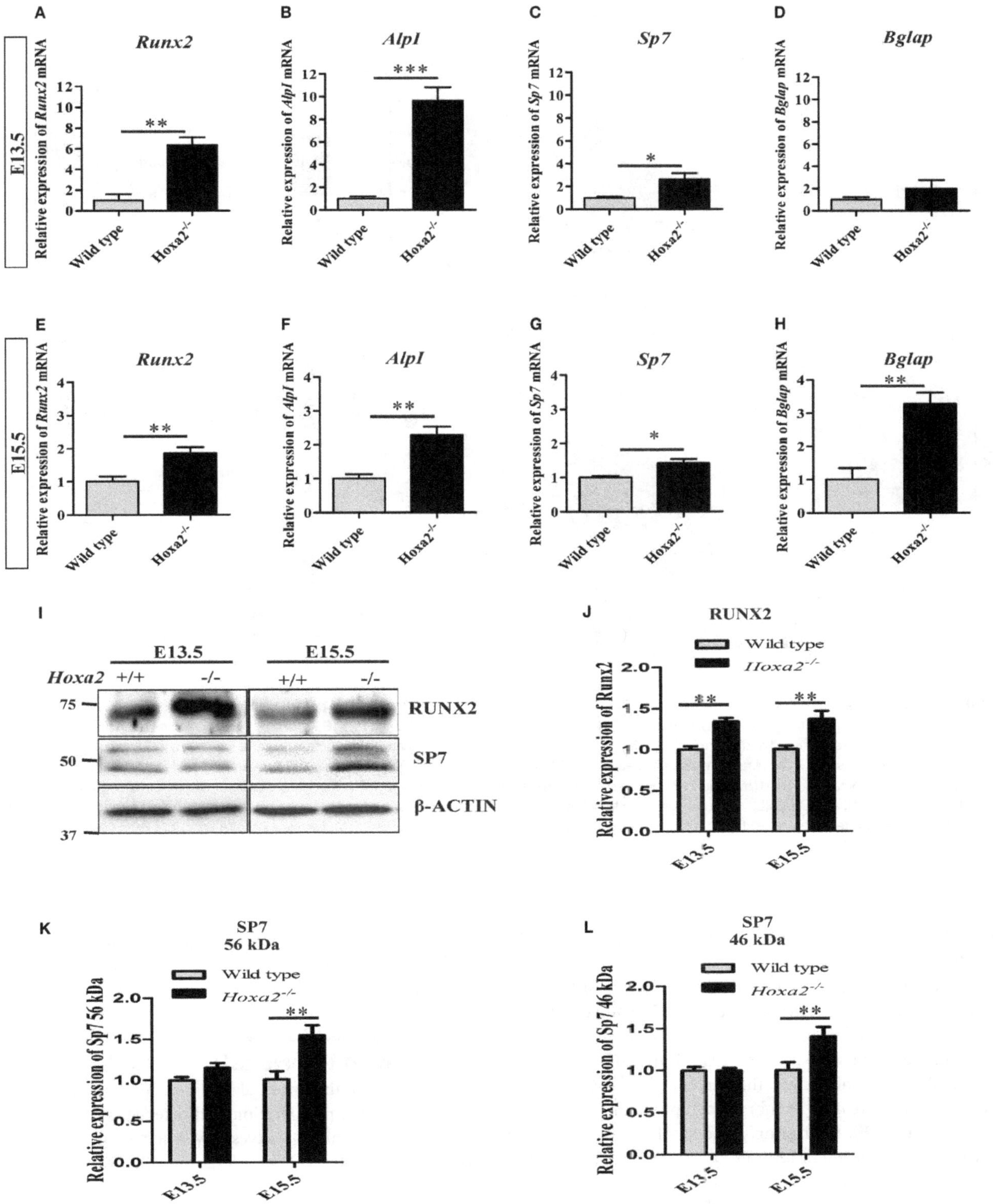

FIGURE 2 | Loss of *Hoxa2* leads to increased expression of osteogenic markers in the developing palate at E13.5 and E15.5. Quantitative real-time PCR (qRT-PCR) analyses indicate that the gene expression profile of osteogenic markers such as *Runx2* **(A,E)**, *Alpl* **(B,F)**, and *Sp7* **(C,G)** were upregulated in the developing *Hoxa2*$^{-/-}$ palatal shelves at E13.5 **(A–C)** and E15.5 **(E–G)**. Gene expression of *Bglap* was upregulated at E15.5 **(H)** but not at E13.5 **(D)**. qRT-PCR data ($n = 5$ biological replicates) were normalized to *β-actin* and represented relative to wild-type (mean ± S.E.M; unpaired *t*-test, $^{*}p < 0.05$; $^{**}p < 0.01$; $^{***}p < 0.001$). Western blot analyses of RUNX2 **(I,J)** and SP7 **(I,K,L)** were carried out using the microdissected palatal shelves from wild-type and *Hoxa2*$^{-/-}$ mice at E13.5 and E15.5. RUNX2 protein expression was upregulated in the *Hoxa2*$^{-/-}$ palate at E13.5 and E15.5 **(I,J)**, whereas SP7 isoforms were upregulated at E15.5 **(I,K,L)**. Densitometric analyses ($n = 4$ biological replicates) were normalized to β-ACTIN and represented relative to wild-type (mean ± S.E.M; unpaired *t*-test, $^{**}p < 0.01$).

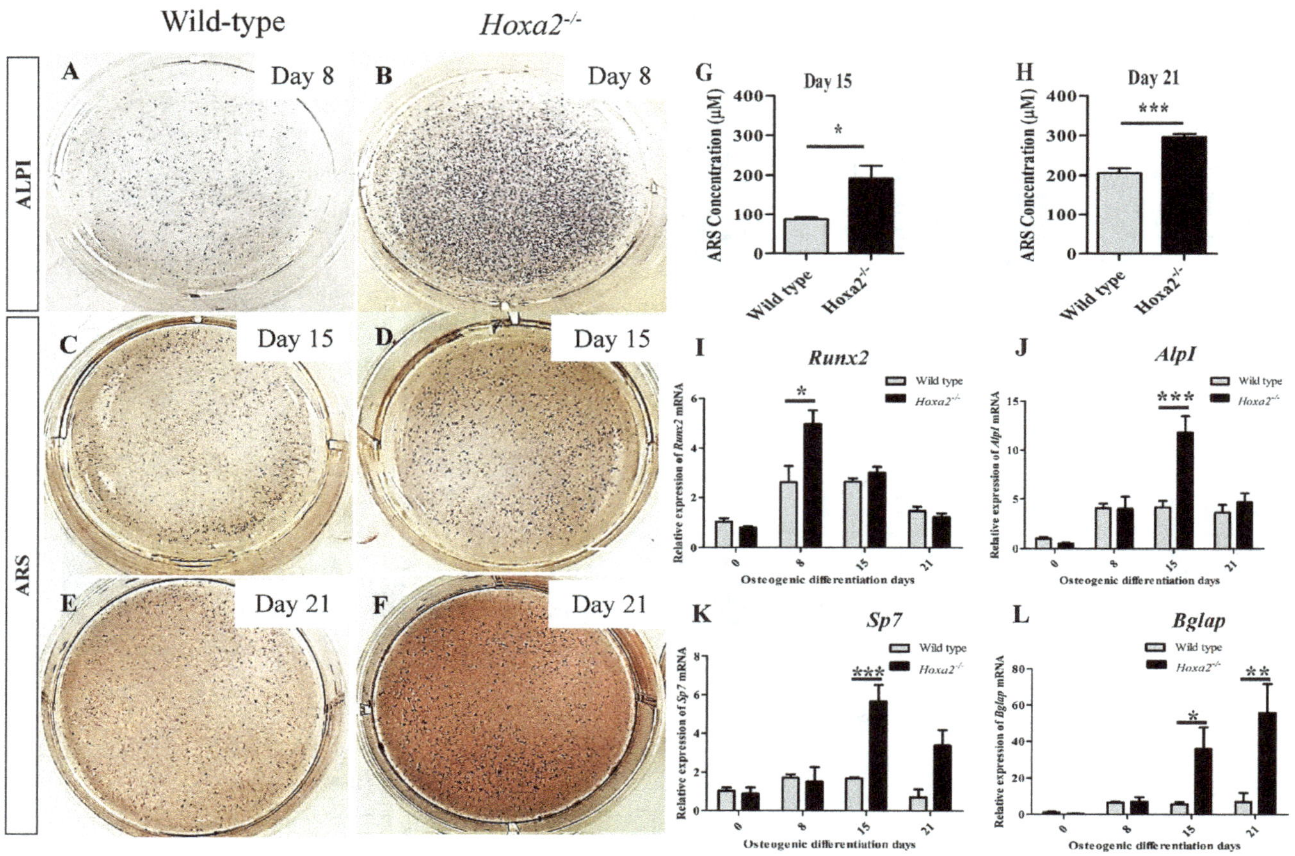

FIGURE 3 | *Hoxa2* inhibits osteoblast differentiation of MEPM cells *in vitro*. Wild-type and *Hoxa2*$^{-/-}$ MEPM cells were subjected to osteogenic differentiation *in vitro* for up to 21 days (d). The differentiated cells were stained for ALPl at d8 **(A,B)**, ARS at d15 **(C,D)**, and d21 **(E,F)**. ARS stained osteocyte matrices from wild-type and *Hoxa2*$^{-/-}$ MEPM cells were extracted and quantified at d15 **(G)** and d21 **(H)**. Experiment was carried out three times and the data shown here are from a representative experiment with $n = 3$ biological replicates; mean ± S.E.M; unpaired *t*-test, $^{*}p < 0.05$; $^{***}p < 0.001$). *Hoxa2*$^{-/-}$ MEPM cells displayed increased matrix deposition and mineralization at d15 **(G)** and d21 **(H)**, respectively. **(I–L)** qRT-PCR analyses revealed that gene expression profile of osteogenic markers such as *Runx2* **(I)**, *Alpl* **(J)**, *Sp7* **(K)**, and *Bglap* **(L)** were upregulated in the *Hoxa2*$^{-/-}$ MEPM cells in a stage-specific manner during osteoblast differentiation. Data was normalized to *β-actin* and represented relative to wild-type at d0 ($n = 3$ biological replicates; mean ± S.E.M; two-way ANOVA with Bonferroni post-hoc test, $^{*}p < 0.05$; $^{**}p < 0.01$; $^{***}p < 0.001$).

the *Hoxa2*$^{-/-}$ mutants (∼64%) compared to wild-type (∼33%; **Figure 4C**).

Next, the rate of cell proliferation was assessed at E13.5 using Ki67 immunostaining. The percentage of Ki67-positive cells was significantly increased in the *Hoxa2*$^{-/-}$ palatal mesenchyme (∼50%) compared to wild-type (∼26%; **Figures 4D–F**). In the nasal side of the palatal shelves, the percentage of Ki67-positive cells was ∼53% in *Hoxa2*$^{-/-}$ embryos compared to ∼26% in the wild-type (**Figure 4F**). Interestingly, the nasal side mesenchyme displayed a higher proliferation rate of ∼53% compared to the oral side of ∼23% in *Hoxa2*$^{-/-}$ palatal shelves (**Figure 4F**). In addition, the percentage of proliferating osteoprogenitor cells (RUNX2-positive/Ki67-positive) in the nasal side of the *Hoxa2*$^{-/-}$ palatal shelves was higher (∼20%) compared to ∼11% in wild-type (**Figures 4G–I**). Furthermore, mRNA expression of cyclin D1 (*Ccnd1*), a critical G1 phase cell cycle regulator was also upregulated in the *Hoxa2*$^{-/-}$ palatal shelves from E12.5 to E14.5 (**Figure 4J**). These results indicate that *Hoxa2* plays a critical role by inhibiting osteoprogenitor commitment and osteoprogenitor proliferation prior to the elevation and fusion of the palatal shelves.

Increased Canonical BMP Signaling Pathway in the *Hoxa2*$^{-/-}$ Palatal Shelves

To understand the molecular signaling pathways underlying the aberrant cell proliferation and osteogenic differentiation in the *Hoxa2*$^{-/-}$ palatal shelves, BMP signaling was investigated as it is critical for cell proliferation (Zhang et al., 2002) and expression of osteogenic markers in the developing palate (Baek et al., 2011). First, the mRNA expression of BMP ligands critical for osteoblast differentiation such as *Bmp2* and *Bmp4* in the developing palatal shelves was examined. *Bmp2* expression was upregulated to ∼3.57-fold at E13.5 and ∼1.96-fold at E15.5 in *Hoxa2*$^{-/-}$ palatal shelves compared to wild-type (**Figure 5A**). Similarly, *Bmp4* expression was upregulated to ∼3.42-fold at E13.5 and to ∼1.81-fold at E15.5

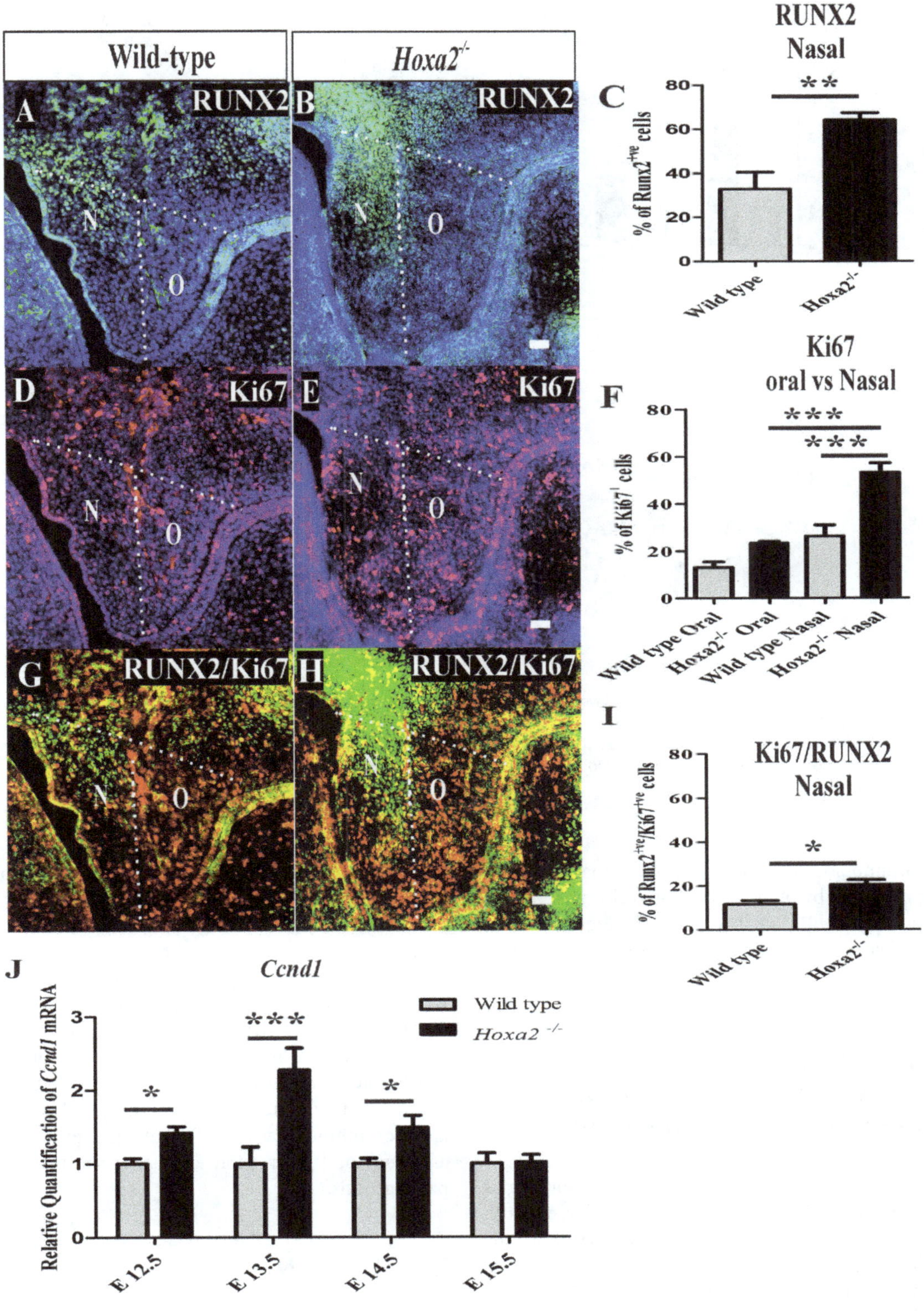

FIGURE 4 | *Hoxa2*$^{-/-}$ palatal shelves exhibit increased osteoprogenitor proliferation and commitment at E13.5. Osteoprogenitor cells in the developing palatal shelves of wild-type and *Hoxa2*$^{-/-}$ embryos were evaluated using RUNX2 immunostaining **(A,B)** and RUNX2-positive cells were counted manually using ImageJ platform **(C)**. Proliferation rate was assessed using Ki67 immunostaining **(D–F)** at E13.5. Scale bar, 50 μm; N, nasal; O, oral. Proliferating osteoprogenitor cells (cellspositive for both RUNX2 and Ki67) (Runx2 /Ki67) **(G,H)** relative to the total number of mesenchymal cells (DAPI-positive) from wild-type and *Hoxa2*$^{-/-}$ palatal shelves were counted in the nasal side **(I)**. *Hoxa2*$^{-/-}$ embryos exhibited increased RUNX2-positive **(C)**, Ki67-positive **(F)** and RUNX2/Ki67-double positive **(I)** cells in the nasal side of the palatal shelves ($n = 5$ biological replicates; mean ± S.E.M; unpaired *t*-test, $^{*}p < 0.05$; $^{**}p < 0.01$; $^{***}p < 0.001$). Expression of cell cycle regulator *Cyclin D1* (*Ccnd1*) mRNA was upregulated in the *Hoxa2*$^{-/-}$ palatal shelves **(J)** from E12.5 to E14.5. qRT-PCR data was normalized to *β-actin* and represented relative to wild-type at respective embryonic stages ($n = 6$ biological replicates; mean ± S.E.M; unpaired *t*-test, $^{*}p < 0.05$; $^{***}p < 0.001$).

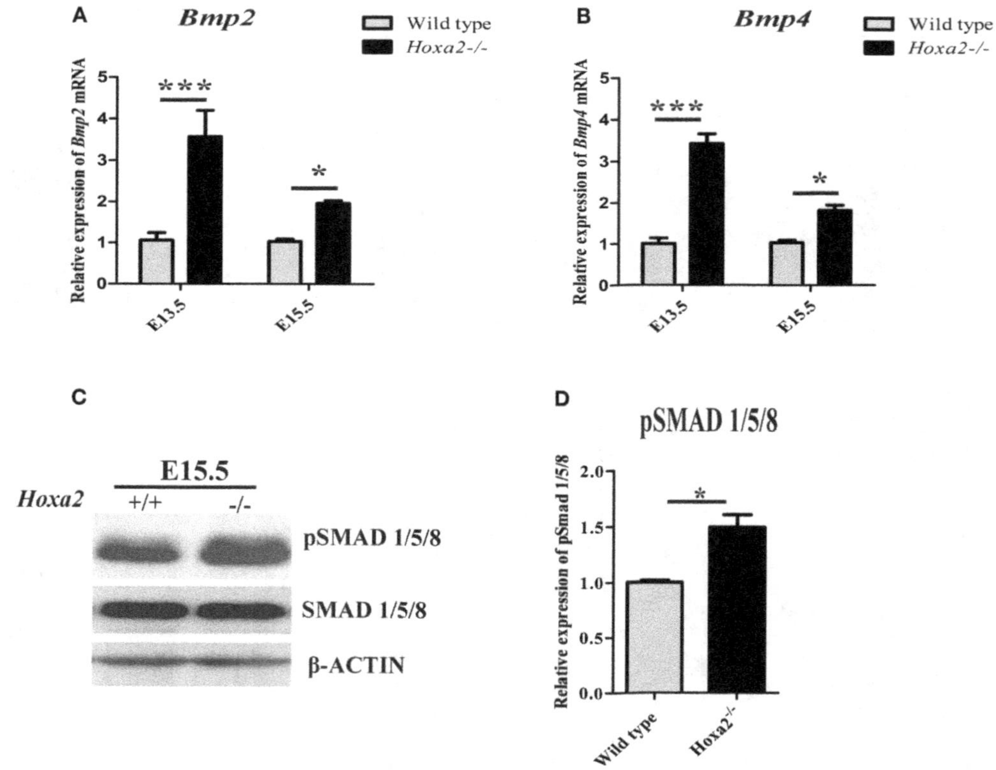

FIGURE 5 | *Hoxa2* regulates canonical BMP signaling in the developing palate. Gene expression of BMP ligands, *Bmp2* **(A)** and *Bmp4* **(B)** were upregulated in *Hoxa2*$^{-/-}$ palatal shelves at E13.5 and E15.5. qRT-PCR data ($n = 4$ biological replicates) were normalized to *β-actin* (mean ± S.E.M; unpaired *t*-test, $^{*}p < 0.05$; $^{***}p < 0.001$). Representative immunoblot **(C)** of pSMAD 1/5/8 from the developing palate of wild-type and *Hoxa2*$^{-/-}$ embryos at E15.5. **(D)** Densitometric analysis represents the relative expression of pSMAD 1/5/8 normalized to SMAD 1/5/8 and represented relative to wild-type ($n = 4$ biological replicates; mean ± S.E.M; unpaired *t*-test, $^{*}p < 0.05$).

(**Figure 5B**). Immunoblotting analyses revealed that canonical BMP signaling mediated by pSMAD 1/5/8 was also upregulated to ~1.5-fold in the *Hoxa2*$^{-/-}$ palate at E15.5 (**Figures 5C,D**). These results indicate that canonical BMP signaling pathway may be downstream of the *Hoxa2* gene network in palate development.

Blocking Canonical BMP Signaling Rescues the Aberrant Cell Proliferation and Osteogenic Differentiation in *Hoxa2*$^{-/-}$ MEPM Cells

To determine if the upregulated canonical BMP signaling is functionally responsible for the increased mesenchymal cell proliferation and osteogenic differentiation observed in the *Hoxa2*$^{-/-}$ palate, dorsomorphin was used to inhibit BMP signaling during osteogenic differentiation of MEPM cells *in vitro*. Although at higher doses dorsomorphin (10–20 μM) inhibits AMPK signaling (Zhou et al., 2001) and mTOR signaling (Vucicevic et al., 2011), it selectively inhibits BMP signaling at lower doses (Yu et al., 2008). Upon 5 μM dorsomorphin treatment, upregulated mRNA expressions of *Bmp2* (**Figure 6A**), *Bmp4* (**Figure 6B**) and *Runx2* (**Figure 6C**) in the *Hoxa2*$^{-/-}$ MEPM cells were restored to the wild-type levels. Moreover, increased protein expression of RUNX2 and pSMAD 1/5/8 (**Figure 6D**) in the *Hoxa2*$^{-/-}$ MEPM cells were reduced after dorsomorphin treatment. The increased cell proliferation (**Figure 6E**) and osteogenic differentiation (**Figure 6F**) in the *Hoxa2*$^{-/-}$ MEPM cells were also reduced after dorsomorphin treatment. These results indicate that the upregulated canonical BMP signaling is functionally responsible for the increased cell proliferation and osteogenic differentiation during palate development in *Hoxa2*$^{-/-}$ embryos. Altogether, the findings reveal that *Hoxa2* inhibits osteoprogenitor proliferation and commitment, via BMP signaling, to control the spatial and temporal expression of osteoblast markers for proper palatogenesis.

DISCUSSION

Mice lacking *Hoxa2* exhibit cleft palate (Gendron-Maguire et al., 1993; Rijli et al., 1993; Barrow and Capecchi, 1999) and microtia (Minoux et al., 2013), which are consistent with *Hoxa2* mutations in humans (Alasti et al., 2008). We have previously shown that *Hoxa2* is expressed in the palatal shelves during development (Nazarali et al., 2000) reaching a maximal expression at E13.5 and regulates cell proliferation in the

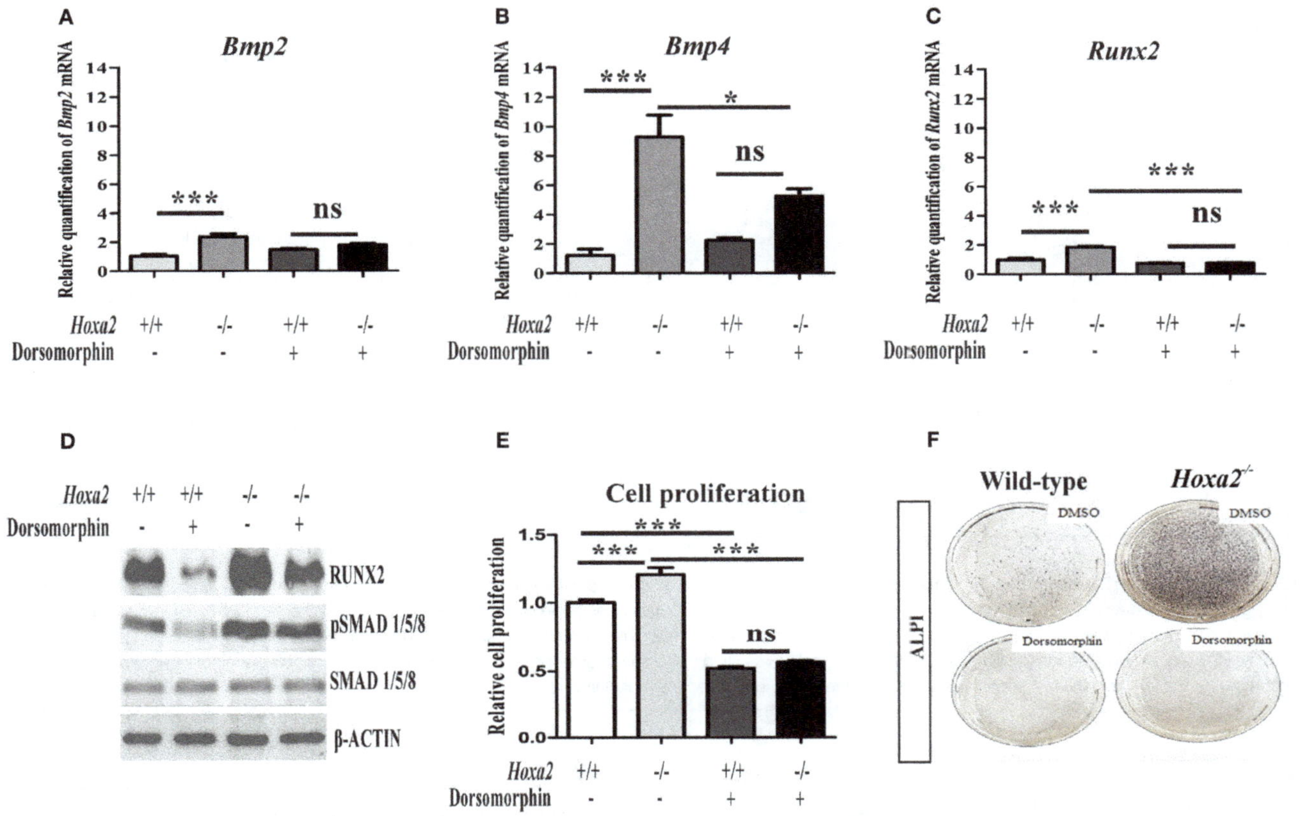

FIGURE 6 | Blocking canonical BMP signaling with dorsomorphin rescues the aberrant osteoprogenitor cell proliferation and osteogenic differentiation in the *Hoxa2*$^{-/-}$ MEPM cells. Dorsomorphin treatment restored gene expressions of *Bmp2* **(A)**, *Bmp4* **(B)**, and *Runx2* **(C)** in the *Hoxa2*$^{-/-}$ MEPM cells close to wild-type levels during osteogenic differentiation *in vitro* at d8. Data represented relative to wild-type MEPM cells treated with DMSO ($n = 4$ biological replicates; mean ± S.E.M; one-way ANOVA followed by Bonferroni *post-hoc* test, $^{*}p < 0.05$; $^{***}p < 0.001$; ns, not significant). **(D)** Representative immunoblots showing restoration of RUNX2 and pSMAD 1/5/8 in *Hoxa2*$^{-/-}$ MEPM cells treated with dorsomorphin during osteogenic differentiation *in vitro* at d8 ($n = 3$ biological replicates). **(E)** Cell proliferation analysis in the wild-type and *Hoxa2*$^{-/-}$ MEPM cells treated with DMSO or dorsomorphin during osteogenic differentiation at d3 ($n = 5$ biological replicates; mean ± S.E.M; one-way ANOVA followed by Bonferroni *post-hoc* test, $^{***}p < 0.001$; ns, not significant). **(F)** ALPI staining revealed that treatment with dorsomorphin nullified the aberrant osteogenic differentiation in *Hoxa2*$^{-/-}$ MEPM cells *in vitro* at d8.

developing palate (Smith et al., 2009). There are several lines of evidence that *Hoxa2* regulates palate development intrinsically (Smith et al., 2009), yet the mechanism is largely unknown. In this study, we have found that *Hoxa2* inhibits BMP signaling dependent osteogenic differentiation spatially and temporally to regulate palate formation. The present study deepens the current understanding of the role of *Hoxa2* in palate formation and the mechanisms underlying the cleft palate phenotype in *Hoxa2*$^{-/-}$ mice linking *Hoxa2*, BMP signaling and osteogenesis.

Our findings here reveal that *Hoxa2* controls the temporal and spatial expression pattern of osteoblast markers in the developing palatal mesenchyme. Ossifying domains characterized by RUNX2 and ALPI were increased in the palatal process of the maxilla and in the palatal process of the palatine bone in *Hoxa2*$^{-/-}$ mice. In contrast, SP7 a marker of mature osteoblasts was expanded only in the palatal process of the maxilla and not in the palatal process of the palatine bone at E16.5. This suggests that cells toward the oral side of the palatal process of the palatine bone are at immature osteoblast stage and may not have developed bone matrix by E16.5. Patterning of the palatal process of the palatine bone and of the maxilla are through independent skeletogenic processes (Baek et al., 2011). The palatal process of the palatine bone ossifies at E13.5, whereas the ossification of the palatal process of the maxilla begins only at E15.5. Consistent with this, qRT-PCR and immunoblot analyses revealed a corresponding upregulation of osteogenic markers in the *Hoxa2*$^{-/-}$ palate at these two critical stages E13.5 and E15.5. In addition, primary *Hoxa2*$^{-/-}$ MEPM cells displayed an increase in osteogenic differentiation and a stage-specific increase in the expressions of the osteoblast-specific transcripts indicating that *Hoxa2* regulates temporal differentiation of mesenchyme cells to osteoblasts in the palate. Together, our results reveal that *Hoxa2* functions as an inhibitor of osteogenic differentiation in the palatal mesenchyme during development. Our findings are in agreement with previous studies showing the role of *Hoxa2* as an inhibitor of bone formation in other craniofacial regions (Kanzler et al., 1998; Dobreva et al., 2006).

Very little is known about the signaling network downstream of *Hoxa2* during palatogenesis. Here, we have demonstrated that *Hoxa2*$^{-/-}$ palatal shelves exhibit upregulated canonical

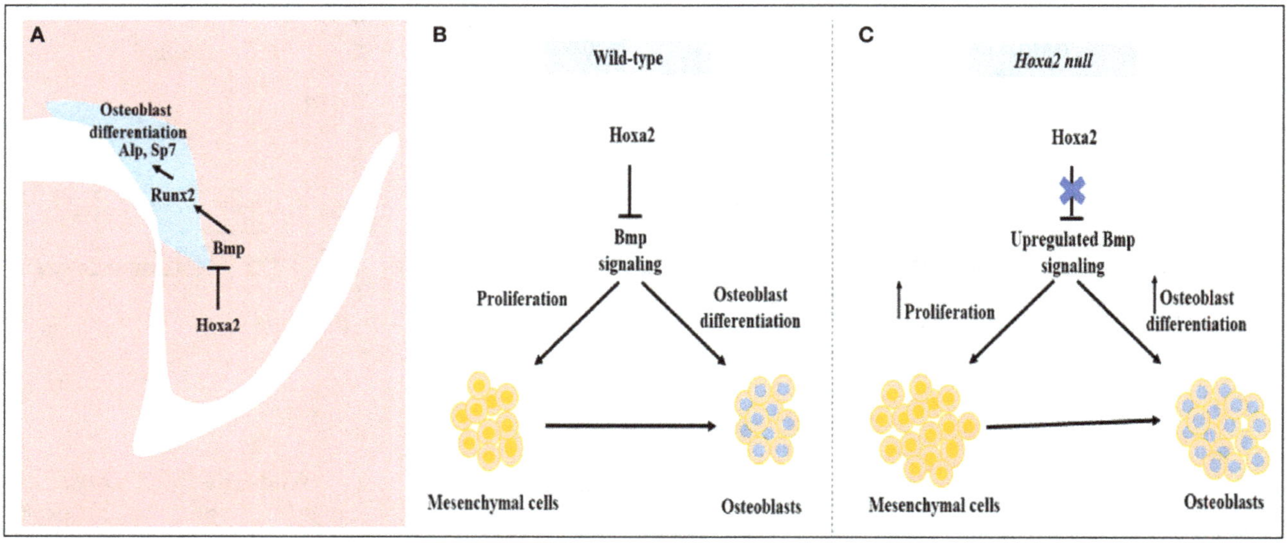

FIGURE 7 | Schematic diagram depicting the role of *Hoxa2* in proliferation and osteogenic differentiation of the palatal mesenchyme. **(A)** *Hoxa2* inhibits canonical BMP signaling in the developing palate, which in turn restricts the expression domain of osteogenic markers such as *Runx2*, *Alpl*, and *Sp7*. **(B)** In wild-type, *Hoxa2* expression peaks during early palatogenesis to control cell proliferation and to maintain mesenchymal cells in an undifferentiated stage by regulating BMP signaling pathway. **(C)** Loss of *Hoxa2* leads to upregulation of BMP signaling resulting in increased osteoprogenitor cell proliferation and osteogenic differentiation, possibly accounting for the failure in the elevation of palatal shelves resulting in manifestation of cleft palate.

BMP signaling mediated by pSMAD 1/5/8. In addition, the expression of BMP ligands such as *Bmp2* and *Bmp4* are upregulated in *Hoxa2*$^{-/-}$ palatal shelves *in vivo* and in *Hoxa2*$^{-/-}$ MEPM cells *in vitro*. BMP signaling plays a critical role in proliferation (Zhang et al., 2002; Baek et al., 2011) and osteogenic differentiation of the palatal mesenchyme (Wu et al., 2008; Han et al., 2009; Baek et al., 2011). Importantly, abnormal BMP signaling in the palatal mesenchyme leads to cleft palate manifestation (Zhang et al., 2002; He et al., 2008). Inactivation of *Bmpr1a* in the palatal mesenchyme (*Osr2-IresCre; Bmpr1a*$^{f/f}$) results in submucous cleft palate, absence in the patterning of the palatal process of the maxilla and defective palatal process of the palatine bone (Baek et al., 2011). Genome-wide mapping revealed that *Bmp2*, *Bmp4* and *Bmpr1a* are possible targets of *Hoxa2* (Donaldson et al., 2012) and HOXA2 protein binds to the intronic region of *Bmp4* (Minoux et al., 2013) in the developing pharyngeal arch2. In this study, dorsomorphin was used to inhibit BMP signaling in the wild-type and *Hoxa2*$^{-/-}$ primary palatal mesenchymal cells during osteogenic differentiation. Dorsomorphin selectively inhibits BMP signaling at lower doses (Yu et al., 2008) and at higher doses dorsomorphin (10–20 μM) also inhibits AMPK signaling (Zhou et al., 2001) and mTOR signaling (Vucicevic et al., 2011). In our study, dorsomorphin treatment not only rescued the upregulated gene expression of osteogenic factors such as *Bmp2*, *Bmp4*, and *Runx2* but also the aberrant cell proliferation and osteogenic differentiation in the *Hoxa2*$^{-/-}$ MEPM cells. These experiments highlight the involvement of BMP signaling in the abnormal osteoprogenitor cell proliferation and osteogenic differentiation in the *Hoxa2*$^{-/-}$ palate, which could attribute to the cleft palate phenotype in these mutants.

To our knowledge, there is no report available on the characterization of osteoprogenitor cell proliferation and commitment in the palatal mesenchyme during development. In this study, we have unraveled the role of *Hoxa2* in maintaining the palatal mesenchymal cells in an undifferentiated stage by inhibiting osteoprogenitor proliferation and commitment preventing abnormal ossification in the developing palate. Palatal mesenchymal cells derived from CNCC undergo osteogenic proliferation and commit to form osteoblasts (Iwata et al., 2010). Double immunolabeling analyses of RUNX2 and Ki67 at E13.5 revealed that among the total population of mesenchyme cells, there was a significantly higher number of (i) proliferating cells (Ki67-positive cells), (ii) osteoprogenitor cells (RUNX2-positive cells), and (iii) proliferating osteoprogenitor cells (RUNX2-positive /Ki67-positive cells) in the nasal side of the *Hoxa2*$^{-/-}$ palatal shelves compared to the wild-type. In the palatal mesenchyme, increased or decreased cell proliferation could result in failure of the palatal shelves to elevate and reorient above the tongue leading to cleft palate (Bush and Jiang, 2012; Smith et al., 2013). Recent studies show evidence for abnormal osteogenic signaling prior to the elevation of palatal shelves in several well-studied cleft palate mutant mice models including *Pax9*$^{-/-}$ mice (Jia et al., 2017a,b) and *Osr2*$^{-/-}$ mice (Fu et al., 2017). Consistent with our findings here in the *Hoxa2*$^{-/-}$ mice, *Osr2*$^{-/-}$ exhibit increased osteogenic centers of the palatal process of the palatine bone prior to the elevation of the palatal shelves at E13.5 and in addition to defective cell proliferation, enhanced osteogenesis could contribute to cleft palate phenotype in *Osr2*$^{-/-}$ mice (Fu et al., 2017). In addition, RNA-Seq data from *Osr2*$^{-/-}$ palatal shelves revealed upregulation of several positive regulators of osteogenesis including *Runx2*, *Runx3*,

Sp7, and Bmp ligands- *Bmp3*, *Bmp5*, and *Bmp7*. Furthermore, *Pax9*$^{-/-}$ mice exhibit reduced cell proliferation and osteogenesis in the developing palate (Jia et al., 2017a). Restoration of reduced cell proliferation and osteogenesis by Wnt agonists (Dkk inhibitors) rescued the cleft palate phenotype in *Pax9*$^{-/-}$ mice (Jia et al., 2017a). The increase in cell proliferation in the nasal side of the *Hoxa2*$^{-/-}$palate indicates a strong role for *Hoxa2* in the spatial maintenance of mesenchymal cells in an undifferentiated state for temporal coordination of osteoblast differentiation (**Figure 7**). Our findings here exemplify the regional heterogeneity in proliferation and osteogenic differentiation by *Hoxa2* along the oral-nasal axis in the palatal mesenchyme prior to the elevation of palatal shelves. Our data argue that improper BMP signaling leading to the increased osteoprogenitor cell proliferation and commitment could be a reason for the cleft palate pathogenesis in the *Hoxa2*$^{-/-}$ mice. Further studies are needed to address if the cleft palate phenotype in the *Hoxa2*$^{-/-}$ mice could be rescued using other mutant mice with impaired osteogenesis.

Our data demonstrate that *Hoxa2* inhibits osteoprogenitor cell proliferation and osteogenic commitment via modulating BMP signaling in the mouse embryonic palatal mesenchyme. *Hoxa2* regulates spatial and temporal programs of osteogenesis by maintaining mesenchymal cells in an undifferentiated stage until osteogenic clues arrive. In conclusion, our findings provide new insights into the signaling mechanism underlying the role of *Hoxa2* during embryonic palate development.

AUTHOR CONTRIBUTIONS

AN conceived and coordinated the study. PI designed the study, performed experiments, analyzed data and wrote the manuscript. AN and PI proofed, revised the manuscript for critical content and interpretation of data.

ACKNOWLEDGMENTS

PI acknowledges the Apotex Graduate Scholarship Award from the College of Pharmacy and Nutrition, University of Saskatchewan; Graduate Research fellowship and Saskatchewan Innovation and Opportunity Scholarships from the College of Graduate and Postdoctoral studies, University of Saskatchewan. Authors thank Drs. Brian F. Eames and Kendra L. Furber for critical suggestions on the manuscript and Larhonda Sobchishin for providing technical expertise. This manuscript is dedicated to the memory of our colleague and mentor, Dr. Adil J. Nazarali, who passed away before the submission of the manuscript.

REFERENCES

Alasti, F., Sadeghi, A., Sanati, M. H., Farhadi, M., Stollar, E., Somers, T., et al. (2008). A mutation in HOXA2 is responsible for autosomal-recessive microtia in an Iranian family. *Am. J. Hum. Genet.* 82, 982–991. doi: 10.1016/j.ajhg.2008.02.015

Baek, J., Lan, Y., Liu, H., Maltby, K. M., Mishina, Y., and Jiang, R. (2011). Bmpr1a signaling plays critical roles in palatal shelf growth and palatal bone formation. *Dev. Biol.* 350, 520–531. doi: 10.1016/j.ydbio.2010.12.028

Barrow, J. R., and Capecchi, M. R. (1999). Compensatory defects associated with mutations in Hoxa1 restore normal palatogenesis to Hoxa2 mutants. *Development* 126, 5011–5026. Available online at: http://dev.biologists.org/content/126/22/5011.abstract

Brown, G. D., and Nazarali, A. J. (2010). Matrix metalloproteinase-25 has a functional role in mouse secondary palate development and is a downstream target of TGF-β3. *BMC Dev. Biol.* 10:93. doi: 10.1186/1471-213X-10-93

Bush, J. O., and Jiang, R. (2012). Palatogenesis: morphogenetic and molecular mechanisms of secondary palate development. *Development* 139, 231–243. doi: 10.1242/dev.067082

Dixon, M. J., Marazita, M. L., Beaty, T. H., and Murray, J. C. (2011). Cleft lip and palate: understanding genetic and environmental influences. *Nat. Rev. Genet.* 12, 167–178. doi: 10.1038/nrg2933

Donaldson, I. J., Amin, S., Hensman, J. J., Kutejova, E., Rattray, M., Lawrence, N., et al. (2012). Genome-wide occupancy links Hoxa2 to Wnt-β-catenin signaling in mouse embryonic development. *Nucleic Acids Res.* 40, 3990–4001. doi: 10.1093/nar/gkr1240

Dobreva, G., Chahrour, M., Dautzenberg, M., Chirivella, L., Kanzler, B., Karsenty, G., et al. (2006). SATB2 is a multifunctional determinant of craniofacial patterning and osteoblast differentiation. *Cell* 125, 971–986. doi: 10.1016/j.cell.2006.05.012

Ferguson, M. W. J. (1988). Palate development. *Development* 103(Suppl.), 41–60.

Fu, X., Xu, J., Chaturvedi, P., Liu, H., Jiang, R., and Lan, Y. (2017). Identification of Osr2 transcriptional target genes in palate development. *J. Dent. Res.* 96, 1451–1458. doi: 10.1177/0022034517719749

Funato, N., Nakamura, M., and Yanagisawa, H. (2015). Molecular basis of cleft palates in mice. *World J. Biol. Chem.* 6, 121–138. doi: 10.4331/wjbc.v6.i3.121

Gendron-Maguire, M., Mallo, M., Zhang, M., and Gridley, T. (1993). Hoxa-2 mutant mice exhibit homeotic transformation of skeletal elements derived from cranial neural crest. *Cell* 75, 1317–1331. doi: 10.1016/0092-8674(93)90619-2

Gordon, J. A., Hassan, M. Q., Saini, S., Montecino, M., van Wijnen, A. J., Stein, G. S., et al. (2010). Pbx1 represses osteoblastogenesis by blocking Hoxa10-mediated recruitment of chromatin remodeling factors. *Mol. Cell. Biol.* 30, 3531–3541. doi: 10.1128/MCB.00889-09

Gregory, C. A., Grady Gunn, W., Peister, A., and Prockop, D. J. (2004). An Alizarin red-based assay of mineralization by adherent cells in culture: comparison with cetylpyridinium chloride extraction. *Anal. Biochem.* 329, 77–84. doi: 10.1016/j.ab.2004.02.002

Han, J., Mayo, J., Xu, X., Li, J., Bringas, P., Maas, R. L., et al. (2009). Indirect modulation of Shh signaling by Dlx5 affects the oral-nasal patterning of palate and rescues cleft palate in Msx1 -null mice. *Development* 136, 4225–4233. doi: 10.1242/dev.036723

He, F., Xiong, W., Yu, X., Espinoza-Lewis, R., Liu, C., Gu, S., et al. (2008). Wnt5a regulates directional cell migration and cell proliferation via Ror2-mediated noncanonical pathway in mammalian palate development. *Development* 135, 3871–3879. doi: 10.1242/dev.025767

Hill, C. R., Yuasa, M., Schoenecker, J., and Goudy, S. L. (2014). Jagged1 is essential for osteoblast development during maxillary ossification. *Bone* 62, 10–21. doi: 10.1016/j.bone.2014.01.019

Iwata, J., Hosokawa, R., Sanchez-lara, P. A., Urata, M., Slavkin, H., and Chai, Y. (2010). Transforming growth factor- β regulates basal transcriptional regulatory machinery to control cell proliferation and differentiation in cranial neural crest-derived osteoprogenitor cells. *J. Biol. Chem.* 285, 4975–4982. doi: 10.1074/jbc.M109.035105

Iwata, J., Tung, L., Urata, M., Hacia, G., Pelikan, R., Suzuki, A., et al. (2012). Fibroblast Growth Factor 9 (FGF9) -Pituitary Homeobox 2 (PITX2) pathway mediates Transforming Growth Factor β (TGFβ) signaling to regulate cell proliferation in palatal mesenchyme during mouse palatogenesis. *J. Biol. Chem.* 287, 2353–2363. doi: 10.1074/jbc.M111.280974

Jia, S., Zhou, J., Fanelli, C., Wee, Y., Bonds, J., Schneider, P., et al. (2017a). Small-molecule Wnt agonists correct cleft palates in Pax9 mutant mice in utero. *Development* 144, 3819–3828. doi: 10.1242/dev.157750

Jia, S., Zhou, J., Wee, Y., Mikkola, M. L., Schneider, P., and Souza, R. N. D. (2017b). Anti-EDAR agonist antibody therapy resolves palate defects in Pax9$^{-/-}$ Mice. *J. Dent. Res.* 96, 1282–1289. doi: 10.1177/0022034517726073

Kanzler, B., Kuschert, S. J., Liu, Y., and Mallo, M. (1998). Hoxa-2 restricts the chondrogenic domain and inhibits bone formation during development of the branchial area. *Development* 125, 2587–2597.

Kaufman, M. H. (1992). *The Atlas of Mouse Development.* Academic Press. Available online at: https://books.google.ca/books?id=Lo5pAAAAMAAJ

Komori, T., Yagi, H., Nomura, S., Yamaguchi, A., Sasaki, K., Deguchi, K., et al. (1997). Targeted disruption of Cbfa1 results in a complete lack of bone formation owing to maturational arrest of osteoblasts. *Cell* 89, 755–764. doi: 10.1016/S0092-8674(00)80258-5

Kwong, F. N., Richardson, S. M., and Evans, C. H. (2008). Chordin knockdown enhances the osteogenic differentiation of human mesenchymal stem cells. *Arthritis Res. Ther.* 10:R65. doi: 10.1186/ar2436

Minoux, M., Kratochwil, C. F., Ducret, S., Amin, S., Kitazawa, T., Kurihara, H., et al. (2013). Mouse Hoxa2 mutations provide a model for microtia and auricle duplication. *Development* 140, 4386–4397. doi: 10.1242/dev.098046

Nakashima, K., Zhou, X., Kunkel, G., Zhang, Z., Deng, J. M., Behringer, R. R., et al. (2002). The novel zinc finger-containing transcription factor osterix is required for osteoblast differentiation and bone formation. *Cell* 108, 17–29. doi: 10.1016/S0092-8674(01)00622-5

Nazarali, A., Puthucode, R., Leung, V., Wolf, L., Hao, Z., and Yeung, J. (2000). Temporal and spatial expression of Hoxa-2 during murine palatogenesis. *Cell. Mol. Neurobiol.* 20, 269–290. doi: 10.1023/A:1007006024407

Rijli, F. M., Mark, M., Lakkaraju, S., Dierich, A., Doll, P., Chambon, P., et al. (1993). A homeotic transformation is generated in the rostral branchial region of the head by disruption of Hoxa-2, which acts as a selector gene. *Cell* 75, 1333–1349. doi: 10.1016/0092-8674(93)90620-6

Smith, T. M., Lozanoff, S., Iyyanar, P. P., and Nazarali, A. J. (2013). Molecular signaling along the anterior-posterior axis of early palate development. *Front. Physiol.* 3:488. doi: 10.3389/fphys.2012.00488

Smith, T. M., Wang, X., Zhang, W., Kulyk, W., and Nazarali, A. J. (2009). Hoxa2 plays a direct role in murine palate development. *Dev. Dyn.* 238, 2364–2373. doi: 10.1002/dvdy.22040

Thangaraj, M. P., Furber, K. L., Gan, J. K., Ji, S., Sobchishin, L., Doucette, J. R., et al. (2017). RNA binding protein Quaking stabilizes Sirt2 mRNA during oligodendroglial differentiation. *J. Biol. Chem.* 292, 5166–5182. doi: 10.1074/jbc.M117.775544

Vucicevic, L., Misirkic, M., Janjetovic, K., Vilimanovich, U., Sudar, E., Isenovic, E., et al. (2011). Compound C induces protective autophagy in cancer cells through AMPK inhibition-independent blockade of Akt/mTOR pathway. *Autophagy* 7, 40–50. doi: 10.4161/auto.7.1.13883

Wu, M., Li, J., Engleka, K. A., Zhou, B., Lu, M. M., Plotkin, J. B., et al. (2008). Persistent expression of Pax3 in the neural crest causes cleft palate and defective osteogenesis in mice. *J. Clin. Invest.* 118, 2076–2087. doi: 10.1172/JCI33715

Xiong, W., He, F., Morikawa, Y., Yu, X., Zhang, Z., Lan, Y., et al. (2009). Hand2 is required in the epithelium for palatogenesis in mice. *Dev. Biol.* 330, 131–141. doi: 10.1016/j.ydbio.2009.03.021

Yu, K., Deng, M., Naluai-cecchini, T., Glass, I. A., and Cox, T. C. (2017). Differences in oral structure and tissue interactions during mouse vs. Human palatogenesis: implications for the translation of findings from mice. *Front. Physiol.* 8:154. doi: 10.3389/fphys.2017.00154

Yu, P. B., Hong, C. C., Sachidanandan, C., Babitt, J. L., Deng, D. Y., Hoyng, S. A., et al. (2008). Dorsomorphin inhibits BMP signals required for embryogenesis and iron metabolism. *Nat. Chem. Biol.* 4, 33–41. doi: 10.1038/nchembio.2007.54

Zhang, Z., Song, Y., Zhao, X., Zhang, X., Fermin, C., and Chen, Y. (2002). Rescue of cleft palate in Msx1-deficient mice by transgenic Bmp4 reveals a network of BMP and Shh signaling in the regulation of mammalian palatogenesis. *Development* 129, 4135–4146.

Zhou, G., Myers, R., Li, Y., Chen, Y., Shen, X., Fenyk-melody, J., et al. (2001). Role of AMP-activated protein kinase in mechanism of metformin action role of AMP-activated protein kinase in mechanism of metformin action. *J. Clin. Invest.* 108, 1167–1174. doi: 10.1172/JCI13505

Zhou, J., Gao, Y., Lan, Y., Jia, S., and Jiang, R. (2013). Pax9 regulates a molecular network involving Bmp4, Fgf10, Shh signaling and the Osr2 transcription factor to control palate morphogenesis. *Development* 140, 4709–4718. doi: 10.1242/dev.099028

4

Monitoring Notch Signaling-Associated Activation of Stem Cell Niches within Injured Dental Pulp

Thimios A. Mitsiadis[1], Javier Catón[2], Pierfrancesco Pagella[1], Giovanna Orsini[3] and Lucia Jimenez-Rojo[1]*

[1] Orofacial Development and Regeneration, Faculty of Medicine, Institute of Oral Biology, ZZM, University of Zurich, Zurich, Switzerland, [2] Department of Medical Basic Sciences, Faculty of Medicine, University CEU-San Pablo, Madrid, Spain, [3] Department of Clinical Sciences and Stomatology, Polytechnic University of Marche, Ancona, Italy

***Correspondence:**
Thimios A. Mitsiadis
thimios.mitsiadis@zzm.uzh.ch

Dental pulp stem/progenitor cells guarantee tooth homeostasis, repair and regeneration throughout life. The decision between renewal and differentiation of these cells is influenced by physical and molecular interactions with stromal cells and extracellular matrix molecules forming the specialized microenvironment of dental pulp stem cell niches. Here we study the activation of putative pulp niches after tooth injury through the upregulation of Notch signaling pathway. Notch1, Notch2, and Notch3 molecules were used as markers of dental pulp stem/progenitor cells. Upon dental injury, Notch1 and Notch3 are detected in cells related to vascular structures suggesting a role of these proteins in the activation of specific pulpal perivascular niches. In contrast, a population of Notch2-positive cells that are actively proliferative is observed in the apical part of the pulp. Kinetics of these cells is followed up with a lipophilic DiI labeling, showing that apical pulp cells migrate toward the injury site where dynamic regenerative/repair events occur. The knowledge of the activation and regulation of dental pulp stem/progenitor cells within their niches in pathologic conditions may be helpful for the realization of innovative dental treatments in the near future.

Keywords: stem cells, dental pulp, niches, tooth injury, regeneration, cell proliferation, Notch signaling, Notch2

INTRODUCTION

Biological repair and regeneration is an attractive alternative and/or complement to prosthetic replacement of tissues and organs. Cell-based therapeutic approaches consist of *in vitro* manipulation of stem cells and their consequent administration to patients (Passier et al., 2008; Segers and Lee, 2008; Djouad et al., 2009; Robinton and Daley, 2012; Shevde, 2012; Bender, 2016). Stem cells are defined by their dual capacity of self-renewal and multipotency (referred to as stemness) (Thomson et al., 1998; Shevde, 2012). These properties make stem cells extremely interesting for clinical tissue engineering applications (Bianco and Robey, 2001; Mitsiadis et al., 2012; Aurrekoetxea et al., 2015; Mele et al., 2016). Stem cells have been identified in the pulp of deciduous and adult permanent teeth (Mitsiadis et al., 2015; Miran et al., 2016). These cells are able to differentiate both *in vivo* and *in vitro* into many cell types such as odontoblasts, osteoblasts, chondrocytes, adipocytes, and neuronal cells (Bluteau et al., 2008; Mitsiadis et al., 2015). There is increasing evidence for the existence of more than one stem/progenitor cell populations within the dental pulp (Mitsiadis et al., 2011; Ducret et al., 2016).

Dental injuries are often lethal for the odontoblasts at the proximity of the lesion site, an event that triggers activation of dental pulp stem/progenitor cells. These cells proliferate, migrate, and finally differentiate into odontoblast-like cells that elaborate the reparative dentin (Mitsiadis and Rahiotis, 2004). However, the nature and exact location of these mesenchymal cell populations are not yet known. Niches consist of specific and protected anatomic locations housing stem/progenitor cells and enabling them to self-renew. Stromal cells belonging to a niche control stem cell behavior through cell-cell interactions, soluble factors, and specialized extracellular matrices (Scadden, 2006; Djouad et al., 2009; Shaker and Rubin, 2010; Oh and Nör, 2015; Pagella et al., 2015). This particular microenvironment permits stem/progenitor cells to survive, to change their number and fate, regulating thus their participation in tissue maintenance, repair and/or regeneration. Therefore, it is essential to identify stem cell niches within the dental pulp in order to understand the mechanisms and the microenvironment that support the survival of stem/progenitor cells in teeth.

Notch molecules are important regulators of the stem cell fate, with capacity to induce cell proliferation and/or differentiation (Hori et al., 2013). The close association of dental pulp mesenchymal cells and neo-vessels in dental diseases (e.g., carious lesions, injuries) and their relation to Notch signaling pathway may be critical in the regulation of stem cells to differentiate into odontoblast-like cells (Lovschall et al., 2007; Mitsiadis et al., 2011; Oh and Nör, 2015). Notch proteins form a family of evolutionary conserved transmembrane receptors that determine cell fate (Artavanis-Tsakonas and Muskavitch, 2010). In mammals, the four Notch receptors (i.e., Notch1, Notch2, Notch3, Notch4) are activated following direct contact with their five ligands: Jagged1 (Jag1), Jag2, Delta-like1 (Dll1), Dll3, Dll4. Upon ligand-receptor binding, the Notch protein is cleaved and its intracellular domain (NICD) translocates to the nucleus, where it associates with the DNA binding protein RBP-Jk to activate transcription (Artavanis-Tsakonas and Muskavitch, 2010; Hori et al., 2013). It has been reported that Notch activation promotes stem cell maintenance (Androutsellis-Theotokis et al., 2006; Artavanis-Tsakonas and Muskavitch, 2010).

Although Notch signaling has been exhaustively studied during tooth development, pathology and repair, its role in regulating the behavior of dental pulp stem/progenitor cells after injury remains elusive (Mitsiadis et al., 1999, 2003; Sun et al., 2014). To address such questions, experiments using loss- and/or gain-of-function transgenic animal models are necessary. In the present manuscript, as a first attempt to investigate this issue, we studied the correlation between the expression of Notch receptors and migration of apical pulp cells upon injury at the tooth crown.

MATERIALS AND METHODS

Tissue Preparation and Dental Explant Cultures

All mice (C57Bl/6; postnatal day 6–8) were maintained and handled according to the Swiss Animal Welfare Law and in compliance with the regulations of the Cantonal Veterinary office, Zurich (License 11/2014). The licensing committee of the Gesundheltsdirektion Kanton Zürich approved all experimental protocols (Versuch Nr. 11/2014 "Study of the function and potency of human and mouse dental stem cells after *in vitro* culture"). Mice were sacrificed by cervical dislocation and their mandibles were dissected out and cultured *in vitro*. Cavity preparations were performed in 20 first mandibular mouse molars using a 20-gauge drill, while 4 intact molars were used as a control. Four hours after the operation, the first molars were carefully extracted from the mandibles. Mandibles and dental explants were cultured in a medium consisted of Dulbecco's Modified Eagle Medium (DMEM; GibcoBRL), 20% fetal calf serum (FCS; GibcoBRL), 20 units/ml penicillin/streptomycin (GibcoBRL), and glutamine at 37°C/5% CO_2. Most of the molars were used for DiI labeling experiments, cell proliferation essays, and whole mount immunohistochemistry, while other molars were sectioned with a cryostat (12–14 μm sections) and used for immunohistochemistry and cell proliferation essays. Molars from more aged mice could not be used, as it was impossible to remove the hard mineralized tissues (i.e., dentin, enamel) without causing sparse damage to the pulp tissue. Cultures were maintained for at most 4 days, since pulps cultured for longer periods showed clear signs of pulp necrosis.

Immunohistochemistry and Immunofluorescence

Polyclonal antibodies against the mouse Notch1, Notch2, and Notch3 proteins were used (Mitsiadis et al., 1995, 1999, 2003). Immunohistochemistry on sections were performed as described previously (Mitsiadis et al., 1995, 1999, 2003). Briefly, the antibodies were applied for 2 h at 37°C, thereafter the sections were incubated with the biotinylated secondary antibody for 1 h and finally with peroxidase-conjugated streptavidine for 10 min. Peroxidase was revealed with 3-amino-9-ethylcarbazole (AEC) reaction solution. In control sections the primary antibodies were omitted.

For immunofluorescence on the entire dental pulp, tissues were first fixed in 1% paraformaldehyde (PFA) at 4°C overnight and then washed with phosphate-buffered saline (PBS)/0.2% bovine serum albumin (BSA)/0.3% Triton X-100 overnight. Samples were then incubated with Notch2 primary antibody during 5 days at 4°C. Thereafter, tissues were washed with PBS and post-fixed 30 min at RT in 4%PFA and incubated in HCl (2 M) for 30 min at 37°C prior to the incubation with the anti-BrdU antibody for 7 days at 4°C. Secondary antibodies were added separately and each of them incubated during 3 days at 4°C. Samples were then mounted with 2.5% 1,4-diazobicyclo-[2.2.2]-octane (DABCO, Sigma, D2522) mounting medium and analyzed using a Leica SP5 confocal microscope.

Cell Proliferation Analysis

Cell proliferation in cultured dental explants was analyzed by using a bromodeoxyuridine (BrdU) cell proliferation kit (Boehringer Mannheim). The explants were cultured for an additional time (i.e., 2–4 h) with BrdU, according to the manufacturer's instructions. BrdU-positive cells were monitored after staining with an anti-BrdU antibody and detected by means of a Vectastain ABC kit (Vector). Whole mount immunohistochemistry was performed as earlier described (Mitsiadis et al., 1995).

DiI Labeling and Fate Mapping of Dental Cells

Immediately after extraction, cells located at the apical part of dental pulp of both intact and injured first molars were labeled with DiI (Molecular probes cell tracker CM-DiI, C-7000). DiI is a lipophilic dye that intercalates in the cell membrane marking small groups of cells. DiI was prepared in ethanol (EtOH) at 2.5 μg/μl. This stock solution was then diluted 1–9 in 0.2 M sucrose and warmed. DiI was injected by a mouth-controlled borosilicate glass micropipette. After DiI labeling, dental explants were cultured for 4 days. Thereafter, explants were fixed with 4%PFA in Dulbecco's PBS at 4°C for 2 h. After fixation, the mineralized part of the majority of the teeth was carefully removed in order to obtain dental pulp tissues free of dentin and enamel. The fate of the labeled cells was assessed in transmitted light and fluorescence images, which were captured with a Zeiss Axioscope equipped with a CCD camera. The transmitted light and fluorescence images were finally merged.

RESULTS

Distribution of Notch Proteins in Injured Teeth

Upon injury of developing first molars (**Figure 1A**), immunohistochemistry on sections showed that Notch1 and Notch3 expression in the central part of the dental pulp is confined to cells forming vascular structures (**Figures 1B,C**). In contrast, Notch2 staining is detected in cells of the apical pulp (**Figure 1D**). This was confirmed by whole mount immunohistochemistry, clearly showing Notch2-positive cells at the apical part of the pulp (**Figures 1E,F**). Immunostaining against the three Notch proteins was not detected in the pulp of intact teeth (data not shown) that is in accordance with our previous results (Mitsiadis et al., 1999, 2003; Sun et al., 2014).

Correlation of Notch2 Protein Distribution and Cell Proliferation at the Apical Part of the Injured Pulp

In an attempt to ascertain whether Notch2 protein expression in the apical pulp was correlated with cell proliferation, healthy and injured dental pulp explants were cultured in presence of BrdU for up to 4 h before fixation. BrdU whole mount immunostaining revealed that while in the intact teeth only few cells proliferate at the apical part of the pulp (**Figure 2A**), cell divisions significantly enhance in this area upon tooth crown injury (**Figure 2B**). Double immunofluorescence on sections of injured pulp explants, analyzed in confocal microscopy, revealed that proliferating cells at the apical pulp part also express the Notch2 protein (**Figures 2C–E**).

Lineage Tracing of Apical Dental Pulp Cells in Intact and Injured Teeth

We then monitored the movement of dental pulp cells located at the apical part of the forming root in cultured first

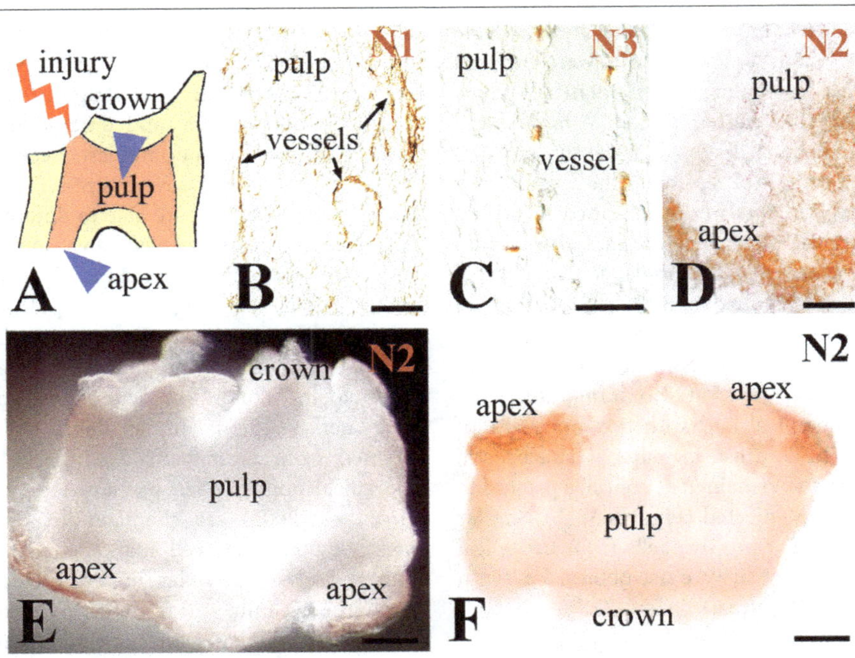

FIGURE 1 | Distribution of Notch proteins in the injured dental pulp. **(A)** Schematic illustration showing dental pulp injury after cavity preparation. Arrowheads indicate the areas of Notch activation within the pulp. **(B)** Notch1 (N1) staining is visible in cells lining blood vessels within the central part of the pulp. **(C)** Notch3 (N3) labeling is detected in perivascular cells of the central part of the pulp. **(D)** Notch2 (N2) staining is mainly found in apical pulp cells at the tooth apex. **(E,F)** Whole mount immunostaining showing Notch2 protein distribution at the apical part of an injured pulp. Scale bars: 50 μm **(B–D)**, 200 μm **(E,F)**.

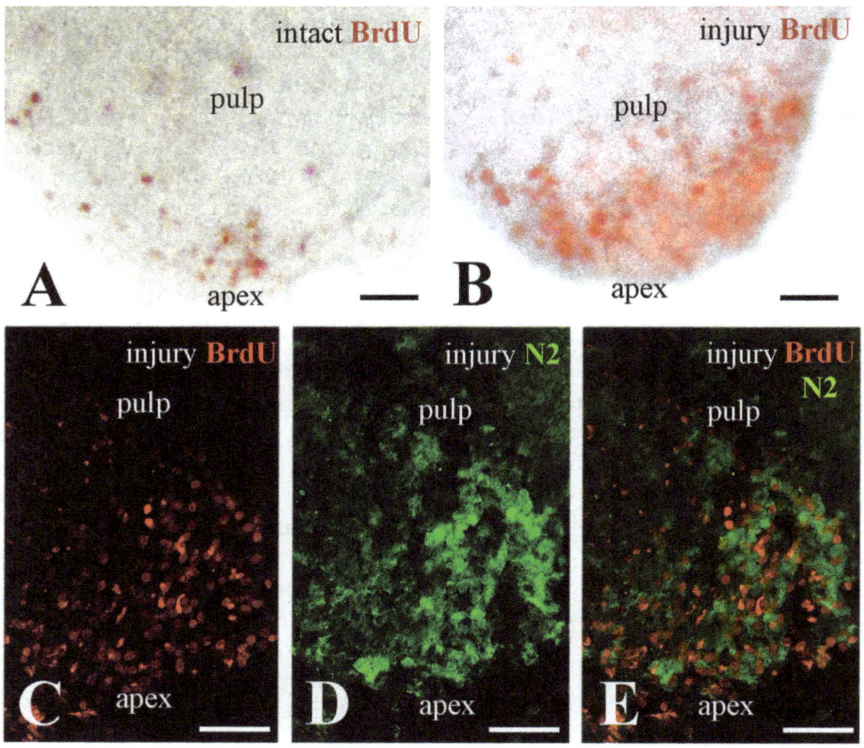

FIGURE 2 | Proliferation of dental pulp cells correlates with Notch2 protein expression in the apex of injured molar teeth. BrdU in red color, Notch2 (N2) staining in green color. **(A)** Proliferating dental pulp cells in intact teeth. **(B)** Proliferating pulp cells in injured teeth. Note that cell proliferation increases upon injury. **(C–E)** Confocal microscope analysis showing co-expression of BrdU **(C)** and Notch2 **(D)** in the apical part of the pulp after merging of the pictures **(E)**. Scale bars: 50 μm **(A–E)**.

molars. For this purpose, DiI was injected in apical pulp cells (**Figures 3A–C,G–I, 4A–C**) of injured and intact molars (time of injection indicated as T0) and then the molars were cultured for up to 4 days (T4). The development of the dental explants proceeded normally during the culture period. After fixation of the dental explants, their hard tissues (i.e., dentin, enamel) were carefully removed in order to keep intact the morphology of the pulp tissue. The experiments were performed in molars from postnatal day 6–8 mouse pups since the integrity of pulp tissues from older mice was severely impaired upon removal of the dental hard tissues. Dental pulps were then photographed using a fluorescence microscope. After merging fluorescence and bright-field images, DiI-positive cells in injured teeth were observed not only in apical pulp cells but also in migrating cells that form a line joining the apical part with the injury site of the tooth (**Figures 3D–F**). In contrast, in pulps of intact teeth, labeled cells did not migrate and remained as cohesive patches in the apical pulp, where DiI was injected (**Figures 3J–L**). Similar results showing migration of DiI-positive cells from the apical part of the pulp toward the injury site were also obtained in tooth explants after 1 day of culture (**Figure 4**).

DISCUSSION

Severe dental injuries (i.e., deep cavity preparations) induce apoptosis of odontoblasts and activation of complex regenerative mechanisms within the dental pulp (Tziafas et al., 2000; Mitsiadis and Rahiotis, 2004; Mitsiadis et al., 2008, 2011). Cells of the sub-odontoblastic layer, which express the Notch2 receptor (Mitsiadis et al., 2003; Mitsiadis and Rahiotis, 2004), could replace the apoptotic odontoblasts and differentiate into odontoblast-like cells. However, sub-odontoblastic cells are equally eliminated by apoptosis after a severe stress. Therefore, the number of neighboring cells that are able to differentiate into odontoblast-like cells decreases considerably and alternative sources of pulp stem/progenitor cells should be activated to ensure dental tissue repair. Although dental pulp contains a significant amount of stem cells (Bluteau et al., 2008; Catón et al., 2011), severe injury might induce stemness in cells that in physiological conditions do not behave as stem cells (Potten and Loeffler, 1990). Human dental pulp stem cells (hDPSCs) isolated from permanent teeth (Gronthos et al., 2000) and the apical pulp of shed primary teeth (called SCAP) (Shi and Gronthos, 2003) are characterized by expression of several mesenchymal stem cell markers (e.g., CD29, CD73, CD105, CD44) and extracellular matrix molecules such as collagen, vimentin, laminin, and fibronectin (Bluteau et al., 2008; Pagella et al., 2015). hDPSCs are multipotent and have shown a great potential for repair and regeneration since they can differentiate into various cell types such as adipocytes (Waddington et al., 2009), chondroblasts/chondrocytes (Waddington et al., 2009), osteoblasts/osteocytes (de Mendonça Costa et al., 2008; Graziano et al., 2008), myocytes (Kerkis et al., 2008), cardiomyocytes

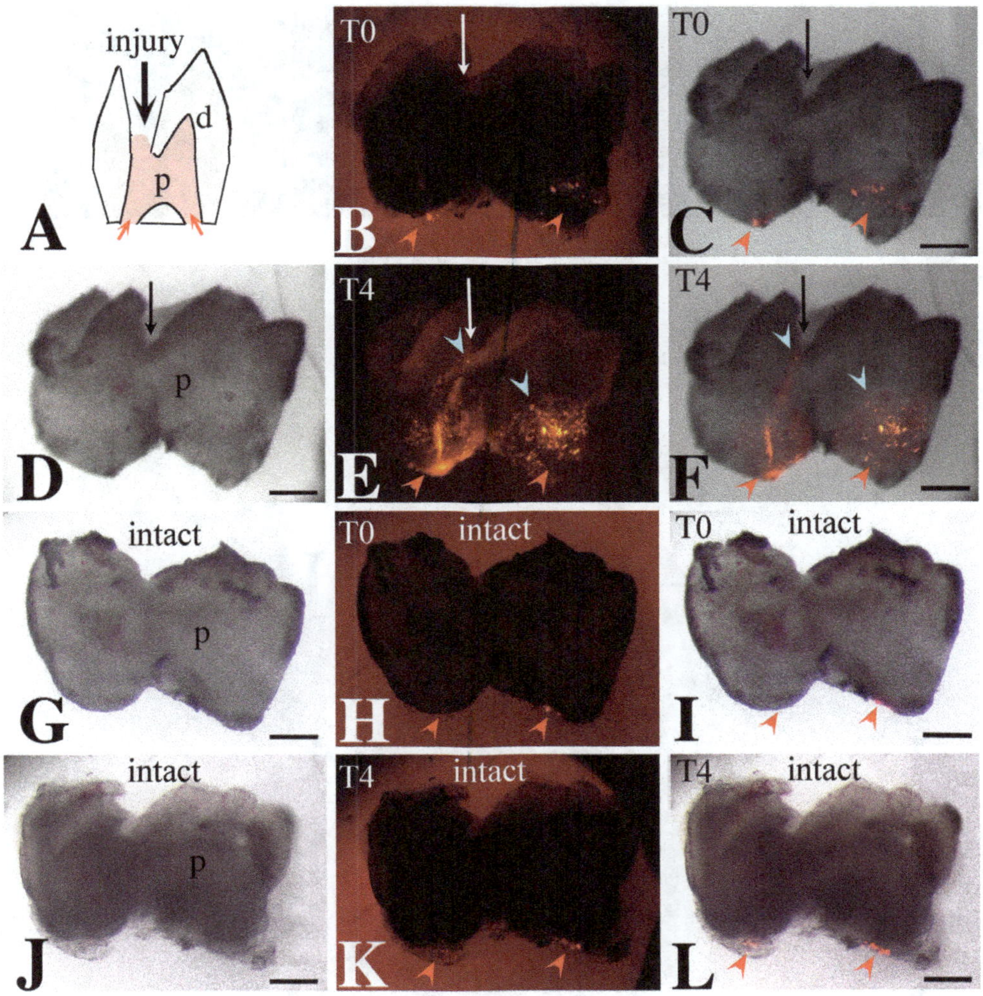

FIGURE 3 | Migration of DiI-labeled cells from the apical part of the pulp toward the injury site. Bright-field pictures **(D,G,J)**, dark-field pictures **(B,E,H,K)**, merged pictures **(C,F,I,L)**. Red arrows and arrowheads indicate the areas of DiI (red color) injection. Light blue arrowheads indicate the final location of migrating DiI-positive cells. Black and white arrows indicate injured teeth. **(A)** Schematic illustration showing dental pulp injury after cavity preparation. **(B,C)** Dental pulps immediately after injury and DiI injection (T0). **(D–F)** Dental pulps 4 days after cavity preparation and DiI injection (T4). **(G–I)** Intact dental pulps immediately after DiI injection (T0). **(J–L)** Intact dental pulps 4 days after DiI injection. Abbreviations: d, dentin; p, pulp; T0, time zero days; T4, time 4 days. Scale bars: 200 μm **(B–L)**.

(Gandia et al., 2008), and odontoblasts (Cordeiro et al., 2008; Nedel et al., 2009). This potential has made hDPSCs an attractive choice for tissue engineering, especially when they can be used as autologous transplants (Mitsiadis et al., 2015). The best example showing the success of such strategies is the first clinical trial using hDPSCs in patients for alveolar bone reconstruction (d'Aquino et al., 2009).

hDPSCs are thought to reside in one or more distinct storage sites, also called stem cell niches (Mitsiadis et al., 2015; Pagella et al., 2015). The concept of stem cell niches refers to defined anatomical compartments that include cellular and acellular (e.g., extracellular matrix) components. The niches provide highly specialized microenvironments, enabling stem cells to survive, self-renew, change their number and fate, and finally to participate in tissue repair (Scadden, 2006; Pagella et al., 2015). Similarly, niche-derived signals influence the function of dental pulp stem/progenitor cells. In addition, intercellular signaling pathways such as bone morphogenetic proteins (BMPs), Wnt, epidermal growth factor (EGF) and Notch are important regulators of stem cell function (Artavanis-Tsakonas and Muskavitch, 2010). Under the influence of these signaling pathways, dental stem cell might migrate from nearby or distant niches to the area of injury, where they will engraft and participate in the regeneration process. These cells will give rise to odontoblast-like cells that form the reparative dentin (Mitsiadis et al., 2015; Miran et al., 2016).

Significant molecular changes accompany dental pulp regeneration. For example, BMPs and transforming growth factor beta (TGFβ) are released from dentin after injury and contribute to reparative dentin formation (Tziafas et al., 2000; About and Mitsiadis, 2001; Mitsiadis and Rahiotis, 2004; Mitsiadis and Graf, 2009). Similarly, although Notch

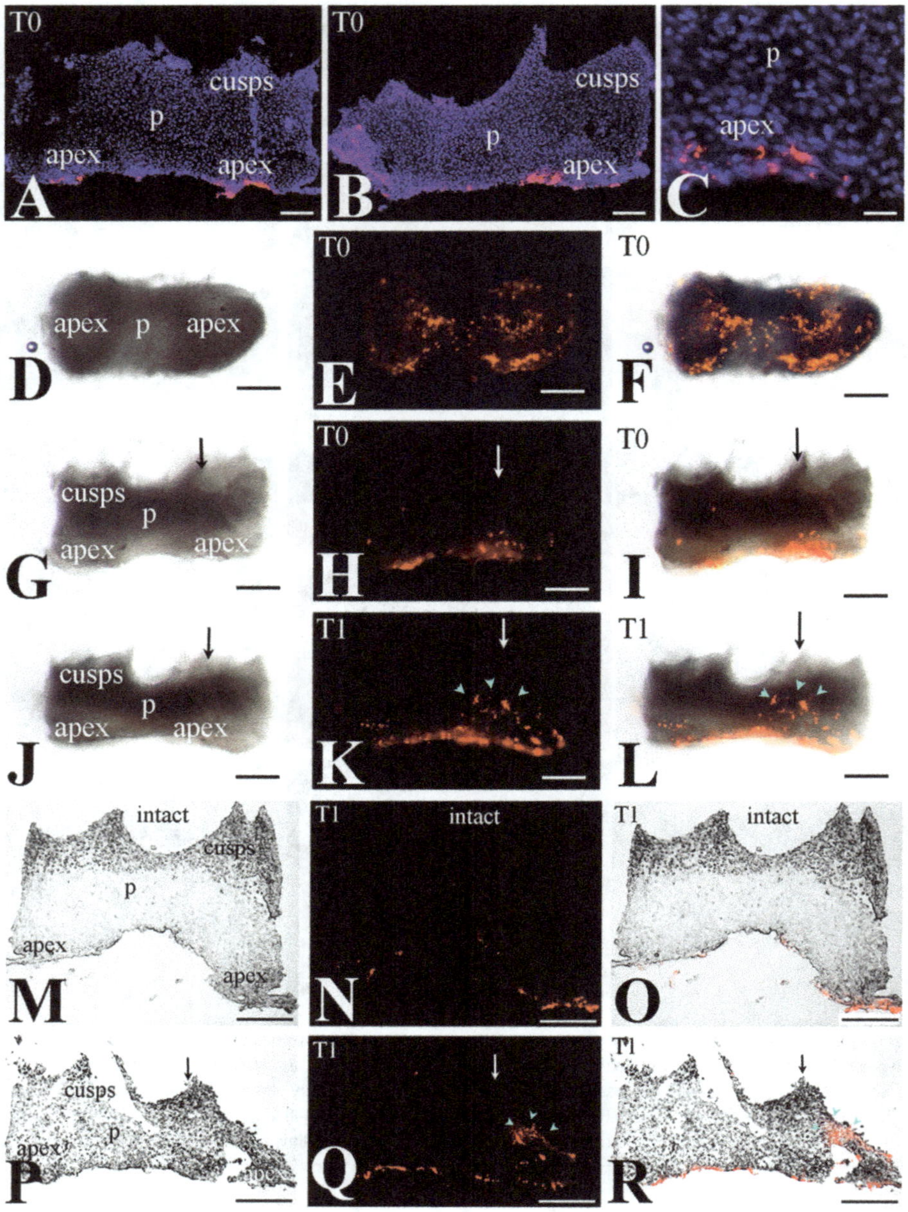

FIGURE 4 | Migration of DiI-labeled cells from the apical part of the pulp toward the injury site. **(A–C)** DiI labeled cells at the apical part of the pulp (T0). Dark-field pictures. DiI labels cells in red color while DAPI stains in blue color the nuclei of pulp cells in cryosections. **(D–L)** Migration of DiI-labeled cells from the root apex toward the injury site - whole pulp view. Bright-field pictures **(D,G,J)**, dark-field pictures **(E,H,K)**, merged pictures **(F,I,L)**. **(D–I)** Dental pulps immediately after injury and DiI injection (T0). **(J–L)** Dental pulps 1 day after cavity preparation and DiI injection (T1). Black and white arrows indicate the area of the tooth injury. DiI-positive pulp cells are seen in red color. Light blue arrowheads indicate the final location of migrating. **(M–R)** Migration of DiI-labeled cells from the apical part of the pulp toward the injury site—cryostat sections. DiI-labeled cells in red color. Bright-field pictures **(M,P)**, dark-field pictures **(N,Q)**, merged pictures **(O,R)**. Black and white arrows indicate injured teeth. **(M–N)** Intact dental pulps 1 day after DiI injection (T1). Note that in DiI-positive cells remain in the apical part of the pulp. **(P–R)** Dental pulps 1day after cavity preparation and DiI injection (T1). Light blue arrowheads indicate the final location of migrating DiI-positive cells. Abbreviations: p, pulp; T0, time zero days; T1, time 1 day. Scale bars: 100 μm **(A,B,D–R)**, 20 μm **(C)**.

receptors are absent in adult dental pulps, their expression is re-activated after injury (Mitsiadis et al., 1999, 2003; Lovschall et al., 2007). In injured rodent teeth, the Notch1 and Notch3 receptors, as well as the Delta-1 ligand are expressed in cells related to vascular structures, either near or far away of the injury site, while Notch2 is strongly expressed in dental pulp mesenchymal cells at the root apex (Mitsiadis et al., 1999). A similar pattern of Notch2 expression was observed in injured human permanent teeth (Mitsiadis et al., 2003), suggesting the existence of a pool of putative stem/progenitor cells at the apical part of the pulp. Previous findings in injured teeth showed reactivation of Notch3 in pericytes that might be another

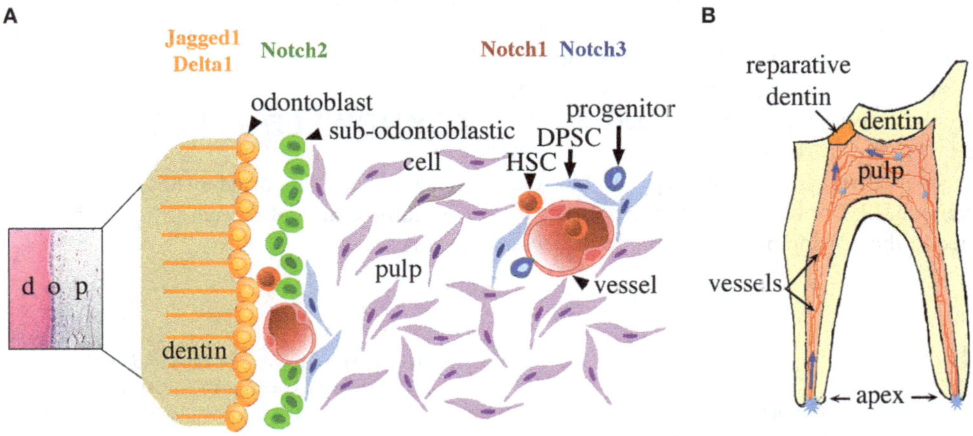

FIGURE 5 | Schematic representation of the suggested relationship between Notch signaling, dental pulp stem cell niches, and their activation upon tooth injury. **(A)** Potential stem/progenitor cells within the dental pulp at the crown level. Cells related to perivascular niches and odontoblast progenitors (i.e., sub-odontoblastic cells) will express a specific Notch receptor after dental injury at the crown level. **(B)** A model summarizing the cellular events after dental injury. Cavity preparation activates stem cell niches located in different parts of the dental pulp (light blue asterisks). Stem/progenitor cells start to migrate toward the injury site (blue arrows) and once on place might differentiate into odontoblast-like cells and participate to the formation of reparative dentin. Abbreviations: d, dentin; DPSC, dental pulp stem cells; HSC, hematopoietic stem cells; o, odontoblasts; p, pulp.

source for dental pulp stem cells (Lovschall et al., 2007). This is in line with previous findings indicating the existence of putative dental pulp perivascular niches (Shi and Gronthos, 2003; Oh and Nör, 2015). However, it has not yet proven that these Notch expressing cell populations participate to the process of dentin/pulp regeneration and can differentiate into odontoblast-like cells after injury. The activation of Notch signaling in human dental pulp stem/progenitor cells *in vitro* by either Jagged1 or the intracellular domain of Notch1 leads to inhibition of odontoblast differentiation without affecting cell proliferation (Zhang et al., 2008). In contrast, the activation of Notch signaling by Delta1 stimulates both cell differentiation and proliferation (He et al., 2009). Together these results suggest that Notch receptors may act as both positive and negative regulators of DPSCs depending on the ligand that they bind. Proliferative events in the apical pulp correlate to Notch2 expression after tooth crown injury. Our results are in line with recent findings showing that Notch2 signaling controls proliferation of various stem cell populations (e.g., bone marrow stem cells) and cancer cells (Huang et al., 2015; Sato et al., 2016; Wu et al., 2016).

In intact teeth, no obvious movement of the DiI-labeled apical pulp cells was observed. In contrast, in injured teeth, these cells migrate from the apex toward to the wounded area, a site where the reparative dentin will form. The migrating cells were seen in the line unifying the apex with the injury site. These results indicate that the apical part of the pulp contains a pool of putative stem/progenitor cells capable of migrating toward the injured site of the tooth. Our findings show a correlation between DiI-labeled cells, proliferating cells and Notch2-positive cells at the apical part of the injured dental pulp, thus suggesting a regulatory role for Notch2 signaling in proliferation and migration of pulp stem/progenitor cells. Loss- and gain-of-function experiments will be needed to investigate the functional role of Notch2 signaling in this process.

Although cells located at the apical pulp can end up far away (i.e., tooth crown) and participate in healing, other pulp stem/progenitor cell populations may also participate in tooth repair (e.g., cells derived from the perivascular niches), either concomitantly with apical pulp cells or at different time points (Mitsiadis et al., 2011, 2015; Oh and Nör, 2015; Ducret et al., 2016). A hypothetical schematic model of the pulp stem cell niches, their activation upon tooth injury, and stem cell kinetics within the pulp during repair is shown in **Figure 5**. To determine whether Notch2-positive cells directly contribute to these cellular events upon tooth injury, genetic lineage tracing experiments using a Notch2-creERT driver (Fre et al., 2011), combined with immunostaining for odontoblast differentiation markers, have to be undertaken. The present findings highlight the importance and dynamic nature of the apical pulp cells for tooth repair. These cells can reach the injury site and may participate in the formation of reparative dentin. Here we establish a conceptual framework where important cellular and molecular mechanisms operating during dental regenerative processes start to be elucidated. Such knowledge might be helpful for the realization of innovative dental treatments.

AUTHOR CONTRIBUTIONS

TM, Contributed to the conception of the hypothesis of the study and in the development of the model, involved in the evaluation of the results and preparation of the manuscript. He also provided approval for the publication of this version. JC, Contributed to the conception of the hypothesis of the study and to the development of the model, the acquisition and the analysis of data for the work. He was also involved in the preparation of the manuscript and provided approval for the publication of this version. PP, Contributed to the analysis and the interpretation of data for the work. He was also involved in the preparation of the manuscript and sanctioned the publication of this version. GO, Contributed to the development of the model and the interpretation of data for the work. She was also involved in the preparation of the manuscript and provided approval for the publication of this version. LJ, Contributed to the hypothesis of the study, collaborated in the development of the model and was involved in the evaluation of the results and preparation of the manuscript. She also provided approval for the publication of this version.

ACKNOWLEDGMENTS

This work was supported by funds from the University of Zürich. The authors did not receive any grant from commercial or profit sectors.

REFERENCES

About, I., and Mitsiadis, T. A. (2001). Molecular aspects of tooth pathogenesis and repair: *in vivo* and *in vitro* models. *Adv. Dent. Res.* 15, 59–62. doi: 10.1177/08959374010150011501

Androutsellis-Theotokis, A., Leker, R. R., Soldner, F., Hoeppner, D. J., Ravin, R., Poser, S. W., et al. (2006). Notch signalling regulates stem cell numbers *in vitro* and *in vivo*. *Nature* 442, 823–826. doi: 10.1038/nature04940

Artavanis-Tsakonas, S., and Muskavitch, M. A. (2010). "Notch: the past, the present, and the future," in *Current Topics in Developmental Biology*, ed R. Kopan (Amsterdam: Elsevier Inc.), 1–29.

Aurrekoetxea, M., Garcia-Gallastegui, P., Irastorza, I., Luzuriaga, J., Uribe-Etxebarria, V., Unda, F., et al. (2015). Dental pulp stem cells as a multifaceted tool for bioengineering and the regeneration of craniomaxillofacial tissues. *Front. Physiol.* 6:289. doi: 10.3389/fphys.2015.00289

Bender, E. (2016). Cell-based therapy: cells on trial. *Nature* 540, S106–S108. doi: 10.1038/540S106a

Bianco, P., and Robey, P. G. (2001). Stem cells in tissue engineering. *Nature* 414, 118–121. doi: 10.1038/35102181

Bluteau, G., Luder, H. U., De Bari, C., and Mitsiadis, T. A. (2008). Stem cells for tooth engineering. *Eur. Cell. Mater.* 16, 1–9. doi: 10.22203/eCM.v016a01

Catón, J., Bostanci, N., Remboutsika, E., De Bari, C., and Mitsiadis, T. A. (2011). Future dentistry: cell therapy meets tooth and periodontal repair and regeneration. *J. Cell. Mol. Med.* 15, 1054–1065. doi: 10.1111/j.1582-4934.2010.01251.x

Cordeiro, M. M., Dong, Z., Kaneko, T., Zhang, Z., Miyazawa, M., Shi, S., et al. (2008). Dental pulp tissue engineering with stem cells from exfoliated deciduous teeth. *J. Endod.* 34, 962–969. doi: 10.1016/j.joen.2008.04.009

d'Aquino, R., De Rosa, A., Lanza, V., Tirino, V., Laino, L., Graziano, A., et al. (2009). Human mandible bone defect repair by the grafting of dental pulp stem/progenitor cells and collagen sponge biocomplexes. *Eur. Cells Mater.* 18, 75–83. doi: 10.22203/eCM.v018a07

de Mendonça Costa, A., Bueno, D. F., Martins, M. T., Kerkis, I., Kerkis, A., Fanganiello, R. D., et al. (2008). Reconstruction of large cranial defects in nonimmunosuppressed experimental design with human dental pulp stem cells. *J. Craniofac. Surg.* 19, 204–210. doi: 10.1097/scs.0b013e31815c8a54

Djouad, F., Bouffi, C., Ghannam, S., Noël, D., and Jorgensen, C. (2009). Mesenchymal stem cells: innovative therapeutic tools for rheumatic diseases. *Nat. Rev. Rheumatol.* 5, 392–399. doi: 10.1038/nrrheum.2009.104

Ducret, M., Fabre, H., Degoul, O., Atzeni, G., McGuckin, C., Forraz, N., et al. (2016). Immunophenotyping reveals the diversity of human dental pulp mesenchymal stromal cells *in vivo* and their evolution upon *in vitro* amplification. *Front. Physiol.* 71:512. doi: 10.3389/fphys.2016.00512

Fre, S., Hannezo, E., Sale, S., Huyghe, M., Lafkas, D., Kissel, H., et al. (2011). Notch lineages and activity in intestinal stem cells determined by a new set of knock-in mice. *PLoS ONE* 6:e25785. doi: 10.1371/journal.pone.0025785

Gandia, C., Armiñan, A., García-Verdugo, J. M., Lledó, E., Ruiz, A., Miñana, M. D., et al. (2008). Human dental pulp stem cells improve left ventricular function, induce angiogenesis, and reduce infarct size in rats with acute myocardial infarction. *Stem Cells* 26, 638–645. doi: 10.1634/stemcells.2007-0484

Graziano, A., d'Aquino, R., Laino, G., and Papaccio, G. (2008). Dental pulp stem cells: a promising tool for bone regeneration. *Stem Cell Rev.* 4, 21–26. doi: 10.1007/s12015-008-9013-5

Gronthos, S., Mankani, M., Brahim, J., Robey, P. G., and Shi, S. (2000). Postnatal human dental pulp stem cells (DPSCs) *in vitro* and *in vivo*. *Proc. Natl. Acad. Sci. U.S.A.* 97, 13625–13630. doi: 10.1073/pnas.240309797

He, F., Yang, Z., Tan, Y., Yu, N., Wang, X., Yao, N., et al. (2009). Effects of Notch ligand Delta1 on the proliferation and differentiation of human dental pulp stem cells *in vitro*. *Arch. Oral Biol.* 54, 216–222. doi: 10.1016/j.archoralbio.2008.10.003

Hori, K., Sen, A., and Artavanis-Tsakonas, S. (2013). Notch signaling at a glance. *J. Cell Sci.* 126, 2135–2140. doi: 10.1242/jcs.127308

Huang, T. T., Ping, Y. H., Wang, A. M., Ke, C. C., Fang, W. L., and Huang, K. H. (2015). The reciprocal regulation loop of Notch2 pathway and miR-23b in controlling gastric carcinogenesis. *Oncotarget* 6, 18012–18026. doi: 10.18632/oncotarget.4000

Kerkis, I., Ambrosio, C. E., Kerkis, A., Martins, D. S., Zucconi, E., Fonseca, S. A. S., et al. (2008). Early transplantation of human immature dental pulp stem cells from baby teeth to golden retriever muscular dystrophy (GRMD) dogs: local or systemic? *J. Transl. Med.* 6:35. doi: 10.1186/1479-5876-6-35

Lovschall, H., Mitsiadis, T. A., Poulsen, K., Jensen, K. H., and Kjeldsen, A. L. (2007). Coexpression of Notch3 and Rgs5 in the pericyte-vascular smooth muscle cell axis in response to pulp injury. *Int. J. Dev. Biol.* 51, 715–721. doi: 10.1387/ijdb.072393hl

Mele, L., Vitiello, P. P., Tirino, V., Paino, F., De Rosa, A., Liccardo, D., et al. (2016). Changing paradigms in cranio-facial regeneration: current and new strategies for the activation of endogenous stem cells. *Front. Physiol.* 7:62. doi: 10.3389/fphys.2016.00062

Miran, S., Mitsiadis, T. A., and Pagella, P. (2016). Innovative dental stem cell-based research approaches: the future of dentistry. *Stem Cells Int.* 2016:7231038. doi: 10.1155/2016/7231038

Mitsiadis, T. A., De Bari, C., and About, I. (2008). Apoptosis in developmental and repair-related human tooth remodeling: a view from the inside. *Exp. Cell Res.* 314, 869–877. doi: 10.1016/j.yexcr.2007.11.001

Mitsiadis, T. A., Feki, A., Papaccio, G., and Catón, J. (2011). Dental pulp stem cells, niches, and notch signaling in tooth injury. *Adv. Dent. Res.* 23, 275–279. doi: 10.1177/0022034511405386

Mitsiadis, T. A., Fried, K., and Goridis, C. (1999). Reactivation of Delta-Notch signaling after injury: complementary expression patterns of ligand and receptor in dental pulp. *Exp. Cell Res.* 246, 312–318. doi: 10.1006/excr.1998.4285

Mitsiadis, T. A., and Graf, D. (2009). Cell fate determination during tooth development and regeneration. *Birth Defects Res. C Embryo Today* 87, 199–211. doi: 10.1002/bdrc.20160

Mitsiadis, T. A., Lardelli, M., Lendahl, U., and Thesleff, I. (1995). Expression of Notch 1, 2, and 3 is regulated by epithelial-mesenchymal interactions and retinoic acid in the developing mouse tooth and associated with determination of ameloblast cell fate. *J. Cell Biol.* 130, 407–418. doi: 10.1083/jcb.130.2.407

Mitsiadis, T. A., Orsini, G., and Jimenez-Rojo, L. (2015). Stem cell-based approaches in dentistry. *Eur. Cells Mater.* 30, 248–257. doi: 10.22203/eCM.v030a17

Mitsiadis, T. A., and Rahiotis, C. (2004). Parallels between tooth development and repair: conserved molecular mechanisms following carious and dental injury. *J. Dent. Res.* 83, 896–902. doi: 10.1177/154405910408301202

Mitsiadis, T. A., Roméas, A., Lendahl, U., Sharpe, P. T., and Farges, J. C. (2003). Notch2 protein distribution in human teeth under normal and pathological conditions. *Exp. Cell Res.* 282, 101–109. doi: 10.1016/S0014-4827(02)00012-5

Mitsiadis, T. A., Woloszyk, A., and Jiménez-Rojo, L. (2012). Nanodentistry: combining nanostructured materials and stem cells for dental tissue regeneration. *Nanomedicine* 7, 1743–1753. doi: 10.2217/nnm.12.146

Nedel, F., André Dde, A., de Oliveira, I. O., Cordeiro, M. M., Casagrande, L., Tarquinio, S. B., et al. (2009). Stem cells: therapeutic potential in dentistry. *J. Contemp. Dent. Pract.* 10, 90–96.

Oh, M., and Nör, J. E. (2015). The perivascular niche and self-renewal of stem cells. *Front. Physiol.* 6:367. doi: 10.3389/fphys.2015.00367

Pagella, P., Neto, E., Lamghari, M., and Mitsiadis, T. A. (2015). Investigation of orofacial stem cell niches and their innervation through microfluidic devices. *Eur. Cells Mater.* 29, 213–223. doi: 10.22203/eCM.v029a16

Passier, R., van Laake, L. W., and Mummery, C. L. (2008). Stem-cell-based therapy and lessons from the heart. *Nature* 453, 322–329. doi: 10.1038/nature07040

Potten, C. S., and Loeffler, M. (1990). Stem cells: attributes, cycles, spirals, pitfalls and uncertainties. Lessons for and from the crypt. *Development* 110, 1001–1020.

Robinton, D. A., and Daley, G. Q. (2012). The promise of induced pluripotent stem cells in research and therapy. *Nature* 481, 295–305. doi: 10.1038/nature 10761

Sato, Y., Mabuchi, Y., Miyamoto, K., Araki, D., Niibe, K., Houlihan, D. D., et al. (2016). Notch2 signaling regulates the proliferation of murine bone marrow-derived mesenchymal stem/stromal cells via c-Myc expression. *PLoS ONE* 11:e0165946. doi: 10.1371/journal.pone.0165946

Scadden, D. T. (2006). The stem-cell niche as an entity of action. *Nature* 441, 1075–1079. doi: 10.1038/nature04957

Segers, V. F., and Lee, R. T. (2008). Stem-cell therapy for cardiac disease. *Nature* 451, 937–942. doi: 10.1038/nature06800

Shaker, A., and Rubin, D. C. (2010). Intestinal stem cells and epithelial-mesenchymal interactions in the crypt and stem cell niche. *Transl. Res.* 156, 180–187. doi: 10.1016/j.trsl.2010.06.003

Shevde, N. (2012). Stem cells: flexible friends. *Nature* 483, S22–S26. doi: 10.1038/483S22a

Shi, S., and Gronthos, S. (2003). Perivascular niche of postnatal mesenchymal stem cells in human bone marrow and dental pulp. *J. Bone Miner. Res.* 18, 696–704. doi: 10.1359/jbmr.2003.18.4.696

Sun, F., Wan, M., Xu, X., Gao, B., Zhou, Y., Sun, J., et al. (2014). Crosstalk between miR-34a and notch signaling promotes differentiation in apical papilla stem cells (SCAPs). *J. Dent. Res.* 93, 589–595. doi: 10.1177/0022034514531146

Thomson, J. A., Itskovitz-eldor, J., Shapiro, S. S., Waknitz, M. A., Swiergiel, J. J., Marshall, V. S., et al. (1998). Embryonic stem cell lines derived from human blastocysts. *Adv. Sci.* 282, 1145–1147. doi: 10.1126/science.282.5391.1145

Tziafas, D., Smith, A. J., and Lesot, H. (2000). Designing new treatment strategies in vital pulp therapy. *J. Dent.* 28, 77–92. doi: 10.1016/S0300-5712(99)00047-0

Waddington, R. J., Youde, S. J., Lee, C. P., and Sloan, A. J. (2009). Isolation of distinct progenitor stem cell populations from dental pulp. *Cells. Tissues Organs* 189, 268–274. doi: 10.1159/000151447

Wu, W. R., Zhang, R., Shi, X. D., Yi, C., Xu, L. B., and Liu, C. (2016). Notch2 is a crucial regulator of self-renewal and tumorigenicity in human hepatocellular carcinoma cells. *Oncol. Rep.* 36, 181–188. doi: 10.3892/or.2016.4831

Zhang, C., Chang, J., Sonoyama, W., Shi, S., and Wang, C. Y. (2008). Inhibition of human dental pulp stem cell differentiation by Notch signaling. *J. Dent. Res.* 87, 250–255. doi: 10.1177/154405910808700312

5

Understanding Mechanisms of GLI-Mediated Transcription during Craniofacial Development and Disease Using the Ciliopathy Mutant, *talpid*²

Ya-Ting Chang[1,2], *Praneet Chaturvedi*[2], *Elizabeth N. Schock*[1,2] *and Samantha A. Brugmann*[1,2]*

[1] *Division of Plastic Surgery, Department of Surgery, Cincinnati Children's Hospital Medical Center, Cincinnati, OH, USA,*
[2] *Division of Developmental Biology, Department of Pediatrics, Cincinnati Children's Hospital Medical Center, Cincinnati, OH, USA*

***Correspondence:**
Samantha A. Brugmann
samantha.brugmann@cchmc.org

The primary cilium is a ubiquitous, microtubule-based organelle that cells utilize to transduce molecular signals. Ciliopathies are a group of diseases that are caused by a disruption in the structure or function of the primary cilium. Over 30% of all ciliopathies are primarily defined by their craniofacial phenotypes, which typically include midfacial defects, cleft lip/palate, micrognathia, aglossia, and craniosynostosis. The frequency and severity of craniofacial phenotypes in ciliopathies emphasizes the importance of the cilium during development of the craniofacial complex. Molecularly, many ciliopathic mutants, including the avian *talpid*² (*ta*²), report pathologically high levels of full-length GLI3 ($GLI3_{FL}$), which can go on to function as an activator (GLI_A), and reduced production of truncated GLI3 ($GLI3_T$), which can go on to function as a repressor (GLI_R). These observations suggest that the craniofacial phenotypes of ciliary mutants like *ta*² are caused either by excessive activity of the GLI_A or reduced activity of GLI_R. To decipher between these two scenarios, we examined GLI3 occupation at the regulatory regions of target genes and subsequent target gene expression. Using *in silico* strategies we identified consensus GLI binding regions (GBRs) in the avian genome and confirmed GLI3 binding to the regulatory regions of its targets by chromatin immunoprecipitation (ChIP). In *ta*² mutants, there was a strikingly low number of GLI3 target genes that had significantly increased expression in facial prominences compared to the control embryo and GLI3 occupancy at GBRs associated with target genes was largely reduced. *In vitro* DNA binding assays, further supported ChIP results, indicated that the excessive $GLI3_{FL}$ generated in *ta*² mutants did not bind to GBRs. In light of these results, we explored the possibility of GLI co-regulator proteins playing a role in regulatory mechanism of GLI-mediated transcription. Taken together our studies suggest that craniofacial ciliopathic phenotypes are produced via reduced GLI_T production, allowing for target gene transcription to be mediated by the combinatorial code of GLI co-regulators.

Keywords: primary cilia, craniofacial, *talpid*², *c2cd3*, ciliopathies, GLI

INTRODUCTION

Primary cilia are ubiquitous organelles that serve as cellular hubs for transduction of numerous signaling pathways. Most notably, cilia have been identified as transducers of the Hedgehog (Hh) pathway. Identification of the primary cilium as a signaling hub for the Hh pathway came from seminal experiments reporting that anterograde and retrograde intraflagellar transport (IFT) proteins in the cilium are required for Sonic Hedgehog (SHH) signal propagation (Huangfu et al., 2003; Huangfu and Anderson, 2005). When SHH ligand is present, it binds to its receptor Patched (PTCH), thus allowing Smoothened (SMO) to localize and accumulate in the primary cilium (Corbit et al., 2005; Rohatgi et al., 2007). Activated, ciliary SMO, in concert with Kif7, then promotes the dissociation of GLI from Suppressor of Fused (SUFU) (Humke et al., 2010; Tukachinsky et al., 2010; Li et al., 2012) and the subsequent post-translational processing of GLI proteins necessary for their function as activators and repressors (Goetz and Anderson, 2010).

In vertebrates, there are three members of the GLI transcription factor family: GLI1, GLI2, and GLI3. GLI1 and GLI2 are considered transcriptional activators, whereas GLI3 mostly behaves as a repressor. However, there have been examples of GLI2 functioning as a repressor in the absence of GLI3, and GLI3 functioning as an activator in the absence of GLI2 (Mo et al., 1997; Theil et al., 1999; Tole et al., 2000; Bai and Joyner, 2001; Persson et al., 2002; Rallu et al., 2002; Buttitta et al., 2003; Motoyama et al., 2003; Bai et al., 2004; Lei et al., 2004; McDermott et al., 2005; Pan et al., 2009). Full-length GLI2 and GLI3 can be processed via phosphorylation and other post-translational modifications into the activator isoform (GLI_A) or truncated into the repressor isoform (GLI_R) (Wang et al., 2000; Pan et al., 2006). Inhibition of GLI processing prevents production of GLI_A and GLI_R isoforms. Thus, an essential role of primary cilia is to establish the ratio of GLI_A to GLI_R proteins (Haycraft et al., 2005; Liu et al., 2005), which in turn controls transcription of SHH target genes.

Three basic models have been proposed to depict the potential mechanism of how SHH target genes are activated by a gradient of GLI isoforms: (1) the ratio sensing model, (2) the threshold repression model and (3) the threshold activation model (Falkenstein and Vokes, 2014). Ratio sensing, as the name implies, is based on the ratio of GLI_A and GLI_R rather than concentration of either. The net balance of GLI_A to GLI_R then determines if, and the extent to which, a target is activated or repressed. The other two models suggest threshold-specific mechanisms. The threshold activation model suggests that SHH targets are activated when GLI_A reaches a threshold-specific concentration. On the other hand, in the threshold repression model (de-repression), the activation of SHH target genes is dictated by the alleviation of repression via loss of GLI_R.

The *talpid*^{2} (*ta*^{2}) is a naturally occurring avian mutant that is best characterized by severe polydactyly and its oral-facial phenotype (Abbott et al., 1959, 1960; Dvorak and Fallon, 1991; Schneider et al., 1999). The face of affected *ta*^{2} embryos is characterized by a dysmorphic frontonasal prominence, facial clefting, hypoplastic maxillary prominences, incomplete fusion of the primary palate and hypoglossia (Chang et al., 2014). Our recent work determined that the *ta*^{2} mutation affected ciliogenesis via a 19 bp deletion in *C2CD3* (Brugmann et al., 2010; Chang et al., 2014), a centriolar protein required for ciliogenesis (Hoover et al., 2008). Our studies also determined that the *ta*^{2} mutant genetically, biochemically and phenotypically phenocopied the human craniofacial ciliopathy, Oral-facial-digital syndrome 14 (OFD14) (Schock et al., 2015). *ta*^{2} embryos, similar to many other ciliopathies, have a significant increase in $GLI3_{FL}$ and a reduction in the amount GLI_T (Chang et al., 2014). However, the mechanism by which this disruption in GLI isoform production affects expression of GLI targets in the developing craniofacial complex remains unknown.

Herein, we utilize a combination of several biochemical techniques to determine the impact loss of cilia has on GLI function. Specifically, we examine the expression of GLI target genes and occupation of GLI binding regions (GBRs) associated with those targets in the developing frontonasal, maxillary and mandibular prominences (FNP, MXP, and MNP, respectively) in order to uncover the mechanism by which GLI mediated transcription is being impacted in *ta*^{2} mutants. Understanding the full extent of molecular disruptions in *ta*^{2} mutants will hopefully guide future therapeutic strategies for craniofacial ciliopathies, a rapidly growing group of disorders that currently have little to no therapeutic treatment.

MATERIALS AND METHODS

Embryo Preparation

talpid^2 (*ta*^{2}) heterozygous carriers were mated, eggs were collected and shipped from the UC Davis Avian Sciences Department. Embryos were incubated at 37°C for approximately 5–7 days when embryos reached Hamburger Hamilton stage 25–31 (HH25-31).

Quantitative RT-PCR of GLI Targets

FNPs, MXPs, and MNPs were harvested from day 5 chick embryos. mRNA was prepared with TRIzol reagent (Thermo Fisher Scientific), and then converted to complementary DNA through reverse transcription reaction (High-Capacity cDNA Reverse Transcription Kit, Applied Biosystems™). Different amounts of cDNA (40, 20, 10 and 5 ng) was used for quantitative PCR to test PCR efficiency and a linear range of duplication (SsoAdvanced™ Universal SYBR® Green Supermix, BioRad). Expression of genes known to play a role in craniofacial development were examined with the following primer sets: *ALX4* (105 bp) F: GTTACGGTAAGGAGAGCAGTTT, R:CTTTCACTCCAGCCTCCTTC, *BMPR1A* (100 bp) F: GTGCTGTCGGACTGATTTCT, R:TGCCATCCAACGAATGCT, *WIF1* (100 bp) F: CAACCTGTTTCAATGGAGGAAC, R: GGCTGATGGCATTTACTGATTT, *OSR2* (140 pb) F: CCACTTCACCAAGTCCTACAA, R: TCTCTTTGGAATGGATGTACCG. The statistical significance of the data was evaluated through two-tailed Student's *t*-test. *p*-values less than or equal to 0.05 (95% confidence level) were considered as statistically significant differences.

Western Blotting of GLI2/3 Proteins

FNPs, MXPs, or MNPs were pooled and lysed in RIPA buffer containing protease inhibitors and phosphatase inhibitors (1 mM Phenylmethylsulfonyl fluoride, 1 mM $NaVO_4$, 1X complete protease inhibitor cocktail, EDTA-free), and slightly sonicated with a microprobe to recover chromosome bound GLI2 and GLI3 proteins. BCA assay (Pierce) was used to measure protein concentration of cell lysates. Proteins were boiled with 1X Laemmli sample buffer and run on 6% SDS-PAGE for GLI2 and GLI3, or 12% SDS-PAGE for GAPDH, which later were wet-transferred to Polyvinylidene difluoride (PVDF) membrane. Anti-GLI2, anti-GLI3 (Polyclonal goat IgG 1:500, R&D systems) and anti-GAPDH (FL-335, polyclonal rabbit IgG 1:4000, Santa Cruz Biotechnology) were prepared in 1X TBST (0.1% Tween-20)/6% nonfat milk, as well as secondary antibodies (anti-goat and anti-rabbit, 1:10,000). Proteins were detected by Electrochemiluminescence assay (Amersham ECL Prime, GE Healthcare Life Science).

DNA Binding Affinity Assay

PATCHED 1 promoter oligonucleotides were designed according to the location of a Gli binding region (GBR) at −2549 from the TSS site (GGAAGAAGTGTCAGTGTAAG AGTCTCCACGTGGGTGGTCAAGGCCATGGCTGCCTCAC GG). 100 pmole of biotin-conjugated positive oligonucleotides and complementary oligonucleotides (Integrated DNA Technologies) were annealed in 1X TE/50 mM NaCl buffer in a PCR cycler and incubated with Dynabeads Streptavidin (M280, Invitrogen). FNPs, MXPs, or MNPs from day 5 control or ta^2 embryos were pooled and processed as described for Western blotting. Cell lysates were incubated with oligonucleotides-bound Dynabeads at 4°C for 2 h. Beads were washed with 1 ml RIPA buffer three times and processed for Western Blotting analysis.

Chromatin Immunoprecipitation

FNPs, MXPs, or MNPs from day 5 control or ta^2 embryos were harvested, pooled and crosslinked in 1% formaldehyde. Tissue was homogenized in RIPA buffer and sonicated (Bioruptor® Pico, Diagenode) at 5 cycles of 30 s on/45 s off. Sheared DNA was distributed around 0.3 kb to 1 kb on 1% agarose gel. Cell lysates were pre-cleaned with Dynabeads protein G (ThermoFisher Scientific) and quantified by BCA assay. Dynabeads for immunoprecipitation were blocked with 20 μg/ml Glycogen, 20 μg/ml BSA, 20 μg/ml yeast RNA in RIPA buffer at 4°C for an hour. GLI3 antibody (AF3690, R&D systems) and pre-blocked Dynabeads Protein G were incubated with 90% of cell lysates at 4°C overnight. 10% of cell lysates were kept as Input. Beads were washed with IP wash buffer I (low salt; 50 mM HEPES-KOH pH 7.5, 150 mM NaCl, 1 mM EDTA, 0.1% sodium deoxycholate, 1% Triton X-100), IP wash buffer II (high salt; 50 mM HEPES-KOH pH 7.5, 500 mM NaCl, 1 mM EDTA, 0.1% sodium deoxycholate, 1% Triton X-100), IP Wash Buffer III (LiCl containing buffer; 10 mM Tris-Cl pH 8.0, 250 mM LiCl, 1 mM EDTA, 0.5% Sodium deoxycholate, 0.5% NP-40) and TE buffer (10 mM Tris-HCl pH 8.0, 1 mM EDTA). ChIP samples were reverse-crosslinked by boiling with 10% Chelex-100 (BioRad), and treated with 0.2 mg/ml Proteinase K at 55°C for 30 min. Immunoprecipitated DNA samples were analyzed with quantitative real-time PCR (BioRad) with primers to GBR of target genes. Error bars in all figures represent standard error of the mean (S.E.M.) from five to seven independent experiments. The statistical significance of the data was evaluated through two-tailed Student's t-test. p-values less than or equal to 0.05 (95% confidence level) were considered as statistically significant differences.

GBR Analysis

Sequences for GBRs from previous publications (Vokes et al., 2007, 2008) were used with a custom perl script to search for all the exact matches of the various possible sequences of the consensus GBRs in the chicken genome. Acquired positions of the motifs in the genome were run through a second custom perl script to search for genes that encompass these motif sites at a distance of 20 kb from either end. Potential GLI targets were confirmed using chromatin-immunoprecipitation (ChIP) assays.

RESULTS

The Avian Ciliopathic Mutant, *talpid²*, has Craniofacial Anomalies Characteristic of a Ciliopathy

To understand the transcriptional networks affected in craniofacial ciliopathies we analyzed the *talpid*^{2} (ta^2) mutant, a naturally occurring avian ciliopathic mutant that has been established as a model for the human craniofacial ciliopathy, Oral-facial-digital syndrome 14 (Chang et al., 2014; Schock et al., 2015). The ta^2 craniofacial phenotype characterized by facial and palatal clefting, micrognathia, and hypoglossia, is fully evident at day 7 (**Figure 1**). Although our previous work has characterized this phenotype (Chang et al., 2014; Schock et al., 2015), to determine the transcriptional networks that contribute, we first needed to identify when phenotypic onset occurred. At day 7 the frontonasal prominence (FNP) is shorter and wider and frequently does not fuse to adjacent prominences (**Figures 1A–B'**). Two days earlier at day 5, the MXPs were medially rotated, the nasal pits were larger, thus preventing the proper juxtapositioning of the FNP with adjacent prominences (**Figures 1C–D'**). Palatal views showed increased patency of the naturally cleft avian secondary palate in ta^2 embryos relative to controls at day 7 (**Figures 1E–F'**, dotted white lines). Two days earlier, at day 5, the dysmorphology and malposition of the MXPs is just becoming apparent (**Figures 1G–H'**). Dorsal views of the developing lower beak showed the MNP of ta^2 embryos failed to fuse completely and had a hypoplastic tongue (hypoglossia, dotted black line) (**Figures 1I–J'**, white arrow). At day 5 there was little difference in mandibular growth between control and ta^2 MNPs (**Figures 1K–L'**). From phenotypic evaluations, taken together with the fact that these anomalies were not readily identifiable at day 4, we determined that craniofacial anomalies were initiated at approximately day 5 of development. Thus, to determine the molecular networks responsible for these

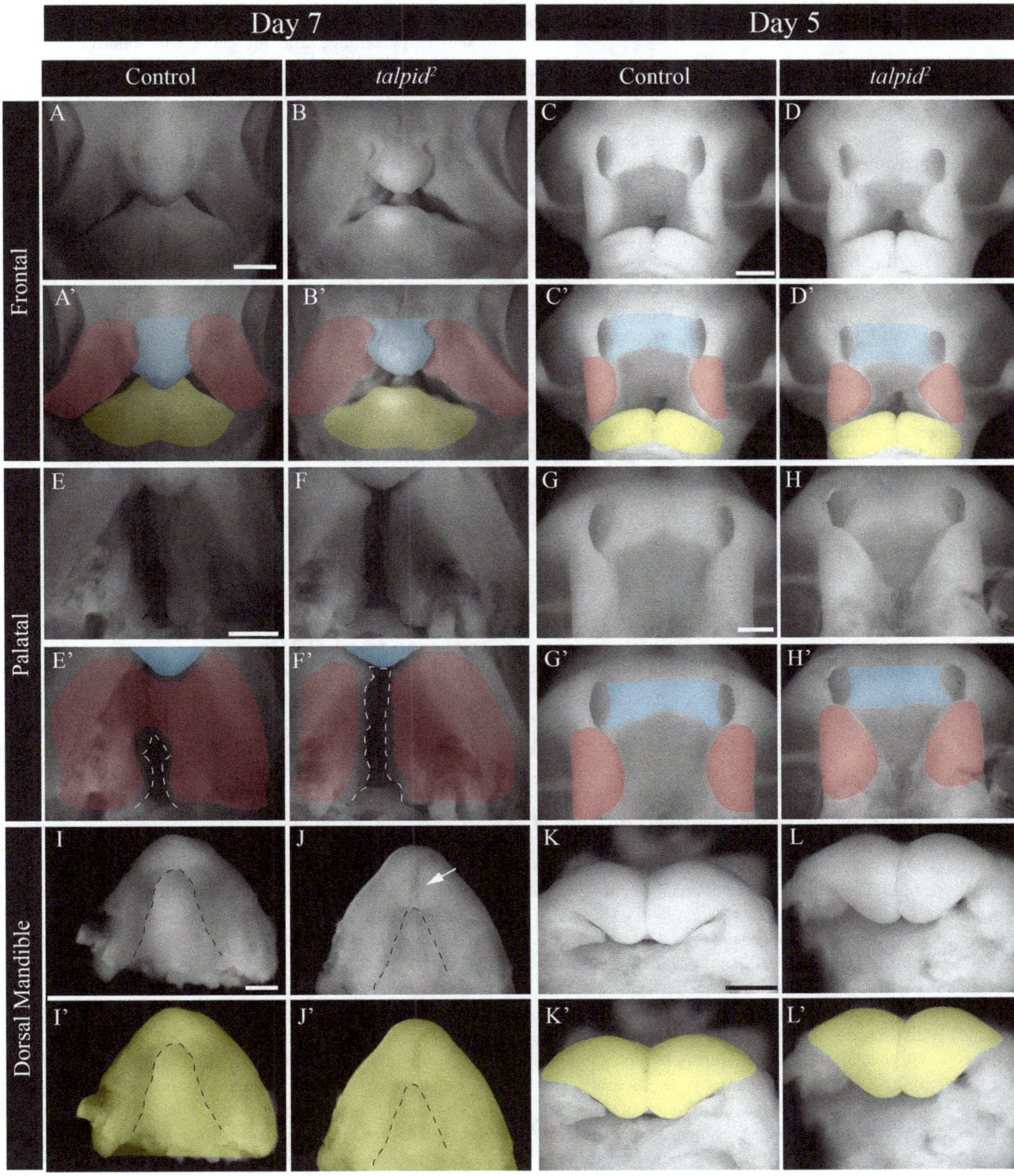

FIGURE 1 | ta^2 embryos have craniofacial anomalies common to craniofacial ciliopathies. (A–B') Frontal view of whole-mount day 7 control and ta^2 embryos. **(C,D')** Frontal view of whole-mount day 5 control and ta^2 embryos. **(E–F')** Palatal view of day 7 control and ta^2 embryo with the forming secondary palate outlined (white dotted line). **(G–H')** Palatal view of day 5 control and ta^2 embryo. **(I–J')** Dorsal view of day 7 control and ta^2 mandibles with tongue outlined (black dotted line). **(K–L')** Dorsal view of day 5 control and ta^2 mandibles. Facial prominences have been pseudocolored as follows: frontonasal prominence (FNP, blue), maxillary prominence (MXP, red), and mandibular prominence (MNP, yellow). Scale bars: 1 mm **(A–J')** and 650 μm **(K–L')**.

phenotypes we carried out our analyses in the facial prominences of day 5 embryos.

Loss of Cilia Results in Aberrant GLI Isoform Production

Our previous work determined that aberrant ciliogenesis in *ta*^{2} embryos disrupted the production of GLI proteins in such a manner that there was increased GLI_{FL} production and decreased GLI_T production (Chang et al., 2014). The GLI_{FL} isoform typically goes on to function as an activator, whereas the GLI_T isoform goes on the function as a repressor. The excessive production of GLI_{FL} is an extraordinarily common molecular phenotype in ciliopathies, including those with craniofacial phenotypes (Huangfu and Anderson, 2005; Davey et al., 2006; Tran et al., 2008; Tabler et al., 2013). To carefully exam the differences of GLI_{FL} and GLI_T protein levels in control and *ta*^{2} mutants, we performed Western blot analysis of GLI2 and GLI3 in the three facial prominences affected in the *ta*^{2} at day 5. We detected a very low level of $GLI2_{FL}$ and a substantial amount of $GLI2_T$ isoforms in the control facial prominences (**Figure 2A**). The loss of cilia in *ta*^{2} embryos disrupted GLI processing and altered the production of GLI2 protein isoforms. In *ta*^{2} facial prominences, we detected dramatically increased levels of $GLI2_{FL}$, and low levels of $GLI2_T$, relative to control prominences. We next examined the production of GLI3 isoforms. Western blot analyses showed that, similar to $GLI2_{FL}$, $GLI3_{FL}$ was increased in *ta*^{2} prominences relative to controls. Contrary to what was observed with the $GLI2_T$, $GLI3_T$ was readily detectable in both control and *ta*^{2} facial prominences. Specifically, *ta*^{2} MNP had less $GLI3_T$ than control MNP. These data suggested that disrupted ciliogenesis affected the processing of GLI2 and GLI3 in distinct manners, yet the net result was an increase in GLI_{FL} production. We did not observe a change in GLI1 protein levels between control and mutant embryos (Data not shown).

Since the GLI_{FL} isoform typically goes on to act as an activator, these results suggest that craniofacial phenotypes in the *ta*^{2} mutant could be caused by increased GLI activator function leading to increased expression of GLI target genes. To test this hypothesis, we utilized an *in silico* approach to look for potential GLI target genes within the avian genome. Using previously published sequences of GBRs (Vokes et al., 2007, 2008) we scanned the chicken genome for possible GLI targets. GBR positions were run through a custom perl script to search for genes that encompass these motif sites at a distance of 100 kb from the 5′ or 3′ end of the gene. From this list we identified several genes known to play a role in craniofacial development (**Supplemental Table 1**). Confirmation of our *in silico* approach was carried out on selected genes using ChIP assays (**Supplemental Figures 1 A–D**). Through these analyses, we selected four GLI3 target genes known to be expressed during, and have a role in, craniofacial development: *ALX4* (Beverdam et al., 2001; Mavrogiannis et al., 2001), *BMPR1A* (Li et al., 2011, 2013; Saito et al., 2012), *OSR2* (Lan et al., 2001), and *WIF1* (Hsieh et al., 1999; Darnell et al., 2007). *PTCH1*, a known GLI target, was used as a positive control (**Supplemental Figure 1E**) and IgG IP as an antibody background control. The data were all normalized to IgG IP percentage, and the genes with relative enrichment >1 were considered positive for GLI3 binding. To determine if increased production of $GLI3_{FL}$ in *ta*^{2} facial prominences correlated with increased expression of these target genes, we performed quantitative RT-PCR (qPCR) with mRNA from facial prominences of day 5 control and *ta*^{2} embryos (**Figures 2B–E**). There was not an increase in *ALX4* expression in any of the facial prominences (**Figure 2B**); however, we detected a significant decrease in *ALX4* expression in the MXP. *BMPR1A* expression was also not significantly increased in any of the developing prominences (**Figure 2C**). No significant changes in *OSR2* expression were detected in the FNP or MNP; however, a significant increase in expression was observed in the MXP (**Figure 2D**). Finally, *WIF1* expression was not changed in the FNP, yet was significantly increased in the MXP and significantly decreased in the MNP (**Figure 2E**). Taken together, these data do not support the idea that increased production of $GLI3_{FL}$ directly and uniformly results in increased expression of GLI targets throughout the facial prominences. Additionally, these data suggest that each facial prominence interprets aberrant GLI production in a unique manner.

Excess Production of GLI_{FL} Does Not Correlate with an Increase of GLI_{FL} Occupancy at GBRs

For GLI_{FL} to function as an activator, it has to occupy the regulatory regions of GLI targets. We wondered if lack of uniform increases of target gene expression in *ta*^{2} embryos was due to failure of GLI_{FL} to recognize and occupy GBRs of target genes. To test this hypothesis, we performed an *in vitro* DNA binding assay using the *PATCHED 1* (*PTCH1*) promoter. We synthesized a 60 base pair biotin-labeled oligonucleotide of the *PTCH1* promoter containing an endogenous GLI binding motif found at position −2549 proximally upstream of the transcription start site (TSS). Through high affinity of Biotin-Streptavidin interaction, we were able to evaluate the DNA binding ability of GLI3 isoforms by Western blot. Pre-incubation of non-labeled *PTCH1* oligonucleotides depleted GLI3 protein signals, which confirmed the specificity of the GLI3-GBR interaction. Under the same exposure, the affinity based pull-down assay showed that $GLI3_T$ predominantly bound to the biotin-labeled oligonucleotides in both control and *ta*^{2} mutants. Interestingly, despite the high level of $GLI3_{FL}$ production in *ta*^{2} embryos, $GLI3_{FL}$ failed to bind to the biotin-labeled oligonucleotides (**Figures 3A,B**). On the contrary, comparison between control and *ta*^{2} embryos indicated that the amount of $GLI3_T$ binding to the oligonucleotides correlates with the protein concentration (**Figures 3A,B**). Taken together these data suggest that despite increased $GLI3_{FL}$ production, target gene expression is not increased via increased GLI activator function because $GLI3_{FL}$ does not occupy the GBRs of target genes. In addition, the predominant binding of the $GLI3_T$ repressor at GBRs supports the idea of the threshold repression model, in which GLI targets underwent de-repression due to the removal of GLI_T repressor.

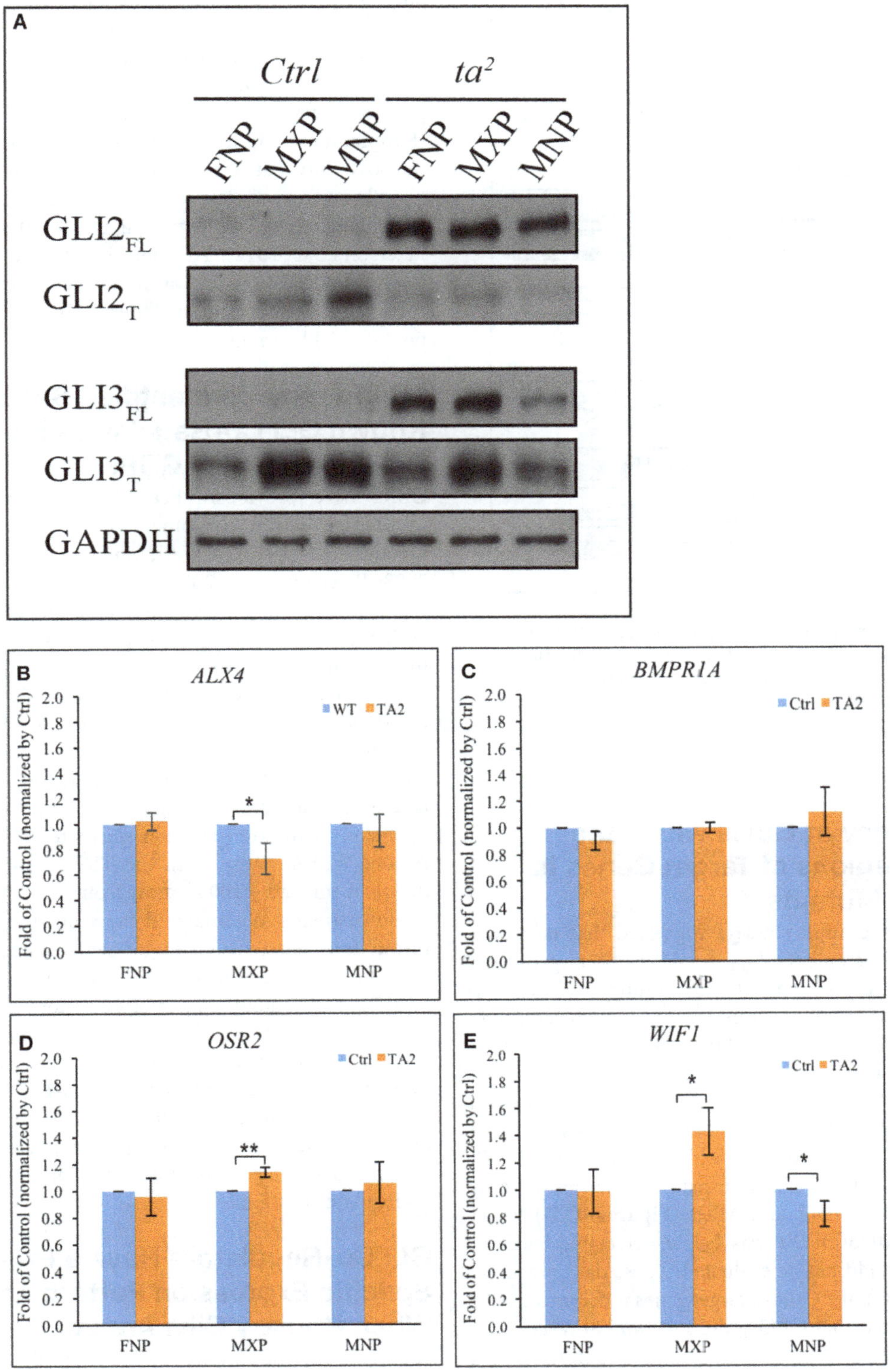

FIGURE 2 | Excessive GLI$_{FL}$ production in ta^2 embryo does not correlate with increased gene activation of GLI targets. (A) Western blot of GLI2 and GLI3 proteins from the frontonasal prominence (FNP), maxillary prominence (MXP) and mandibular prominence (MNP) of day 5 control and ta^2 embryos. GAPDH was used as a loading control. **(B–E)** mRNA-qPCR analyses of *ALX4*, *BMPR1A*, *OSR2*, *WIF1* from FNP, MXP, and MNP of day 5 control and ta^2 embryos. The data was normalized by the individual facial prominences of control and ta^2 embryos. The asterisks indicate statistically significant differences and are assigned as followed: $^*P < 0.05$, $^{**}P < 0.01$. Error bars are based on the standard error of the means (S.E.M.). $n = 4$.

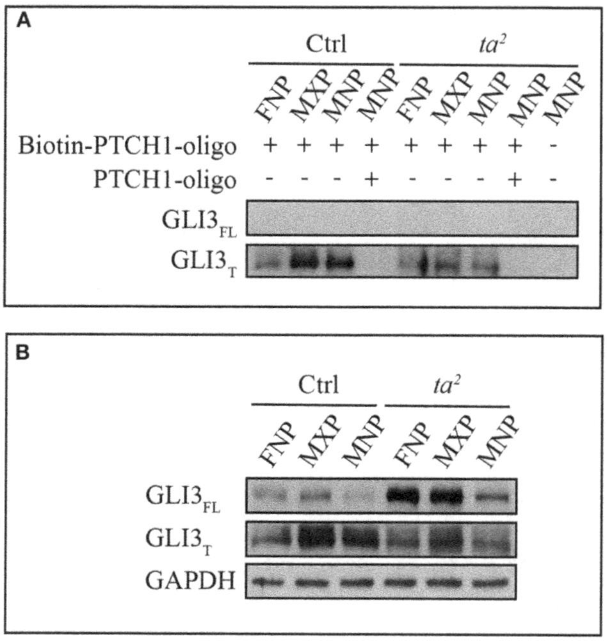

FIGURE 3 | $GLI3_T$ isoform is predominantly recruited to GBR motif of *PTCH1* promoter *in vitro*. (A) DNA binding affinity assay of GLI3 proteins with frontonasal prominence (FNP), maxillary prominence (MXP), and mandibular prominence (MNP) in day 5 control and ta^2 embryos. **(B)** Western blot of GLI3 proteins from the same lysates as **(A)**. GAPDH as loading control of cell lysates.

GLI3 Occupancy at GBRs within the Regulatory Regions of Target Genes Is Altered in ta^2 Mutants

In vitro DNA binding affinity assays suggested that there was not an increase of ectopic $GLI3_{FL}$ at GBRs of target genes in ta^2 mutants. To determine if GLI3 binding to GBRs was altered *in vivo* in ta^2 mutants compared to control embryos, we next performed ChIP-qPCR (**Figure 4**). In ta^2 mutants, GLI3 enrichment at GBRs associated with the craniofacial genes *ALX4* and *OSR2* was reduced in all facial prominences, yet only significantly in the MXP and MNP (**Figures 4A,B**). GLI3 enrichment at the GBRs associated with *BMPR1A* and *WIF1*, was also overwhelmingly reduced in facial prominences, yet only significantly in the ta^2 FNP and MXP (**Figures 4C,D**). GLI3 binding in the MNP of *WIF1* was below detectable levels in controls, and thus could not be evaluated. These data suggested that GLI3 occupancy at the GBR of target genes is decreased. Our *in vitro* data suggested that $GLI3_{FL}$ did not bind at target gene GBRs (**Figure 3**). Thus, taken together these data indicate that the observed reduction of GLI3 binding is indicative of reduced $GLI3_T$ binding at the regulatory regions of target genes.

Reduced GLI3 binding at GBRs of GLI target genes appeared to be a general trend in ta^2 mutants, as several other target genes expressed in the craniofacial complex also exhibited reduced enrichment of GLI3 at associated GBRs (**Supplemental Figure 2**). Thus, these data suggested that altered expression of GLI targets could be caused by aberrant $GLI3_T$ binding in ta^2 mutants. Interestingly, there was not always a direct correlation with loss of $GLI3_T$ repressor binding and increased gene expression. Furthermore, different results among the three facial prominences examined pointed to context—and tissue-specific regulation of GLI targets (**Supplemental Figures 1A–D**). Several studies have proposed the possibility that GLI proteins work together with co-regulators to influence expression of targets genes (Brewster et al., 1998; Koyabu et al., 2001; Mizugishi et al., 2001; Lee et al., 2010; Peterson et al., 2012). To determine if target gene expression in the craniofacial complex was influenced by the action of GLI co-regulators, we next examined the proximity of GBRs to motifs for potential GLI co-regulators.

Motif Analyses Identified Sequences for Known GLI Co-Regulators Frequently Co-Localize with GBRs

GBRs have previously been identified in close proximity to binding motifs for other transcription factors, including members of the bHLH, SP, and Sox families (Vokes et al., 2008; Peterson et al., 2012; Aberger and Ruiz I Altaba, 2014). Furthermore, the co-occupancy and cooperativity of GLI with SOX transcription factors was previously shown to be essential for activating neural gene expression signatures (Peterson et al., 2012). To determine if expression of our identified GLI targets could be influenced by the presence or absence of GLI co-regulators, we first examined the genomic sequence around the GBRs of our target genes for E-box, SP, and SOX binding motifs. (**Figure 5**, **Supplemental Figure 3**). We defined the area <1 kb upstream of the transcription start site (TSS) as the promoter region, <20 kb away from the TSS as proximal upstream or downstream, and <100 kb away from the TSS as distal upstream or downstream. We analyzed the sequence surrounding GBRs in our four selected GLI target genes for sequences predictive of E-box, SP, and SOX binding. All four of our identified GLI target genes contained at least one motif cluster containing a GBR, E-box, SP, and SOX binding site within 1 kb of each other (**Figures 5A–D**). Several other clusters containing three of the four motifs were also identified (**Figures 5A–C**; red box). The close proximity of these binding motifs suggested that expression of GLI targets in the developing craniofacial complex could be influenced by the cooperative function of GLI isoforms and co-regulator proteins.

GLI Co-Regulators Have a Prominence Specific Expression Pattern That Changes When Primary Cilia Are Lost

Several transcription factors synergistically cooperate with GLI proteins to influence GLI target gene expression (Aberger and Ruiz I Altaba, 2014). Their co-occupancy at the promoter of GLI targets is required for the optimal activation/repressor. ChIP-based, high-throughput analyses uncovered several transcription factor motifs located close to GBRs in the cis-regulatory modules of GLI targets. Specifically, binding sequences for Sox (Peterson et al., 2012), bHLH (Lee et al., 2010), and SP proteins (Vokes et al., 2008) have been shown to exist in very close proximity

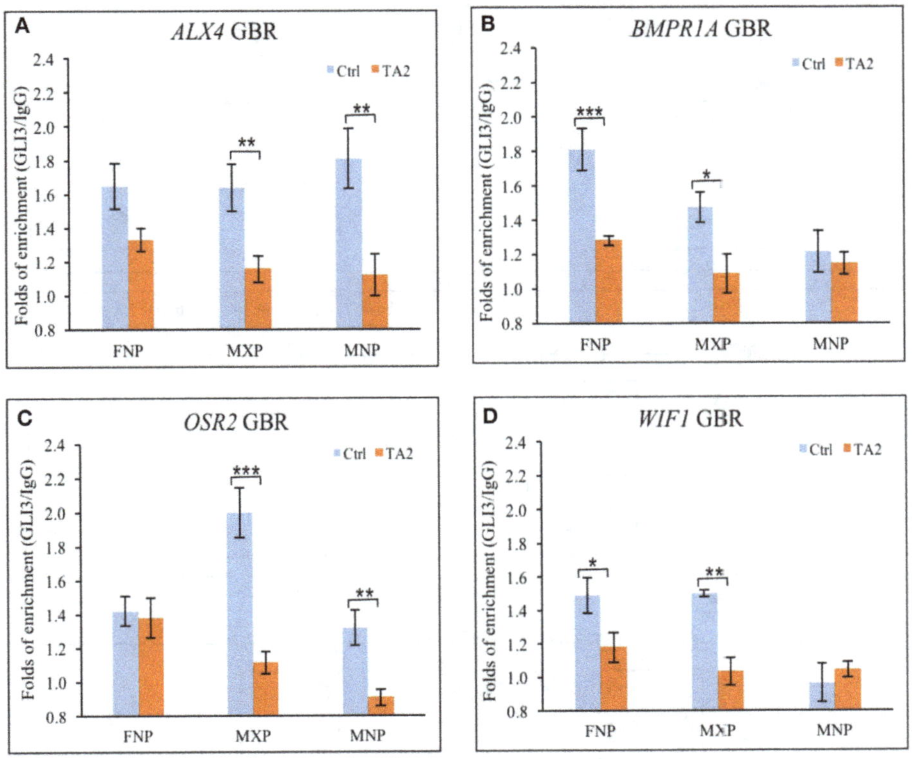

FIGURE 4 | GLI3 occupancies at the GBRs of GLI targets is reduced in *ta*^{2} mutant. (A–D) ChIP-qPCR analyses of GLI3 precipitated with GLI binding regions of **(A)** *ALX4*, **(B)** *BMPR1A*, **(C)** *OSR2*, and **(D)** *WIF1* in control and *ta*^{2} facial prominences. The asterisks indicate statistic significant difference and are labeled as followed: $^*P < 0.05$, $^{**}P < 0.01$, $^{***}P < 0.001$. Error bars are based on the standard error of the means (S.E.M.). $n = 5$.

to GBRs. Our *in silico* analyses confirmed these sequences exist in near GBRs in four previously identified GLI-targets. We hypothesized that differential expression of these co-regulators could contribute to the differential gene expression of GLI targets in both control and *ta*^{2} mutant embryos. We first investigated the expression of genes that could bind to motifs found in close proximity to GBRs, specifically *SOX8*, *SP3*, and *HAND2* (**Figures 6A–C**). *SOX8* expression was significantly reduced in the FNP and MXP of *ta*^{2} mutants, yet was not significantly altered in the MNP (**Figure 6A**). *SP3* expression was significantly increased in *ta*^{2} MNP, yet not changed in the FNP and MXP (**Figure 6B**). *HAND2* expression was reduced in the MXP, but not significantly changed between control and *ta*^{2} FNPs and MNPs (**Figure 6C**). Thus, differential expression of GLI co-regulators could possibly contribute to altered target gene expression in *ta*^{2} mutants and explain why changes in GLI_{FL} and GLI_T isoforms do not uniformly or directly correlate with changes in target gene expression.

Our previous analyses indicate that GLI target gene expression changed in a prominence specific manner (Chang et al., 2014). We wondered if differential expression of potential GLI co-regulators could contribute to this prominence-specific expression changes. *SOX8* was robustly expressed within the FNP, with levels significantly higher than those in the MXP or MNP (**Figure 6A'**). *SP3* was more robustly expressed in the MXP and MNP, relative to the FNP (**Figure 6B'**). *HAND2* was robustly and exclusively expressed in the MNP (**Figure 6C'**). Thus, each of these potential co-regulators has a prominences specific expression pattern that could differentially influence GLI target gene expression. Collectively, the proximity of binding motifs, coupled with the differential expression of these co-regulators could possibly contribute to altered expression of GLI targets in *ta*^{2} embryos.

DISCUSSION

Craniofacial ciliopathies are a rapidly growing group of disorders that severely impact craniofacial growth and development. Currently, there are little to no therapeutic options for these conditions. Although the molecular mechanism behind these disorders remains nebulous, many ciliopathies have aberrant production of GLI_{FL} and GLI_T isoforms. (Huangfu and Anderson, 2005; Davey et al., 2006; Tran et al., 2008; Tabler et al., 2013; Chang et al., 2014). Herein, we attempted to identify the mechanism by which aberrant GLI protein production impacts craniofacial development. To do so we used the avian *ta*^{2} model, which has recently been characterized as a bona fide model for the human craniofacial ciliopathy Orofacial-digital syndrome 14 (Schock et al., 2015). *In silico* and ChIP assays identified GLI target genes in the avian genome that play a role in craniofacial development. RT-qPCR of mRNA levels verified some significant

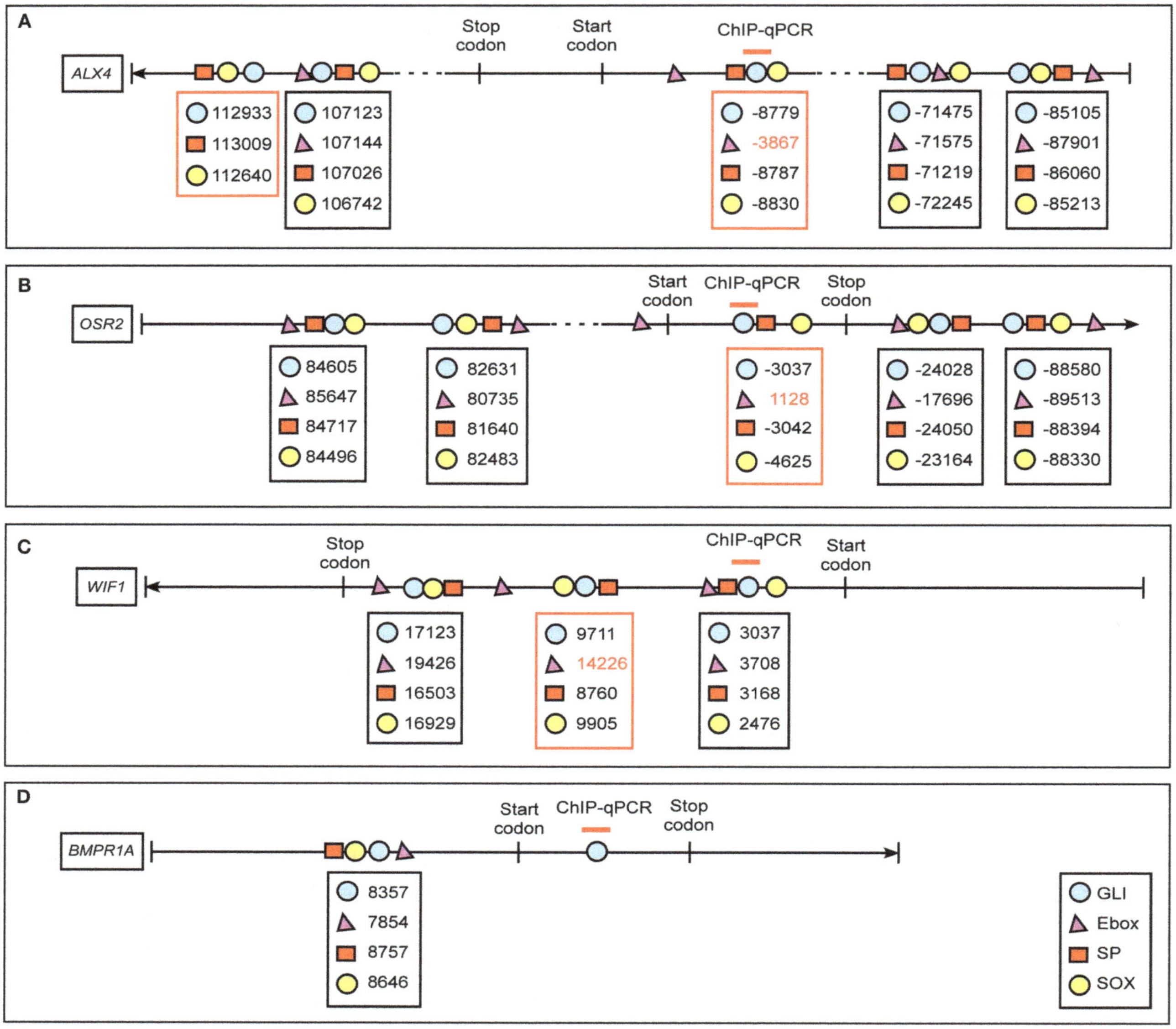

FIGURE 5 | Schematic diagram of co-regulator motif clusters near GBRs of *ALX4, OSR2, WIF1* and *BMPR1A*. *In silico* analyses predict location of GLI (blue circle), E-box (magenta triangle), SP (red rectangle), and SOX (yellow circle) sites in GLI target genes **(A)** *ALX4*, **(B)** *OSR2*, **(C)** *WIF1*, **(D)** *BMPR1A*. We defined 5′-untranslated region (UTR), gene and 3′-UTR as intragenic region, <1 kb upstream of transcription start site (TSS) is promoter region, 1–20 kb away from TSS as proximal regulatory region, and <100 kb away from TSS as distal regulatory region. The numbers labeled below the symbols indicate the positions of the motifs according to the distance away from TSS sites. The position upstream of TSS site is assigned a negative symbol. The area amplified by primer sets used for ChIP-quantitative PCRs are labeled above the specific GLI binding motif (red line). Clusters of four motifs are highlighted in a black box, clusters of three motifs are highlighted in a red box.

changes in the expression of these GLI targets in the developing facial prominences, yet there was not a clear, linear relationship between changes in GLI isoform production and target gene expression. Motif cluster analysis supported the hypothesis that GLI proteins work in concert with co-regulators. GBRs associated with GLI target genes were found to be situated within 1000 bp of binding motifs for several, previously identified GLI co-regulators. Differential expression within developing facial prominences of predicted co-regulators supported a hypothesis in which expression of GLI target genes is dependent upon the cooperative function of GLI isoforms and co-regulator proteins. Together, these data provide a better understanding of the complex nature of GLI-mediated transcription that occurs in normal and ciliopathic craniofacial development.

GLI Binding Regions Are Present throughout the Avian Genome in Genes That Affect Craniofacial Development

Work in other species has identified GBRs and examined the role of GLI proteins as transcription factors that affect gene expression in numerous signaling pathways (Vokes et al., 2007, 2008).

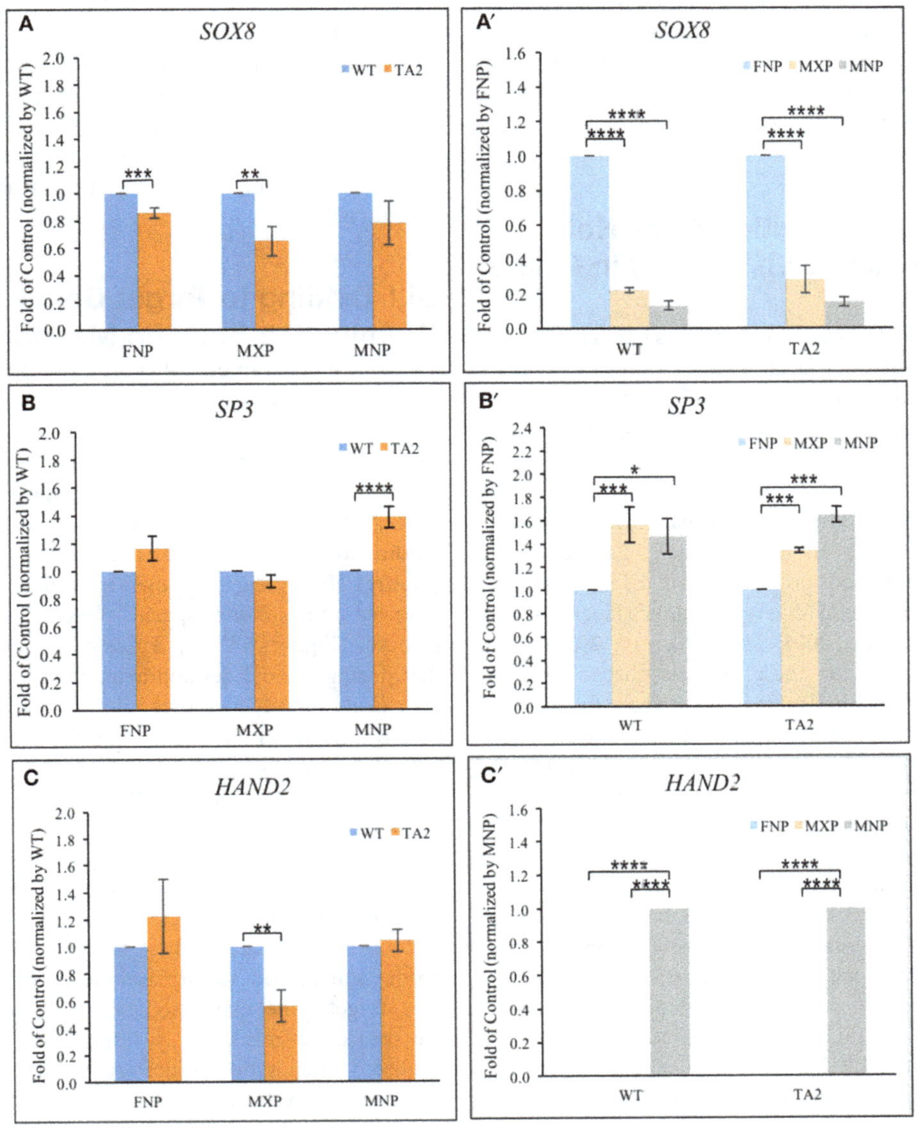

FIGURE 6 | Prominence-specific expression of *SOX8*, *SP3*, and *Hand2*. Quantitative RT-PCR analyses of transcription factors (*SOX8*, *SP3* and *Hand2*) based on the comparison between control and ta^2 embryos **(A–C)** or individual facial prominences **(A′–C′)**. The asterisks indicate statistical significance and are labeled as followed: *$P < 0.05$, **$P < 0.01$, ***$P < 0.001$, ****$P < 0.0001$. Error bars are based on the standard error of the means (S.E.M.). $n = 4$.

Three models currently exist to explain GLI_{FL}/GLI_{T} function (Falkenstein and Vokes, 2014). First the GLI_{FL}::GLI_{T} ratio sensing model suggest that the relative levels of GLI_{FL} to GLI_{T} is integrated and results in graded levels of transcription of targets. This model suggests that response to changes in ratio, rather than concentration, affect target gene expression. The threshold activation model suggests that, rather than ratio of GLI_{FL}::GLI_{T}, a threshold-specific concentration of GLI_{FL} activates target gene expression (Oosterveen et al., 2012). The threshold repression model depends on the removal of the GLI_{T} repressor from target genes, allowing for transcriptional activation by other target genes, allowing for transcriptional activation by other transcription factors to initiate gene expression. From our results, mRNA expression of most target genes was not dramatically altered despite excessive GLI_{FL} production in ta^2 mutant, indicating that the ratio sensing model cannot explain our observation in ta^2 mutant. Secondly, the accumulated $GLI3_{FL}$ in the nucleus was expected to bind and activate target gene in the threshold activation model; however, instead we found reduced occupancy of GLI3 at target genes, along with lack of detectable GLI_{FL} binding to GBRs (**Figures 3, 4**), suggesting that a dysfunctional GLI_{FL} that fails to promote GLI_{A}-mediated activation is produced under ciliopathic conditions. Thus, these data do not support the threshold activation model for GLI_{FL} function. Conversely, our results showed that reduced GLI_{T} production could lead to a de-repression of target genes and potentially a gene activation, when the required transcription factors are available. The threshold repression model seems to be more applicable to the observation owing to less GLI3 occupancy and the failure of GLI_{FL} to GLI_T conversion. A more in depth understanding of GLI mechanisms of action will require tools with the ability to definitively decipher between GLI_{FL} and GLI_T *in vivo*.

Excessive GLI_{FL} Production Does Not Equate to Increased GLI_A Activity in Ciliary Mutants

A number of disorders identified as ciliopathies have craniofacial abnormalities including Oral-facial-digital syndrome, Joubert syndrome, Bardet-Biedl syndrome, Meckel-Gruber syndrome, Ellis-van Creveld syndrome (Zaghloul and Brugmann, 2011). The phenotypes for syndromes such as these, while not identical, do have several phenotypes indicative of aberrant SHH signaling including widening of the midface, cleft lip/palate, micrognathia, craniosynostosis and oral/dental anomalies (Zaghloul and Brugmann, 2011). Increased production of GLI_{FL} isoforms has been observed in several ciliary mutants (Huangfu and Anderson, 2005; Liu et al., 2005; Humke et al., 2010), thus a common interpretation of these data is that ciliopathic phenotypes were due to either increased activator function or skewed GLI_{FL}::GLI_T ratio in favor of GLI_{FL}. Despite these common interpretation regarding the molecular mechanism causing ciliopathic phenotypes, examination of subsequent levels of GLI processing, binding, and transcriptional function in ciliary mutants has not been performed.

Our studies are among the first to examine how and if GLI proteins function in the developing craniofacial complex of ciliary mutants; however, some questions remain regarding the mechanistic reasons as to why GLI_{FL} appears not to function in ciliary mutants. Prior to processing, GLI proteins associate with Suppressor of Fused (SUFU), a conserved protein known to regulate the activity of GLI proteins via modulating GLI processing, stabilization and subcellular localization (Barnfield et al., 2005; Humke et al., 2010; Tukachinsky et al., 2010; Wang et al., 2010). In the presence of a SHH signal, the SUFU-GLI_{FL} complex traffics through the cilium (Eggenschwiler and Anderson, 2007). Activated ciliary SMO then works through KIF7 to promote the dissociation of the inhibitory SUFU-GLI_{FL} complex (Humke et al., 2010; Tukachinsky et al., 2010; Li et al., 2012). Free GLI_{FL} is then processed into an activator and moves to the nucleus to activate downstream targets. In the absence of the SHH ligand, SMO is not translocated into the cilium and thus cannot antagonize SUFU. SUFU remains in complex with GLI_{FL}, GLI_{FL} is proteolytically processed into GLI_T and the SUFU-GLI_T complex moves to the nucleus where it recruits the Sap18-Sin3 co-repressor complex to repress GLI target genes (Ding et al., 1999; Kogerman et al., 1999; Cheng and Bishop, 2002; Paces-Fessy et al., 2004). Furthermore, our recent work with the murine ciliary mutant, *Kif3$^{fl/fl}$;Wnt1-Cre* shows increased SUFU production and nuclear localization, as well as enhanced association of SUFU with GLI3 (Chang et al., in press). We hypothesize a similar mechanism is at play in *ta*^{2} mutants. Specifically, excessive GLI_{FL} produced in *ta*^{2} mutants cannot dissociate from SUFU because the complex cannot undergo ciliary trafficking. We further hypothesize that lack of dissociation prevents GLI_{FL} from occupying GBRs and directly activating target gene transcription. Our future studies will address the association of GLI_{FL} and SUFU in *ta*^{2} mutants and determine if their maintained association contributes to ciliopathic phenotypes.

GLI-Binding to Target Genes Occurs in a Prominence Specific Manner

Frequently the craniofacial complex is thought of as a singular organ system; however, the prominences that make up the face develop independently prior to their fusion. There is evidence to support that these prominences have distinct molecular profiles and develop as separate developmental fields (Brugmann et al., 2007). Our ChIP-qPCR results detected differential GLI binding to target genes in facial prominences of control embryos (**Figures 2B–D**). Further, the expression of co-regulators also followed a prominence specific pattern in both control and *ta*^{2} embryos (**Figures 6A'–C'**). These data supported the hypothesis that during normal development, as well as when cilia are lost, each facial prominence uses a unique mechanism to transduce a SHH-dependent GLI signal. Based on our examination of co-regulators, we hypothesize that there is a combinatorial code of GLI isoforms and co-regulators that work together to precisely regulate target gene expression. Thus, when cilia are lost and GLI production is altered, target gene expression is dictated by how the combinatorial code of remaining GLI isoforms and co-regulators function together.

In sum, our data suggest that the increased or decreased production of GLI isoforms alone is not sufficient to explain how target gene expression will be altered. To understand the molecular mechanisms responsible for ciliopathic, GLI-mediated phenotypes, future studies will have to account for tissue specificity, the presence or absence of co-regulators and the mode of GLI function (activation or de-repression) to begin to address this process.

AUTHOR CONTRIBUTIONS

YC designed and tested all primers, and performed and interpreted all ChIP and qPCR experiments, PC performed *in silico* GBR analysis, ES harvested and photographed embryos, SB conceived the project, analyzed data and wrote the manuscript with input from all authors.

FUNDING

This work was funded by the National Institutes of Health, National Institute of Dental and Craniofacial Research (NIDCR) [R00-DE01985 and [R01-DE023804] to SB] and by C.T.O. and Research in Progress (RIP) funds from the Cincinnati Children's Research Foundation to SB.

ACKNOWLEDGMENTS

We thank the UC Davis Avian Facility and Jackie Pisenti for husbandry of the *talpid*^{2} line and providing *talpid*^{2} eggs for this study.

SUPPLEMENTARY MATERIAL

Supplementary Figure 1 | GLI3 binding to GLI targets is confirmed by ChIP. ChIP-qPCR analyses of GLI3 precipitated with GLI binding regions of *ALX4* **(A)**, *BMPR1A* **(B)**, *OSR2* **(C)**, *WIF1* **(D)**, and *PTCH1* **(E)** in facial prominences of control embryo. Error bars are based on the standard error of the means (S.E.M.). $n = 3$.

Supplementary Figure 2 | ChIP-qPCR analyses of GLI3 precipitated with GLI binding regions of *PTCH1* (A), *TFAP2A* (B), *CTNNB1* (C), *WNT2B* (D), *DKK1* (E), *FGFR* (F), *BMP2* (G), *BMP4* (H), *BMP7* (I), and *EPHA4* (J) in control and *ta*^{2} facial prominences. Error bars are based on the standard error of the means (S.E.M.). $n = 3$.

Supplementary Figure 3 | The schematic of the clusters of transcription factor motifs in GBRs of GLI targets. The *in silico* analyses of GLI (blue circle), E-box (magenta triangle), SP site (red rectangle), and SOX site (yellow circle) in the GBRs of GLI targets. We defined 5′-untranslated region (UTR), gene and 3′-UTR as intragenic region, <1 kb upstream of transcription start site (TSS) is promoter region, 1–20 kb away from TSS as proximal regulatory region, and <100 kb away from TSS as distal regulatory region. The numbers labeled below the symbols indicate the positions of the motifs according to the distance away from TSS sites. The position at the upstream of TSS site is assigned a negative symbol. The primer sets used for ChIP-quantitative PCRs are labeled above the specific GLI binding motif (red line). Clusters of four motifs are highlighted in a black box, clusters of three motifs are highlighted in a red box.

Supplementary Table 1 | Identified Gli target genes.

REFERENCES

Abbott, U. K., Taylor, L. W., and Abplanalp, H. (1959). A second talpid-like mutation in the fowl. *Poult. Sci.* 38:1185.

Abbott, U. K., Taylor, L. W., and Abplanalp, H. (1960). Studies with *talpid*^{2}, an embryonic lethal of the fowl. *J. Hered.* 51, 195–202.

Aberger, F., and Ruiz I Altaba, A. (2014). Context-dependent signal integration by the GLI code, the oncogenic load, pathways, modifiers and implications for cancer therapy. *Semin. Cell Dev. Biol.* 33, 93–104. doi: 10.1016/j.semcdb.2014.05.003

Bai, C. B., and Joyner, A. L. (2001). Gli1 can rescue the *in vivo* function of Gli2. *Development* 128, 5161–5172.

Bai, C. B., Stephen, D., and Joyner, A. L. (2004). All mouse ventral spinal cord patterning by hedgehog is Gli dependent and involves an activator function of Gli3. *Dev. Cell* 6, 103–115. doi: 10.1016/S1534-5807(03)00394-0

Barnfield, P. C., Zhang, X., Thanabalasingham, V., Yoshida, M., and Hui, C. C. (2005). Negative regulation of Gli1 and Gli2 activator function by Suppressor of fused through multiple mechanisms. *Differentiation* 73, 397–405. doi: 10.1111/j.1432-0436.2005.00042.x

Beverdam, A., Brouwer, A., Reijnen, M., Korving, J., and Meijlink, F. (2001). Severe nasal clefting and abnormal embryonic apoptosis in Alx3/Alx4 double mutant mice. *Development* 128, 3975–3986.

Brewster, R., Lee, J., and Ruiz i Altaba, A. (1998). Gli/Zic factors patternt the neural plate by defining domains of cell differentiation. *Nature* 393, 579–583. doi: 10.1038/31242

Brugmann, S. A., Allen, N. C., James, A. W., Mekonnen, Z., Madan, E., and Helms, J. A. (2010). A primary cilia-dependent etiology for midline facial disorders. *Hum. Mol. Genet.* 19, 1577–1592. doi: 10.1093/hmg/ddq030

Brugmann, S. A., Goodnough, L. H., Gregorieff, A., Leucht, P., ten Berge, D., Fuerer, C., et al. (2007). Wnt signaling mediates regional specification in the vertebrate face. *Development* 134, 3283–3295. doi: 10.1242/dev.005132

Buttitta, L., Mo, R., Hui, C. C., and Fan, C. M. (2003). Interplays of Gli2 and Gli3 and their requirement in mediating Shh-dependent sclerotome induction. *Development* 130, 6233–6243. doi: 10.1242/dev.00851

Chang, C. F., Chang, Y. T., Millington, G., and Brugmann, S. A. (in press). Craniofacial ciliopathies reveal specific requirements for Gli proteins during development of the facial midline. *PLoS Genet.*

Chang, C. F., Schock, E. N., O'Hare, E. A., Dodgson, J., Cheng, H. H., Muir, W. M., et al. (2014). The cellular and molecular etiology of the craniofacial defects in the avian ciliopathic mutant *talpid*^{2}. *Development* 141, 3003–3012. doi: 10.1242/dev.105924

Cheng, S. Y., and Bishop, J. M. (2002). Suppressor of Fused represses Gli-mediated transcription by recruiting the SAP18-mSin3 corepressor complex. *Proc. Natl. Acad. Sci. U.S.A.* 99, 5442–5447. doi: 10.1073/pnas.082096999

Corbit, K. C., Aanstad, P., Singla, V., Norman, A. R., Stainier, D. Y., and Reiter, J. F. (2005). Vertebrate Smoothened functions at the primary cilium. *Nature* 437, 1018–1021. doi: 10.1038/nature04117

Darnell, D. K., Kaur, S., Stanislaw, S., Davey, S., Konieczka, J. H., Yatskievych, T. A., et al. (2007). GEISHA: an *in situ* hybridization gene expression resource for the chicken embryo. *Cytogenet. Genome Res.* 117, 30–35. doi: 10.1159/000103162

Davey, M. G., Paton, I. R., Yin, Y., Schmidt, M., Bangs, F. K., Morrice, D. R., et al. (2006). The chicken *talpid*^{3} gene encodes a novel protein essential for Hedgehog signaling. *Genes Dev.* 20, 1365–1377. doi: 10.1101/gad.369106

Ding, Q., Fukami, Si., Meng, X., Nishizaki, Y., Zhang, X., Sasaki, H., et al. (1999). Mouse suppressor of fused is a negative regulator of sonic hedgehog signaling and alters the subcellular distribution of Gli1. *Curr. Biol.* 9, 1119–1122. doi: 10.1016/S0960-9822(99)80482-5

Dvorak, L., and Fallon, J. F. (1991). *Talpid*^{2} mutant chick limb has anteroposterior polarity and altered patterns of programmed cell death. *Anat. Rec.* 231, 251–260. doi: 10.1002/ar.1092310213

Eggenschwiler, J. T., and Anderson, K. V. (2007). Cilia and developmental signaling. *Annu. Rev. Cell Dev. Biol.* 23, 345–373. doi: 10.1146/annurev.cellbio.23.090506.123249

Falkenstein, K. N., and Vokes, S. A. (2014). Transcriptional regulation of graded Hedgehog signaling. *Semin. Cell Dev. Biol.* 33, 73–80. doi: 10.1016/j.semcdb.2014.05.010

Goetz, S. C., and Anderson, K V. (2010). The primary cilium: a signalling centre during vertebrate development. *Nat. Rev. Genet.* 11, 331–344. doi: 10.1038/nrg2774

Haycraft, C. J., Banizs, B., Aydin-Son, Y., Zhang, Q., Michaud, E. J., and Yoder, B. K. (2005). Gli2 and Gli3 localize to cilia and require the intraflagellar transport protein polaris for processing and function. *PLoS Genet.* 1:e53. doi: 10.1371/journal.pgen.0010053

Hoover, A. N., Wynkoop, A., Zeng, H., Jia, J., Niswander, L. A., and Liu, A. (2008). C2cd3 is required for cilia formation and Hedgehog signaling in mouse. *Development* 135, 4049–4058. doi: 10.1242/dev.029835

Hsieh, J. C., Kodjabachian, L., Rebbert, M. L., Rattner, A., Smallwood, P. M., Samos, C. H., et al. (1999). A new secreted protein that binds to Wnt proteins and inhibits their activities. *Nature* 398, 431–436. doi: 10.1038/18899

Huangfu, D., and Anderson, K. V. (2005). Cilia and Hedgehog responsiveness in the mouse. *Proc. Natl. Acad. Sci. U.S.A.* 102, 11325–11330. doi: 10.1073/pnas.0505328102

Huangfu, D., Liu, A., Rakeman, A. S., Murcia, N. S., Niswander, L., and Anderson, K. V. (2003). Hedgehog signalling in the mouse requires intraflagellar transport proteins. *Nature* 426, 83–87. doi: 10.1038/nature02061

Humke, E. W., Dorn, K. V., Milenkovic, L., Scott, M. P., and Rohatgi, R. (2010). The output of Hedgehog signaling is controlled by the dynamic association between Suppressor of Fused and the Gli proteins. *Genes Dev.* 24, 670–682. doi: 10.1101/gad.1902910

Kogerman, P., Grimm, T., Kogerman, L., Krause, D., Undén, A. B., Sandstedt, B., et al. (1999). Mammalian suppressor-of-fused modulates nuclear-cytoplasmic shuttling of Gli-1. *Nat. Cell Biol.* 1, 312–319. doi: 10.1038/13031

Koyabu, Y., Nakata, K., Mizugishi, K., Aruga, J., and Mikoshiba, K. (2001). Physical and functional interactions between Zic and Gli proteins. *J. Biol. Chem.* 276, 6889–6892. doi: 10.1074/jbc.C000773200

Lan, Y., Kingsley, P. D., Cho, E. S., and Jiang, R. (2001). Osr2, a new mouse gene related to Drosophila odd-skipped, exhibits dynamic expression patterns during craniofacial, limb, and kidney development. *Mech. Dev.* 107, 175–179. doi: 10.1016/S0925-4773(01)00457-9

Lee, E. Y., Ji, H., Ouyang, Z., Zhou, B., Ma, W., Vokes, S. A., et al. (2010). Hedgehog pathway-regulated gene networks in cerebellum development and tumorigenesis. *Proc. Natl. Acad. Sci. U.S.A.* 107, 9736–9741. doi: 10.1073/pnas.1004602107

Lei, Q., Zelman, A. K., Kuang, E., Li, S., and Matise, M. P. (2004). Transduction of graded Hedgehog signaling by a combination of Gli2 and Gli3 activator functions in the developing spinal cord. *Development* 131, 3593–3604. doi: 10.1242/dev.01230

Li, L., Lin, M., Wang, Y., Cserjesi, P., Chen, Z., and Chen, Y. (2011). Bmprla is required in mesenchymal tissue and has limited redundant function with Bmprlb in tooth and palate development. *Dev. Biol.* 349, 451–461. doi: 10.1016/j.ydbio.2010.10.023

Li, L., Wang, Y., Lin, M., Yuan, G., Yang, G., Zheng, Y., et al. (2013). Augmented BMPRIA-mediated BMP signaling in cranial neural crest lineage leads to cleft palate formation and delayed tooth differentiation. *PLoS ONE* 8:e66107. doi: 10.1371/journal.pone.0066107

Li, Z. J., Nieuwenhuis, E., Nien, W., Zhang, X., Zhang, J., Puviindran, V., et al. (2012). Kif7 regulates Gli2 through Sufu-dependent and -independent functions during skin development and tumorigenesis. *Development* 139, 4152–4161. doi: 10.1242/dev.081190

Liu, A., Wang, B., and Niswander, L. A. (2005). Mouse intraflagellar transport proteins regulate both the activator and repressor functions of Gli transcription factors. *Development* 132, 3103–3111. doi: 10.1242/dev.01894

Mavrogiannis, L. A., Antonopoulou, I., Baxová, A., Kutílek, S., Kim, C. A., Sugayama, S. M., et al. (2001). Haploinsufficiency of the human homeobox gene ALX4 causes skull ossification defects. *Nat. Genet.* 27, 17–18. doi: 10.1038/83703

McDermott, A., Gustafsson, M., Elsam, T., Hui, C. C., Emerson, C. P. Jr., and Borycki, A. G. (2005). Gli2 and Gli3 have redundant and context-dependent function in skeletal muscle formation. *Development* 132, 345–357. doi: 10.1242/dev.01537

Mizugishi, K., Aruga, J., Nakata, K., and Mikoshiba, K. (2001). Molecular properties of Zic proteins as transcriptional regulators and their relationship to GLI proteins. *J. Biol. Chem.* 276, 2180–2188. doi: 10.1074/jbc.M004430200

Mo, R., Freer, A. M., Zinyk, D. L., Crackower, M. A., Michaud, J., Heng, H. H., et al. (1997). Specific and redundant functions of Gli2 and Gli3 zinc finger genes in skeletal patterning and development. *Development* 124, 113–123.

Motoyama, J., Milenkovic, L., Iwama, M., Shikata, Y., Scott, M. P., and Hui, C. C. (2003). Differential requirement for Gli2 and Gli3 in ventral neural cell fate specification. *Dev. Biol.* 259, 150–161. doi: 10.1016/S0012-1606(03)00159-3

Oosterveen, T., Kurdija, S., Alekseenko, Z., Uhde, C. W., Bergsland, M., Sandberg, M., et al. (2012). Mechanistic differences in the transcriptional interpretation of local and long-range Shh morphogen signaling. *Dev. Cell* 23, 1006–1019. doi: 10.1016/j.devcel.2012.09.015

Paces-Fessy, M., Boucher, D., Petit, E., Paute-Briand, S., and Blanchet-Tournier, M. F. (2004). The negative regulator of Gli, Suppressor of fused (Sufu), interacts with SAP18, Galectin3 and other nuclear proteins. *Biochem. J.* 378, 353–362. doi: 10.1042/bj20030786

Pan, Y., Bai, C. B., Joyner, A. L., and Wang, B. (2006). Sonic hedgehog signaling regulates Gli2 transcriptional activity by suppressing its processing and degradation. *Mol. Cell. Biol.* 26, 3365–3377. doi: 10.1128/MCB.26.9.3365-3377.2006

Pan, Y., Wang, C., and Wang, B. (2009). Phosphorylation of Gli2 by protein kinase A is required for Gli2 processing and degradation and the Sonic Hedgehog-regulated mouse development. *Dev. Biol.* 326, 177–189. doi: 10.1016/j.ydbio.2008.11.009

Persson, M., Stamataki, D., te Welscher, P., Andersson, E., Böse, J., Rüther, U., et al. (2002). Dorsal-ventral patterning of the spinal cord requires Gli3 transcriptional repressor activity. *Genes Dev.* 16, 2865–2878. doi: 10.1101/gad.243402

Peterson, K. A., Nishi, Y., Ma, W., Vedenko, A., Shokri, L., Zhang, X., et al. (2012). Neural-specific Sox2 input and differential Gli-binding affinity provide context and positional information in Shh-directed neural patterning. *Genes Dev.* 26, 2802–2816. doi: 10.1101/gad.207142.112

Rallu, M., Machold, R., Gaiano, N., Corbin, J. G., McMahon, A. P., and Fishell, G. (2002). Dorsoventral patterning is established in the telencephalon of mutants lacking both Gli3 and Hedgehog signaling. *Development* 129, 4963–4974.

Rohatgi, R., Milenkovic, L., and Scott, M. P. (2007). Patched1 regulates hedgehog signaling at the primary cilium. *Science* 317, 372–376. doi: 10.1126/science.1139740

Saito, H., Yamamura, K., and Suzuki, N. (2012). Reduced bone morphogenetic protein receptor type 1A signaling in neural-crest-derived cells causes facial dysmorphism. *Dis. Model. Mech.* 5, 948–955. doi: 10.1242/dmm.009274

Schneider, R. A., Hu, D., and Helms, J. A. (1999). From head to toe: conservation of molecular signals regulating limb and craniofacial morphogenesis. *Cell Tissue Res.* 296, 103–109. doi: 10.1007/s004410051271

Schock, E. N., Chang, C. F., Struve, J. N., Chang, Y. T., Chang, J., Delany, M. E., et al. (2015). Using the avian mutant *talpid*^{2} as a disease model for understanding the oral-facial phenotypes of oral-facial-digital syndrome. *Dis. Model. Mech.* 8, 855–866. doi: 10.1242/dmm.020222

Tabler, J. M., Barrell, W. B., Szabo-Rogers, H. L., Healy, C., Yeung, Y., Perdiguero, E. G., et al. (2013). Fuz mutant mice reveal shared mechanisms between ciliopathies and FGF-related syndromes. *Dev. Cell* 25, 623–635. doi: 10.1016/j.devcel.2013.05.021

Theil, T., Alvarez-Bolado, G., Walter, A., and Rüther, U. (1999). Gli3 is required for Emx gene expression during dorsal telencephalon development. *Development* 126, 3561–3571.

Tole, S., Ragsdale, C. W., and Grove, E. A. (2000). Dorsoventral patterning of the telencephalon is disrupted in the mouse mutant extra-toes(J). *Dev. Biol.* 217, 254–265. doi: 10.1006/dbio.1999.9509

Tran, P. V., Haycraft, C. J., Besschetnova, T. Y., Turbe-Doan, A., Stottmann, R. W., Herron, B. J., et al. (2008). THM1 negatively modulates mouse sonic hedgehog signal transduction and affects retrograde intraflagellar transport in cilia. *Nat. Genet.* 40, 403–410. doi: 10.1038/ng.105

Tukachinsky, H., Lopez, L. V., and Salic, A. (2010). A mechanism for vertebrate Hedgehog signaling: recruitment to cilia and dissociation of SuFu-Gli protein complexes. *J. Cell Biol.* 191, 415–428. doi: 10.1083/jcb.201004108

Vokes, S. A., Ji, H., McCuine, S., Tenzen, T., Giles, S., Zhong, S., et al. (2007). Genomic characterization of Gli-activator targets in sonic hedgehog-mediated neural patterning. *Development* 134, 1977–1989. doi: 10.1242/dev.001966

Vokes, S. A., Ji, H., Wong, W. H., and McMahon, A. P. (2008). A genome-scale analysis of the cis-regulatory circuitry underlying sonic hedgehog-mediated patterning of the mammalian limb. *Genes Dev.* 22, 2651–2663. doi: 10.1101/gad.1693008

Wang, B., Fallon, J. F., and Beachy, P. A. (2000). Hedgehog-regulated processing of Gli3 produces an anterior/posterior repressor gradient in the developing vertebrate limb. *Cell* 100, 423–434. doi: 10.1016/S0092-8674(00)80678-9

Wang, C., Pan, Y., and Wang, B. (2010). Suppressor of fused and Spop regulate the stability, processing and function of Gli2 and Gli3 full-length activators but not their repressors. *Development* 137, 2001–2009. doi: 10.1242/dev.052126

Zaghloul, N. A., and Brugmann, S. A. (2011). The emerging face of primary cilia. *Genesis* 49, 231–246. doi: 10.1002/dvg.20728

6

Ephrin Ligands and Eph Receptors Show Regionally Restricted Expression in the Developing Palate and Tongue

Guilherme M. Xavier[1,2], *Isabelle Miletich*[1] *and Martyn T. Cobourne*[1,2*]

[1] *Department of Craniofacial Development and Stem Cell Biology, King's College London Dental Institute, Guy's Hospital, London, UK,*

[2] *Department of Orthodontics, King's College London Dental Institute, Guy's Hospital, London, UK*

Correspondence:
Martyn T. Cobourne
martyn.cobourne@kcl.ac.uk

The Eph family receptor-interacting (ephrin) ligands and erythropoietin-producing hepatocellular carcinoma (Eph) receptors constitute the largest known family of receptor tyrosine kinases. Ephrin ligands and their receptors form an important cell communication system with widespread roles in normal physiology and disease pathogenesis. In order to investigate potential roles of the ephrin-Eph system during palatogenesis and tongue development, we have characterized the cellular mRNA expression of family members *EphrinA1*-A3, *EphA1–A8,* and *EphrinB2, EphB1*, *EphB4* during murine embryogenesis between embryonic day 13.5–16.5 using radioactive *in situ* hybridization. With the exception of *EphA6* and *ephrinA3,* all genes were regionally expressed during the process of palatogenesis, with restricted and often overlapping domains. Transcripts were identified in the palate epithelium, localized at the tip of the palatal shelves, in the mesenchyme and also confined to the medial epithelium seam. Numerous Eph transcripts were also identified during tongue development. In particular, *EphA1* and *EphA2* demonstrated a highly restricted and specific expression in the tongue epithelium at all stages examined, whereas *EphA3* was strongly expressed in the lateral tongue mesenchyme. These results suggest regulatory roles for ephrin-EphA signaling in development of the murine palate and tongue.

Keywords: palatogenesis, tongue development, ephrin, Eph, gene expression, *in situ* hybridization

INTRODUCTION

The formation of a palate separating the oral and nasal cavities is a developmental process characteristic of higher vertebrates and requires complex and highly coordinated molecular interactions (reviewed in Ferguson, 1988; Cobourne, 2004; Dudas et al., 2007; Gritli-Linde, 2007). In the embryo, the primary palate is a derivative of the frontonasal process, whilst the secondary palate forms from the paired palatal shelves of the maxillary process, themselves a derivative of the first pharyngeal arch. The palate is formed by elevation and fusion of the maxillary palatal shelves, with each other posteriorly, with the primary palate anteriorly and the nasal septum superiorly (reviewed in Dudas et al., 2007). The palatal structures are built from cranial neural crest (CNC)-derived ectomesenchyme, mesoderm and the oro-pharyngeal ectoderm (reviewed in Ferguson, 1988). In mice, the palate is formed relatively late in organogenesis, with the palatal shelves initially appearing at embryonic day (E) 11.5 and growing vertically adjacent to the developing tongue from E12.5 to E14.0. However, by E14.5 the shelves have elevated above the tongue and grown to meet their counterpart at the midline, where the layers of epithelium adhere and then fuse with each other to achieve continuity in the roof of the oral cavity (**Figures 1A–L**).

Palatal shelf elevation is a rapid process, accompanied and facilitated by changes within the extracellular matrix of the palatal shelf mesenchyme and the coordinated movement of other craniofacial structures. It is generally accepted that elevation of the palatal shelves above the tongue and their associated change in orientation from a vertical to horizontal position, arises from a combination of intrinsic and extrinsic forces, including descent of the tongue (Ferguson, 1988). The complexity of palatogenesis means that in humans it is frequently disturbed, resulting in the birth defect of cleft palate (reviewed in Ferguson, 1988; Cobourne, 2004). The causes of cleft palate as a malformation can be broadly categorized on an embryological basis as a lack of adequate growth in the palatal shelves, failure to elevate above the tongue or a breakdown in the mechanism of fusion between the shelves. In addition, cleft palate can also arise secondary to other craniofacial malformations, such as micrognathia and basoccipital or basisphenoid fusion, craniosynostosis and both muscle and tongue abnormalities

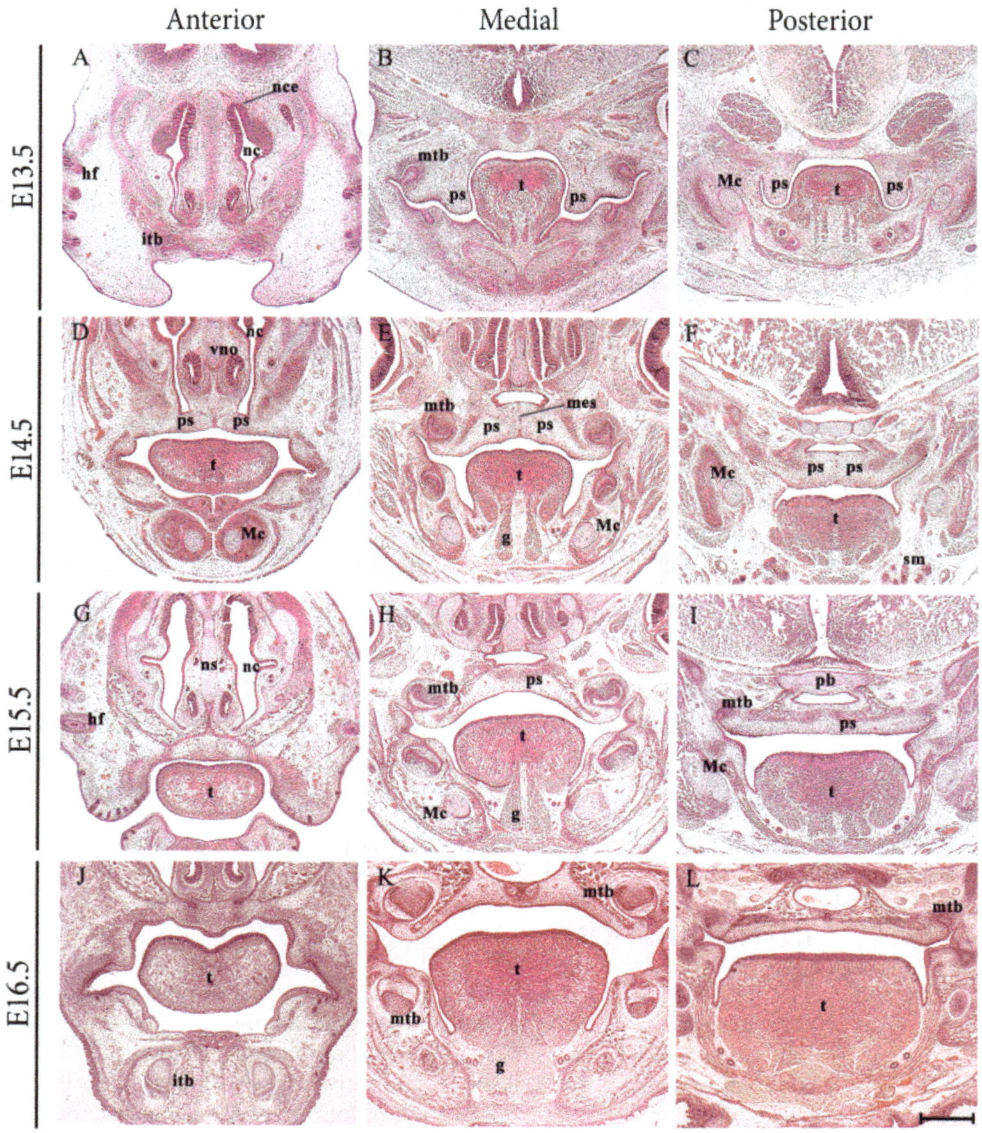

FIGURE 1 | Frontal sections through the developing craniofacial region of the early mouse embryo between E13.5 and E16.5. At E13.5, the palatal shelves are positioned vertically adjacent to the developing tongue. At E14.5 the shelves have elevated above the tongue and grown to meet their counterpart at the midline, where the layers of epithelium adhere and begin to fuse with each other. At E15.5, continuity has been achieved and the palate separates the oral and nasal cavities. At E16.5, palatogenesis is essentially complete. g, genioglossus; hf, hair follicle; itb, incisor tooth bud; Mc, Meckel's cartilage; mes, medial epithelium seam; mtb molar tooth bud; nc, nasal cavity; ns, nasal septum; pb, presphenoid bone; ps, palatal shelves; sm, submandibular gland; t, tongue. Scale bar in L = 500 μm for **(A–L)**.

(reviewed in Ferguson, 1988; Rice et al., 2004; Casey et al., 2006; Chai and Maxson, 2006; Gritli-Linde, 2007; Xiong et al., 2009).

Development of the vertebrate tongue involves contributions from CNC cells derived from pharyngeal arches 1–3 and the somitic myoblasts (Parada and Chai, 2015). The oral portion or anterior two thirds of the murine tongue emerges from the floor of the early oral cavity as a set of mesenchymal swellings derived from the first branchial arch. A medial lingual swelling initially forms, but this is rapidly engulfed by two lateral lingual swellings that will form the anterior two thirds proper. The posterior third or pharyngeal component is derived from two further swellings within the third branchial arch, the copula and hypopharyngeal eminence (Noden and Francis-West, 2006; Hosokawa et al., 2010). In the mouse embryo, the process of tongue development begins around E10.5, with a noticeable tongue bud evident by E12.5, which undergoes rapid enlargement and differentiation to form a large muscular organ by E16.5 (Parada et al., 2012; **Figures 1A–L**).

The Eph family receptor-interacting (ephrin) ligands and erythropoietin-producing hepatocellular carcinoma (Eph) receptors have been extensively studied since their discovery (Hirai et al., 1987). Ephs constitute the largest known family of receptor tyrosine kinases, comprising at least 16 distinct receptors that are highly conserved (Hirai et al., 1987; Jones et al., 1995; Scales et al., 1995; Lackmann and Boyd, 2008; Islam et al., 2010). Based on structural features in their ligand-binding domains and their ephrin-binding preferences, Ephs are classified into 10 EphA and 6 EphB receptors. The EphA group preferentially bind glycosylphosphatidylinositol (GPI)-linked ligands of the ephrin-A subclass; whilst the EphB group preferentially interact with transmembrane ligands of the ephrin-B subclass (reviewed in Lackmann and Boyd, 2008). However, EphA4 binds both classes of ephrin and EphB2 can bind ephrinA5 (Himanen et al., 2004; Dravis and Henkemeyer, 2011).

Together, Eph receptors and their ligands, form an important cell communication system with widespread roles in normal physiology and disease pathogenesis (Pasquale, 2005, 2010). Eph–ephrin complexes emanate bidirectional signals, forward signals that depend on Eph kinase activity propagated in the receptor-expressing cell and reverse signals, that depend on Src family kinases propagated in the ephrin-expressing cell. Ephrin-dependent but kinase-independent Eph signals can also occur (Gu and Park, 2001; Matsuoka et al., 2005; Miao et al., 2005). Eph signaling is known to control cell morphology, adhesion, migration, and invasion by modifying organization of the actin cytoskeleton and influencing the activities of integrins and intercellular adhesion molecules (Pasquale, 2005, 2010; Klein, 2012).

There is evidence from both humans and mice for the potential involvement of specific ephrin and Eph family members during palate development. In the human craniofrontonasal syndrome, mutations in *EPHRINB1* give rise to a range of cranial defects, including cleft lip and palate (Twigg et al., 2004; Wieland et al., 2004; Torii et al., 2007); whilst targeted disruption of *EphrinB1* in mice results in craniofacial and other skeletal defects, including cleft palate (Orioli et al., 1996; Compagni et al., 2003; Davy et al., 2004). Additionally, engineering of compound transgenic mice for *EphB2* and *EphB3* leads to cleft palate; suggesting that a combination of EphB3 protein and EphB2 forward signaling is important for palate development (Risley et al., 2009).

EphA-family receptor expression patterns have previously been described in the developing palate (Agrawal et al., 2014); however, only limited tongue expression data was shown. On the basis of this previous data and a rudimentary PCR-based screen of EphA transcriptional activity in the developing palate (data not shown) we have investigated expression of EphA-family members and their ephrin-A ligands during murine palate and tongue development. We also mapped *ephrinb2* expression in these regions, given that this ligand interacts with EphA4, and ephrinB2 reverse signaling is known to be important for normal closure of the secondary palate (Dravis and Henkemeyer, 2011). In addition, *EphB1* and *EphB4* expression was analyzed. EphB1 has also been associated with cleft lip and palate in human populations (Watanabe et al., 2006) and previously identified as the preferred receptor of ephrinB2 in the mechanism of axonal pathfinding (Chenaux and Henkemeyer, 2011); whilst EphB4 only binds ephrinB2 amongst all the ephrin-B family ligands (Sakano et al., 1996).

We find widespread expression of these family members during murine palatogenesis. In addition, regionally-restricted expression of many members in the developing tongue, suggests some commonalities during the coordinated development of the palate and tongue.

MATERIALS AND METHODS

Mouse plasmids containing cDNA were linearized with the appropriate restriction enzymes and antisense ^{35}S-UTP radio-labeled riboprobes generated using specific RNA polymerases (**Table 1**).

CD-1 mice were time-mated and pregnant females sacrificed with cervical dislocation. Matings were set up such that noon of the day on which vaginal plugs were detected was considered as E0.5. Embryos were collected between E13.5 and E16.5, fixed in 4% (w/v) paraformaldehyde at 4°C overnight, washed in PBS, dehydrated through a graded series of ethanols, embedded in paraffin wax and sectioned at 7 μm, prior to section *in situ* hybridisation.

Radioactive section *in situ* hybridisation was carried out as previously described (Xavier et al., 2009). Light and dark-field images of sections were photographed using a Zeiss Axioscop microscope and merged in Adobe Photoshop CS2.

RESULTS AND DISCUSSION

EphrinA1 transcripts were identified in the palate epithelium from E13.5 to E16.5 (**Figures 2A–D**), particularly at the tip of the palatal shelf at E13.5 (**Figure 2A**, highlighted) with strong expression throughout the oral surface of the palatal shelf epithelium at E14.5 (**Figure 2B**, highlighted). In contrast,

TABLE 1 | Plasmids used for the generation of riboprobes.

Gene	Source	Sequence length	Restriction enzyme	Polymerase
ephrinA1	David Wilkinson	1.5 kb	SalI	T3
ephrinA2	David Wilkinson	1.6 kb	HindIII	T3
ephrinA3	David Wilkinson	1.2 kb	NotI	T7
EphA1	RZPD-IMAGE 4196138	3.2 kb—Full length	EcorV	T7
EphA2	David Wilkinson	1.3 kb—3′ coding	HindIII	T7
EphA3	Tyler Cutforth	1.7 kb—extracell dom	XBal	T3
EphA4	David Wilkinson	1.5 kb—3′UTR	HindIII	T7
EphA5	Andrea Ballabio	0.6 kb—3′UTR	EcoRI	T3
EphA6	David Feldheim	4.4 kb	BamHI	T7
EphA7	RZPD-IMAGE 3991628	3.5 kb—Full length	EcoRV	T7
EphA8	Tyler Cutforth	0.5 kb	EcorV	T3
ephrinB2	Andrea Ballabio	1 kb—Full length ORF	NotI	T3
EphB1	Mark Henkemeyer	0.6 kb—Exon 3	SacII	SP6
EphB4	David Anderson	1 kb—kinase frag	EcoRI	T7

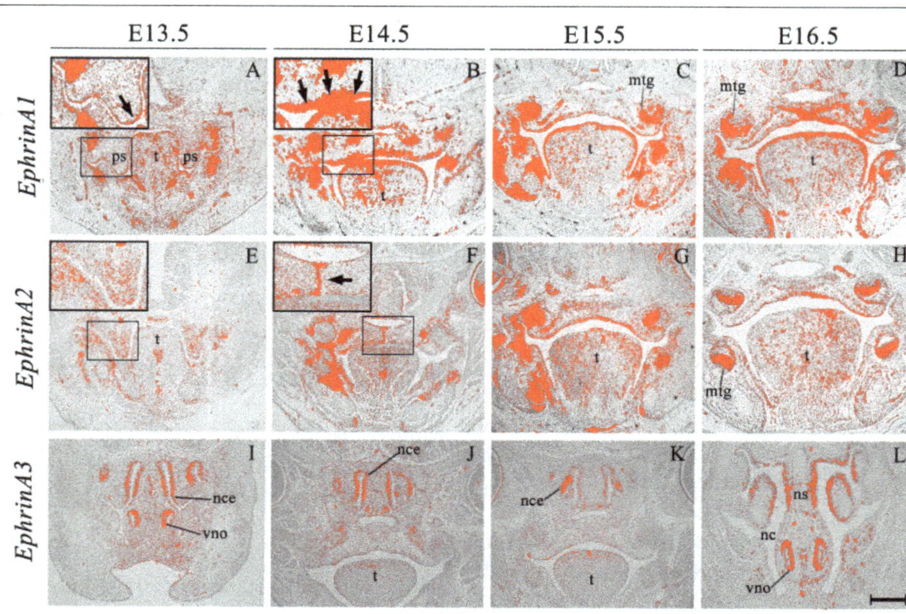

FIGURE 2 | *EphrinA1, EphrinA2, and EphrinA3* expression in the craniofacial region of the mouse embryo between E13.5 and E16.5. Radioactive *in situ* hybridization of frontal sections of embryos. Regions of *EphrinA1* and *EphrinA2* expression in the palatal shelf are highlighted at E13.5 and E14.5, respectively in **(A, E)** and **(B, F)** for each gene. At E13.5, *EphrinA1* expression was intensified in epithelium at the tip of the palatal shelf (arrow in **A**), and strongly expressed throughout the epithelium at E14.5 (arrow in **B**). *EphrinA2* was localized to the medial epithelial seam of the palate during fusion of the shelves at E14.5 (arrow in **F**). *EphrinA3* expression was confined to epithelium of the developing nasal cavity and vomeronasal organ as shown in sections **(I–L)**. mtg, molar tooth germ; nc, nasal cavity; nce, nasal cavity epithelium; ns, nasal septum; ps, palatal shelves; t, tongue; vno, vomeronasal organ. Scale bar in L = 500 μm for **(A–L)**.

EphrinA1 was only expressed at background levels between E13.5 and E16.5 (**Figures 2A–D**). *EphrinA2* showed no specific epithelial expression in the palate at E13.5, although transcripts were present in the mesenchyme (**Figure 2E**, highlighted); however, by E14.5 distinct transcriptional activity was observed in the MES (**Figure 2F**, highlighted). During subsequent development at E15.5–E16.5 *EphrinA2* upregulated in the palatal shelf epithelium (**Figures 2G,H**). *EphrinA3* was not detected above low-level background signal in the developing palate between E13.5 and E16.5 (data not shown). However, at E13.5 transcripts were identified in epithelium of the developing vomeronasal organ and nasal cavity (**Figure 2I**), expression domains that were maintained between E14.5 and E16.5 (**Figures 2J–L**).

EphA1 was generally expressed in the palatal shelf mesenchyme at E13.5, and in a complementary manner to its ligand EphrinA1 (see **Figure 2A**), was upregulated in mesenchyme at the tip of the shelves (**Figure 3A**, highlighted). Lower-level expression was maintained in the palatal mesenchyme at later stages (**Figures 3B–D**), but at E15.5–E16.5

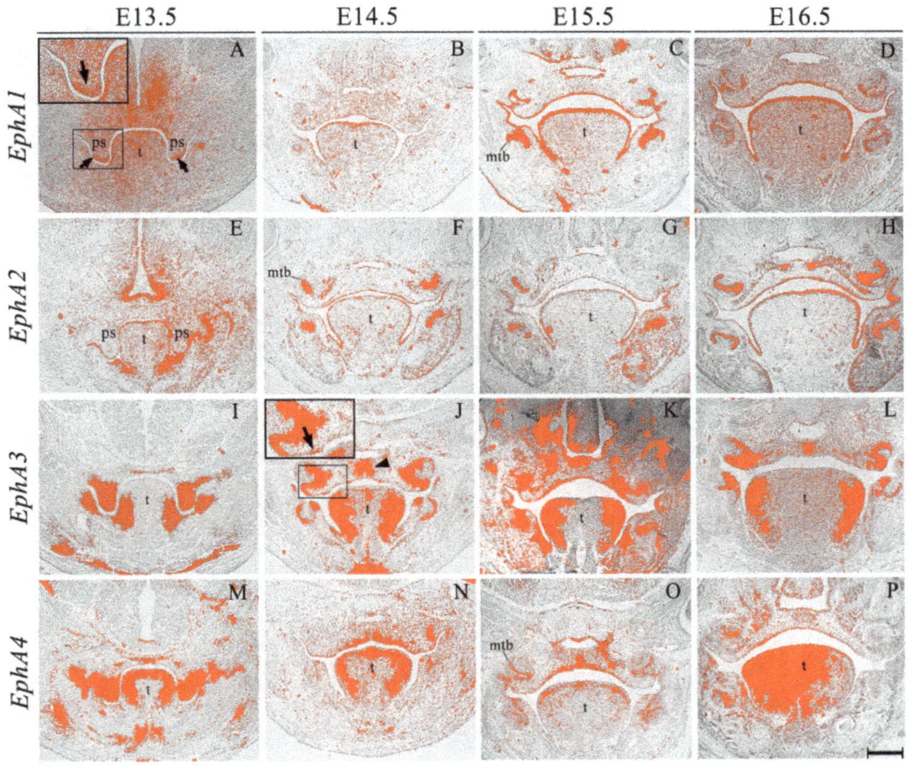

FIGURE 3 | *EphA1*, *EphA2*, *EphA3*, and *EphA4* expression in the craniofacial region of the mouse embryo between E13.5 and E16.5. Radioactive *in situ* hybridization of frontal sections of embryos. Regions of *EphA1* and *EphA3* expression are highlighted at E13.5 and E14.5 in **(A,J)**, respectively. At E13.5, *EphA1* expression was intensified in mesenchyme at the tip of the palatal shelf (arrows in **A**). *EphA3* expression was localized to regions of the epithelium and a broad region of epithelium and mesenchyme across the midline of the palate during fusion at E14.5 (arrow and arrowhead in **J**, respectively). *EphA4* expression was strong in the palatal shelves prior to elevation **(M)**, and localized to the oral epithelium and MES at later stages **(N–P)**. mtb, molar tooth bud; ps, palatal shelves; t, tongue. Scale bar in P = 500 μm for **(A–P)**.

EphA1 was clearly upregulated in the oral epithelium after palatal shelf fusion (**Figures 3C,D**). In contrast, no expression was detected in epithelium of the MES (**Figure 3B**), which is in agreement with previous findings (Agrawal et al., 2014). *EphA2* was detected in the palatal shelf epithelium from E13.5–E16.5 (**Figures 3E–H**); although no transcriptional activity was observed in the MES (**Figure 3F**). *EphA2* has been shown to function as a positive regulator of mammary epithelial proliferation and branching (Vaught et al., 2009; Park J. E. et al., 2013) and it is known that growth of the palatal shelves is controlled by reciprocal epithelial-mesenchymal interactions along the antero-posterior axis (Bush and Jiang, 2012; Economou et al., 2013). Based on the distinctive expression pattern within the epithelium, *EphA2* may be important for normal growth of the early palatal shelves.

EphA3 was intensely expressed throughout the palatal shelves at E13.5 (**Figure 3I**), although this expression became localized to regions of epithelium at E14.5 (**Figure 3J**, highlighted) in contrast to previous observations, transcripts were also detected in the midline during the process of fusion, including the MES and regions of adjacent mesenchyme (**Figure 3J**, arrowhead). *EphA3* remained enriched in these regions of the palate epithelium and mesenchyme during subsequent stages of palatogenesis between E15.5 and E16.5 (**Figures 3K,L**; Agrawal et al., 2014). *EphA4* was also strongly expressed throughout the palatal shelves prior to elevation at E13.5 (**Figure 3M**), progressively localizing to the oral epithelium and MES during later development (**Figures 3N–P**). Despite this dynamic expression pattern, an absence of both *EphA3* and *EphA4* function does not result in any overt developmental phenotype in the mouse, including the palate. Redundant roles played by other family members may explain the lack of palate phenotype in compound *EphA3*$^{-/-}$; *EphA4*$^{-/-}$ mutant embryos (Agrawal et al., 2014). *EphA5* hybridization signals were present in a patchy distribution within the mesenchymal component of the palatal shelves at E13.5, (**Figure 4A**, highlight); whilst during later stages, expression was detected throughout the epithelium and very strongly in mesenchyme at the lateral edges of the palate, with this strong expression also observed in the nasal cavity epithelium (**Figure 4B**). Following fusion at E15.5, *EphA5* was localized to the palatal epithelium (**Figure 4C**, arrowed); however, at E16.5, marked up-regulation was observed in the mesenchyme, but restricted to medial regions of the fused shelves (**Figure 4D**). *EphA6* transcripts were not detected at any significant level in the palatal shelves at E13.5 (data not shown) although some upregulation was seen in mesenchyme of the nasal cavity

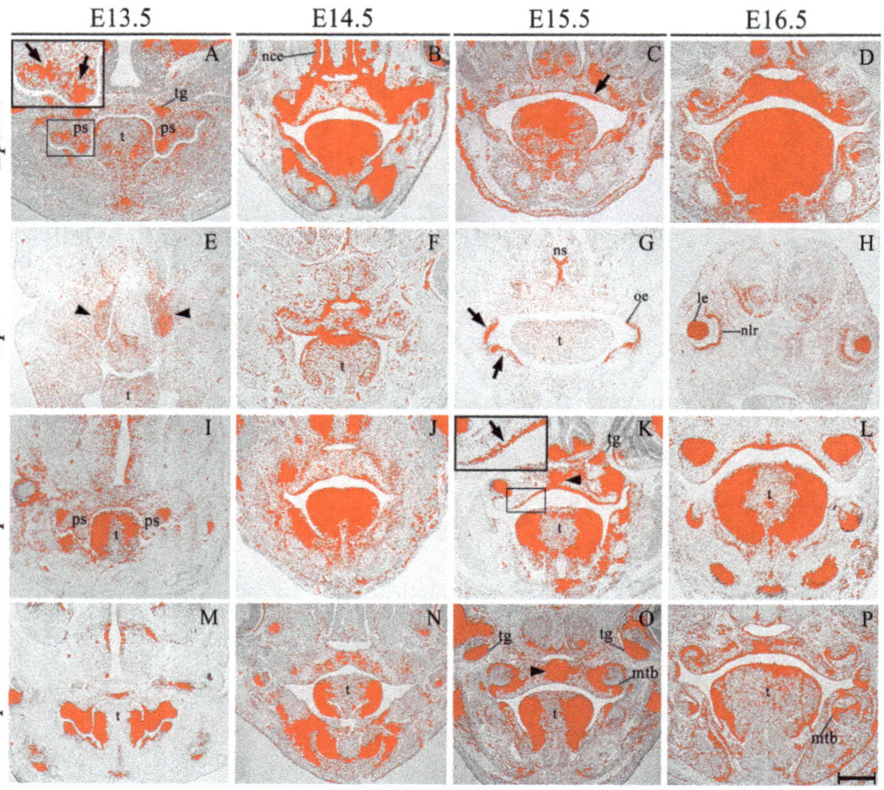

FIGURE 4 | *EphA5, EphA6, EphA7*, and *EphA8* expression in the craniofacial region of the mouse embryo between E13.5 and E16.5. Radioactive *in situ* hybridization of frontal sections of embryos. Regions of *EphA5* and *EphA7* expression are highlighted at E13.5 and E15.5 in **(A,K)**, respectively. At E13.5, there was patchy expression of *EphA5* in the palatal shelf mesenchyme (arrow in **A**), whilst at E15.5, expression was detected in the palatal shelf epithelium (arrow in **C**). *EphA6* expression was confined to mesenchyme of the developing nasal cavity at E13.5 (arrowheads in **E**) but upregulated in oral epithelium at E15.5 (arrows in **G**). *EphA7* was strongly expressed in the epithelium throughout palatogenesis, but was upregulated in the palatal midline at E15.5 (arrow and arrowhead in **K**, respectively). *EphA8* was also strongly expressed in the mid-palatal region at E15.5 (arrowhead in **O**). le, lens; mtb, molar tooth bud; nce, nasal cavity epithelium; nlr, neural layer of the retina; oe, oral epithelium; ps, palatal shelves; t, tongue; tg, trigeminal ganglion. Scale bar in P = 500 μm for **(A–P)**.

(**Figure 4E**, arrowheads). Transcripts were detected in palatal epithelium of the oral cavity during fusion at E14.5, but they were absent from the MES (**Figure 4F**) and no expression was observed following fusion of the palatal shelves at E15.5 (**Figure 4G**) and E16.5 (data not shown). Interestingly, there was strong localized expression of *EphA6* in epithelium of the oral commissure at E15.5 (**Figure 4G**, arrowed) and intense expression also identified in the lens and neural layer of the retina at E16.5 (**Figure 4H**). *EphA7* was consistently detected in the palatal shelf epithelium throughout palatogenesis, but only weakly in the mesenchyme (**Figures 4I–L**, highlight in **Figure 4K**). However, at E15.5 strong midline expression was detected (**Figure 4K**, arrowhead). This expression pattern was different from that described in previously published data, where *EphA7* was mainly observed in the mesenchyme (Agrawal et al., 2014). *EphA8* showed intense expression in both the epithelium and mesenchyme of the palatal shelves at E13.5 (**Figure 4M**), with lower-level expression at later stages; again, with the exception at E15.5, where strong expression was detected in the midline mesenchymal region (**Figures 4N–P**, arrowhead in **Figure 4O**), which also differs from that previously reported (Agrawal et al., 2014). Recently, *in vivo* expression of EphA8-Fc was reported to result in neuroepithelial cell apoptosis and a subsequent decrease in brain size (Kim et al., 2013). These findings are in agreement with previous studies that demonstrated that Ephrin-Eph signaling plays a critical role in determining the size of the neuroepithelial cell population during early embryonic brain development (Holmberg et al., 2000; Park E. et al., 2013). *EphA8* may therefore have a role in mediating epithelial apoptosis during the process of palatal shelf fusion.

EphrinB2 was expressed in the epithelium and (more weakly) in the mesenchyme during palatogenesis, particularly at the tip of the palatal shelves at E13.5 and in the MES at E14.5 (**Figures 5A–D**, highlighted in **Figure 5A**). *EphB1* transcriptional activity was weak but widespread in the palatal shelf mesenchyme at E13.5–E14.5; however, by E15.5 expression was up-regulated in the midline of the embryonic palate, returning to previous levels by E16.5 (**Figures 5E–H**). *EphB4* was also weakly expressed in the palatal shelf mesenchyme throughout palatogenesis, but with strong midline expression at E14.5 in the MES during shelf fusion (**Figures 5I–L**, arrow in **Figure 5J**). *EphB1* expression has been previously reported in the venous vasculature throughout embryonic development to adulthood (Li and Mukouyama, 2013). Additionally, *EphB1*

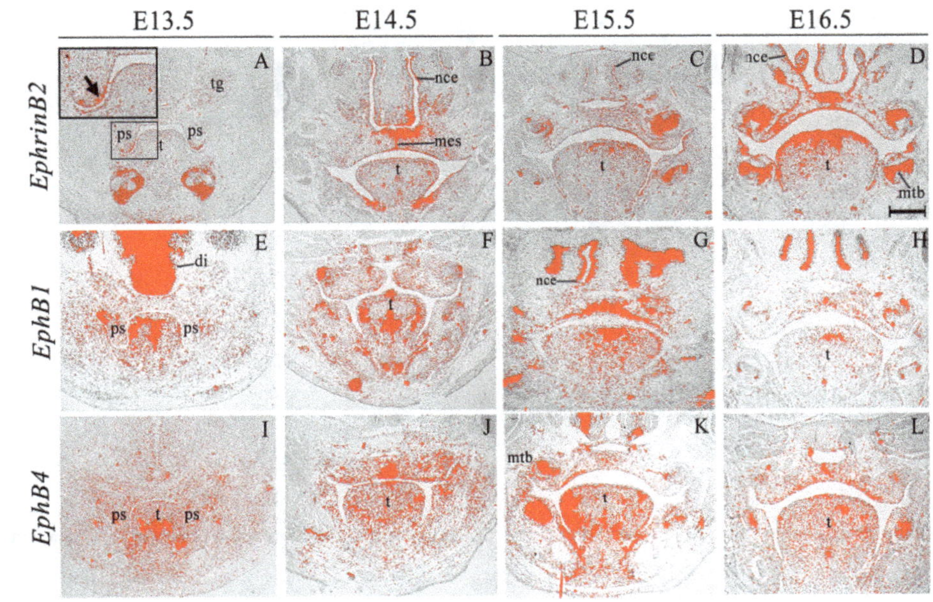

FIGURE 5 | *EphrinB2, EphB1, EphB4* expression in the craniofacial region of the mouse embryo between E13.5 and E16.5. Radioactive *in situ* hybridization of frontal sections of embryos. *EphrinB2* expression is highlighted in **A** (arrowed). di, diencephalon; mes, medial epithelium seam; mtb, molar tooth bud; nce, nasal cavity epithelium; ps, palatal shelves; t, tongue; tg, trigeminal ganglion. Scale bar in D = 500 μm for **(A–L)**.

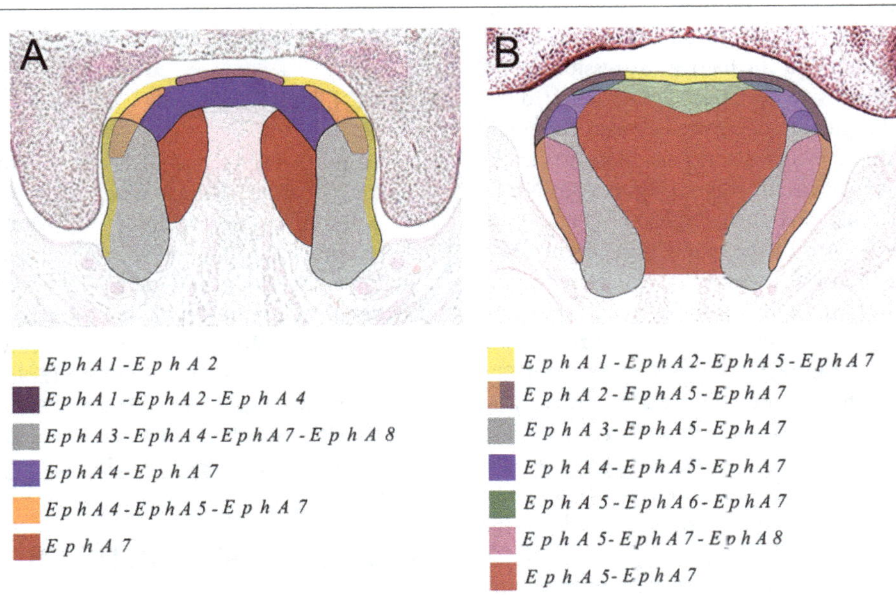

FIGURE 6 | The main domains of expression associated with the EphA family of receptors in the developing tongue at (A) E13.5 and (B) E14.5. Diagrams not drawn to scale.

has been observed in the mouse retina (Birgbauer et al., 2000), during the early stages of embryonic rat spinal cord development (Jevince et al., 2006) and in the basal ganglia nuclei (Richards et al., 2007). Interestingly, behavioral evaluation of *EphB1* null mice in an open-field environment has revealed the presence of spontaneous locomotor hyperactivity (Richards et al., 2007). During palatogenesis streams of directional cell migration (both in the anterior and posterior aspect) have been demonstrated to occur and are thought to be of importance for palate patterning (shaping) and elevation (He et al., 2008). Interestingly, a cellular migration system solely dependent on EphrinB2–EphB4 signal transduction has demonstrated that EphB4 is capable of triggering the regulation of cell migration (Sturz et al., 2004). Taken together, these results suggest that these genes could also be involved in cell migration events that take place during palate development.

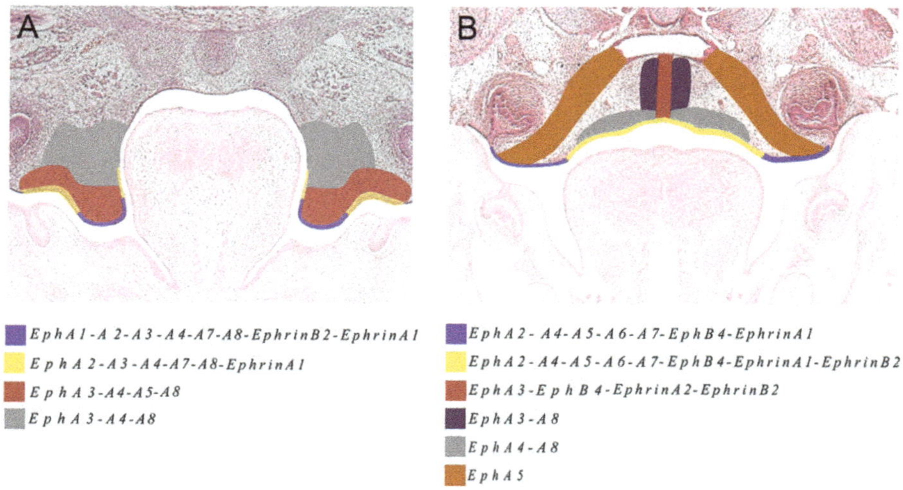

FIGURE 7 | The main domains of expression associated with ephrins and Eph receptors in the developing palate at (A) E13.5 and (B) E14.5. Diagrams not drawn to scale.

We also identified the expression of numerous Ephs during murine tongue development between E13.5 and E16.5. The main domains of expression associated with the EphA group in the tongue at E13.5 and E14.5 are summarized in **Figures 6A,B**. *EphA5* and *EphA7* presented with ubiquitous expression at E14.5 (see **Figures 4B,J**, respectively). During all stages examined, *EphA1* and *EphA2* demonstrated distinctive expression in the tongue epithelium (**Figures 3A–H**), whereas *EphA3* was strongly expressed in the lateral tongue mesenchyme between E13.5 and E16.5 (**Figures 3I–L**). Although *EphA4* was also detected in the lateral tongue mesenchyme at earlier stages (**Figures 3M,N**); by E15.5, transcriptional activity was down-regulated (**Figure 3O**) and restricted to patchy regions of the epithelium (**Figure 3O**), although at E16.5, expression was increased in the mesenchyme (**Figure 3P**). *EphA6* presented weak and widespread expression in the mesenchyme during tongue development (**Figures 3E–G**). However, at E14.5, a marked upregulation was observed in the inter-molar eminence of the tongue (**Figure 4F**). Similarly to *EphA3*, *EphA7*, and *EphA8* transcriptional activity were also markedly increased in the lateral mesenchyme of the tongue during development (**Figures 4I–O**). However, by E16.5 *EphA8* expression was down-regulated and more restricted to the epithelial compartment (**Figure 4P**). Rapid depression of the tongue in embryogenesis is critical for proper palatogenesis. Any delay in this process can disturb palatal shelf elevation and hence, lead to cleft palate (Nie, 2005). For these events to take place a coordinated balance between apoptosis and proliferation is essential (Parada et al., 2012; Parada and Chai, 2015).

The Eph and ephrin family-member gene expression in the developing palate and tongue described here is summarized in **Figures 6, 7**. These dynamic domains suggest important potential roles for these molecules in both epithelium and mesenchyme during development of these regions. Further analysis using animal models will be required to delineate the precise requirements during these developmental processes. However, the co-expression of *EphA3, A4,* and *A8* in the palatal shelves makes it difficult to test the hypothesis that these genes are involved in palatogenesis. Considering the known promiscuous interactions between Ephs and ephrins, it is likely EphA3, A4, and A8 may also play redundant roles during palate development. Analysis of a triple loss-of-function mouse model may be required to definitively address this question.

CONCLUSIONS

Eph receptors A3, A4, and A8 are very strongly expressed within palatal shelf mesenchyme during early palatogenesis and both EphA1 and A5 are up-regulated at the shelf tip during this stage. Eph receptors A3, A4, and A8 are also strongly expressed in lateral regions of the tongue at these stages, suggesting some co-ordination in the regulation of palatogenesis and tongue development. EphA and ephrinA-family members are also expressed in palatal shelf epithelium (*EphA2, EphA7, ephrinA1*) and mesenchyme (*EphA1, A3, A4, A5, A6, A8,* and *ephrinA2, A3*) suggesting the possibility of epithelial-mesenchymal interactions being mediated by these proteins during development of the palate.

AUTHOR CONTRIBUTIONS

MC and IM conceived the experiments, GX and IM conducted the experiments and undertook data acquisition, GX, IM, and MC wrote the manuscript.

ACKNOWLEDGMENTS

GMX is the recipient of a National Institute of Health Research, UK Clinical Lectureship. GMX is supported by the Academy of Medical Sciences (Wellcome Trust, British Heart Foundation, Arthritis Research, UK). We thank David Anderson, Andrea Ballabio, Tyler Cutforth, David Feldheim, Mark Henkemeyer, and David Wilkinson for kindly providing plasmid cDNA.

REFERENCES

Agrawal, P., Wang, M., Kim, S., Lewis, A. E., and Bush, J. O. (2014). Embryonic expression of EphA receptor genes in mice supports their candidacy for involvement in cleft lip and palate. *Dev. Dyn.* 243, 1470–1476. doi: 10.1002/dvdy.24170

Birgbauer, E., Cowan, C. A., Sretavan, D. W., and Henkemeyer, M. (2000). Kinase independent function of EphB receptors in retinal axon pathfinding to the optic disc from dorsal but not ventral retina. *Development* 127, 1231–1241.

Bush, J. O., and Jiang, R. (2012). Palatogenesis: morphogenetic and molecular mechanisms of secondary palate development. *Development* 139, 231–243. doi: 10.1242/dev.067082

Casey, L. M., Lan, Y., Cho, E. S., Maltby, K. M., Gridley, T., and Jiang, R. (2006). Jag2-Notch1 signaling regulates oral epithelial differentiation and palate development. *Dev. Dyn.* 235, 1830–1844. doi: 10.1002/dvdy.20821

Chai, Y., and Maxson, R. E. Jr. (2006). Recent advances in craniofacial morphogenesis. *Dev. Dyn.* 235, 2353–2375. doi: 10.1002/dvdy.20833

Chenaux, G., and Henkemeyer, M. (2011). Forward signaling by EphB1/EphB2 interacting with ephrin-B ligands at the optic chiasm is required to form the ipsilateral projection. *Eur. J. Neurosci.* 34, 1620–1633. doi: 10.1111/j.1460-9568.2011.07845.x

Cobourne, M. T. (2004). The complex genetics of cleft lip and palate. *Eur. J. Orthod.* 26, 7–16. doi: 10.1093/ejo/26.1.7

Compagni, A., Logan, M., Klein, R., and Adams, R. H. (2003). Control of skeletal patterning by ephrinB1-EphB interactions. *Dev. Cell* 5, 217–230. doi: 10.1016/S1534-5807(03)00198-9

Davy, A., Aubin, J., and Soriano, P. (2004). Ephrin-B1 forward and reverse signaling are required during mouse development. *Genes Dev.* 18, 572–583. doi: 10.1101/gad.1171704

Dravis, C., and Henkemeyer, M. (2011). Ephrin-B reverse signaling controls septation events at the embryonic midline through separate tyrosine phosphorylation-independent signaling avenues. *Dev. Biol.* 355, 138–151. doi: 10.1016/j.ydbio.2011.04.020

Dudas, M., Li, W. Y., Kim, J., Yang, A., and Kaartinen, V. (2007). Palatal fusion - where do the midline cells go? A review on cleft palate, a major human birth defect. *Acta Histochem.* 109, 1–14. doi: 10.1016/j.acthis.2006.05.009

Economou, A. D., Brock, L. J., Cobourne, M. T., and Green, J. B. (2013). Whole population cell analysis of a landmark-rich mammalian epithelium reveals multiple elongation mechanisms. *Development* 140, 4740–4750. doi: 10.1242/dev.096545

Ferguson, M. W. (1988). Palate development. *Development* 103(Suppl.) 41–60.

Gritli-Linde, A. (2007). Molecular control of secondary palate development. *Dev. Biol.* 301, 309–326. doi: 10.1016/j.ydbio.2006.07.042

Gu, C., and Park, S. (2001). The EphA8 receptor regulates integrin activity through p110gamma phosphatidylinositol-3 kinase in a tyrosine kinase activity-independent manner. *Mol. Cell. Biol.* 21, 4579–4597. doi: 10.1128/MCB.21.14.4579-4597.2001

He, F., Xiong, W., Yu, X., Espinoza-Lewis, R., Liu, C., Gu, S., et al. (2008). Wnt5a regulates directional cell migration and cell proliferation via Ror2-mediated noncanonical pathway in mammalian palate development. *Development* 135, 3871–3879. doi: 10.1242/dev.025767

Himanen, J. P., Chumley, M. J., Lackmann, M., Li, C., Barton, W. A., Jeffrey, P. D., et al. (2004). Repelling class discrimination: ephrin-A5 binds to and activates EphB2 receptor signaling. *Nat. Neurosci.* 7, 501–509. doi: 10.1038/nn1237

Hirai, H., Maru, Y., Hagiwara, K., Nishida, J., and Takaku, F. (1987). A novel putative tyrosine kinase receptor encoded by the eph gene. *Science* 238, 1717–1720. doi: 10.1126/science.2825356

Holmberg, J., Clarke, D. L., and Frisén, J. (2000). Regulation of repulsion versus adhesion by different splice forms of an Eph receptor. *Nature* 408, 203–206. doi: 10.1038/35041577

Hosokawa, R., Oka, K., Yamaza, T., Iwata, J., Urata, M., Xu, X., et al. (2010). TGF-beta mediated FGF10 signaling in cranial neural crest cells controls development of myogenic progenitor cells through tissue-tissue interactions during tongue morphogenesis. *Dev. Biol.* 341, 186–195. doi: 10.1016/j.ydbio.2010.02.030

Islam, S., Loizides, A. M., Fialkovich, J. J., Grand, R. J., and Montgomery, R. K. (2010). Developmental expression of Eph and ephrin family genes in mammalian small intestine. *Dig. Dis. Sci.* 55, 2478–2488. doi: 10.1007/s10620-009-1102-z

Jevince, A. R., Kadison, S. R., Pittman, A. J., Chien, C. B., and Kaprielian, Z. (2006). Distribution of EphB receptors and ephrin-B1 in the developing vertebrate spinal cord. *J. Comp. Neurol.* 497, 734–750. doi: 10.1002/cne.21001

Jones, T. L., Karavanova, I., Maéno, M., Ong, R. C., Kung, H. F., and Daar, I. O. (1995). Expression of an amphibian homolog of the Eph family of receptor tyrosine kinases is developmentally regulated. *Oncogene* 10, 1111–1117.

Kim, Y., Park, E., Noh, H., and Park, S. (2013). Expression of EphA8-Fc in transgenic mouse embryos induces apoptosis of neural epithelial cells during brain development. *Dev. Neurobiol.* 73, 702–712. doi: 10.1002/dneu.22092

Klein, R. (2012). Eph/ephrin signalling during development. *Development* 139, 4105–4109. doi: 10.1242/dev.074997

Lackmann, M., and Boyd, A. W. (2008). Eph, a protein family coming of age: more confusion, insight, or complexity? *Sci Signal* 1:re2. doi: 10.1126/stke.115re2

Li, W., and Mukouyama, Y. S. (2013). Tissue-specific venous expression of the EPH family receptor EphB1 in the skin vasculature. *Dev. Dyn.* 242, 976–988. doi: 10.1002/dvdy.23985

Matsuoka, H., Obama, H., Kelly, M. L., Matsui, T., and Nakamoto, M. (2005). Biphasic functions of the kinase-defective Ephb6 receptor in cell adhesion and migration. *J. Biol. Chem.* 280, 29355–29363. doi: 10.1074/jbc.M500010200

Miao, H., Strebhardt, K., Pasquale, E. B., Shen, T. L., Guan, J. L., and Wang, B. (2005). Inhibition of integrin-mediated cell adhesion but not directional cell migration requires catalytic activity of EphB3 receptor tyrosine kinase. Role of Rho family small GTPases. *J. Biol. Chem.* 280, 923–932. doi: 10.1074/jbc.M411383200

Nie, X. (2005). Apoptosis, proliferation and gene expression patterns in mouse developing tongue. *Anat. Embryol.* 210, 125–132. doi: 10.1007/s00429-005-0009-5

Noden, D. M., and Francis-West, P. (2006). The differentiation and morphogenesis of craniofacial muscles. *Dev. Dyn.* 235, 1194–1218. doi: 10.1002/dvdy.20697

Orioli, D., Henkemeyer, M., Lemke, G., Klein, R., and Pawson, T. (1996). Sek4 and Nuk receptors cooperate in guidance of commissural axons and in palate formation. *EMBO J.* 15, 6035–6049.

Parada, C., and Chai, Y. (2015). Mandible and Tongue Development. *Curr. Top. Dev. Biol.* 115, 31–58. doi: 10.1016/bs.ctdb.2015.07.023

Parada, C., Han, D., and Chai, Y. (2012). Molecular and cellular regulatory mechanisms of tongue myogenesis. *J. Dent. Res.* 91, 528–535. doi: 10.1177/0022034511434055

Park, E., Kim, Y., Noh, H., Lee, H., Yoo, S., and Park, S. (2013). EphA/ephrin-A signaling is critically involved in region-specific apoptosis during early brain development. *Cell Death Differ.* 20, 169–180. doi: 10.1038/cdd.2012.121

Park, J. E., Son, A. I., and Zhou, R. (2013). Roles of EphA2 in development and disease. *Genes (Basel)* 4, 334–357. doi: 10.3390/genes4030334

Pasquale, E. B. (2005). Eph receptor signalling casts a wide net on cell behaviour. *Nat. Rev. Mol. Cell Biol.* 6, 462–475. doi: 10.1038/nrm1662

Pasquale, E. B. (2010). Eph receptors and ephrins in cancer: bidirectional signalling and beyond. *Nat. Rev. Cancer* 10, 165–180. doi: 10.1038/nrc2806

Rice, R., Spencer-Dene, B., Connor, E. C., Gritli-Linde, A., McMahon, A. P., Dickson, C., et al. (2004). Disruption of Fgf10/Fgfr2b-coordinated epithelial-mesenchymal interactions causes cleft palate. *J. Clin. Invest.* 113, 1692–1700. doi: 10.1172/JCI20384

Richards, A. B., Scheel, T. A., Wang, K., Henkemeyer, M., and Kromer, L. F. (2007). EphB1 null mice exhibit neuronal loss in substantia nigra pars reticulata and spontaneous locomotor hyperactivity. *Eur. J. Neurosci.* 25, 2619–2628. doi: 10.1111/j.1460-9568.2007.05523.x

Risley, M., Garrod, D., Henkemeyer, M., and McLean, W. (2009). EphB2 and EphB3 forward signalling are required for palate development. *Mech. Dev.* 126, 230–239. doi: 10.1016/j.mod.2008.10.009

Sakano, S., Serizawa, R., Inada, T., Iwama, A., Itoh, A., Kato, C., et al. (1996). Characterization of a ligand for receptor protein-tyrosine kinase HTK expressed in immature hematopoietic cells. *Oncogene* 13, 813–822.

Scales, J. B., Winning, R. S., Renaud, C. S., Shea, L. J., and Sargent, T. D. (1995). Novel members of the eph receptor tyrosine kinase subfamily expressed during Xenopus development. *Oncogene* 11, 1745–1752.

Sturz, A., Bader, B., Thierauch, K. H., and Glienke, J. (2004). EphB4 signaling is capable of mediating ephrinB2-induced inhibition of cell migration. *Biochem. Biophys. Res. Commun.* 313, 80–88. doi: 10.1016/j.bbrc.2003.11.092

Torii, C., Izumi, K., Nakajima, H., Takahashi, T., and Kosaki, K. (2007). EFNB1 mutation at the ephrin ligand-receptor dimerization interface in a patient with craniofrontonasal syndrome. *Congenit. Anom. (Kyoto).* 47, 49–52. doi: 10.1111/j.1741-4520.2006.00140.x

Twigg, S. R., Kan, R., Babbs, C., Bochukova, E. G., Robertson, S. P., Wall, S. A., et al. (2004). Mutations of ephrin-B1 (EFNB1), a marker of tissue boundary formation, cause craniofrontonasal syndrome. *Proc. Natl. Acad. Sci. U.S.A.* 101, 8652–8657. doi: 10.1073/pnas.0402819101

Vaught, D., Chen, J., and Brantley-Sieders, D. M. (2009). Regulation of mammary gland branching morphogenesis by EphA2 receptor tyrosine kinase. *Mol. Biol. Cell* 20, 2572–2581. doi: 10.1091/mbc.E08-04-0378

Watanabe, A., Akita, S., Tin, N. T., Natsume, N., Nakano, Y., Niikawa, N., et al. (2006). A mutation in RYK is a genetic factor for nonsyndromic cleft lip and palate. *Cleft Palate Craniofac. J.* 43, 310–316. doi: 10.1597/04-145.1

Wieland, I., Jakubiczka, S., Muschke, P., Cohen, M., Thiele, H., Gerlach, K. L., et al. (2004). Mutations of the ephrin-B1 gene cause craniofrontonasal syndrome. *Am. J. Hum. Genet.* 74, 1209–1215. doi: 10.1086/421532

Xavier, G. M., Sharpe, P. T., and Cobourne, M. T. (2009). Scube1 is expressed during facial development in the mouse. *J. Exp. Zoolog. B Mol. Dev. Evol.* 312B, 518–524. doi: 10.1002/jez.b.21260

Xiong, W., He, F., Morikawa, Y., Yu, X., Zhang, Z., Lan, Y., et al. (2009). Hand2 is required in the epithelium for palatogenesis in mice. *Dev. Biol.* 330, 131–141. doi: 10.1016/j.ydbio.2009.03.021

7

Intermittent Hypoxia Influences Alveolar Bone Proper Microstructure via Hypoxia-Inducible Factor and VEGF Expression in Periodontal Ligaments of Growing Rats

Shuji Oishi[1], Yasuhiro Shimizu[1], Jun Hosomichi[1], Yoichiro Kuma[1], Hideyuki Maeda[2], Hisashi Nagai[3], Risa Usumi-Fujita[1], Sawa Kaneko[1], Naoki Shibutani[1], Jun-ichi Suzuki[4], Ken-ichi Yoshida[2] and Takashi Ono[1]*

[1] Department of Orthodontic Science, Graduate School of Medical and Dental Sciences, Tokyo Medical and Dental University, Tokyo, Japan, [2] Department of Forensic Medicine, Graduate School of Medicine, Tokyo Medical University, Tokyo, Japan, [3] Department of Legal Medicine (Forensic Medicine), Keio University School of Medicine, Tokyo, Japan, [4] Department of Advanced Clinical Science and Therapeutics, The University of Tokyo, Tokyo, Japan

***Correspondence:**
Jun Hosomichi
hosomichi.orts@tmd.ac.jp

Intermittent hypoxia (IH) recapitulates morphological changes in the maxillofacial bones in children with obstructive sleep apnea (OSA). Recently, we found that IH increased bone mineral density (BMD) in the inter-radicular alveolar bone (reflecting enhanced osteogenesis) in the mandibular first molar (M1) region in the growing rats, but the underlying mechanism remains unknown. In this study, we focused on the hypoxia-inducible factor (HIF) pathway to assess the effect of IH by testing the null hypothesis of no significant differences in the mRNA-expression levels of relevant factors associated with the HIF pathway, between control rats and growing rats with IH. To test the null hypothesis, we investigated how IH enhances mandibular osteogenesis in the alveolar bone proper with respect to HIF-1α and vascular endothelial growth factor (VEGF) in periodontal ligament (PDL) tissues. Seven-week-old male Sprague–Dawley rats were exposed to IH for 3 weeks. The microstructure and BMD in the alveolar bone proper of the distal root of the mandibular M1 were evaluated using micro-computed tomography (micro-CT). Expression of HIF-1α and VEGF mRNA in PDL tissues were measured, whereas osteogenesis was evaluated by measuring mRNA levels for alkaline phosphatase (ALP) and bone morphogenetic protein-2 (BMP-2). The null hypothesis was rejected: we found an increase in the expression of all of these markers after IH exposure. The results provided the first indication that IH enhanced osteogenesis of the mandibular M1 region in association with PDL angiogenesis during growth via HIF-1α in an animal model.

Keywords: bone mineral density, hypoxia inducible factor, intermittent hypoxia, periodontal ligament, vascular endothelial growth factor

INTRODUCTION

Intermittent hypoxia (IH) during sleep has been implicated in the pathogenesis of obstructive sleep apnea (OSA; Noda et al., 1998; Lal et al., 2012), although the role of IH in the growth of children with OSA has not been clarified. In particular, it has been reported that pediatric OSA is frequently associated with impairment in the growth and development of craniofacial and otolaryngological tissues, as well as with neuromuscular diseases (Balbani et al., 2005; Huang and Guilleminault, 2012). Hypertension, cardiac remodeling, and other complications of OSA have been studied using rodent models of IH induced by short cycles of hypoxia–normoxia (Skelly et al., 2012; Maeda et al., 2013; Nagai et al., 2015). Previously, we demonstrated that IH exposure induces a decrease in the volume of the nasal cavity, reflecting impaired development of maxillofacial bones (Kuma et al., 2014). Other researchers showed that IH increased the bone mineral density (BMD) in the inter-radicular alveolar bone in the mandibular first molar (M1) region during growth (Oishi et al., 2015), but the underlying mechanism remains unknown.

Hypoxia is critical to the remodeling and repair of damaged bones via hypoxia-inducible factor (HIF; Maes et al., 2012), the key stimulator of vessel formation and angiogenesis. The gene encoding the prominent angiogenic factor vascular endothelial growth factor (VEGF) is the primary target for HIF-1α (Riddle et al., 2009). A recent study provided evidence supporting the view that HIFs and VEGF play essential roles in coupling between angiogenesis and osteogenesis during bone formation and repair (Schipani et al., 2009).

Alveolar bone proper is covered with collagen fibers in the periodontal ligament (PDL; Shimizu et al., 2014). The PDL is a specialized soft connective tissue that connects the tooth with the alveolar bone socket, thereby promoting the development and maintenance of periodontium (Kaku and Yamauchi, 2014). PDL tissues are comprised of PDL cells (Shimizu et al., 2014), collagen fibers (Kaku and Yamauchi, 2014), blood vessels (Muramoto et al., 2000), nerve elements (Muramoto et al., 2000), extracellular substances (Kaneko et al., 2001), osteoclasts (Kaneko et al., 2001), and osteoblasts (Mayahara et al., 2012), and provides progenitor cells for bone formation and remodeling. Alkaline phosphatase (ALP) and bone morphogenetic protein-2 (BMP-2) are known to induce osteogenesis and the osteogenic transformation of PDL cells (Kuru et al., 1999; Selvig et al., 2002). ALP activity reflects early osteogenic differentiation in the presence of osteoblasts (Kuru et al., 1999). Previous data showed that ALP activation and BMP-2 upregulation in PDL cells induce periodontium osteogenesis in response to growth hormones (Li et al., 2001) or matrix Gla proteins (Li et al., 2012). In addition, mechanical forces such as moderate occlusal stimuli and dissipation of masticatory force are transmitted from the teeth through the PDL to the progenitor cells, thereby promoting bone remodeling in the periodontal tissue (Chen et al., 2005). As such, PDL tissues maintain proper alveolar bone homeostasis via ALP and BMP-2.

Bone remodeling, a complex process by which old bone is continuously replaced by new tissue, is affected by a variety of biochemical and mechanical factors (Hadjidakis and Androulakis, 2006). With regard to signaling pathways, the Wnt (Wang et al., 2014), OPG/RANKL/RANK (Hsu et al., 2006), and HIF pathways (Mamalis and Cochran, 2011) are well-known in the control of bone remodeling. In this study, we specifically focused on the HIF pathway to assess the effect of IH by testing the null hypothesis that no significant differences in the mRNA-expression levels of relevant factors associated with the HIF pathway in PDL occur between control rats and growing rats with IH. To this end, we analyzed the microarchitecture and mineral density of the alveolar bone proper around the mandibular M1 after 3 weeks of IH in growing rats, with reference to HIF1-α, VEGF, ALP, and BMP-2 mRNA expression.

MATERIALS AND METHODS

Experimental IH Model

Experiments were conducted on twelve 7-week-old male Sprague–Dawley rats randomly divided into two groups. Experimental rats were exposed to IH at a rate of 20 cycles per h (nadir, 4% oxygen; peak, 21% oxygen; 0% carbon dioxide) for 3 weeks (IH group), and control rats breathed room air (C group). The control cage was placed next to the cage equipped with the IH apparatus, and all rats underwent their respective treatments for 8 h per day during the 12-h "lights on" period (Maeda et al., 2013; Nagai et al., 2015). The experiments were conducted while the rats were 7 to 10 weeks of age, when craniofacial bones actively develop (puberty), as documented by studies of craniofacial growth (Spence, 1940) and puberty onset (Cheung et al., 2001) in male rats. All rats were allowed free access to food and water throughout the experimental period, as previously described (Skelly et al., 2012; Maeda et al., 2013; Nagai et al., 2015). Immediately after the IH-exposure period, all rats were anesthetized by a sodium pentobarbital injection and sacrificed. All experimental procedures were performed according to the Guide for the Care and Use of Laboratory Animals published by the US National Institutes of Health (NIH publication 85-23, revised 1996). The animal protocol was approved by the Animal Experimental Committee of Tokyo Medical University (approval number S-26063).

Three-Dimensional Microcomputed Tomography (Micro-CT) Analysis

Changes in the bony microstructure of the alveolar bone proper around roots of the mandibular M1 and in the PDL space were investigated using micro-CT with a desktop X-ray micro-CT system (SMX-100CT; Shimadzu, Kyoto, Japan) with a scanning resolution of 20-μm intervals on individual images. The region of interest (ROI) for structural morphometry was enlarged to a 40-μm radius around the distal root (**Figure 1A**; Shimizu et al., 2014). Each ROI was analyzed with respect to BMD, bone volume/tissue volume (BV/TV), trabecular thickness (Tb.Th), and trabecular number (Tb.N) using three-dimensional image-analysis software (TRI/3D-BON; Ratoc System Engineering, Tokyo, Japan). Additionally, to evaluate changes from mechanical stimuli in the PDL space, tissue volume (TV) around the distal root of the mandibular M1 was computed (**Figure 1B**; Shimizu et al., 2014).

Reverse Transcription Quantitative Real-Time PCR (RT-qPCR) Analysis

PDL tissues were removed from extracted roots of the mandibular M1. Total RNA was isolated from PDL tissues using the PureLink™ FFPE Total RNA Isolation Kit (Invitrogen, CA, USA) according to instructions provided by the manufacturer (Afanador et al., 2005; Luan et al., 2007). cDNA was synthesized from total RNA with reverse transcription random primers using High-Capacity cDNA Reverse Transcription Kits (Applied Biosystems, Foster City, CA, USA). Quantitative PCR assays were carried out in triplicate for each sample using a 7500 Real-Time PCR System (Applied Biosystems, Foster City, CA, USA). PCR analyses were conducted with gene-specific primers and fluorescently labeled TaqMan probes (Takara Bio, Shiga, Japan). Appropriate primers were chosen for real-time PCR amplification of VEGF (forward primer: 5′-ccttgctgctctacctccac-3′, reverse primer: 5′-ccacttcgtgatgattctgc-3′), HIF-1α (forward primer: 5′-ctaccagaagggcaggatacag-3′, reverse primer: 5′-gcaggcagatgaaataccagtc-3′), ALP (forward primer: 5′-acgtggctaagaatgtcatc-3′, reverse primer: 5′-ctggtaggcgatgtcctta-3′), BMP-2 (forward primer: 5′-tcaagccaaacacaaacagc-3′, reverse primer: 5′-acgtctgaacaatggcatga-3′), and Hprt-1 (forward primer: 5′-cagactttgctttccttgg-3′, reverse primer: 5′-tccactttcgctgatgacac-3′). The thermocycling conditions used were 95°C for 30 s, followed by 40 cycles of 95°C for 5 s and 60°C for 34 s. Gene expression levels were calculated according to the ΔΔCT method of relative quantification. The threshold cycle (Ct) value of the target mRNAs (VEGF, HIF1α, ALP, or BMP-2) was normalized to the Ct values of the internal control (Hprt-1) in the same sample ($\Delta Ct = Ct_{target} - Ct_{Hprt-1}$), followed by normalization to the control ($\Delta\Delta Ct = \Delta Ct_{IHgroup} - \Delta Ct_{Cgroup}$). The fold change in expression was calculated as the relative quantification value (RQ; $2^{-\Delta\Delta Ct}$; Livak and Schmittgen, 2001).

Statistical Analysis

Statistical calculations were performed using statistical analysis software (IBM SPSS Statistics Version 20.0 Chicago, IL, USA). We first examined the normality and variance of the data using the F-test. The control and experimental groups were compared using the Mann–Whitney U-test for nonparametric data, and statistical significance was established at a p level of less than 0.05.

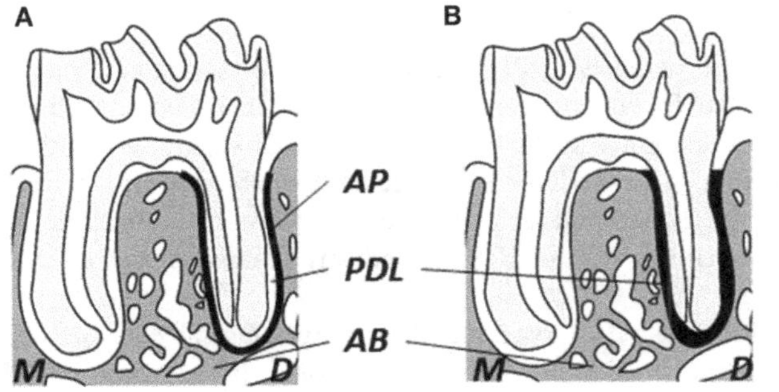

FIGURE 1 | Schematic drawing of observational area of micro-CT. (A) Observational area for alveolar bone proper (heavy black line). **(B)** Observational area for the periodontal ligament (heavy black area). M, Mesial; D, distal; AB, inter-radicular alveolar bone; AP, alveolar bone proper; PDL, periodontal ligament.

RESULTS

Body Weight Changes in Rats after IH

The median body weight (mean ± standard error) of rats exposed to IH for 3 weeks (277.5 ± 3.8 g) was significantly lower than that of control (C) rats (356.0 ± 9.8 g). Previous reports using this animal model showed that the correlation between the body weight and whole-body growth in this IH model was low (Maeda et al., 2013; Kuma et al., 2014; Oishi et al., 2015).

Three-Dimensional Micro-CT Analysis

We investigated changes in the bony microstructure of the alveolar bone proper around the distal roots of mandibular M1 using micro-CT. Micro-CT images of alveolar bone proper around the distal root of mandibular M1 showed higher bone volume (BV) density in the IH rats than in the C rats (**Figure 2**). In addition, micro-CT analyses demonstrated significant increases in the BMD, BV/TV, Tb.Th, and Tb.N in the distal root alveolar bone proper of IH rats, compared with those of C rats (**Figure 3**).

Quantitative Real-Time PCR

We evaluated the relative expression levels of osteogenesis–angiogenesis coupling markers (**Figure 4**) and osteogenic markers (**Figure 5**) in PDL tissues by RT-qPCR analysis. IH

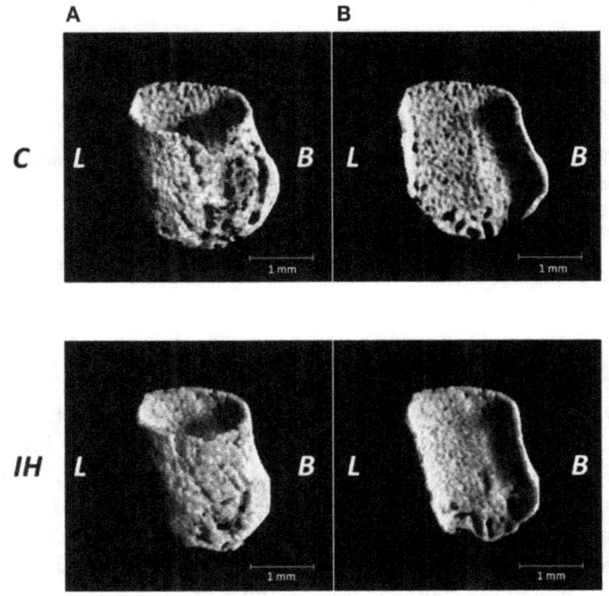

FIGURE 2 | Microarchitecture of the alveolar bone proper of the distal roots in the mandibular first molar region in the C and IH groups. Representative micro-CT images of alveolar bone proper in the distal root of mandibular first molar region **(A)** and half of mesial surface **(B)**. Scale bar: 1.0 mm. C, control group; IH, IH group; L, lingual; B, buccal.

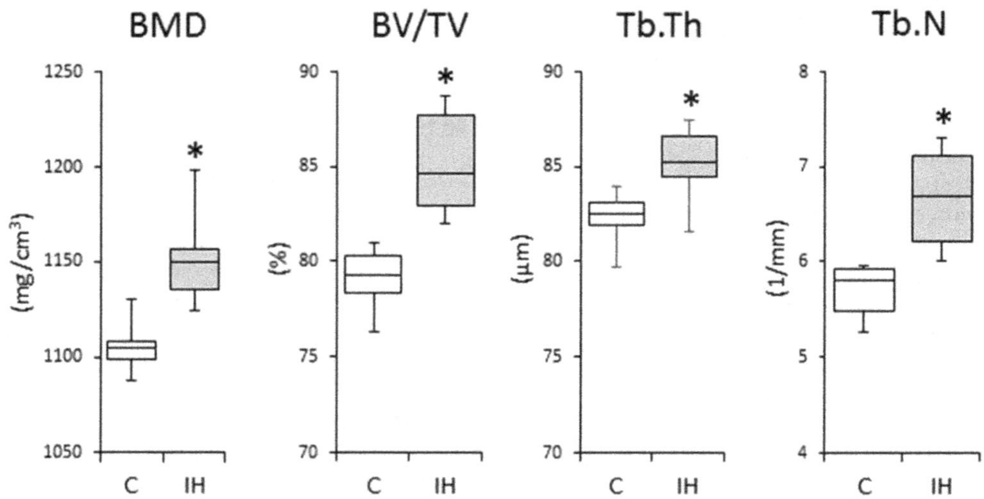

FIGURE 3 | Comparisons of bone morphology between the C and IH groups by micro-CT analysis. Cancellous bone of the alveolar bone proper of the distal roots in the mandibular first molar region was compared between the C and IH groups. Box edges represent the upper and lower quantiles, the middle lines in the boxes represent the medians, and the whiskers represent the maxima and minima. BMD, bone mineral density; BV/TV, bone volume/tissue volume; Tb.Th, trabecular thickness; Tb.N, trabecular number. $^{*}p < 0.05$ by the Mann–Whitney *U*-test.

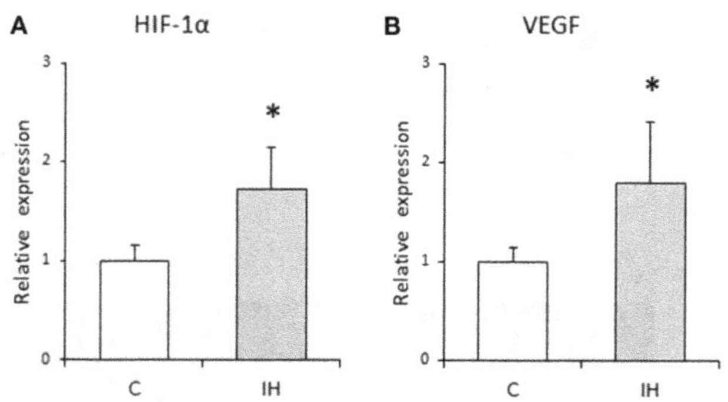

FIGURE 4 | Relative expression levels of osteogenesis–angiogenesis coupling markers. Relative HIF-1α **(A)** and VEGF **(B)** expression in the PDL tissues was compared between the C and IH rat groups by RT-qPCR. The mRNA-expression levels measured in C rats were set to a value of 1. Data are shown as the mean ± standard deviation for each group. $^{*}p < 0.05$ by the Mann–Whitney *U*-test.

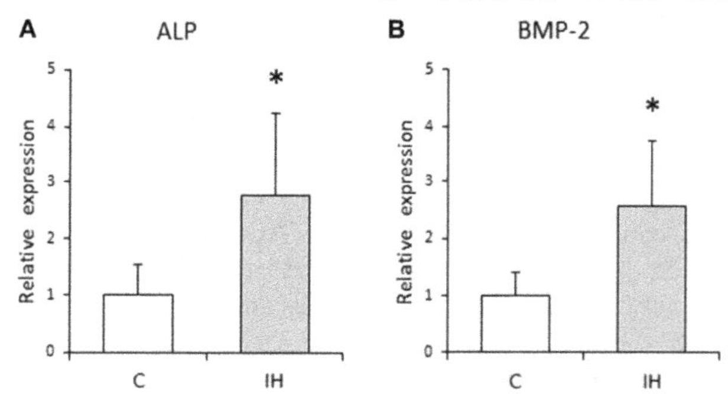

FIGURE 5 | Relative expression levels of osteogenic markers. Relative ALP **(A)** and BMP-2 **(B)** expression in the PDL tissues was compared between the C and IH rat groups by RT-qPCR. The mRNA-expression levels measured in C rats were set to a value of 1. Data are shown as the mean ± standard deviation for each group. $^{*}p < 0.05$ by the Mann–Whitney *U*-test.

increased the mRNA levels of HIF-1α and VEGF by 1.71- and 1.97-fold, respectively, in PDL tissues compared with those observed in C rats (**Figure 4**). Similarly, ALP and BMP-2 mRNA levels were increased 2.75- and 2.57-fold in PDL tissues compared to the corresponding levels in C rats (**Figure 5**). These changes are not likely to have been mediated by mechanical forces, as IH had no effect on the PDL space surrounding the distal root of the mandibular M1 (**Figure 6**).

DISCUSSION

The null hypothesis that no significant differences would occur in the mRNA-expression levels of some factors associated with the HIF pathway in PDL between control rats and IH rats was rejected: IH enhanced osteogenesis in the mandibular M1 region in association with VEGF, ALP, and BMP-2 gene up-regulation in PDL tissues. These molecules are abundantly expressed in osteoblasts and promote angiogenesis in association with osteogenesis via the HIF-1α pathway (Mamalis and Cochran, 2011).

Previously, we reported that morphological changes occur in craniofacial bone after IH exposure in growing rats. IH suppressed development of the nasal cavity and decreased the size of the mandibular and viscerocranial bones, which could have disturbed nasal breathing (Kuma et al., 2014; Oishi et al., 2015). Oxygen is indispensable for enzymatic reactions to promote tissue development, whereas HIF and VEGF play pivotal survival roles under hypoxic conditions (Maes et al., 2012). In the elderly,

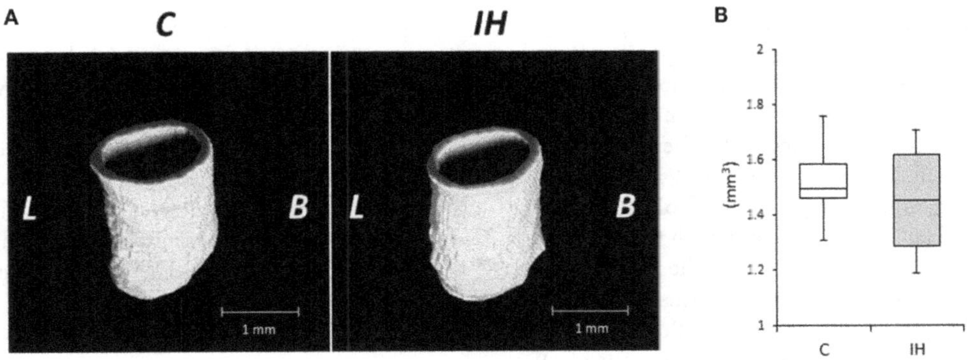

FIGURE 6 | Micro-CT analysis of the periodontal ligament (PDL) space around the distal roots in the mandibular first molar. (A) Three-dimensional reconstructed images of the periodontal ligament (PDL) space. Scale bar: 1.0 mm. C, control group; IH, IH group; L, lingual; B, buccal. **(B)** Comparison of tissue volume (TV) of the PDL around the distal root of the mandibular first molar. Box edges represent the upper and lower quantiles with the median values shown by the middle line in each box. The whiskers represent the maxima and minima. There was no significant difference in TV in the PDL between the 2 groups. $^*p < 0.05$ by the Mann–Whitney *U*-test.

it was reported that OSA is associated with an increase in BMD, which suggests that IH can stimulate bone remodeling (Sforza et al., 2013). Moreover, activation of the HIF pathway by hypoxia-mimicking agents prevents bone loss in estrogen-deficient mice, but increases BMD and trabecular microarchitecture (Peng et al., 2014). Data from the present study revealed enhanced BMD and bone development in the alveolar bone proper in the mandibular M1 region after IH exposure (**Figures 2, 3**). The 3 weeks of IH exposure starting at the age of 7 weeks in rats reflects pre-puberal development (Sengupta, 2013). Given that remodeling of inter-radicular alveolar bone, such as alveolar bone proper, in the mandibular M1 region is promoted by signals from PDL tissues (Kaku and Yamauchi, 2014), we considered that IH induced the peri-M1 changes via enhanced coupling in the signaling pathways for osteogenesis and angiogenesis in the PDL.

HIF-1α, a member of the HIF subfamily, is a ubiquitously expressed transcription factor that regulates cellular adaptation under hypoxia (Liu and Simon, 2004). VEGF is transcriptionally activated by HIF and positively regulates angiogenesis (Miyagawa et al., 2009; Wan et al., 2010). Previous findings have indicated that HIF-1α promotes both angiogenesis and osteogenesis via VEGF upregulation in osteoblasts (Wang et al., 2007). In addition, it was reported that VEGF stimulates the differentiation and chemotactic migration of osteoblastic cells (Hankenson et al., 2015), whereas HIFs and VEGF are involved in skeletal development and bone homeostasis (Wan et al., 2010; Maes et al., 2012). IH stimulates vessel network formation and VEGF production in a highly correlated fashion (Ehsan and George, 2015). The vascular system not only supplies nutrients and oxygen to developing bones, but also delivers critical signals that stimulate mesenchymal cell differentiation toward an osteogenic phenotype, whereas HIF triggers the initiation and promotion of angiogenic-osteogenic cascade events (Mamalis and Cochran, 2011). It was also shown that hypoxia promotes VEGF production in PDL cells (Motohira et al., 2007) and that the PDL plays an important role in tooth eruption (Kaku and Yamauchi, 2014). Consistent with these findings, we found increased HIF-1α and VEGF mRNA expression in peri-M1 PDL tissues after IH exposure (**Figure 4**), and the lack of change observed in the PDL space (**Figure 6**) suggests that, not mechanical force, but chemical stimulation related to HIF-1α from PDL tissues induced peri-M1 osteogenesis. Collectively, our findings indicate that HIF-1α mediated VEGF induction in PDL tissues and that VEGF induced peri-M1 osteogenesis.

We evaluated osteogenesis by studying ALP and BMP-2 expression. Given that ALP is a well-known indicator of osteoblastic differentiation, ALP expression indicates the presence of osteoblasts and osteogenic activity (Kuru et al., 1999; Nettelhoff et al., 2016). BMP-2, a member of the transforming growth factor beta superfamily, induces osteogenesis from PDL cells and the regeneration of alveolar bone by promoting osteoblastic differentiation (Selvig et al., 2002). We found significantly higher ALP and BMP-2 expression levels in PDL tissues in rats after IH exposure (**Figure 5**), which are thought to induce osteogenesis in the alveolar bone proper.

Cephalometric analysis indicated small mandibular sizes and posterior displacements in patients with OSA (Rivlin et al., 1984). Children with OSA present with increased over jet, reduced over bite, narrowed upper dental arches, and shorter lower dental arches (Pirilä-Parkkinen et al., 2009). Oral appliances and mandibular-advancement devices have been used to treat abnormal craniofacial development, such as morphological changes and intermaxillary relations in patients with OSA (Almeida et al., 2006; Hou et al., 2006). It has been suggested that a priori changes in craniofacial bones induce pathogenesis in patients with OSA.

Data from previous reports have indicated that the morphologies of mandibular and dental changes play primary roles in the development of OSA pathophysiology, whereas the present data indicated that the changes of molecular mechanism about PDL tissues in IH rat model. The osteogenesis–angiogenesis coupling phenomenon with HIF-1α and VEGF was involved in the increased BMD observed in developing alveolar bone under IH. Collectively, our data demonstrated for the first time that short periods of IH exposure can enhance peri-M1 abnormally osteogenesis via the HIF-1α-VEGF pathway in growing rats. Similar mechanisms may occur in the craniofacial bones in young children under IH exposure. Our results suggested the necessity of early treatment in children with OSA to maintain normal bone growth. Furthermore, we also demonstrated the usefulness of this IH model in studying the molecular mechanism underlying the morphological changes occurring in craniofacial bones in children with OSA. Although IH has been strongly implicated in OSA pathogenesis, OSA is associated with multifactorial pathogenesis, such as hypercapnia, intrathoracic negative pressure, and sympathetic overactivation (Fletcher, 2001). IH exposure as a single pathogenesis of OSA, a limitation of this study, is that the morphological changes observed in rats may differ somewhat from those that occur in children with OSA; thus, further morphological studies on pediatric OSA are required. Further study is also expected under different experimental settings, involving differences in IH exposure and age.

In conclusion, we demonstrated that IH increases BMD in alveolar bone proper around the roots of the first mandibular molar. Our data suggest the involvement of an osteogenesis–angiogenesis coupling phenomenon with HIF-1α and VEGF in PDL tissues. IH was found to significantly increase BMD and alter bone microstructure, potential risk factors for homeostasis disturbance in alveolar bone proper in growing IH rats. The expression levels of HIF-1α, VEGF, ALP, and BMP-2 transcripts were up-regulated in PDL tissues subjected to IH exposure for 3 weeks. Although the signaling pathway underlying IH-induced changes in the bony microstructure is not yet fully elucidated, these findings improve our current understanding of the molecular mechanisms underlying the impacts of IH on bone homeostasis.

AUTHOR CONTRIBUTIONS

SO, YS, JH, YK, HM, HN, RU, SK, NS, JS, KY, and TO conceived of and designed the study; SO performed the experiments; SO, YS, JH, and TO analyzed the data; SO, YS, JH, YK, HM, HN, RU, SK, NS, JS, KY, and TO interpreted the results of the experiments; SO and YS prepared the figures; SO drafted the manuscript; YS, JH, JS, and TO edited the manuscript; All authors approved the final version of the manuscript.

REFERENCES

Afanador, E., Yokozeki, M., Oba, Y., Kitase, Y., Takahashi, T., Kudo, A., et al. (2005). Messenger RNA expression of periostin and Twist transiently decrease by occlusal hypofunction in mouse periodontal ligament. *Arch. Oral Biol.* 50, 1023–1031. doi: 10.1016/j.archoralbio.2005.04.002

Almeida, F. R., Lowe, A. A., Sung, J. O., Tsuiki, S., and Otsuka, R. (2006). Long-term sequellae of oral appliance therapy in obstructive sleep apnea patients: part 1. Cephalometric analysis. *Am. J. Orthod. Dentofacial. Orthop.* 129, 195–204. doi: 10.1016/j.ajodo.2005.10.001

Balbani, A. P., Weber, S. A., and Montovani, J. C. (2005). Update in obstructive sleep apnea syndrome in children. *Braz. J. Otorhinolaryngol.* 71, 74–80. doi: 10.1016/S1808-8694(15)31288-X

Chen, C. C., Kanno, Z., and Soma, K. (2005). Occlusal forces promote periodontal healing of transplanted teeth with enhanced nitric oxide synthesis. *J. Med. Dent. Sci.* 52, 59–64.

Cheung, C. C., Thornton, J. E., Nurani, S. D., Clifton, D. K., and Steiner, R. A. (2001). A reassessment of leptin's role in triggering the onset of puberty in the rat and mouse. *Neuroendocrinology* 74, 12–21. doi: 10.1159/000054666

Ehsan, S. M., and George, S. C. (2015). Vessel network formation in response to intermittent hypoxia is frequency dependent. *J. Biosci. Bioeng.* 120, 347–350. doi: 10.1016/j.jbiosc.2015.01.017

Fletcher, E. C. (2001). Invited review: physiological consequences of intermittent hypoxia: systemic blood pressure. *J. Appl. Physiol.* 90, 1600–1605.

Hadjidakis, D. J., and Androulakis, I. I. (2006). Bone remodeling. *Ann. N. Y. Acad. Sci.* 1092, 385–396. doi: 10.1196/annals.1365.035

Hankenson, K. D., Gagne, K., and Shaughnessy, M. (2015). Extracellular signaling molecules to promote fracture healing and bone regeneration. *Adv. Drug Deliv. Rev.* 94, 3–12. doi: 10.1016/j.addr.2015.09.008

Hou, H. M., Sam, K., Hägg, U., Rabie, A. B., Bendeus, M., Yam, L. Y., et al. (2006). Long-term dentofacial changes in Chinese obstructive sleep apnea patients after treatment with a mandibular advancement device. *Angle Orthod.* 76, 432–440. doi: 10.1043/0003-3219(2006)076[0432:LDCICO]2.0.CO;2

Hsu, Y. H., Niu, T., Terwedow, H. A., Xu, X., Feng, Y., Li, Z., et al. (2006). Variation in genes involved in the RANKL/RANK/OPG bone remodeling pathway are associated with bone mineral density at different skeletal sites in men. *Hum. Genet.* 118, 568–577. doi: 10.1007/s00439-005-0062-4

Huang, Y. S., and Guilleminault, C. (2012). Pediatric obstructive sleep apnea and the critical role of oral-facial growth: evidences. *Front. Neurol.* 3:184. doi: 10.3389/fneur.2012.00184

Kaku, M., and Yamauchi, M. (2014). Mechano-regulation of collagen biosynthesis in periodontal ligament. *J. Prosthodont. Res.* 58, 193–207. doi: 10.1016/j.jpor.2014.08.003

Kaneko, S., Ohashi, K., Soma, K., and Yanagishita, M. (2001). Occlusal hypofunction causes changes of proteoglycan content in the rat periodontal ligament. *J. Periodontal. Res.* 36, 9–17. doi: 10.1034/j.1600-0765.2001.00607.x

Kuma, Y., Usumi-Fujita, R., Hosomichi, J., Oishi, S., Maeda, H., Nagai, H., et al. (2014). Impairment of nasal airway under intermittent hypoxia during growth period in rats. *Arch. Oral Biol.* 59, 1139–1145. doi: 10.1016/j.archoralbio.2014.06.005

Kuru, L., Griffiths, G. S., Petrie, A., and Olsen, I. (1999). Alkaline phosphatase activity is upregulated in regenerating human periodontal cells. *J. Periodontal. Res.* 34, 123–127. doi: 10.1111/j.1600-0765.1999.tb02231.x

Lal, C., Strange, C., and Bachman, D. (2012). Neurocognitive impairment in obstructive sleep apnea. *Chest* 141, 1601–1610. doi: 10.1378/chest.11-2214

Li, H., Bartold, P. M., Young, W. G., Xiao, Y., and Waters, M. J. (2001). Growth hormone induces bone morphogenetic proteins and bone-related proteins in the developing rat periodontium. *J. Bone Miner. Res.* 16, 1068–1076. doi: 10.1359/jbmr.2001.16.6.1068

Li, R., Li, X., Zhou, M., Han, N., and Zhang, Q. (2012). Quantitative determination of matrix Gla protein (MGP) and BMP-2 during the osteogenic differentiation of human periodontal ligament cells. *Arch. Oral Biol.* 57, 1408–1417. doi: 10.1016/j.archoralbio.2012.07.005

Liu, L., and Simon, M. C. (2004). Regulation of transcription and translation by hypoxia. *Cancer. Biol. Ther.* 3, 492–497. doi: 10.4161/cbt.3.6.1010

Livak, K. J., and Schmittgen, T. D. (2001). Analysis of relative gene expression data using real-time quantitative PCR and the 2(-Delta Delta C(T)) method. *Methods* 25, 402–408. doi: 10.1006/meth.2001.1262

Luan, X., Ito, Y., Holliday, S., Walker, C., Daniel, J., Galang, T. M., et al. (2007). Extracellular matrix-mediated tissue remodeling following axial movement of teeth. *J. Histochem. Cytochem.* 55, 127–140. doi: 10.1369/jhc.6A70 18.2006

Maeda, H., Nagai, H., Takemura, G., Shintani-Ishida, K., Komatsu, M., Ogura, S., et al. (2013). Intermittent-hypoxia induced autophagy attenuates contractile dysfunction and myocardial injury in rat heart. *Biochim. Biophys. Acta* 1832, 1159–1166. doi: 10.1016/j.bbadis.2013.02.014

Maes, C., Carmeliet, G., and Schipani, E. (2012). Hypoxia-driven pathways in bone development, regeneration and disease. *Nat. Rev. Rheumatol.* 8, 358–366. doi: 10.1038/nrrheum.2012.36

Mamalis, A. A., and Cochran, D. L. (2011). The therapeutic potential of oxygen tension manipulation via hypoxia inducible factors and mimicking agents in guided bone regeneration. *A review. Arch. Oral. Biol.* 56, 1466–1475. doi: 10.1016/j.archoralbio.2011.05.001

Mayahara, K., Yamaguchi, A., Takenouchi, H., Kariya, T., Taguchi, H., and Shimizu, N. (2012). Osteoblasts stimulate osteoclastogenesis via RANKL expression more strongly than periodontal ligament cells do in response to PGE(2). *Arch. Oral Biol.* 57, 1377–1384. doi: 10.1016/j.archoralbio.2012.07.009

Miyagawa, A., Chiba, M., Hayashi, H., and Igarashi, K. (2009). Compressive force induces VEGF production in periodontal tissues. *J. Dent. Res.* 88, 752–756. doi: 10.1177/0022034509341637

Motohira, H., Hayashi, J., Tatsumi, J., Tajima, M., Sakagami, H., and Shin, K. (2007). Hypoxia and reoxygenation augment bone-resorbing factor production from human periodontal ligament cells. *J. Periodontol.* 78, 1803–1809. doi: 10.1902/jop.2007.060519

Muramoto, T., Takano, Y., and Soma, K. (2000). Time-related changes in periodontal mechanoreceptors in rat molars after the loss of occlusal stimuli. *Arch. Histol. Cytol.* 63, 369–380. doi: 10.1679/aohc.63.369

Nagai, H., Kuwahira, I., Schwenke, D. O., Tsuchimochi, H., Nara, A., Ogura, S., et al. (2015). Pulmonary macrophages attenuate hypoxic pulmonary vasoconstriction via beta3AR/iNOS pathway in rats exposed to chronic intermittent hypoxia. *PLoS ONE* 10:e0131923. doi: 10.1371/journal.pone.0131923

Nettelhoff, L., Grimm, S., Jacobs, C., Walter, C., Pabst, A. M., Goldschmitt, J., et al. (2016). Influence of mechanical compression on human periodontal ligament fibroblasts and osteoblasts. *Clin. Oral Investig.* 20, 621–629. doi: 10.1007/s00784-015-1542-0

Noda, A., Ito, R., Okada, T., Yasuma, F., Nakashima, N., and Yokota, M. (1998). Twenty-four-hour ambulatory oxygen desaturation and electrocardiographic recording in obstructive sleep apnea syndrome. *Clin. Cardiol.* 21, 506–510. doi: 10.1002/clc.4960210710

Oishi, S., Shimizu, Y., Hosomichi, J., Kuma, Y., Nagai, H., Maeda, H., et al. (2015). Intermittent hypoxia induces disturbances in craniofacial growth and defects in craniofacial morphology. *Arch. Oral Biol.* 61, 115–124. doi: 10.1016/j.archoralbio.2015.10.017

Peng, J., Lai, Z. G., Fang, Z. L., Xing, S., Hui, K., Hao, C., et al. (2014). Dimethyloxalylglycine prevents bone loss in ovariectomized C57BL/6J mice through enhanced angiogenesis and osteogenesis. *PLoS ONE* 9:e112744. doi: 10.1371/journal.pone.0112744

Pirilä-Parkkinen, K., Pirttiniemi, P., Nieminen, P., Tolonen, U., Pelttari, U., and Löppönen, H. (2009). Dental arch morphology in children with sleep-disordered breathing. *Eur. J. Orthod.* 31, 160–167. doi: 10.1093/ejo/cjn061

Riddle, R. C., Khatri, R., Schipani, E., and Clemens, T. L. (2009). Role of hypoxia-inducible factor-1alpha in angiogenic-osteogenic coupling. *J. Mol. Med.* 87, 583–590. doi: 10.1007/s00109-009-0477-9

Rivlin, J., Hoffstein, V., Kalbfleisch, J., McNicholas, W., Zamel, N., and Bryan, A. C. (1984). Upper airway morphology in patients with idiopathic obstructive sleep apnea. *Am. Rev. Respir. Dis.* 129, 355–360.

Schipani, E., Maes, C., Carmeliet, G., and Semenza, G. L. (2009). Regulation of osteogenesis-angiogenesis coupling by HIFs and VEGF. *J. Bone Miner. Res.* 24, 1347–1353. doi: 10.1359/jbmr.090602

Selvig, K. A., Sorensen, R. G., Wozney, J. M., and Wikesjö, U. M. (2002). Bone repair following recombinant human bone morphogenetic protein-2 stimulated periodontal regeneration. *J. Periodontol.* 73, 1020–1029. doi: 10.1902/jop.2002.73.9.1020

Sengupta, P. (2013). The Laboratory rat: relating its age with human's. *Int. J. Prev. Med.* 4, 624–630.

Sforza, E., Thomas, T., Barthélémy, J. C., Collet, P., and Roche, F. (2013). Obstructive sleep apnea is associated with preserved bone mineral density in healthy elderly subjects. *Sleep* 36, 1509–1515. doi: 10.5665/sleep.3046

Shimizu, Y., Hosomichi, J., Nakamura, S., and Ono, T. (2014). Micro-computed tomography analysis of changes in the periodontal ligament and alveolar bone proper induced by occlusal hypofunction of rat molars. *Korean J. Orthod.* 44, 263–267. doi: 10.4041/kjod.2014.44.5.263

Skelly, J. R., Edge, D., Shortt, C. M., Jones, J. F., Bradford, A., and O'Halloran, K. D. (2012). Respiratory control and sternohyoid muscle structure and function in aged male rats: decreased susceptibility to chronic intermittent hypoxia. *Respir. Physiol. Neurobiol.* 180, 175–182. doi: 10.1016/j.resp.2011.11.004

Spence, J. M. (1940). Method of studying the skull development of the living rat by serial cephalometric roentgenograms. *Angle. Orthod.* 10, 127–139.

Wan, C., Shao, J., Gilbert, S. R., Riddle, R. C., Long, F., Johnson, R. S., et al. (2010). Role of HIF-1alpha in skeletal development. *Ann. N. Y. Acad. Sci.* 1192, 322–326. doi: 10.1111/j.1749-6632.2009.05238.x

Wang, Y., Li, Y. P., Paulson, C., Shao, J. Z., Zhang, X., Wu, M., et al. (2014). Wnt and the Wnt signaling pathway in bone development and disease. *Front. Biosci.* 19, 379–407. doi: 10.2741/4214

Wang, Y., Wan, C., Deng, L., Liu, X., Cao, X., Gilbert, S. R., et al. (2007). The hypoxia-inducible factor alpha pathway couples angiogenesis to osteogenesis during skeletal development. *J. Clin. Invest.* 117, 1616–1626. doi: 10.1172/JCI31581

8

MicroRNA Profiling during Craniofacial Development: Potential Roles for *Mir23b* and *Mir133b*

Hai-Lei Ding[1†], Joan E. Hooper[2], Peter Batzel[3], B. Frank Eames[3,4], John H. Postlethwait[3], Kristin B. Artinger[1] and David E. Clouthier[1*]*

[1] Department of Craniofacial Biology, School of Dental Medicine, University of Colorado Anschutz Medical Campus, Aurora, CO, USA, [2] Department of Cell and Developmental Biology, School of Medicine, University of Colorado Anschutz Medical Campus, Aurora, CO, USA, [3] Department of Neuroscience, University of Oregon, Eugene, OR, USA, [4] Department of Anatomy and Cell Biology, University of Saskatchewan, Saskatoon, SK, Canada

***Correspondence:**
Kristin B. Artinger
kristin.artinger@ucdenver.edu;
David E. Clouthier
david.clouthier@ucdenver.edu

†Present Address:
Hai-Lei Ding,
Laboratory of Anesthesiology, Xuzhou Medical College, Xuzhou, Jiangsu, China

Defects in mid-facial development, including cleft lip/palate, account for a large number of human birth defects annually. In many cases, aberrant gene expression results in either a reduction in the number of neural crest cells (NCCs) that reach the frontonasal region and form much of the facial skeleton or subsequent failure of NCC patterning and differentiation into bone and cartilage. While loss of gene expression is often associated with developmental defects, aberrant upregulation of expression can also be detrimental. microRNAs (miRNAs) are a class of non-coding RNAs that normally repress gene expression by binding to recognition sequences located in the 3′ UTR of target mRNAs. miRNAs play important roles in many developmental systems, including midfacial development. Here, we take advantage of high throughput RNA sequencing (RNA-seq) from different tissues of the developing mouse midface to interrogate the miRs that are expressed in the midface and select a subset for further expression analysis. Among those examined, we focused on four that showed the highest expression level in *in situ* hybridization analysis. *Mir23b* and *Mir24.1* are specifically expressed in the developing mouse frontonasal region, in addition to areas in the perichondrium, tongue musculature and cranial ganglia. *Mir23b* is also expressed in the palatal shelves and in anterior epithelium of the palate. In contrast, *Mir133b* and *Mir128.2* are mainly expressed in head and trunk musculature. Expression analysis of *mir23b* and *mir133b* in zebrafish suggests that *mir23b* is expressed in the pharyngeal arch, otic vesicle, and trunk muscle while *mir133b* is similarly expressed in head and trunk muscle. Functional analysis by overexpression of *mir23b* in zebrafish leads to broadening of the ethmoid plate and aberrant cartilage structures in the viscerocranium, while overexpression of *mir133b* causes a reduction in ethmoid plate size and a significant midfacial cleft. These data illustrate that *miRs* are expressed in the developing midface and that *Mir23b and Mir133b* may have roles in this developmental process.

Keywords: craniofacial development, neural crest cell, mouse, zebrafish, RNA duplex, facebase

INTRODUCTION

Morphogenesis of the vertebrate face is a complex event requiring coordination among a variety of signaling cascades. Human craniofacial birth defects occur at a world-wide rate of 1:800 births (Schutte and Murray, 1999; Spritz, 2001), with structural defects often resulting from failure of spatio-temporal integration of these signaling cascades. While the vertebrate mid-face has a complex embryonic origin, most facial birth defects result from disruption of cranial neural crest cell (NCC) patterning and differentiation (Chai and Maxson, 2006; Knight and Schilling, 2006; Walker and Trainor, 2006; Dixon et al., 2011; Clouthier et al., 2013). Cranial NCCs arise at the border between the neural and non-neural ectoderm and subsequently migrate to the frontonasal region (Le Douarin, 1982; Bronner-Fraser, 1995). These cells eventually give rise to most of the bone, cartilage, and connective tissue of the mid-face and neck (Couly et al., 1996; Köntges and Lumsden, 1996). NCC development relies on intricate regulation of patterning cues within specific boundaries of the head. While boundaries are established through continuous refinement of gene expression, the mechanisms required for this refinement are less clear.

MicroRNAs (miRNAs) are a class of small, noncoding RNAs that inhibit translation of target mRNAs by binding to a recognition sequence almost always in the 3′ untranslated region (UTR) of the target mRNA (Lee et al., 1993; Wightman et al., 1993; Lai, 2002; Lewis et al., 2003). This binding results in decreased mRNA translation through a number of mechanisms that can include cleavage and degradation of the target mRNA, translational repression, deadenylation of the 3′-poly(A) tail and thus mRNA decay and miRNA sponging (Hutvágner et al., 2001; Zheng and Cullen, 2003; Wu et al., 2006; Hausser and Zavolan, 2014; Jens and Rajewsky, 2015). miRNAs have been implicated in many clinically relevant processes, including development, cancer, and stem cell maintenance and differentiation (Chen et al., 2012; Fernández-Hernando et al., 2013; Kuppusamy et al., 2013; Morceau et al., 2013; Parpart and Wang, 2013). miRNAs are also involved in numerous aspects of craniofacial development, including palatogenesis, odontogenesis, and upper and lower jaw development (Tavares et al., 2015). One of the first examples of miRNA action in facial development is *mir140*, whose regulation of *pdgfra* is required for NCCs to migrate past the optic stalk on their way from the hindbrain to the future palate (Eberhart et al., 2008). A SNP in the human *MIR140* gene leads to reduced *Mir140* expression in murine palatal mesenchymal cells (Li et al., 2011). In addition, this SNP is associated with increased risk of nonsyndromic cleft palate in mothers who smoke during pregnancy (Li et al., 2010). These findings suggest that miRNA function is evolutionarily conserved and illustrates a role for miRNAs in human palate development. Another miRNA family involved in craniofacial development is the *MIR17* and *MIR92* family, which has been linked to Feingold syndrome in human patients (Kannu et al., 2013; Tassano et al., 2013). Targeted knockouts of *Mir17 and Mir92* in mice results in hypoplasia of most skull bones, including reduced ossification and cleft palate, similar to human patients (Ventura et al., 2008; de Pontual et al., 2011; Li et al., 2012; Wang et al., 2013). In addition, others, such as *Mir196*, *Mir199*, and *Mir200* have likely roles in determining craniofacial size, bone and cartilage formation, and cartilage size, respectively (Watanabe et al., 2008; Desvignes et al., 2014). However, targeted deletion of the miRNA processing enzyme DICER in NCCs results in hypoplasia of most craniofacial structures, suggesting that numerous other miRNAs are also likely involved in this process (Huang et al., 2010; Zehir et al., 2010; Nie et al., 2011; Oommen et al., 2012).

Here, we use data from a high-throughput miRNA sequencing project of developing mouse facial structures to identify many miRNAs that are potentially involved in craniofacial development. We have examined the expression of a number of these miRNAs in both mouse and zebrafish. Further, we have performed functional analysis of four of these miRNAs in zebrafish. Our *in situ* hybridization and overexpression analyses provide evidence that *Mir23b* and *Mir133b* are important regulators of craniofacial development.

MATERIALS AND METHODS

miRNA-Seq Differential Expression Analysis

RNA-Seq count data with gene assignments have been deposited in the FaceBase repository for craniofacial research (www.facebase.org). Specific FaceBase accession numbers are: E10.5 FB00000662.01, E11.5 FB00000663.01, E12.5 FB00000664.01, FB00000664.01, E13.5 FB00000665.01, E14.5 FB00000666.01. Counts of overlapping and nested sequences assigned to each mature (1035 sequences) or hairpin (306 sequences) mouse miRNA were summed to obtain consolidated counts per mature or hairpin miRNA (724 and 255, respectively). A threshold of 1 was used for the RNA-seq analysis. After low filtering (mean counts per sample >5; 629 mature miRs and 163 hairpin miRNAs), we used DESeq to identify miRNAs differentially expressed by anatomy or age. For principal components analysis and hierarchical clustering, count data was normalized using the regularized log transformation in the DESeq R package. A $p < 0.01$ after multiple testing correction (Benjamini and Hochberg method) was used, as well as no fold-change threshold (Benjamini and Hochberg, 1995).

Mouse and Zebrafish Maintenance

All mouse embryo collection was performed using 129S6 mice (Taconic), with the day of the copulation plug denoted as 0.5 days. Embryo collection and fixation were performed as previously described (Clouthier et al., 1998). Zebrafish were maintained according to common lab practice (Westerfield, 2000), with embryo staging according to established methods (Kimmel et al., 1995). The wild type lines used are AB and an in-cross line maintained between the AB and TL lines (TAB). This study was carried out in accordance with the recommendations of the Institutional Animal Care and Use Committee (IACUC) of the University of Colorado Anschutz Medical Campus as laid out in protocols approved by IACUC. Nomenclature for miRNAs is consistent with that described in Desvignes et al. (2015).

For simplicity, pri-MiR(mouse) and pri-miR (zebrafish) were annotated without the "pri" in the text below.

Cloning and Probe Synthesis

To detect expression of mouse MiRNAs, we used both Locked Nucleic Acid (LNA; Obernosterer et al., 2007) and conventional riboprobes against the primary *pri-MiR* transcripts, both labeled with digoxigenin (He et al., 2011). For LNA-based experiments, Exiqon LNA *Mir133b* (#616614-360) and *Mir23b* (#615366-360) probes were used. To generate *pri-MiR* probes, PCR primers were designed to amplify about 200–600 nt of the primary MiR transcript centered on the mature miRNA sequence for mouse and zebrafish. All primer sequences are given in Supplemental Table 1. To generate mouse *pri-MiRs,* PCR primers were used with genomic tail DNA obtained from tails of 2 month old mice. To generate zebrafish *pri-miRs*, PCR primers were used with 5 day post fertilization (dpf) zebrafish embryos. PCR products were cloned into the pCR®II-TOPO® Vector (Invitrogen). Inserts were validated by sequencing. Plasmids were linearized and transcribed using the DIG Labeling Kit (Roche). Probes were purified as previously described (Clouthier et al., 1998). The opposite stand sense probes were used as controls for specificity for the antisense expression (data not shown).

Mouse and Zebrafish Whole Mount *In situ* Hybridization (ISH)

Whole mount ISH in mouse was performed as previously described (Clouthier et al., 1998). For sectional miRNA ISH, serial 10 μm frontal sections through the head of E12.5 and/or E13.5 mouse embryos were collected on Superfrost Plus slides (Fisher). Subsequent ISH was performed as previously described (Hendershot et al., 2007). Hybridizations were performed at 70°C overnight. Colorimetric detection was performed with BM purple (Roche). Signal detection required an average of 2–3 days in staining solution. After developing, slides were rinsed in TBST, coverslipped and photographed using Nomarski optics on an Olympus BX51 compound microscope fitted with a DP71 digital camera. Whole-mount ISH in zebrafish was performed as previously described (Johnson et al., 2011). BM Purple (Roche) was used as a substrate for the alkaline phosphatase reaction. After staining, embryos were mounted in 80% glycerol or 3% methylcellulose and imaged under Nomarski optics on the Olympus BX51 compound microscope as described for mice.

Overexpression Analysis and Bone and Cartilage Staining

MiRNA duplexes were created by annealing 5p and 3p MiRs together at 95°C and slowly cooling to room temperature (MiR133b-3p: UUUGGUCCCCUUCAACCA; MiR133b-5p: GCUGGUCAAAUGGAACCA; MiR23b-3p: AUCACAUUG CCAGGGAUU; MiR23b-5p: GGUUCUUGGCAUGCUGA). Thirty-three micrometers of MiR23b duplex (5′—3′), 6.25 μM of MiR133b (5′—3′), and 33 μM of standard control miRNA (5′- CTTACCTCAGTTACAATTTATA -3 duplexed with 5′-TAAATTGTAACTGAGGTAAGAG-3′) were injected into single cell zebrafish embryos and allowed to grow for 6 dpf. Zebrafish embryos were fixed and stained with alizarin red and alcian blue (Birkholz et al., 2009) with minor modifications. Larvae were fixed in 2% PFA/PBS for 1 h at room temperature, washed in 100 mM Tris (pH 7.5)/10 mM $MgCl_2$, and stained overnight in 0.04% alcian blue (Anatech Ltd) in 80% EtOH/100 mM Tris (pH 7.5)/10 mM $MgCl_2$. Larvae were then rehydrated in 80% EtOH/100 mM Tris (pH 7.5)/10 mM $MgCl_2$, followed by 50 and 25% EtOH/100 mM Tris (pH 7.5), cleared in 25% glycerol/0.1% KOH, then stained 30 min with 0.01% alizarin red (Sigma) in 25% glycerol/100 mM Tris (pH 7.5) and stored in 50% glycerol/0.1% KOH. Stained skeletons were dissected, flat-mounted and imaged as previously described (Johnson et al., 2011).

RESULTS

Identification of miRNAs Involved in Midfacial Development from miRNA-Seq Data

We have previously conducted massively parallel miRNA sequencing (miRNA-Seq) on miRNAs extracted from embryonic age (E) 10.5, E11.5, E12.5, E13.5, and E14.5 mouse maxillary prominences, frontonasal prominences, and palatal shelves, with the data deposited in FaceBase (www.facebase.org). Between E10.5 and E11.5, NCC-derived mesenchyme that will give rise to craniofacial structures undergoes significant patterning events that establishes the positional and functional identity of the mesenchyme. Between E12.5 and E14.5, gene expression in the facial region is driving differentiation into the bone and cartilage of the upper and lower face. Because we are interested in the mechanisms that govern this second event, we focused our analysis of miRNA expression between E12.5 and E14.5. Using a combination of biostatical approaches and packages (Section Materials and Methods), we identified 262 differentially expressed mature miRNAs and 71 hairpin miRNAs at a false discovery rate-adjusted $p > 0.01$ (data not shown). Of these, 49 mature miRNAs and 11 hairpin miRNAs were differentially expressed between maxillary prominences, frontonasal prominences, and palatal shelves (**Figure 1A**); some also differed by age (**Figure 2**). **Table 1** shows the top differentially expressed miRNAs as total counts, while **Figure 2** shows the log2fold change in expression of specific miRNAs between facial prominences at E13.5. Total counts of each miRNA are also shown in **Table 1** so that the relative expression of miRNAs can be compared.

Principal Components Analysis of miRNAs Expressed in the Face

Principal Components Analysis (PCA) is a primary quality control assay, with the expectation that replicates will cluster and that principal components might reflect known qualities of the sample conditions (e.g., age, anatomy) or of the experiment (e.g., batch or read depth). After sequence consolidation and low-expression filtering, normalized counts for 979 miRNAs (724 mature miRNAs and 255 hairpin miRNAs) were used to analyze the principal components of the variability among the 24 samples (**Figure 1B**). The first principal component, which

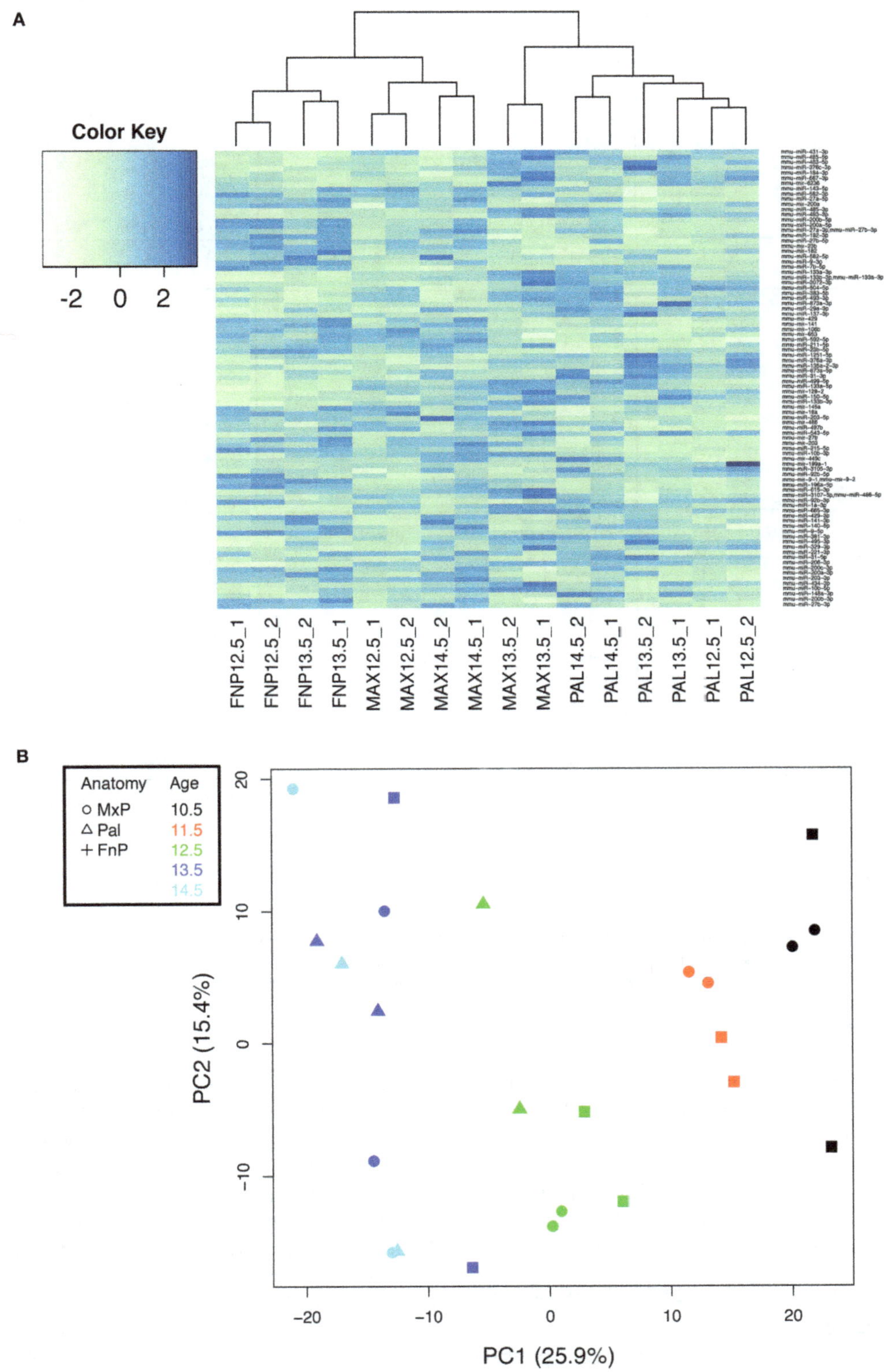

FIGURE 1 | Analysis of miRNA-Seq data defines miRNAs whose expression differs by prominence. (A) 49 mature miRNAs and 11 hairpin miRNAs were differentially expressed by prominence (FDR adjusted $p < 0.01$). Hierarchical clustering of their normalized and scaled expression values (using the R hclust function, ward. D2 method) shows groups of miRNAs enriched in the frontonasal prominence (FnP), palate (Pal), the maxillary prominence (Max), or in combinations thereof. The dendrogram at the top shows the clustering of the samples; the three major divisions correspond to FnP, Pal, and Max, and duplicate samples cluster together. **(B)** Principal Component Analysis (PCA) analysis of data. Data is color coded by age (inset), with tissue source denoted by symbol (inset). Principal Component 1 (PC1) distributes samples by age. Principal Component 2 (PC2) is orthogonal to PC1 but does not correspond to any obvious property of the samples.

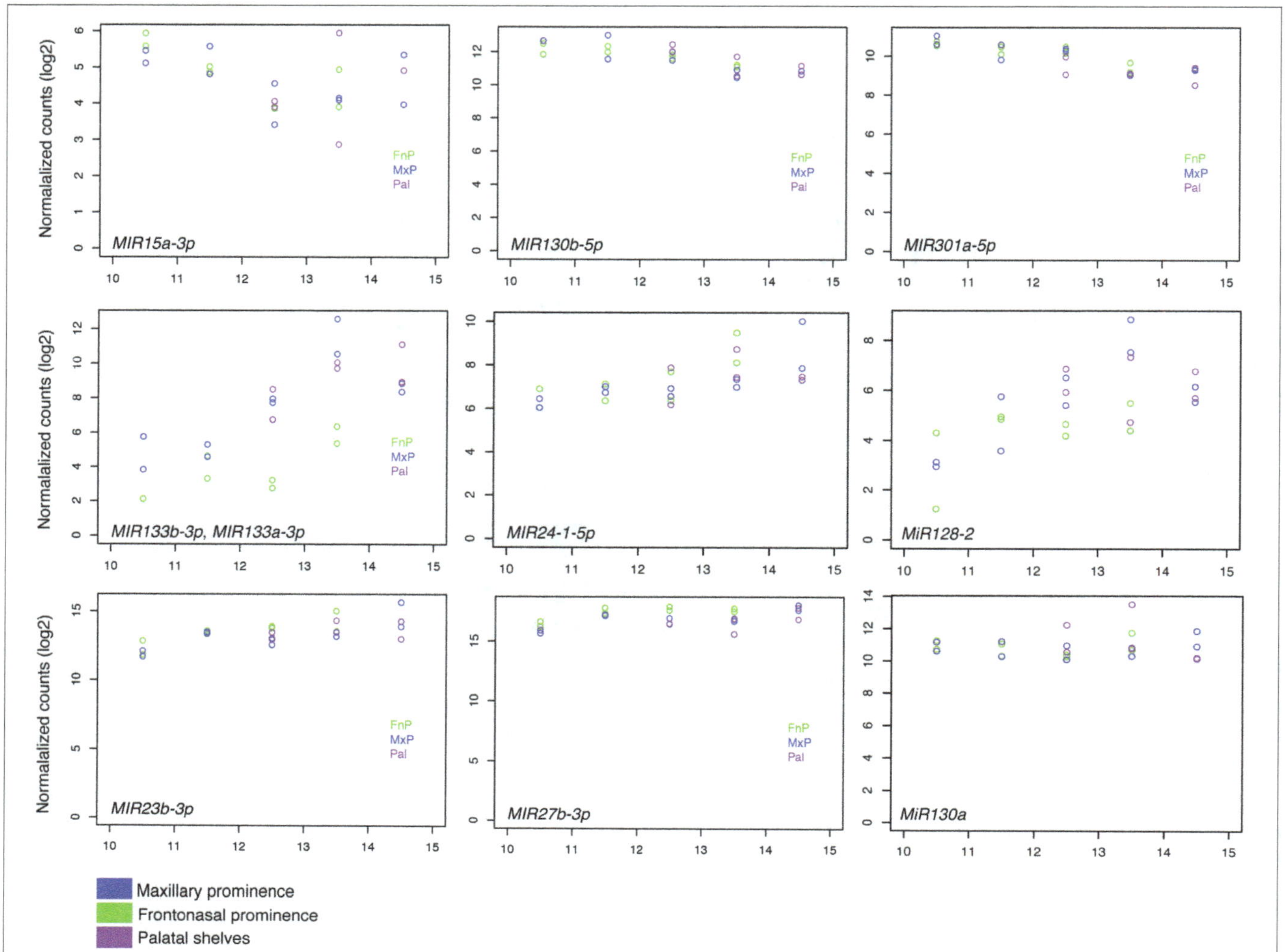

FIGURE 2 | RNAseq values for expression of selected miRNAs. Normalized counts for selected miRNAs from each prominence (see inset) as compared to embryonic age (E10–15). Each row represents a different pattern of expression over time. **(Top)** *Mir15a*, *Mir130b*, and *Mir301a* showed a downward trend of expression over time. **(Middle)** Expression of *Mir133b*, *Mir24.1,* and *Mir1282* increased over time. **(Bottom)** *Mir23b*, *Mir27b*, and *Mir130a* were expressed consistently over time. Blue, Maxillary prominence; Green, Frontonasal prominence; and Purple, Palate.

accounts for 26% of the variability, distributed the samples by age (color-coded). Neither prominence (symbols) nor read depth (not shown) correlated with any of the top five principal components. Biological duplicates from E10.5-E12.5 tended to cluster, indicating biological reproducibility at those ages. Together these demonstrate the biological reproducibility for key miRNAs between replicates and within prominences.

Expression Analysis of Selected miRNAs in the Mouse at E12.5

For our *in situ* hybridization (ISH) analysis of miRNA expression in the developing midface, we focused on E12.5 mouse embryos, as at this stage, the lateral and medial nasal prominences, palatal shelves, and maxilla are well-defined and are undergoing extensive growth. We initially examined miRNA expression in E12.5 mouse embryo using whole mount ISH and LNA probes against *Mir23b*, *Mir24.1,* and *Mir666* (Supplemental Figure 1). LNA probes specifically detect the mature Mir sequence. However, the overall level of expression of these Mir's as detected in whole mount analysis was low (likely due in part to poor probe penetration; Supplemental Figure 1), leading us to examine Mir expression using frozen sectional ISH analysis. When using LNA probes against *Mir23b* and *Mir133b*, robust expression was present in a variety of facial structures, though overall background staining on the sections was high (Supplemental Figure 2). To next assess whether we could improve the signal to noise ratio of the staining, we PCR-generated probes against the pri-miRNA transcript, an approach we have previously used to examine Mir expression in embryos (He et al., 2011). Probes encompassed the pri-miRNA sequence (see (Section) Materials and Methods). These probes detect both pri-miRNAs and mature miRNAs, so expression is expected in both the nucleus and cytoplasm. However, the relative abundance of mature miRNAs for any single species

TABLE 1 | microRNAs that are differentially expressed between prominences at E13.5.

microRNA	Normalized counts						Pattern
	Fn (1)	Fn (2)	Mx (1)	Mx (2)	Pal (1)	Pal (2)	
MIR1a-3p	911.78	711.95	**9059.94**	**11523.71**	**3472.3**	**4385.36**	Pal&Mx
MiR128.2	45.21	20.06	**444.7**	**181.49**	**157.72**	**24.72**	Pal&Mx
MIR133a-3p	67.82	165.42	**3063.12**	**1421.33**	**628.5**	**722.18**	Pal&Mx
MIR133a-5p	11.3	23.03	**225.67**	**249.28**	**47.79**	**186.84**	Pal&Mx
MIRp133b-3p	0	10.9	**560.85**	**203.36**	**109.93**	**186.37**	Pal&Mx
MIR133b-3p, MIR133a-3p	41.44	77.51	**5883.99**	**1478.18**	**1049.1**	**781.84**	pAL&Mx
MIR184-3p	97.96	97.57	**829.67**	**467.95**	**389.53**	**285.26**	Pal&Mx
MIR206-3p	678.18	281.07	**26993.99**	**23655.32**	**13105.35**	**10618**	Pal&Mx
MIR214-3p	14901.2	6127.98	**19507.09**	**17443.01**	**20518.33**	**28066.97**	Pal&Mx
MIR483-3p	331.56	253.33	**1158.21**	**682.24**	**924.83**	**584.54**	Pal&Mx
MIR499-5p	15.07	25.01	**235.62**	**308.32**	**52.57**	**156.18**	Pal&Mx
MIR3099-3p	90.42	48.54	**132.75**	**124.64**	**136.22**	**154.51**	Pal&Mx
MIR137-3p	56.52	67.36	**185.84**	**67.79**	**143.38**	**911.87**	Pal>Mx
MIR483-5p	350.39	151.8	**487.84**	**756.59**	**642.84**	**1184.77**	Pal>Mx
let-7e-5p	3142.25	3950.77	2216.87	5053.38	**4698.23**	**15721.97**	Pal
MIR31-3p	11.3	37.64	19.91	21.87	**64.52**	**221.07**	Pal
MIR31-5p	877.87	1350.11	365.05	531.36	**1464.91**	**4273.87**	Pal
MIR135a-2-3p	18.84	22.29	46.46	54.67	**114.71**	**150.47**	Pal
MIR376c-3p	184.62	181.02	348.46	419.84	**291.55**	**841.27**	Pal
MIR450a-2-3p	3.77	29.22	6.64	4.37	**23.9**	**68.46**	Pal
MIR495-3p	565.15	1077.21	1181.44	1176.42	**996.52**	**2931.26**	Pal
MIR500-3p	470.96	430.88	418.15	750.03	**630.89**	**1213.3**	Pal
MIR873a-3p	94.19	61.91	146.02	67.79	**611.77**	**54.44**	Pal
MIR873a-5p	60.28	75.78	23.23	41.55	**157.72**	**174.24**	Pal
MIR1251-5p	26.37	91.38	89.6	61.23	**133.83**	**434.07**	Pal
MIR7b-5p	**768.61**	**226.09**	49.78	61.23	**1032.37**	**305.46**	Fn>Pal
MIR200a-3p	**13639.02**	**20365.01**	2598.51	3391.51	**3345.64**	**13267.57**	Fn&Pal
MIR9-3p	**968.3**	**1467.98**	89.6	104.96	71.69	139.54	Fn
MIR9-5p	**7490.16**	**4400.23**	726.79	763.15	365.63	487.32	Fn
MiR23b	**380.54**	**244.91**	79.65	104.96	86.03	71.31	Fn
MiR141	**259.97**	**162.7**	26.55	48.11	26.29	51.35	Fn
MiR200a	**862.8**	**569.81**	149.34	150.88	303.5	66.32	Fn
MIR200b-3p	**141254.31**	**59360.85**	7055.47	17631.06	15461.64	23046.91	Fn
MIR200b-5p	**779.91**	**289.98**	73.01	96.21	164.89	87.48	Fn
MIR3085-3p	**3.77**	**29.72**	13.27	8.75	7.17	9.75	Fn
MIR429-3p	**5218.24**	**10519.04**	1085.2	1445.38	1930.91	3339.65	Fn
MiR653	**195.92**	**80.98**	33.19	102.77	69.3	63.71	Fn
Mir19b.1	**184.62**	**198.11**	**59.74**	**170.56**	50.18	146.67	Fn> Mx
MiR27b	**64.05**	**23.77**	**19.91**	**8.75**	4.78	5.94	Fn> Mx
MIR200a-5p	**678.18**	**249.12**	**79.65**	**87.47**	95.59	62.99	Fn> Mx
MiR429	**327.79**	**131.99**	**39.82**	**76.53**	28.68	43.03	Fn> Mx
MIR215-5p	**75.35**	**54.97**	**6.64**	**13.12**	4.78	3.09	Fn> Mx
MiR18a	**33.91**	**36.9**	**26.55**	**15.31**	14.34	28.29	Fn & Mx
MIR18b-5p	**52.75**	**48.29**	**13.27**	**32.8**	9.56	64.9	Fn & Mx
MIR20b-5p	**437.05**	**646.33**	**172.57**	**321.44**	114.71	422.89	Fn & Mx
MIR27b-5p	**440.82**	**129.02**	**73.01**	**181.49**	64.52	78.68	Fn & Mx
MiR92a.2	**832.66**	**1542.27**	**1025.47**	**848.43**	1493.59	657.99	Fn & Mx
MIR106a-5p	**290.11**	**252.84**	**69.69**	**177.12**	33.46	192.07	Fn & Mx
MiR106b	**128.1**	**70.82**	**49.78**	**59.04**	23.9	22.82	Fn & Mx
MIR182-3p	**395.61**	**350.16**	**126.11**	**65.6**	148.16	99.36	Fn & Mx

(Continued)

TABLE 1 | Continued

microRNA	Normalized counts						Pattern
	Fn (1)	Fn (2)	Mx (1)	Mx (2)	Pal (1)	Pal (2)	
MIR293-3p	**11.3**	**11.39**	**13.27**	**13.12**	4.78	10.7	Fn & Mx
MIR302a-5p	**30.14**	**20.06**	**26.55**	**34.99**	11.95	23.77	Fn & Mx
MIR302b-3p	**18.84**	**85.68**	**53.1**	**39.36**	33.46	70.84	Fn & Mx
MIR302d-3p	**48.98**	**84.2**	**46.46**	**72.16**	43.02	117.67	Fn & Mx
MiR326	**26.37**	**26.5**	**29.87**	**26.24**	23.9	7.84	Fn & Mx
MiR3473f	**7.54**	**9.66**	**13.27**	**26.24**	0	5.71	Fn & Mx
MIR582-3p	**391.84**	**241.69**	**574.13**	**301.76**	210.3	69.89	Fn & Mx
MiR6399	**26.37**	**4.46**	**9.96**	**4.37**	2.39	1.19	Fn & Mx
MiR6539	**45.21**	**13.12**	**16.59**	**30.61**	14.34	15.93	Fn & Mx
MIR18b-3p	**0**	**4.21**	**0**	**0**	2.39	0.95	Mx>Fn
MIR128.1-5p	**90.42**	**33.93**	**172.57**	**48.11**	64.52	28.76	Mx>Fn
MIR211-5p	**131.87**	**119.11**	**242.26**	**74.35**	21.51	15.93	Mx>Fn
MIR216b-5p	**26.37**	**52.99**	**33.19**	**8.75**	2.39	19.97	Mx>Fn
MIR217-5p	**22.61**	**21.3**	**13.27**	**30.61**	2.39	7.84	Mx>Fn
MIR363-3p	**252.43**	**832.8**	**504.44**	**284.27**	446.88	173.53	Mx>Fn
MiR486	**26.37**	**6.44**	**132.75**	**83.09**	28.68	6.89	Mx>Fn
MIR741-3p	**3.77**	**2.72**	**23.23**	**0**	0	1.66	Mx>Fn

Colored and bolded areas indicate groups of miRs that are highly expressed within a specific prominence. Green, Frontal nasal prominence (Fn); Brown, Maxilla (Mx); Pink, Palate (Pal).

TABLE 2 | Expression profiles of miRNAs in the developing mouse midface.

miRNA	Embryonic age	Expression profile
Mir15a	E12.5	Tongue, oral and nasal epithelium, nasal mesenchyme
Mir20a	E12.5	Eye, lung, brain
Mir23b	E12.5, E13.5	Naris, vibrissae, TG, DRG, palatal shelf, maxilla, tongue, nasal and tongue epithelium, tongue muscle, incisor, otic capsule, malleus, diencephalon, limb muscle, mesothelium, intervertebral space, foregut, gastrointestinal neurons
Mir24.1	E12.5, E13.5	Vibrissae, TG, DRG, nasal epithelium, maxilla, tongue, incisor, limb muscle, gastrointestinal neurons, mesothelium, intervertebral space, pinna
Mir27b	E12.5	Tongue, limb, rib, pinna, TG, nasal epithelium, eye, vibrissae, brain, facial cartilage, intestinal neuron
Mir128.2	E12.5, E13.5	Maxilla, TG, DRG, tongue, diencephalon, telencephalon, ocular muscles, limb, mesothelium, ribs
Mir130a	E12.5	Tongue, rib, limb, intestine, facial cartilage, nasal epithelium, maxilla
Mir130b	E12.5	Tongue, intestine, facial cartilage, nasal epithelium, maxilla
Mir133b	E12.5, E13.5	Vibrissae, maxilla, TG, tongue, intervertebral space, hyoid, ocular muscles, diencephalon, muscle, mesothelium, ribs
Mir206	E12.5	Tongue, rib, limb, eye, maxilla, nasal epithelium
Mir335	E12.5	Tongue, brain
Mir376	E12.5	Tongue, rib, mandible, vertebrae, lateral nasal prominence
Mir411	E13.5	Tongue, proximal mandible and mesenchyme of the outflow tract, maxillary mesenchyme
Mir666	E12.5, E13.5	FNP, DRG, ocular muscle, tongue, mandible, vertebrae, mesothelium, ribs, liver, spinal cord, limb

compared to that of pri-miRNA species makes it far more likely that these probes detect the mature miRNA. Further, we have shown that the use of pri-miRNA probes for miRNA ISH provides comparable results to those using LNA probes (He et al., 2011). Based on our bioinformatics analysis (**Figures 1, 2**), we examined the expression of 13 pri-miRNAs in E12.5 mouse embryos and found that many were expressed in specific embryonic tissues, including facial structures (**Table 2** and Supplemental Figures 3-9). Based on this initial analysis of ISH data, we focused our subsequent analysis on *MiR23b* and *MiR133b*.

Expression of *MiR23b* and *MiR133b* in Mouse Facial Structures at E12.5

In E12.5 wild type mouse embryos, *MiR23b* expression appeared throughout the facial region including the nasal epithelium, mystacial vibrissae, and vomeronasal nasal organs (**Figures 3A–C**), upper incisors (**Figure 3D**), tongue connective tissue and epithelium (**Figures 3E,F**), and maxillary epithelium (**Figure 3F**). Expression was also observed in the anterior palatal shelves, with expression more prominent on the nasal side of the shelves (**Figures 3E,F**) and in the trigeminal ganglion (**Figure 3G**). In addition, *MiR23b* was expressed along the

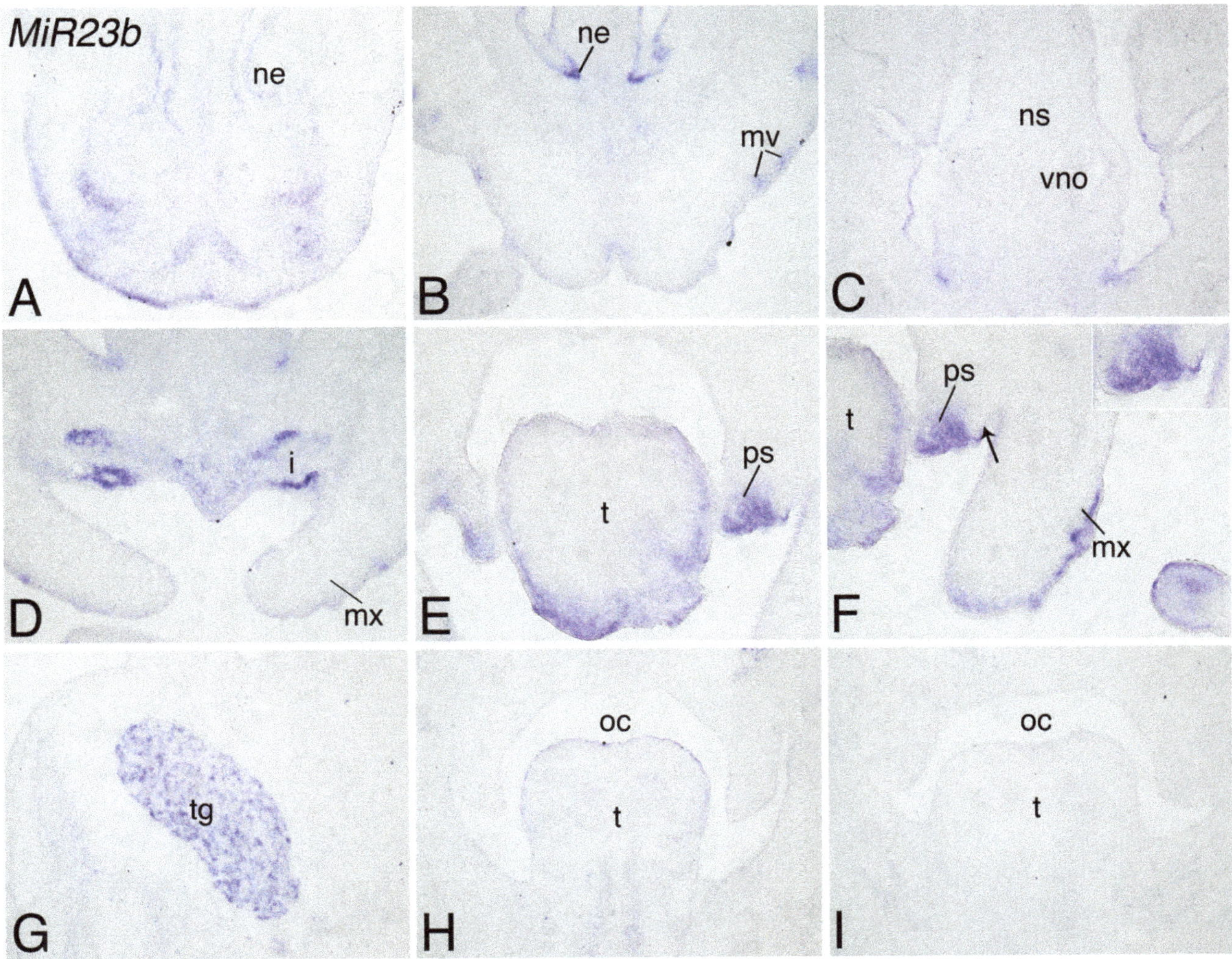

FIGURE 3 | Expression of *Mir23b* in mouse facial structures at E12.5. ISH analysis in frozen frontal sections through the head of E12.5 mouse embryos. **(A–C)** *Mir23b* is moderately expressed in the nasal epithelium epithelium (ne), mystacial vibrissae (mv), nasal septum (ns), and vomeronasal organ (vo). **(D–F)** *Mir23b* is also expressed in the upper incisors (i), tongue (t), maxillary epithelium (te), and palatal shelves (ps). The arrow in **(F)** denotes the epithelium where *Mir23b* expression begins. **(G–I)** More posteriorly, expression is observed in the trigeminal ganglion (tg; **G**), posterior tongue (t; **H,I**). i, incisor; mx, maxilla; oc, oral cavity.

palatal shelf epithelium, again starting at the midline of the shelf and continuing on the oral side (**Figures 3H,I**). Overall, the expression pattern of *MiR23b* supported our analysis (**Figure 1**), though it was difficult to assess the qualitative differences in expression between prominences compared to the quantitative differences of miRNA-seq. In the genome, *MiR23b* is part of the 850 bp *Mirc23* cluster, which contains *Mir23b*, *Mir27b*, and *Mir3074.1*. In addition, *Mir24.1* is 5 kb away from *Mir23b*. As previously described for many clustered miRNAs (Lagos-Quintana et al., 2003; Lim et al., 2003), *Mir24.1* had an expression pattern similar to that observed for *Mir23b*, including expression in the nasal epithelium (Supplemental Figures 3A–C), tongue (Supplemental Figures 3E,F,H,I) and maxillary process epithelium (Supplemental Figure 3D), though expression in the palatal shelf mesenchyme and overlying epithelium (Supplemental Figures 3D,F,H,I) and trigeminal ganglia (Supplemental Figure 3G) was weak.

Like *MiR23b*, *MiR133b* was also strongly expressed in the craniofacial region at E12.5. Weak expression was observed in the nasal epithelium, mystacial vibrissae and maxilla (**Figures 4A–C**), but strong expression was observed in facial musculature, including the intrinsic and extrinsic musculature of the tongue and eye (**Figures 4D–I**) and facial muscles (including the masseter muscle (arrow; **Figure 4F**). Expression of *MiR133b* was not observed in the maxilla or palatal shelves, suggesting that the expression observed by miRNA-seq might reflect presence of other tissue in dissected samples. Like *Mir23b*, *Mir133b* exists in a cluster with *Mir206*, which had a similar pattern of expression to that of *Mir133b*. Message was primarily detected in facial muscles (Supplemental Figures 4E,F), with message also detected in the cornea and lens of the eye (Supplemental Figure 4A). Further, like the comparison between *MiR23b* and *MiR24.1*, expression of *MiR206* was much weaker than the expression observed for *MiR133b*.

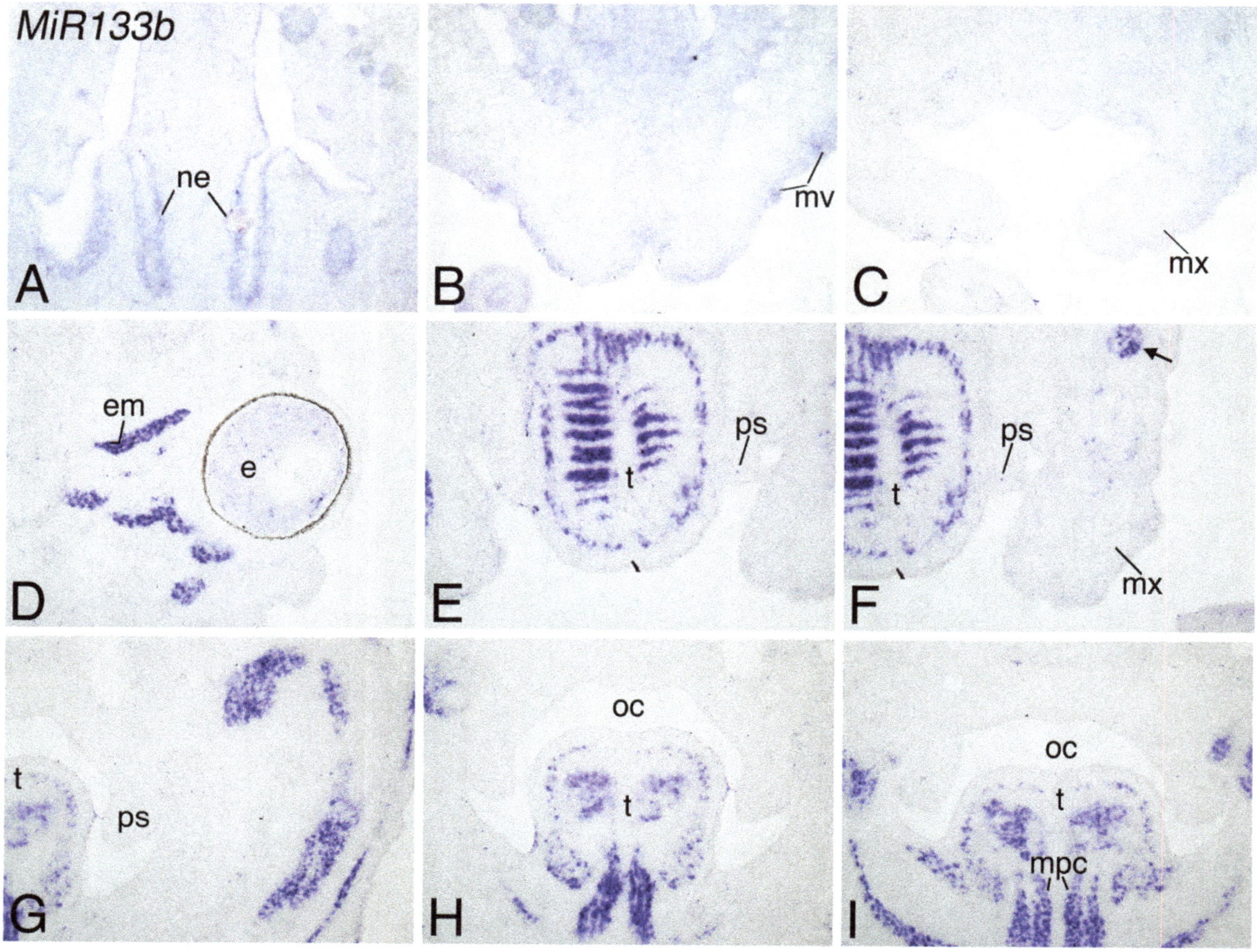

FIGURE 4 | Expression of *Mir133b* in mouse facial muscles at E12.5. ISH analysis in frozen frontal sections through the head of E12.5 mouse embryos. **(A–C)** *Mir133b* is weakly expressed in the nasal epithelium (ne; **A**), mystacial vibrissae (mv; **B**), and maxilla (mx); **(D–F).** (mx); **(D–F).** *Mir133b* is strongly expressed in facial muscles, including the masseter (ma), and in the muscles of the eye (em; **D**) and tongue muscle (t; **E–I**) Expression is not observed in the palatal shelves (ps; **E,F**). **(G–I)** Posterior expression continues continues in the tongue muscles. e, eye; oc, oral cavity.

Expression of *mir23b* and *mir133b* is Conserved in Zebrafish Facial Structures

Based on analysis of *mir140* action, miRNA function during facial development is also present in zebrafish embryos. Similarly, we found that a selected subset of the miRNAs from **Table 1** were also expressed in the head region of 30-hours post fertilization (hpf) zebrafish embryos (**Table 3** and Supplemental Figure 10). To examine whether the pattern of expression of *mir23b* and *mir133b* was also conserved between mouse and zebrafish embryos, we examined expression of both miRNAs in 30–72 hpf embryos. Expression of *mir23b* was detected in the head and pharyngeal arch mesenchyme (**Figure 5A**) and in the somitic mesoderm (**Figure 5D**) at 30 hpf. Diffuse expression was also present in the eye (**Figure 5A**). At 48 hpf, *mir23b* expression was still present in the head and pharyngeal arch mesenchyme while also appearing in the otic vesicle (**Figure 5B**). Expression was also observed in the trunk muscle and notochord (**Figure 5E**). By 72 hpf, expression remained in cranial muscle (**Figures 5C,G**) while also being present in the somite-derived trunk muscle and notochord (**Figure 5F**) and in ceratobranchial structures (arrows, **Figure 5G**).

At 30 hpf, *mir133b* expression was also observed in the head region (around the eye and portions of the brain; **Figure 6A**), though expression was weaker than that of *mir23b*. Expression was quite strong in the developing somites (**Figure 6D**). By 48 hpf, expression around the otic vesicle, eye, and posterior brain was increased (**Figures 6B,G**). As in 30 hpf embryos, *mir133b* was strongly expressed in the somites (**Figure 6E**). By 72 hpf, *mir133b* expression was observed in trunk muscles (**Figure 6F**), otic vesicle and heart (**Figure 6C**). Expression was also present in the facial muscles, including the anterior mandibularis (arrow, **Figure 6H**) and muscles developing near the ceratobranchials, including the stemohyoideus (arrowheads, **Figure 6H**).

TABLE 3 | Expression profiles of miRNAs in the developing zebrafish.

miRNA	Embryonic age	Expression profile
mir15a	48 and 72 hpf	Midbrain, MHB, notochord
mir15b	48 and 72 hpf	Midbrain, neurocranium, notochord
mir23b	30, 48, and 72 hpf	Somites, lens, pharyngeal arches, notochord
mir27b	48 and 72 hpf	
mir30c	48 and 72 hpf	Brain, neurocranium, eye, heart
mir130a	48 and 72 hpf	Brain, gut tube, heart, eye
mir133b	30, 48, and 72 hpf	Notochord
mir301a	48 and 72 hpf	Forming cartilage
		Midbrain, neurocranium, eye, trigeminal ganglia

mir23b and *mir133b* Overexpression Results in Viscerocranial and Neurocranial Defects in Zebrafish

Two potential methods for assessing function of genes in zebrafish are over-expression and gene inactivation. While Crispr-Cas9-mediated gene inactivation is underway, we began our analysis of potential function by injecting 1–2 cell zebrafish embryos with duplex RNA for MiR23b and MiR133b examining cartilage development at 6 dpf. Overexpression of miRNA duplex is more likely to generate a phenotype, as increasing the repressor function will result in reduced gene expression of the miRNA gene targets. In the viscerocranium, MiR23b duplex injection resulted in aberrant development of Meckel's cartilage and the ceratohyal (**Figure 7B**). In addition, ectopic cartilage extended from the basihyal to the medial aspect of Meckel's cartilage (23/128; 18%; **Figure 7B**). Two bilateral ectopic cartilages also extended anteriorly from Meckel's cartilage. Morphological changes were also present in the neurocranium, including a slight increase in the width of the ethmoid plate likely resulting from a shortening of the trabeculae (74/128; 58%; **Figures 7F,I**) as compared to standard control MiR injected embryos ($n = 10$; **Figures 7D,H,I**) and control non-injected embryos (**Figures 7A,E**).

Injection of duplex RNA for MiR133b resulted in the formation of a cleft in the ethmoid plate (40/89; 45%; **Figure 7G**) and a general reduction in the overall size of the neurocranium, with a significant reduction in both the ethmoid plate width and length (46/89; 52%; **Figures 7G,I**). Injected animals also showed a mild change in the viscerocranium, including a reduction in the size of the ceratohyal (**Figure 7C**).

DISCUSSION

miRNAs have well defined roles in numerous developmental process, including craniofacial development (Tavares et al., 2015). We have shown here that numerous miRNAs are expressed within the developing midface, with expression patterns for some of these suggesting distinct functions in a variety of tissues. In addition, we have shown that over-expression of *mir23b* and *mir133b* results in changes in craniofacial cartilage morphogenesis. Together, results from our study illustrate the utility of an approach to quickly assess potential miRNA function during vertebrate morphogenesis.

Identification of miRNAs in Craniofacial Development

In addition to the identification of novel miRNAs expressed in the craniofacial complex, several miRNAs identified in this study as differentially expressed between facial prominences and over time have been identified to play a role in development in other systems. *Mir199a*, which we found to be enriched in the palate as compared to the FNP at E13.5, is involved in aspects of chondrogenesis and osteogenesis (Suomi et al., 2008; Lin et al., 2009). Similarly, *Mir92a* which is in the *Mirc1* cluster on mouse chromosome 14 containing *Mir17, Mir18, Mir19a, Mir20a, Mir19b-1*, and *Mir92a-1*, is required to promote proliferation of orofacial development (Ning et al., 2013). Thus, these data confirm and validate the deep sequencing data. Other groups have performed miRNA expression profiling of the developing mouse orofacial region using microarrays (Mukhopadhyay et al., 2010) and have found similar differential expression across time for miRNAs that included *Mir133a* and *Mir133b*. Interestingly, *Mir23b* was not identified by microarray analysis. This may be due to the retrospective nature of microarray studies, as they are limited by the total number of miRNAs that are present on the microarray chip. This approach may exclude all of the transcribed miRNAs in the genome. By definition, the inclusion of miRNAs on microarray chips means that the miRNA has already been identified and annotated. Furthermore, because microarrays are generally based on genome sequence, they may not assay miRNAs that originate by post-transcriptional editing (de Hoon et al., 2010). In contrast, miRNA-seq is prospective: it identifies all miRNAs present in a sample, regardless of whether they have been annotated or not or whether they have experienced editing. Thus, miRNA-seq has the power to identify novel and edited miRNAs in addition to known miRNAs.

miRNA-seq was recently used on avian embryos, in which dissection of the chick, quail and duck FNPs followed by miRNA-seq identified 170 miRNAs that were differentially expressed between the three species (Powder et al., 2012). Interestingly, several miRNAs were found to be avian-specific, suggesting that miRNAs may have promoted the evolutionary diversification of facial shape and beak formation.

Potential *Mir23b* and *Mir133b* Functions and Targets

Here we have shown that *Mir23b* is expressed in the developing face of mouse embryos and in the head of zebrafish embryos and that its overexpression in zebrafish embryos results in ectopic cartilage structures in the viscerocranium. This may indicate roles for *Mir23b* in regulating either patterning of the NCC-derived mesenchyme or later chondrogenesis. One of the interesting aspects our data analysis (**Figure 1**) is that *Mir27b* expression is also present in the developing midface, with its expression mirroring that of *Mir23b*. In mouse, *Mir23b* is part

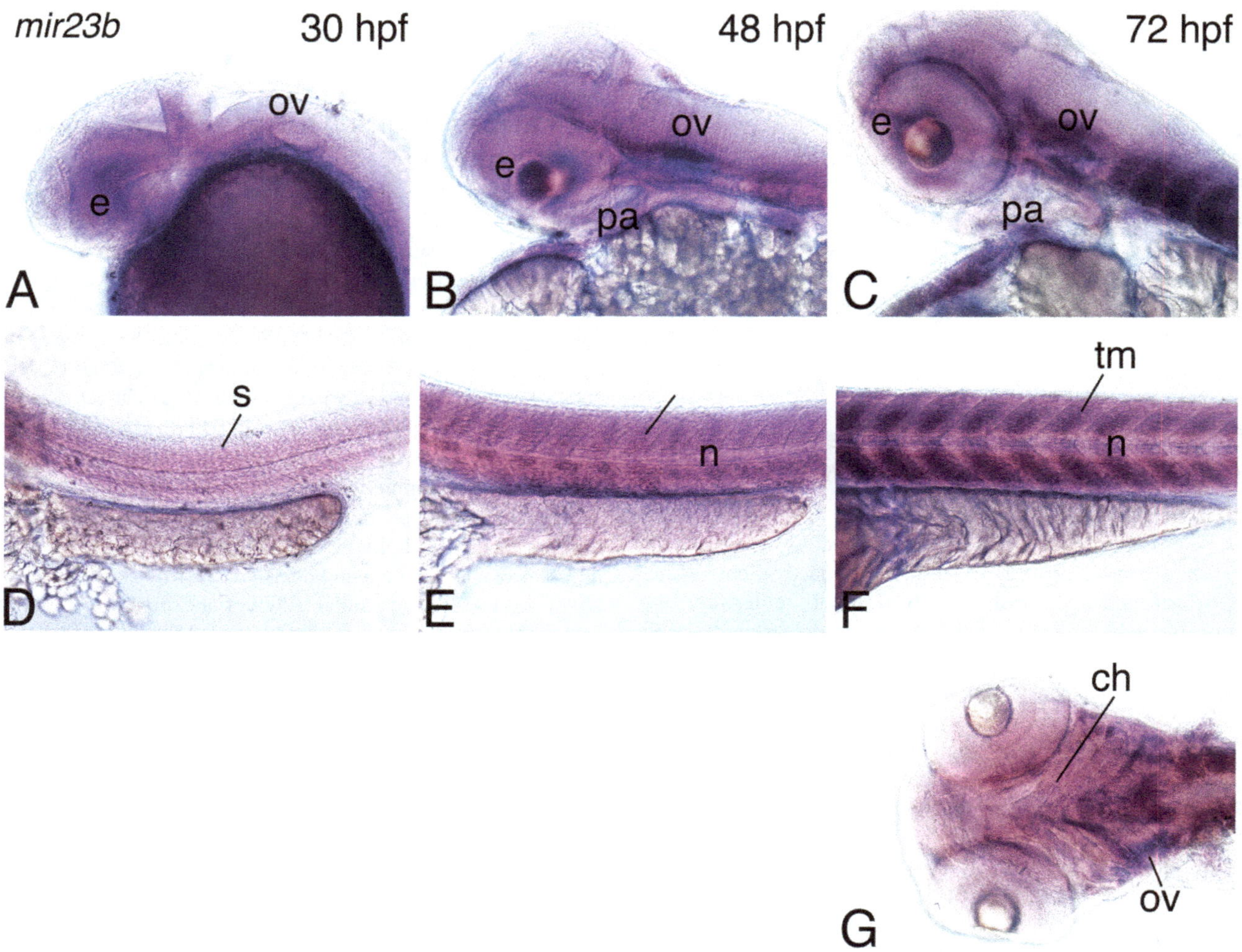

FIGURE 5 | Expression of mir23b in zebrafish embryos. Whole-mount *in situ* hybridization analysis with a digoxigenin-labeled probe against the *mir23b* transcript at 30–72 hpf. **(A–C)** Expression is observed in the otic vesicle (ov; **A**), weakly in the eye (e), and pharyngeal arch **(B,C)**, and palate (pl; **C**). **(D–F)** In the trunk, expression is observed in the trunk muscle the somites (s; **E,D**) at 30, 48 hpf, and trunk muscle (tm; **F**) at 72 hpf. **(G)** Ventral view of expression shows more detailed expression in the cranial muscle including the muscles supporting the craniofacial structures (arrows) and the eye. Anterior is to the left. n, notochord; ch, ceratohyal.

of a miRNA cluster that includes *Mir23b*, *Mir27b*, *Mir3074.1*, and *Mir24.1*. In zebrafish, this corresponds to *mir23b*, *mir27d*, and *mir24.1*. *mir23b* and *mir27b* are separated by less than 200 bp, though it is not clear that their expression is co-regulated. In the fetal mouse liver, the *Mir23b* cluster regulates cell fate switch between hepatocytes and bile duct cells by regulating expression of *Smad3*, *4*, and *5* and thereby repressing TGF-β signaling (Rogler et al., 2009). This negative regulation of TGF-β signaling is interesting, as proper regulation of TGF-β signaling is crucial for proper craniofacial development (Behnan et al., 2005). Marfan syndrome results from aberrant TGF-β signaling due to the failure of fibrullin-1 to bind to and sequester the latent form of TGF-β (Neptune et al., 2003; Chaudhry et al., 2007). Conversely, loss of TGF-β signaling is also detrimental to midfacial development, with loss of numerous TGF family members leading to facial birth defects (Iwata et al., 2011), illustrating the importance of miRNA regulation. While our miRNA-seq data suggests that the two miRNAs are co-expressed, further analysis of embryonic expression and loss-of-function phenotypes for individual miRNAs and the clusters will be required to fully understand their function. This is especially true for *Mir23b* and *Mir27b*, as while both work concurrently to drive cardiomyocyte development from ES cells *in vitro*, *Mir23b* subsequently controls the later beating phenotype of differentiated cells while *Mir27b* functions to inhibit this event (Chinchilla et al., 2011; Wang et al., 2012). Our analysis of expression and function in zebrafish suggest that *mir23b* is expressed in the pharyngeal arch mesenchyme and potentially functions to promote proliferation of chondrocytes, such that when overexpressed, ectopic cartilage arises.

Mir133b resides in a cluster that includes *Mir206* and *Mir133b*. This family is referred to as myomiRs because they regulate genes involved in adult muscle formation. In addition,

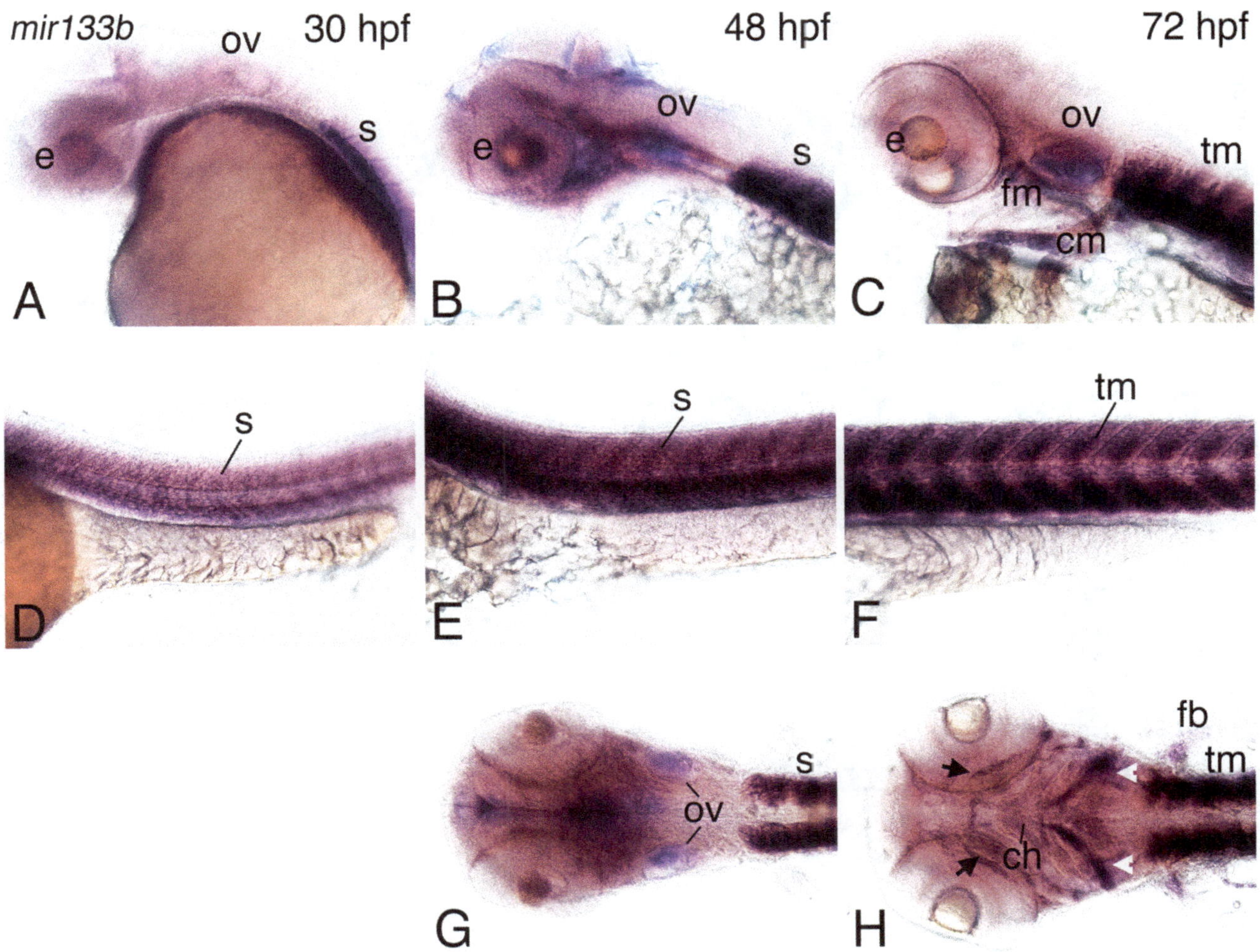

FIGURE 6 | Expression of *mir133b* in zebrafish embryos. Whole-mount *in situ* hybridization analysis with a digoxigenin-labeled probe against *mir133b* at 30–72 hpf. **(A–C)** Expression is observed in the developing pharyngeal region, including at 48 hpf in the facial muscle (fm) and otic vessicle **(B,G)**. **(D–F)** Strong expression of *miR133b* is observed in the somites (s; **D**) at 30 hpf, somites **(E)**, and pectoral fin (pf) at 48 hpf **(H)** and facial muscle (fm; **C**), cardiac muscle (cm; **C**), and trunk muscle (tm; **F**) at 72 hpf, including the anterior mandibularis (arrows) and stemohyoideus (arrowheads) facial muscles muscles. Anterior is to the left. e, eye; tm, trunk muscle; n, notochord; ch, ceratohyal.

Mir133b is down-regulated in several cancers, including muscle rhabdomyosarcoma, osteosarcoma, and prostate, colorectal and gastric cancers (Namløs et al., 2012; Qin et al., 2012; Mo et al., 2013). In these abnormal contexts, *MIR133b* in human cervical carcinoma targets EGFR and FGFR1, similarly acting as a tumor suppressor (Namløs et al., 2012). Interestingly, both EGF and FGF signaling have been implicated in craniofacial development. Mutations in EGF signaling have been implicated in human clefting (Falagan-Lotsch et al., 2015) and cranial suture formation in mice (Rawlins et al., 2008). More roles have been ascribed for FGF signaling in craniofacial development, with FGFR1 specifically linked to skeletal dysplasias and craniosynostosis in both humans and mice, suggesting a mechanism by which *Mir133b* may regulate craniofacial development (Moosa and Wollnik, 2016). Changes in facial muscle can affect development of facial bone and cartilages (Reider et al., 2012). From our expression analysis, it is plausible that overexpression of *Mir133b* may lead to changes in facial muscle which affects subsequent viscerocranium development.

In addition, *Mir133b* is involved in the differentiation of dopaminergic neurons. Zebrafish *mir133b* is expressed in the midbrain at low levels and regulates *pitx3* to control dopaminergic neuron differentiation (Sanchez-Simon et al., 2010). In contrast, mice in which *Mir133b* has been inactivated have normal dopaminergic neuron numbers and normal PITX3 protein levels (Heyer et al., 2012) even though *Mir133b* can target the *Pitx3* message. This suggests the possibility that other *Mir133* family members with the same seed sequence (GGACCAAA; i.e., *Mir133a*, *Mir133c*) can compensate for loss of *Mir133b*. *Mir133b* is clustered in the genome with *Mir 206.1,* which does not have the same seed sequence but is predicted to bind some of the same targets in mouse including

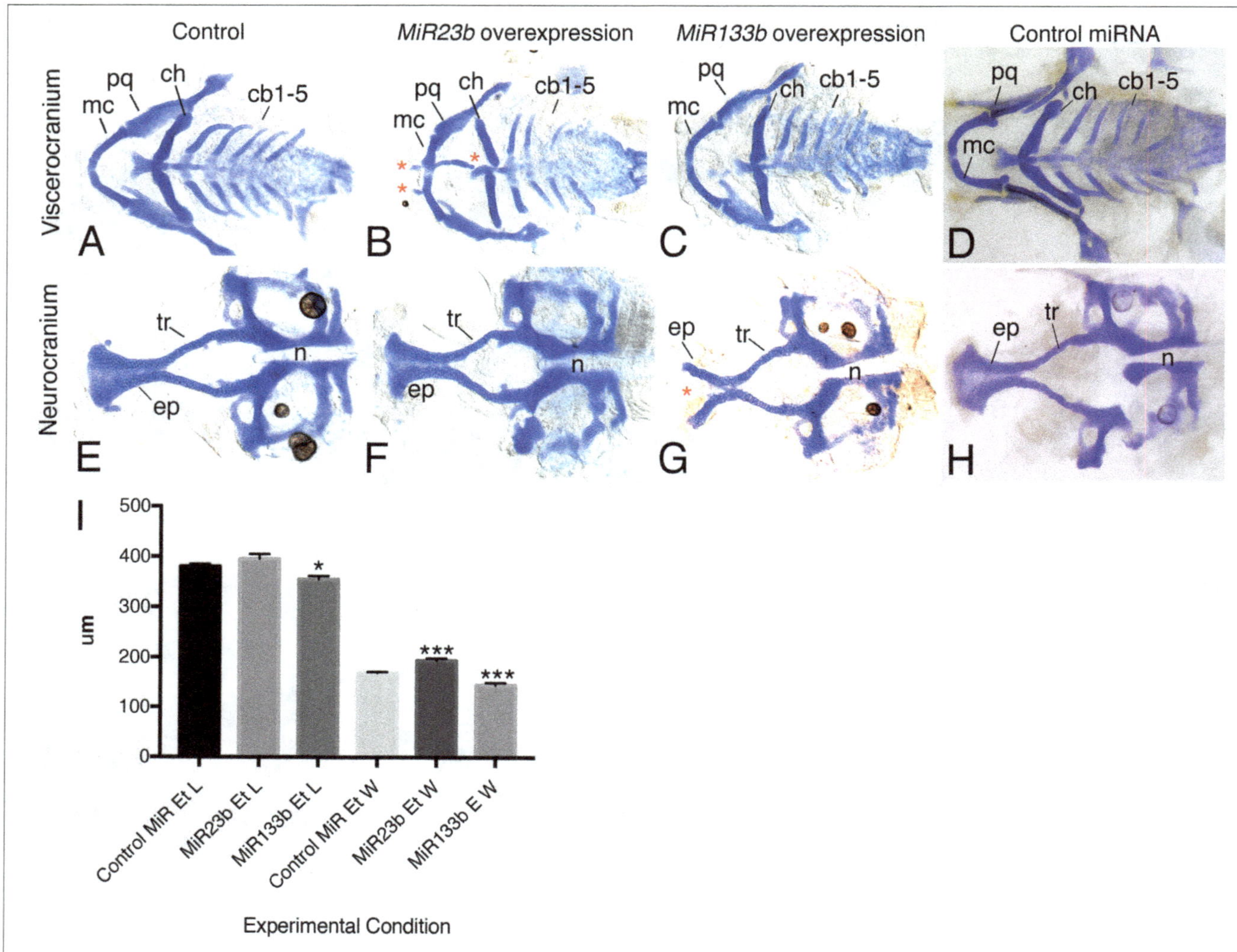

FIGURE 7 | Injection of MiR133b and MiR23b RNA duplexes resulted in facial defects. Alcian blue stain of 6 dpf zebrafish larvae, flat mounted ventral views, anterior is to the left. **(A,D,E,H)** Control embryos, either uninjected or 33 μM control miR-injected, display wild type type craniofacial cartilage in both the viscerocranium and neurocranium. **(B,F)** Injection of 33 μM RNA duplex of MiR23b leds to a slight increase in the width of the ethmoid plate, likely resulting from shortening of the trabeculae (tr) **(F)**, and production of ectopic cartilage (*; **B**) in the **B**) in the viscerocranium. **(C,G)** Injection of 6.25 μM RNA duplex of MiR133b resulted in hypoplastic cartilage structure and a cleft (*) in the ethmoid plate (ep; **G,I**). **(I)** Quantification of ethmoid plate length and width comparing standard control MiR ($n = 10$) injected with 33 μM compared to MiR23b ($n = 9$) and MiR133b ($n = 9$). Elements were measured and the mean and standard deviation for each are: Ethmoid plate length for control MiR, 380 ± 13.23 μm; MiR23b, 396 ± 27.13 μm; and MiR133b, 355 ± 19.27 μm; Ethmoid plate width for control MiR, 169.2 ± 4.92 μm; MiR23b, 193.9 ± 193.9 ± 14.09 μm; and MiR133b: 144.7 ± 14.7μm. Student's (Welsh's) *T*-test was used to compare to the standard control using GraphPad PRISM. $^{*}p < 0.02$ and $^{***}p < 0.0008$. Anterior is to the left. cb, ceratobranchial; ch, ceratohyal; mc, Meckel's cartilage; n, notochord; pq, palatoquadrate.

Histone Deacetylase 4, DNA Polymerase α, and Connexin43 (Anderson et al., 2006; Chen et al., 2006; Kim et al., 2006; Goljanek-Whysall et al., 2012). *mir133b* has the potential to target the same set of myogenic targets in zebrafish, but only Histone Deacetylase 4 contains a seed sequence for *mir133b*. More work is needed to distinguish between these possibilities. While we have not determined the numbers of dopaminergic neurons in zebrafish in which *mir133b* is over-expressed, we do see specific defects in cartilage differentiation, including hypoplasia of the ethmoid plate and specific gaps or missing cartilage in the viscerocranium, suggesting that *mir133b* may act non-cell autonomously to regulate cartilage differentiation. While there is little known about a direct role of *mir133b* on the development of the craniofacial cartilage, these results suggest that it is involved in both muscle and neuronal development, both of which can influence, either directly or indirectly, formation of the craniofacial complex. In summary, our results illustrate multiple MiRNAs are expressed in the developing face. This analysis will allow for more focused analysis of miR function in both zebrafish and mouse craniofacial development.

AUTHOR CONTRIBUTIONS

Experiments were designed by DC and KA in consultation with JP. All mouse and zebrafish experiments were performed by HD with help from BE. The RNA-seq was performed by BE and JP with bioinformatics performed by PB and JH. HD, KA, and DC analyzed and interpreted the data, and wrote the manuscript. All authors commented on the manuscript.

ACKNOWLEDGMENTS

We appreciate the excellent fish care provided by Morgan Singleton.

REFERENCES

Anderson, C., Catoe, H., and Werner, R. (2006). MIR-206 regulates connexin43 expression during skeletal muscle development. *Nucleic Acids Res.* 34, 5863–5871. doi: 10.1093/nar/gkl743

Behnan, S. M., Guo, C., Gong, T. W., Shum, L., and Gong, S. G. (2005). Gene and protein expression of transforming growth factor beta 2 gene during murine primary palatogenesis. *Differentiation* 73, 233–239. doi: 10.1111/j.1432-0436.2005.00022.x

Benjamini, Y., and Hochberg, Y. (1995). Controlling the false discovery rates: a practical and powerful approach to multiple testing. *J. R. Stat. Soc. B* 57, 289–300.

Birkholz, D. A., Olesnicky Killian, E. C., George, K. M., and Artinger, K. B. (2009). Prdm1a is necessary for posterior pharyngeal arch development in zebrafish. *Dev. Dyn.* 238, 2575–2587. doi: 10.1002/dvdy.22090

Bronner-Fraser, M. (1995). Origins and developmental potential of the neural crest. *Exp. Cell Res.* 218, 405–417. doi: 10.1006/excr.1995.1173

Chai, Y., and Maxson, R. E. Jr. (2006). Recent advances in craniofacial morphogenesis. *Dev. Dyn.* 235, 2353–2375. doi: 10.1002/dvdy.20833

Chaudhry, S. S., Cain, S. A., Morgan, A., Dallas, S. L., Shuttleworth, C. A., and Keilty, C. M. (2007). Fibrillin-1 regulates the bioavailability of TGFbeta1. *J. Cell Biol.* 176, 355–367. doi: 10.1083/jcb.200608167

Chen, B., Li, H., Zeng, X., Yang, P., Liu, X., Zhao, X., et al. (2012). Roles of microRNA on cancer cell metabolism. *J. Transl. Med.* 10:228. doi: 10.1186/1479-5876-10-228

Chen, J. F., Mandel, E. M., Thomson, J. M., Wu, Q., Callis, T. E., Hammond, S. M., et al. (2006). The role of microRNA-1 and microRNA-133 in skeletal muscle proliferation and differentiation. *Nat. Genet.* 38, 228–233. doi: 10.1038/ng1725

Chinchilla, A., Lozano, E., Daimi, H., Esteban, F. J., Crist, C., Aranega, A. E., et al. (2011). MicroRNA profiling during mouse ventricular maturation: a role for miR-27 modulating Mef2c expression. *Cardiovasc. Res.* 89, 98–108. doi: 10.1093/cvr/cvq264

Clouthier, D. E., Hosoda, K., Richardson, J. A., Williams, S. C., Yanagisawa, H., Kuwaki, T., et al. (1998). Cranial and cardiac neural crest defects in endothelin-A receptor-deficient mice. *Development* 125, 813–824.

Clouthier, D. E., Passos-Bueno, M. R., Tavares, A. L. P., Lyonnet, S., Amiel, J., and Gordon, C. T. (2013). Understanding the basis of Auriculocondylar syndrome: insights from human, mouse and zebrafish studies. *Am. J. Med. Genet. C Semin. Med. Genet.* 163, 306–317. doi: 10.1002/ajmg.c.31376

Couly, G. F., Grapin-Botton, A., Coltey, P., and Le Douarin, N. M. (1996). The regeneration of the cephalic neural crest, a problem revisited: the regenerating cells originate from the contralateral or from the anterior and posterior neural fold. *Development* 122, 3393–3407.

de Hoon, M. J., Taft, R. J., Hashimoto, T., Kanamori-Katayama, M., Kawaji, H., Kawano, M., et al. (2010). Cross-mapping and the identification of editing sites in mature microRNAs in high-throughput sequencing libraries. *Genome Res.* 20, 257–264. doi: 10.1101/gr.095273.109

de Pontual, L., Yao, E., Callier, P., Faivre, L., Drouin, V., Cariou, S., et al. (2011). Germline deletion of the miR-17 approximately 92 cluster causes skeletal and growth defects in humans. *Nat. Genet.* 43, 1026–1030. doi: 10.1038/ng.915

Desvignes, T., Batzel, P., Berezilkow, E., Eilbeck, K., Eppig, J. T., McAndrews, M. S., et al. (2015). miRNA nomenclature: a view INcorporating genetic orignins, biosynthetic pathways, and sequence varients. *Trends Genet.* 11, 613–626. doi: 10.1016/j.tig.2015.09.002

Desvignes, T., Contreras, A., and Postlethwait, J. H. (2014). Evolution of the miR199-214 cluster and vertebrate skeletal development. *RNA Biol.* 11, 281–294. doi: 10.4161/rna.28141

Dixon, M. J., Marazita, M. L., Beaty, T. H., and Murray, J. C. (2011). Cleft lip and palate: understanding genetic and environmental influences. *Nat. Rev. Genet.* 12, 167–178. doi: 10.1038/nrg2933

Eberhart, J. K., He, X., Swartz, M. E., Yan, Y. L., Song, H., Boling, T. C., et al. (2008). MicroRNA Mirn140 modulates Pdgf signaling during palatogenesis. *Nat. Genet.* 40, 290–298. doi: 10.1038/ng.82

Falagan-Lotsch, P., Lopes, T. S., Küchler, E. C., Tannure, P. N., Costa Mde, C., Amorinm, L. M., et al. (2015). The functional EGF+61 polymorphism and nonsyndromic oral clefts susceptibility in a Brazilian population. *J. Appl. Oral Sci.* 23, 390–396. doi: 10.1590/1678-775720140517

Fernández-Hernando, C., Ramírez, C. M., Goedeke, L., and Suárez, Y. (2013). MicroRNAs in metabolic disease. *Arterioscler. Thromb. Vasc. Biol.* 33, 178–185. doi: 10.1161/ATVBAHA.112.300144

Goljanek-Whysall, K., Sweetman, D., and Münsterberg, A. E. (2012). microRNAs in skeletal muscle differentiation and disease. *Clin. Sci.* 123, 611–625. doi: 10.1042/CS20110634

Hausser, J., and Zavolan, M. (2014). Identification and consequences of miRNA-target interactions–beyond repression of gene expression. *Nat. Rev. Genet.* 15, 599–612. doi: 10.1038/nrg3765

He, X., Yan, Y. L., DeLaurier, A., and Postlethwait, J. H. (2011). Observation of miRNA gene expression in zebrafish embryos by *in situ* hybridization to microRNA primary transcripts. *Zebrafish* 8, 1–8. doi: 10.1089/zeb.2010.0680

Hendershot, T. J., Liu, H., Sarkar, A. A., Giovannucci, D. R., Clouthier, D. E., Abe, M., et al. (2007). Expression of Hand2 is sufficient for neurogenesis and cell type-specific gene expression in the enteric nervous system. *Dev. Dyn.* 236, 93–105. doi: 10.1002/dvdy.20989

Heyer, M. P., Pani, A. K., Smeyne, R. J., Kenny, P. J., and Feng, G. (2012). Normal midbrain dopaminergic neuron development and function in miR-133b mutant mice. *J. Neurosci.* 32, 10887–10894. doi: 10.1523/JNEUROSCI.1732-12.2012

Huang, T., Liu, Y, Huang, M., Zhao, X., and Cheng, L. (2010). Wnt1-cre-mediated conditional loss of Dicer results in malformation of the midbrain and cerebellum and failure of neural crest and dopaminergic differentiation in mice. *J. Mol. Cell Biol.* 2, 152–163. doi: 10.1093/jmcb/mjq008

Hutvágner, G., McLachlan, J., Pasquinelli, A. E., Bálint, E., Tuschi, T., and Zamore, P. D. (2001). A cellular function for the RNA-interference enzyme Dicer in the maturation of the let-7 small temporal RNA. *Science* 293, 834–838. doi: 10.1126/science.1062961

Iwata, J., Parada, C., and Chai, Y. (2011). The mechanism of TGF-b during palate development. *Oral Dis.* 17, 733–744. doi: 10.1111/j.1601-0825.2011.01806.x

Jens, M., and Rajewsky, N. (2015). Competition between target sites of regulators shapes post-transcriptional gene regulation. *Nat. Rev. Genet.* 16, 113–126. doi: 10.1038/nrg3853

Johnson, C. W., Hernandez-Lagunas, L., Feng, W., Melvin, V. S., Williams, T., and Artinger, K. B. (2011). Vgll2a is required for neural crest cell survival during zebrafish craniofacial development. *Dev. Biol.* 357, 269–281. doi: 10.1016/j.ydbio.2011.06.034

Kannu, P., Campos-Xavier, A. B., Hull, D., Martinet, D., Ballhausen, D., and Bonafé, L. (2013). Post-axial polydactyly type A2, overgrowth and autistic traits associated with a chromosome 13q31.3 microduplication encompassing miR-17-92 and GPC5. *Eur. J. Med. Genet.* 56, 452–457. doi: 10.1016/j.ejmg.2013.06.001

Kim, H. K., Lee, Y. S., Sivaprasad, U., Malhotra, A., and Dutta, A. (2006). Muscle-specific microRNA miR-206 promotes muscle differentiation. *J. Cell Biol.* 174, 677–687. doi: 10 1083/jcb.200603008

Kimmel, C. B., Ballard, W. W., Kimmel, S. R., Ullmann, B., and Schilling, T. F. (1995). Stages of embryonic development of the zebrafish. *Dev. Dyn.* 203, 253–310. doi: 10.1002/aja.1002030302

Knight, R. D., and Schilling, T. F. (2006). Cranial neural crest and development of the head skeleton. *Adv. Exp. Med. Biol.* 589, 120–133. doi: 10.1007/978-0-387-46954-6_7

Köntges, G., and Lumsden, A. (1996). Rhombencephalic neural crest segmentation is preserved throughout craniofacial ontogeny. *Development* 122, 3229–3242.

Kuppusamy, K. T., Sperber, H., and Ruohola-Baker, H. (2013). MicroRNA regulation and role in stem cell maintenance, cardiac differentiation and hypertrophy. *Curr. Mol. Med.* 13, 757–764. doi: 10.2174/1566524011313050007

Lagos-Quintana, M., Rauhut, R., Meyer, J., Borkhardt, A., and Tuschl, T. (2003). New microRNAs from mouse and human. *RNA* 9, 175–179. doi: 10.1261/rna.2146903

Lai, E. C. (2002). Micro RNAs are complementary to 3′ UTR sequence motifs that mediate negative post-transcriptional regulation. *Nat. Genet.* 30, 363–364. doi: 10.1038/ng865

Le Douarin, N. M. (1982). *The Neural Crest.* New York, NY: Cambridge University Press.

Lee, R. C., Feinbaum, R. L., and Ambros, V. (1993). The *C. elegans* heterochronic gene lin-4 encodes small RNAs with antisense complementarity to lin-14. *Cell* 75, 843–854.

Lewis, B. P., Shih, I. H., Jones-Rhoades, M. W., Bartel, D. P., and Burge, C. B. (2003). Prediction of mammalian microRNA targets. *Cell* 115, 787–798. doi: 10.1016/S0092-8674(03)01018-3

Li, L., Meng, T., Jia, Z., Zhu, G., and Shi, B. (2010). Single nucleotide polymorphism associated with nonsyndromic cleft palate influences the processing of miR-140. *Am. J. Med. Genet. A* 152A, 856–862. doi: 10.1002/ajmg.a.33236

Li, L., Shi, J. Y., Zhu, G. Q., and Shi, B. (2012). MiR-17-92 cluster regulates cell proliferation and collagen synthesis by targeting TGFB pathway in mouse palatal mesenchymal cells. *J. Cell. Biochem.* 113, 1235–1244. doi: 10.1002/jcb.23457

Li, L., Zhu, G. Q., Meng, T., Shi, J. Y., Wu, J., Xu, X., et al. (2011). Biological and epidemiological evidence of interaction of infant genotypes at Rs7205289 and maternal passive smoking in cleft palate. *Am. J. Med. Genet. A* 155A, 2940–2948. doi: 10.1002/ajmg.a.34254

Lim, L. P., Glasner, M. E., Yekta, S., Burge, C. B., and Bartel, D. P. (2003). Vertebrate microRNA genes. *Science* 299, 1540. doi: 10.1126/science.1080372

Lin, E. A., Kong, L., Bai, X. H., Luan, Y., and Liu, C. J. (2009). miR-199a, a bone morphogenic protein 2-responsive MicroRNA, regulates chondrogenesis via direct targeting to Smad1. *J. Biol. Chem.* 284, 11326–11335. doi: 10.1074/jbc.M807709200

Mo, W., Zhang, J., Li, X., Meng, D., Gao, Y., Yang, S., et al. (2013). Identification of novel AR-targeted microRNAs mediating androgen signalling through critical pathways to regulate cell viability in prostate cancer. *PLoS ONE* 8:e56592. doi: 10.1371/journal.pone.0056592

Moosa, S., and Wollnik, B. (2016). Altered FGF signalling in congenital craniofacial and skeletal disorders. *Semin. Cell Dev. Biol.* 53, 1115–1125. doi: 10.1016/j.semcdb.2015.12.005

Morceau, F., Chateauvieux, S., Gaigneaux, A., Dicato, M., and Diederich, M. (2013). Long and short non-coding RNAs as regulators of hematopoietic differentiation. *Int. J. Mol. Sci.* 14, 14744–14770. doi: 10.3390/ijms1407 14744

Mukhopadhyay, P., Brock, G., Pihur, V., Webb, C., Pisano, M. M., and Greene, R. M. (2010). Developmental microRNA expression profiling of murine embryonic orofacial tissue. *Birth Defects Res. A Clin. Mol. Teratol.* 88, 511–534. doi: 10.1002/bdra.20684

Namløs, H. M., Meza-Zepeda, L. A., Barøy, T., Østensen, I. H., Kresse, S. H., Kuijjer, M. L., et al. (2012). Modulation of the osteosarcoma expression phenotype by microRNAs. *PLoS ONE* 7:e48086. doi: 10.1371/journal.pone.0048086

Neptune, E. R., Frischmeyer, P. A., Arking, D. E., Myers, L., Bunton, T. E., Gayraud, B., et al. (2003). Dysregulation of TGF-beta activation contributes to pathogenesis in Marfan syndrome. *Nat. Genet.* 33, 407–411. doi: 10.1038/ng1116

Nie, X., Wang, Q., and Jiao, K. (2011). Dicer activity in neural crest cells is essential for craniofacial organogenesis and pharyngeal arch artery morphogenesis. *Mech. Dev.* 128, 200–207. doi: 10.1016/j.mod.2010.12.002

Ning, G., Liu, X., Dai, M., Meng, A., and Wang, Q. (2013). MicroRNA-92a upholds Bmp signaling by targeting noggin3 during pharyngeal cartilage formation. *Dev. Cell* 24, 283–295. doi: 10.1016/j.devcel.2012.12.016

Obernosterer, G., Martinez, J., and Alenius, M. (2007). Locked nucleic acid-based *in situ* detection of microRNAs in mouse tissue sections. *Nat. Protoc.* 2, 1508–1514. doi: 10.1038/nprot.2007.153

Oommen, S., Otsuka-Tanaka, Y., Imam, N., Kawasaki, M., Kawasaki, K., Jalani-Ghazani, F., et al. (2012). Distinct roles of microRNAs in epithelium and mesenchyme during tooth development. *Dev. Dyn.* 241, 1465–1472. doi: 10.1002/dvdy.23828

Parpart, S., and Wang, X. W. (2013). microRNA regulation and its consequences in cancer. *Curr. Pathobiol. Rep.* 1, 71–79. doi: 10.1007/s40139-012-0002-7

Powder, K. E., Ku, Y. C., Brugmann, S. A., Veile, R. A., Renaud, N. A., Helms, J. A., et al. (2012). A cross-species analysis of microRNAs in the developing avian face. *PLoS ONE* 7:e35111. doi: 10.1371/journal.pone.0035111

Qin, W., Dong, P., Ma, C., Mitchelson, K., Deng, T., Zhang, L., et al. (2012). MicroRNA-133b is a key promoter of cervical carcinoma development through the activation of the ERK and AKT1 pathways. *Oncogene* 31, 4067–4075. doi: 10.1038/onc.2011.561

Rawlins, J. T., Fernandez, C. R., Cozby, M. E., and Opperman, L. A. (2008). Timing of Egf treatment differentially affects Tgf beta2 induced cranial suture closure. *Exp. Biol. Med. (Maywood).* 233, 1518–1526. doi: 10.3181/0805-RM-151

Reider, M. J., Green, G. E., Park, S. S., Stamper, B. D., Gordon, C. T., Johnson, J. M., et al. (2012). A human homeotic transformation resulting from mutations in *PLCB4* and *GNAI3* causes auriculocondylar syndrome. *Am. J. Hum. Genet.* 90, 907–914. doi: 10.1016/j.ajhg.2012.04.002

Rogler, C. E., Levoci, L., Ader, T., Massimi, A., Tchaikovskaya, T., Norel, R., et al. (2009). MicroRNA-23b cluster microRNAs regulate transforming growth factor-beta/bone morphogenetic protein signaling and liver stem cell differentiation by targeting Smads. *Hepatology* 50, 575–584. doi: 10.1002/hep.22982

Sanchez-Simon, F. M., Zhang, X. X., Loh, H. H., Law, P. Y., and Rodriguez, R. E. (2010). Morphine regulates dopaminergic neuron differentiation via miR-133b. *Mol. Pharmacol.* 78, 935–942. doi: 10.1124/mol.110.066837

Schutte, B. C., and Murray, J. C. (1999). The many faces and factors of orofacial clefts. *Hum. Mol. Genet.* 8, 1853–1859. doi: 10.1093/hmg/8.10.1853

Spritz, R. A. (2001). The genetics and epigenetics of orofacial clefts. *Curr. Opin. Pediatr.* 13, 556–560. doi: 10.1097/00008480-200112000-00011

Suomi, S., Taipaleenmäki, H., Seppänen, A., Ripatti, T., Väänänen, K., Hentunen, T., et al. (2008). MicroRNAs regulate osteogenesis and chondrogenesis of mouse bone marrow stromal cells. *Gene Regul. Syst. Bio.* 2, 177–191.

Tassano, E., Di Rocco, M., Signa, S., and Gimelli, G. (2013). *De novo* 13q31.1-q32.1 interstitial deletion encompassing the miR-17-92 cluster in a patient with Feingold syndrome-2. *Am. J. Med. Genet. A* 161A, 894–896. doi: 10.1002/ajmg.a.35781

Tavares, A. L., Artinger, K. B., and Clouthier, D. E. (2015). Regulating Craniofacial Development at the 3′ end: MicroRNAs and their function in facial morphogenesis. *Curr. Top. Dev. Biol.* 115, 335–375. doi: 10.1016/bs.ctdb.2015.08.001

Ventura, A., Young, A. G., Winslow, M. M., Lintault, L., Meissner, A., Erkeland, S. J., et al. (2008). Targeted deletion reveals essential and overlapping functions of the miR-17w92 family of miRNA clusters. *Cell* 132, 875–886. doi: 10.1016/j.cell.2008.02.019

Walker, M., and Trainor, P. (2006). craniofacial malformations: intrinsic vs extrinsic neural crest cell defects in treacher collins and 22q11 deletion syndromes. *Clin. Genet.* 69, 471–479. doi: 10.1111/j.0009-9163.2006.00615.x

Wang, J., Bai, Y., Li, H., Greene, S. B., Klysik, E., Yu, W., et al. (2013). MicroRNA-17-92, a direct Ap-2alpha transcriptional target, modulates T-box factor activity in orofacial clefting. *PLoS Genet.* 9:e1003785. doi: 10.1371/annotation/90602bc3-5052-49ac-a7fb-33210d7c8b4d

Wang, J., Song, Y., Zhang, Y., Xiao, H., Sun, Q., Hou, N., et al. (2012). Cardiomyocyte overexpression of miR-27b induces cardiac hypertrophy and dysfunction in mice. *Cell Res.* 22, 516–527. doi: 10.1038/cr.2011.132

Watanabe, T., Sato, T., Amano, T., Kawamura, Y., Kawamura, N., Kawaguchi, H., et al. (2008). Dnm3os, a non-coding RNA, is required for normal growth and skeletal development in mice. *Dev. Dyn.* 237, 3738–3748. doi: 10.1002/dvdy.21787

Westerfield, M. (2000). *The Zebrafish Book. A Guide for the Laboratory Use of Zebrafish (Danio rerio).* Eugene, OR: University of Oregon Press.

Wightman, B., Ha, I., and Ruvkun, G. (1993). Posttranscriptional Regulation of the heterochronic gene *lin-14* by *lin-4* mediates temporal pattern formation in *C. elegans. Cell* 75, 855–862. doi: 10.1016/0092-8674(93)90530-4

Wu, L., Fan, J., and Belasco, J. G. (2006). MicroRNAs direct rapid deadenylation of mRNA. *Proc. Natl. Acad. Sci. U.S.A.* 103, 4034–4039. doi: 10.1073/pnas.0510928103

Zehir, A., Hua, L. L., Maska, E. L., Morikawa, Y., and Cserjesi, P. (2010). Dicer is required for survival of differentiating neural crest cells. *Dev. Biol.* 340, 459–467. doi: 10.1016/j.ydbio.2010.01.039

Zheng, Y., and Cullen, B. R. (2003). Sequence requirements for microRNA processing and function in human cells. *RNA* 9, 112–123. doi: 10.1261/rna.2780503

9

Regulation of Calvarial Osteogenesis by Concomitant De-Repression of GLI3 and Activation of IHH Targets

*Lotta K. Veistinen[1], Tuija Mustonen[1,2], Md. Rakibul Hasan[1], Maarit Takatalo[1], Yukiho Kobayashi[1,3], Dörthe A. Kesper[4], Andrea Vortkamp[4] and David P. Rice[1,5]**

[1] Orthodontics, Oral and Maxillofacial Diseases, University of Helsinki, Helsinki, Finland, [2] Minerva Research Institute, Helsinki, Finland, [3] Orthodontics, Tokyo Medical and Dental University, Tokyo, Japan, [4] Center of Medical Biotechnology, University of Duisburg-Essen, Essen, Germany, [5] Orthodontics, Oral and Maxillofacial Diseases, Helsinki University Hospital, Helsinki, Finland

***Correspondence:**
David P. Rice
david.rice@helsinki.fi

Loss-of-function mutations in *GLI3* and *IHH* cause craniosynostosis and reduced osteogenesis, respectively. In this study, we show that *Ihh* ligand, the receptor *Ptch1* and *Gli* transcription factors are differentially expressed in embryonic mouse calvaria osteogenic condensations. We show that in both $Ihh^{-/-}$ and $Gli3^{Xt-J/Xt-J}$ embryonic mice, the normal gene expression architecture is lost and this results in disorganized calvarial bone development. RUNX2 is a master regulatory transcription factor controlling osteogenesis. In the absence of *Gli3*, RUNX2 isoform II and IHH are upregulated, and RUNX2 isoform I downregulated. This is consistent with the expanded and aberrant osteogenesis observed in $Gli3^{Xt-J/Xt-J}$ mice, and consistent with *Runx2-I* expression by relatively immature osteoprogenitors. $Ihh^{-/-}$ mice exhibited small calvarial bones and HH target genes, *Ptch1* and *Gli1*, were absent. This indicates that IHH is the functional HH ligand, and that it is not compensated by another HH ligand. To decipher the roles and potential interaction of Gli3 and Ihh, we generated $Ihh^{-/-};Gli3^{Xt-J/Xt-J}$ compound mutant mice. Even in the absence of *Ihh*, *Gli3* deletion was sufficient to induce aberrant precocious ossification across the developing suture, indicating that the craniosynostosis phenotype of $Gli3^{Xt-J/Xt-J}$ mice is not dependent on IHH ligand. Also, we found that Ihh was not required for *Runx2* expression as the expression of RUNX2 target genes was unaffected by deletion of *Ihh*. To test whether RUNX2 has a role upstream of IHH, we performed RUNX2 siRNA knock down experiments in WT calvarial osteoblasts and explants and found that *Ihh* expression is suppressed. Our results show that IHH is the functional HH ligand in the embryonic mouse calvaria osteogenic condensations, where it regulates the progression of osteoblastic differentiation. As GLI3 represses the expression of *Runx2-II* and *Ihh*, and also elevates the *Runx2-I* expression, and as IHH may be regulated by RUNX2 these results raise the possibility of a regulatory feedback circuit to control calvarial osteogenesis and suture patency. Taken together, RUNX2-controlled osteoblastic cell fate is regulated by IHH through concomitant inhibition of GLI3-repressor formation and activation of downstream targets.

Keywords: calvarial development, hedgehog signaling pathway, osteoblast, cell differentiation, craniosynostosis

INTRODUCTION

The majority of the bones of the face and calvaria are formed by intramembranous ossification. Growth occurs primarily at the bone edges in the sutural joints (Rice and Rice, 2008). We and others have shown that across the suture there is the complete spectrum of osteogenic differentiation from quiescent stem cells through all osteoprogenitor stages to functioning mature osteoblasts. The expansion of each cell population is tightly regulated and dependent on the functional demands of the growing skull (Lana-Elola et al., 2007; Zhao et al., 2015; Maruyama et al., 2016). Osteoprogenitors condense at the osteogenic fronts and in order for osteogenesis to proceed a constant supply of progenitor cells must be available (Rice et al., 2003; Lana-Elola et al., 2007). Mis-regulation of the osteogenic condensations will result in alterations in skull bone shape and size, as well as in the patency of the sutures with consequent effects on skull growth. Within this niche, GLI transcription factors regulate stem cell maintenance, osteoprogenitor proliferation and differentiation (Rice et al., 2010; Veistinen et al., 2012). GLI1-positive cells in the suture mesenchyme are a source of mesenchymal stem cells, and ablation of *Gli1* in postnatal mice results in the premature fusion, or craniosynostosis, of all the calvarial sutures and the consequent secession of growth (Zhao et al., 2015). *GLI3* loss of function mutations cause craniosynostosis resulting in fusion across the interfrontal suture in patients and across the lambdoid and interfrontal sutures in mice (McDonald-McGinn et al., 2010; Rice et al., 2010; Hurst et al., 2011). These differences in phenotypes can, in part, be explained by location-specific differences in mRNA expression. *Gli1* is expressed evenly in all calvarial sutures while *Gli3* transcripts are more highly expressed in the interfrontal and lambdoid sutures compared to other calvarial sutures (Rice et al., 2010; Zhao et al., 2015).

GLI proteins are regulators of Hedgehog (HH) signaling, with GLI3 mainly functioning as a repressor of HH target genes. In the absence of the HH ligand GLI3 is proteolytically cleaved into the truncated repressor isoform, GLI3R (Wang et al., 2000). GLI3 acts as a strong repressor during limb patterning and during endochondral ossification, with SHH regulating limb patterning and IHH regulating cartilage development (Litingtung et al., 2002; Hilton et al., 2005; Koziel et al., 2005).

Indian hedgehog (*Ihh*) is expressed in the embryonic calvaria, and in osteoblastic cells has been shown to upregulate an osteogenic master regulator *Runx2* through GLI2 activator function (GLI2A) (Shimoyama et al., 2007; Rice et al., 2010). It has been proposed that IHH regulates several stages of osteoblast differentiation, either through Gli3R or Gli2A functions (Hilton et al., 2005; Joeng and Long, 2009). Although IHH is essential for osteoblast differentiation during endochondral ossification, it is not essential for intramembranous bone development. Osteoblasts appear to develop normally in calvarial bones of $Ihh^{-/-}$ mice although the bones are reduced in size (St-Jacques et al., 1999; Lenton et al., 2011). By mapping the gene expression of *Ihh* in the developing chick dentary bone and analyzing the retroviral missexpression (gain of function) of *Ihh* in the developing chick frontal bone, it has been proposed that IHH regulates the transition of osteoprogenitors to osteoblasts. It is suggested that IHH does this by restricting the differentiation of preosteoblasts so that they can proliferate for longer which increases the pool of progenitors (Abzhanov et al., 2007). There is also evidence that IHH positively regulates osteoprogenitor recruitment to the osteogenic front possibly by controlling Bone morphogenetic protein (BMP) signaling (Lenton et al., 2011).

We have shown earlier how $Gli3^{Xt-J/Xt-J}$ mice, which produce no functional GLI3 protein, can be used as a model to study craniosynostosis and suture biogenesis, and by genetically reducing the dosage of *Runx2* the calvarial phenotype can be rescued (Rice et al., 2010; Tanimoto et al., 2012; Veistinen et al., 2012). The transcription factor TWIST1 negatively regulates osteogenesis by inhibiting *Runx2* through direct DNA binding (Rice et al., 2000, 2010; Bialek et al., 2004), and in $Gli3^{Xt-J/Xt-J}$ mice the expression of *Twist1* is reduced across the sutures. This aberrant signaling results in an increased pool of osteoprogenitors and enhanced osteogenic differentiation, with consequent ectopic bone formation and suture fusion. Support for this mechanism comes from premature activation of *Runx2* in embryonic day (E) 9.5 mice, as well as from the deletion of one allele of *Twist1* both of which result in enhanced osteogenesis and craniosynostosis (Bourgeois et al., 1998; Maeno et al., 2011). GLI3 repressor reduces RUNX2 activity by competing for the same DNA target sequences, thus negatively regulating osteoblast differentiation (Ohba et al., 2008; Lopez-Rios et al., 2012).

In this study we aimed to elucidate whether GLI3 controls IHH regulated intramembranous osteogenesis, and to test whether IHH, GLI3 and RUNX2 regulate and maintain the different stages of osteogenesis within the patent suture.

We show that IHH is the functional HH ligand in the embryonic mouse calvaria osteogenic condensations, where it regulates the progression of osteoblastic differentiation. We also demonstrate a location specific regulatory role for GLI3 repressor within the suture which is independent of IHH expression, as *Ihh* deletion does not rescue craniosynostosis exhibited by $Gli3^{Xt-J/Xt-J}$ mice. In addition, we show that GLI3 represses the expression of *Runx2-II* and *Ihh*, and elevates *Runx2-I*. And that IHH is regulated by RUNX2 in calvarial osteoblasts. These data raise the possibility of a regulatory feedback circuit to control calvarial osteogenesis and suture patency.

MATERIAL AND METHODS

Mice

The $Ihh^{+/-}$ and $Gli3^{+/Xt-J}$ mice maintenance, breeding and PCR genotyping has been described previously (Koziel et al., 2005). Wild-type (WT) littermates NMRI mice were used as controls. All animal experiments were approved by the University of Helsinki, Helsinki University Hospital and the Southern Finland Council Animal Welfare and Ethics committees.

In Situ Hybridization

E13.5 and E15.5 tissues were fixed in a copious volume of freshly prepared 4% paraformaldehyde overnight at 4°C. They were then washed in PBS before dehydrating in an increasing strength ethanol or methanol series before *in situ* hybridization on either tissue sections or whole mounts, respectively.

Ihh, Ptch1, Gli1-3, Runx2, Osx, Bglap, and *Ibsp* riboprobes were prepared, and *in situ* hybridization was performed as described previously and briefly described below (Rice et al., 2006; Tanimoto et al., 2012).

In Situ Hybridization on Tissue Sections

Sections (7μm) were deparaffinised, rehydrated and permeabilized with proteinase K. Tissues were hybridized overnight at 52°C with ^{35}S-UTP labeled riboprobes. Hybridization was followed by high stringency washes at 50°C and at 65°C. Slides were then washed in NTE at 37° and treated with ribonuclease A to remove non-specifically bound and excess probe. The slides were coated with autoradiography liquid emulsion and exposed in a dark box for 10–18 days at 4°C. The slides were developed, fixed and then counterstained with hematoxylin.

In Situ Hybridization on Whole Mounts

Samples were rehydrated, bleached with H_2O_2 and permeabilized with proteinase K. Tissues were prehybridized in PBST. Tissues were hybridized overnight at 64°C with denatured digoxigenin-labeled probes followed by high stringency washes. Next tissues were washed MABT then pre-blocked at room temperature for 3 h prior to overnight incubation with anti-dig-antibody coupled to alkaline phosphatase 4°C. Following extensive MABT and NTMT washes the color reaction was performed with NBT/BCIP.

Immunohistochemistry

Immunohistochemical staining was performed as described previously (Rice et al., 2016). Briefly tissue sections were permeabilized and blocked, then incubated overnight at 4°C with anti-IHH (AF1705, R&D systems), anti-GLI1 (L42B10, Cell Signaling), anti-GLI3 (AF3690, R&D systems) or anti-PTCH1(G-19, Santa Cruz Biotechnology). Signal visualization was performed using Enzmet HRP detection (Nanoprobes). Sections were counterstained with nuclear fast red.

Skeletal Staining

Heads of mutant mice and WT littermates aged E16.5 and E18.5 were fixed in 95% ethanol overnight and stained with Alcian blue and Alizarin red and then cleared in 1% KOH and transferred to glycerol. For calculations of calvarial bone and suture size, images were captured using AnalySIS software (Soft Imaging System) and Olympus BX41 microscope and analyzed in Adobe® Photoshop CS4.

Western Blot Analysis

Calvaria were dissected from E15.5 WT embryos and tissue samples taken from osteogenic front of the frontal bone and from interfrontal midsutural mesenchyme. Samples were pooled from three calvaria of the same litter and this was repeated 4 times. Age-matched brain tissue was used as control. Western blotting was carried out as described previously (Tanimoto et al., 2012). Briefly, 10 μg of each sample was probed for GLI3 antibody (AF3690, R&D Systems), GLI1 antibody (2643, Cell Signaling Technology), α-tubulin (T6199, Sigma-Aldrich). 20 μg of total protein from siRNA treated calvarial cells was probed for RUNX2 antibody (8486, Cell Signaling Technology), IHH antibody (AF1705, R&D Systems), and normalized against signal by Actin antibody (A2066 Sigma), detected by secondary antibodies goat anti-mouse IRDye 800CW (926-32210, LI-COR) and goat anti-rabbit 680RD (926-68071, LI-COR). Blots were analyzed with an Odyssey CLx infrared imager (model 9120) (Li-Cor) and Image-J (NIH) software. Statistical values were calculated using Student's *t*-test, with *P*-value below 0.05 indicated as significant.

The Effect of Exogenous IHH on Primary Calvaria Derived Cells

Mouse E15.5 wild type (WT) primary calvaria derived cells (CDC) were isolated by trysinization and cultured for several days in DMEM containing high glucose and supplemented with 10% FBS. Cells were pooled from at least 2 calvaria. After 1st passage cells were seeded onto 6-well plates for experiments (100,000 cells per well). After 48 h of culture, cells were treated with recombinant human/mouse IHH protein (1705-HH-025 R&D systems): 50, 100, 250 ng/ml, and control cells with BSA (bovine serum albumin) for 1, 2, 6, and 24 h. RNA isolated from control and IHH treated CDC cells was quantified. 300 ng of RNA was used for cDNA synthesis using reverse transcriptase enzyme and random hexamer primers. Thereafter, RT-qPCR was performed using the primers *Gli1* (FP:CAGCATGGGAACAGAAGGACT, RP:CTCTGGCTGCTC CATAACCC), *Gli2* (FP:AACTTTTGTCTCCTCGGGTCC,RP: CTGCTGTCCTCCAAGAGACC) and *Gli3* (FP:AAGCCCATG ACATCTCAGCC,RP:CTCGAGCCCACTGTTGGAAT). SYBR fast (Kapa Biosystems) qPCR master mix was used for real time quantitative PCR using Quant studio 3 from Thermo scientific. Mouse *18S rRNA* gene was used as the reference gene and negative control with no cDNA was used. The experiment conducted 3 times, each time with different biological samples.

Calvarial Osteoblasts and Explant Cultures

E15.5 mouse calvarial cells were isolated by four sequential trypsin-treatments of whole calvaria separated from the skin and meninges. The first set of cells after 15 min 0.25% trypsin incubation were discarded, and the cells from the following trypsin treatments were pooled and cultured in growth medium (DMEM containing 4,5 g/L glucose supplemented with 1 mM Na-pyruvate, 4 mM L-glutamine, 1% penicillin-streptomycine, and 10% FBS, (Lonza and Gibco).

Analysis of Wt and $Gli3^{Xt-J/Xt-J}$ calvarial cells: At passage 2 the cells were transferred into new growth medium until confluent from which cell lysates were derived. Western blot analyses were carried out with 20 μg of total protein.

siRNA experiments: At passage 2 the cells were transfected either with negative control siRNA (Ambion Silencer Select control #1 siRNA, 4390843, Thermo Fisher) or *Runx2* siRNAs (Ambion 4390771 Runx2 Silencer Select Pre-designed siRNA, Thermo Fisher) using Lipofectamine RNAiMAX (Thermo Fisher). Cells were grown on six well plates with the siRNA transfection complex for 3 days, after which the medium was replaced by osteogenic medium (DMEM, 10 mM β-glycerophosphate, (Sigma), 50 μg/ml ascorbic acid, Sigma, and 100 ng/ml BMP2 (R&D Systems) for 24 h from which cell lysates were derived. Western blot analyses were carried out with 20 μg of total protein. siRNA experiments were carried out 3 times.

E15 mouse calvarias were dissected for Trowell type of organ culture (Rice et al., 2000). Affi-gel agarose beads (Bio-Rad) were washed with PBS, and circa 200 beads were soaked with premixed siRNA—RNAiMAX reagent (Thermo Fisher) at 37°C for 30 min. Several beads were placed on the calvarias that were further cultured for 3 days in osteogenic medium. Efforts were made to place beads onto comparable areas of the calvaria that had endogenous expression of either *Runx2* full length or *Ihh* (Rice et al., 2010). The areas of *Ihh* expression in WT E15.5 calvaria were further identified (**Figure 1B**) and beads impregnated with either negative control or anti-RUNX2 SiRNAs were placed on the parietal bone osteogenic fronts for IHH experiments, which can be identified in bright field microscopy (Kim et al., 1998). Beads placed on the parietal bone or osteogenic fronts for RUNX2 experiments.

RESULTS

Location Specific Regulatory Role of GLI3 Repressor

To determine the specific transcript (**Figures 1A–C**) and protein (**Figure 1D**) expression domains and protein activity of HH pathway members in the developing calvaria *in situ* hybridization and immunohistochemistry were performed. Detailed *in situ* hybridization was performed at different developmental stages of calvarial and suture maturation. In an attempt to get comparable data, at both E13.5 and E15.5 analysis was done on consecutive E15.5 calvarial tissue sections. Also, at E15.5 whole calvarial tissue was analyzed to determine whether all sutures have similar expression patterns.

Ihh mRNA and protein were detected in the osteogenic fronts of all the calvarial bones, in a very restricted group of osteoprogenitors (**Figures 1C,D**). In addition there was weak protein expression across the suture. The cell surface HH receptor *Ptch1* and *Gli1* and *Gli2* expression domains were overlapping with that of *Ihh*. *Ptch1* and *Gli1* are induced by HH ligand and therefore indicate the limit of Hedgehog activation (Lee et al., 2016). In contrast, *Gli3* was diffusely expressed across the sutural mesenchyme.

In general, the calvarial osteogenic fronts (E15.5) have similar expression patterns to the osteogenic condensations (E13.5). Indeed, the osteogenic fronts can be considered analogous to osteogenic condensations with similar steps and regulation of osteoblastic differentiation and development. We also observe a differential expression of *Gli3* in different sutures which may, in part, explain the suture specific phenotype seen in mice and patients with *GLI3* mutations.

To establish if GLI3R is the predominant protein isoform in the calvarial suture, we performed western blotting on tissue samples dissected from either the midsuture or the osteogenic front from WT calvaria (**Figure 1E**). The total amount of GLI3 protein was higher in the midsutural samples. Both isoforms were observed in both samples, but the level of GLI3R was higher in the suture compared to the osteogenic front, and the opposite was true for the GLI3FL (Full length) (**Figures 1F,G**). The ratio of GLI3R/GLI3FL was significantly higher in the suture mesenchyme indicating that GLI3R is predominate in the midsutural tissue.

To verify whether a sample was midsutural or from the osteogenic front, we blotted the samples against GLI1. GLI1 also acts as a read-out for HH signaling, and based on our *in situ* hybridization results, HH signaling is active only in the osteogenic front. The level of GLI1 protein was significantly higher in the osteogenic front samples compared to the samples isolated from the suture (**Figures 1F,G**). Taken together, HH signaling is activated in the osteogenic fronts and GLI3R is predominantly localized in the midsutural mesenchyme.

GLI3 Represses the Expression of Runx2-II and Ihh, and Elevates Runx2-I

RUNX2-I and RUNX2-II isoforms differ in their N-termini due to alternative promoter usage which results in dissimilar functions during bone development (Fujiwara et al., 1999; Zhang et al., 2009). Across developing sutures, *Runx2* isoforms are differentially expressed with *Runx2-I* primarily expressed in relatively undifferentiated osteoprogenitors and *Runx2-II* in cells further along in osteoblastic differentiation (Park et al., 2001). We have previously shown that *Runx2* is ectopically expressed across the $Gli3^{Xt-J/Xt-J}$ suture (Rice et al., 2010). Here we analyzed their protein levels in osteogenic cells isolated from $Gli3^{Xt-J/Xt-J}$ calvaria. We found that RUNX2-II was upregulated and RUNX2-I downregulated, compared to wild type controls indicating that in $Gli3^{Xt-J/Xt-J}$ mice the osteoprogenitors within the suture were more differentiated than their WT littermates (**Figures 2B,C**). These results indicate that GLI3 maintains osteoprogenitors in an undifferentiated state by participating in the regulation of RUNX2. These data help explain the location specific differences seen in mRNA expression in $Gli3^{Xt-J/Xt-J}$ calvaria and the craniosynostosis observed.

As *Runx2* expression is altered in $Gli3^{Xt-J/Xt-J}$ calvaria (**Figure 2**) (Rice et al., 2010), and RUNX2 is known to regulate limb growth through the induction of *Ihh* (Yoshida et al., 2004), we analyzed IHH protein levels in $Gli3^{Xt-J/Xt-J}$ cells. We found IHH to be upregulated (**Figure 2D**). This indicates that the lack of GLI3 has allowed either increased IHH expression or a broader IHH protein expression domain.

Ihh Does Not Alter the Expression of *Gli3* mRNA

In mesenchymal cells of the developing limb bud, Sonic hedgehog is known to up-regulate *Gli* transcription, while down-regulating *Gli3* expression (Marigo et al., 1996). To test whether IHH has a direct effect on the expression of *Gli3* in WT primary calvaria derived cells (CDC) we added recombinant mouse IHH, of varying concentration, to mouse E15.5 calvarial cells and

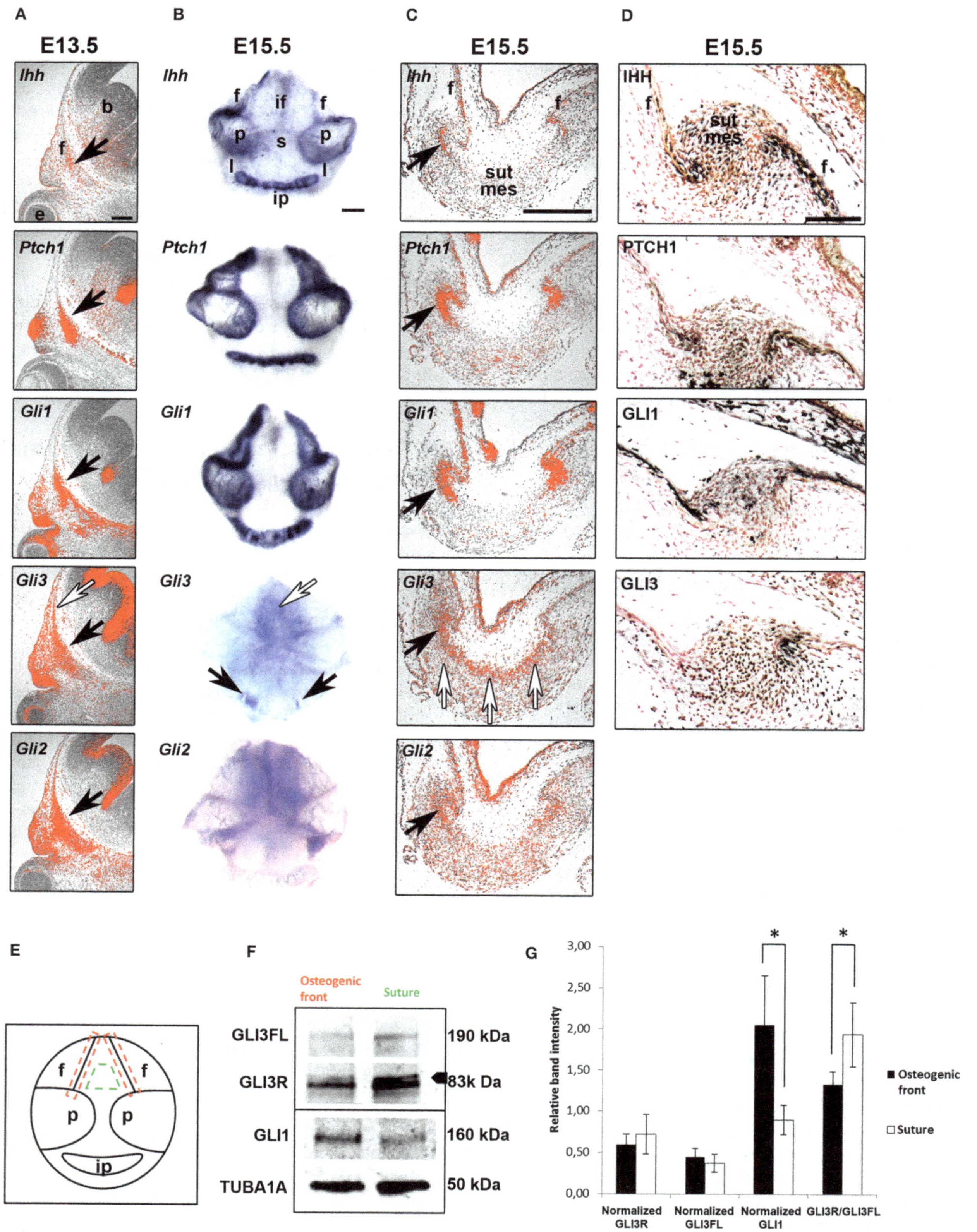

FIGURE 1 | Regulatory role for GLI3R suggested by location-specific expression. **(A–C)** mRNA and protein expression **(D)** of hedgehog ligand, receptor and transcription factors in consecutive paracoronal calvarial tissue sections in E13.5 and E15.5 WT mice (black arrows). Ihh is expressed by a narrow strip of cells in the

(Continued)

FIGURE 1 | osteogenic fronts calvarial bone primordia. Ptch1, Gli1,-2 and−3 are also expressed in the osteogenic fronts but in a wider domain than Ihh. Gli3 is also expressed more distant from the osteogenic fronts in the midsutural mesenchyme (white arrows). **(E)** Schematic to show the areas of tissue sampling from E15.5 WT calvaria interfrontal midsutural mesenchyme (green) and osteogenic fronts of frontal bones (red). **(F)** Western blot analysis (triplicate), GLI3R (83 kDa) is the upper band indicated by the arrowhead. Integrated density values obtained for GLI3; both GLI3 full-length (GLI3FL) (190 kDa) and GLI3R, and GLI1 levels were normalized against those of α-tubulin and compared against the samples **(G)**. GLI3R/GLI3FL ratio is higher in the midsutural mesenchyme compared to the osteogenic front. Conversely, normalized GLI1 intensity is greater in the osteogenic fronts compared to the midsuture. Error bars standard deviation. Statistical values calculated using Student's *t*-test, with $p < 0.05$ considered significant (*$p < 0.05$). b, brain; e, eye; f, frontal bone; if, interfrontal suture, ip, interparietal bone; l, lambdoid suture; p, parietal bone; s, sagittal suture; sut mes, sutural mesenchyme. Scale bars: **(A–C)** 250 μm, **(D)** 100 μm.

investigated *Gli1*, −2 and −3 expression levels RT-qPCR at different time points.

Exogenous IHH did not alter the mRNA levels of *Gli3* or *Gli2* (**Supplementary Figure 1**). At 24 h, IHH exposure resulted in a gradual up-regulation of *Gli1* expression in a dose-dependent manner (not statistically significant) (**Supplementary Figure 1D**). As *Gli1* is a known target of hedgehog signaling activation this response was used as a positive control. This is consistent with previous work in a chondrogenesis model using human bone marrow stromal/stem cells (Handorf et al., 2015).

Ihh Deletion Does Not Rescue the *Gli3*$^{Xt-J/Xt-J}$ Craniosynostosis

GLI transcription factors are effectors of HH signaling, with GLI3 acting as a strong repressor of IHH signals in chondrocyte differentiation with the developmental defects in endochondral ossification observed in *Ihh*$^{-/-}$ mice being partially normalized by the loss of *Gli3* (*Ihh*$^{-/-}$;*Gli3*$^{Xt-J/Xt-J}$ mice) (Koziel et al., 2005). We considered an analogous role during osteoblast development in the calvaria, and compared the calvarial phenotypes of *Ihh*$^{-/-}$, *Gli3*$^{Xt-J/Xt-J}$ and *Ihh*$^{-/-}$;*Gli3*$^{Xt-J/Xt-J}$ mutant mice, E16.5–18.5, to those of WT littermates (**Figure 3**).

Calvarial bones of *Ihh*$^{-/-}$ mice were smaller than WT. The size of the frontal and the interparietal bones was most affected, the difference being the greatest at E16.5 [frontal bone 43% smaller ($p < 0.05$), interparietal bone 33% smaller compared to WT]. Concomitant with the reduced bone size was a widening of all of the calvarial sutures [E16.5: posterior interfrontal suture 32% wider ($p < 0.05$), sagittal suture 43% wider, lambdoid suture 45% wider. E18.5: lambdoid suture comparable to WT, posterior interfrontal suture 47% wider ($p < 0.05$), sagittal suture 71% wider ($p < 0.05$)] (**Figures 3E–H,Q–T**). The posterior part of the frontal bone was reduced in height (in apical direction) and the interfrontal suture was the widest posteriorly. At E18.5, the overall length of *Ihh*$^{-/-}$ skull (nasal bones to the occiput) was slightly reduced (7%, not significant). This was in part due to the short cranial base (12% shorter, $p < 0.05$) (**Figures 3E,G**).

Gli3$^{Xt-J/Xt-J}$ mutant mice showed very specific stage and location differences in bone size and suture width (**Figures 3I–L,Q–T**). Already at E16.5 25% of *Gli3*$^{Xt-J/Xt-J}$ mice showed synostosis of the lambdoid suture. This was primarily due to an increase in the size of the interparietal bone which was enlarged from E16.5 onwards (**Figure 3T**) as opposed to a generalized increase in the size of the parietal bone. At E16.5 the width of the posterior interfrontal suture in *Gli3*$^{Xt-J/Xt-J}$ calvaria was significantly wider (26%, $p < 0.05$). However, the surface area of the frontal bones was only 15% smaller. This mismatch of the widened interfrontal suture in between the near normally sized frontal bones, indicated that frontal bone development was affected from an early stage and that extrinsic factors, for example brain shape and size and may affect frontal bone and interfrontal suture morphology. Later, the size of the frontal bones relative to WT increased. This was in part due to strong heterotopic ossification in the interfrontal suture, which culminated in partial fusion of the suture at E18.5. (**Figure 3K**). At every stage examined the width of sagittal suture was significantly wider ($p < 0.05$) (51% wider compared to WT at E16.5, 87% wider at E18.5), but the size of parietal bones was not significantly smaller compared to WT (15% smaller at E16.5, 12% smaller at E18.5). This sagittal suture widening may be caused also by extrinsic factors. At E16.5 and E18.5 overall length of *Gli3*$^{Xt-J/Xt-J}$ mutant skull was comparable to WT samples (**Figures 3I–L**).

In conclusion, *Gli3*$^{Xt-J/Xt-J}$ calvaria exhibited enlargement of the interparietal bone and heterotopic interfrontal bones with consequent interfrontal and lambdoid suture fusion. In contrast, the same sutures were wider and the bones smaller in *Ihh*$^{-/-}$ mice. These opposite differences led us to test whether *Gli3*$^{Xt-J/Xt-J}$ phenotype could be rescued by deleting *Ihh*. The craniosynostosis phenotype across the interfrontal and lambdoid sutures in *Gli3*$^{Xt-J/Xt-J}$ mice was unaffected by the loss of *Ihh* (**Figures 3M–P**), despite there being a small normalization of interparietal size at E16.5 (not significant) (**Figure 3T**). Thus, even in the absence of IHH ligand, *Gli3* deletion is sufficient to drive precocious ossification of the suture mesenchyme.

Unlike *Ihh*$^{-/-}$ Endochondral Bones, Osteoblastogenesis In *Ihh*$^{-/-}$ Calvaria Progresses Normally

Ihh$^{-/-}$ mice exhibit a severe disruption of endochondral osteogenesis with a complete lack osteoblasts. In contrast *Ihh*$^{-/-}$ mice do form calvarial bones (St-Jacques et al., 1999). Using *Runx2*, *Osterix* (*Osx*, *Sp7*), *Integrin binding sialoprotein* (*Ibsp*), and *Bglap* (*Osteocalcin*) as markers of increasing osteoblastic maturity, we analyzed osteoblastogenesis in *Ihh*$^{-/-}$ embryonic calvaria (**Figure 4**). We found that osteoblastogenesis progressed normally even though the calvarial bones were small and thin, and the sutures wide with marker expression reflecting this phenotype (**Figures 4E–H**).

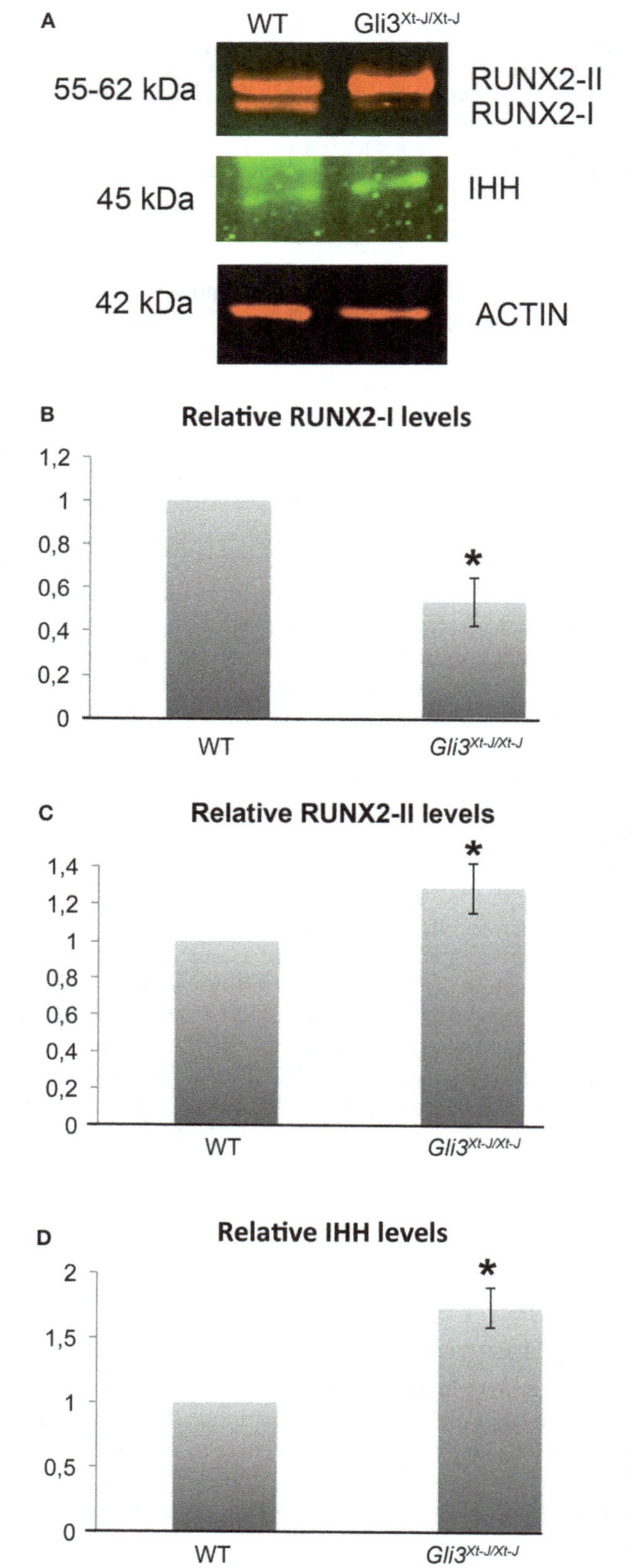

FIGURE 2 | In the absence of *Gli3*, total RUNX2, RUNX2-II and IHH are upregulated and RUNX2-I downregulated. **(A)** Protein samples from

(Continued)

FIGURE 2 | *Gli3*$^{Xt-J/Xt-J}$ calvarial osteoblasts in growth medium without osteogenic supplements show upregulated levels of RUNX2-II and IHH, and downregulated RUNX2-I, for 3 biological samples in each test group by six separate western blot analysis, representative results are shown. **(B,C)** Results are normalized against Actin antibody, and normalized values are shown with 1 representing the WT osteoblasts. (*$p < 0.05$) Error bars standard deviation.

De-repression of GLI3 in *Ihh*$^{-/-}$ Mice Results in a Similar Calvarial Osteoblastic Phenotype to *Gli3*$^{Xt-J/Xt-J}$ Mice

In *Ihh*$^{-/-}$ endochondral bones, we have previously shown that, de-repression of GLI3R (*Ihh*$^{-/-}$;*Gli3*$^{Xt-J/Xt-J}$ mice) is sufficient to restore the RUNX2-positive osteoprogenitor population (Koziel et al., 2005) but the additional action of GLI2A is required to restore the progression of osteoblastogenesis to the RUNX2-positive/Osterix-positive cell stage (Hilton et al., 2005). In *Ihh*$^{-/-}$;*Gli3*$^{Xt-J/Xt-J}$ calvaria the osteoblastic expression pattern was similar to that in *Gli3*$^{Xt-J/Xt-J}$ mice although the heterotopic ossifications were less extensive (**Figures 4M–P**). Interestingly *Gli3*$^{Xt-J/Xt-J}$ mice, which exhibit heterotopic ossifications in the interfrontal suture, showed expression of immature osteoblasts (*Runx2* and *Osx*) extending across the full width of the suture and more mature osteoblastic expression markers (*Ibsp* and *Bglap*) were limited to isolated ossification islands (**Figures 4I-L**).

Ihh Is the Functional HH Ligand in Late Embryonic Mouse Calvaria

Ptch1 and *Gli1* are direct transcriptional targets of HH signaling and both are upregulated by IHH (Lee et al., 2016). In *Gli3*$^{Xt-J/Xt-J}$ mice, *Ptch1* and *Gli1* are expressed in the developing calvarial bones and in the abnormal craniosynostotic sutures. In *Ihh*$^{-/-}$ calvaria however, *Ptch1* and *Gli1* were absent, indicating that no other Hh ligands are functional to compensate for the lack of Ihh (**Figures 5A–F**).

Endochondral ossification defects observed in *Ihh*$^{-/-}$ mice can be partially normalized by deletion of *Gli3* (*Ihh*$^{-/-}$;*Gli3*$^{Xt-J/Xt-J}$ mice). This rescue is accompanied by a concomitant normalization of *Ptch1* expression (Koziel et al., 2005). We therefore decided to test whether *Ptch1* and *Gli1* are normalized in the developing calvaria of *Ihh*$^{-/-}$;*Gli3*$^{Xt-J/Xt-J}$ mice. However, similar to *Ihh*$^{-/-}$ calvaria, *Ptch1* and *Gli1* expression were absent in *Ihh*$^{-/-}$;*Gli3*$^{Xt-J/Xt-J}$ mice (**Figures 5G,H**). This suggests that the mechanism of *Ptch1* and HH signaling activation in the calvarial osteoprogenitors differs compared to that in chondrocytes in the developing growth plate.

Ihh Is Regulated by Runx2 in Calvarial Osteoblasts and Calvarial Explants

In the developing growth plate, it has been shown that Runx2 directly regulates *Ihh* expression in chondrocytes (Yoshida et al., 2004). To test an analogous interaction during intramembranous osteogenesis, we silenced *Runx2* in E15.5 primary calvarial osteoblasts by selective *Runx2* siRNA. Silencing was verified by western blot analysis showing

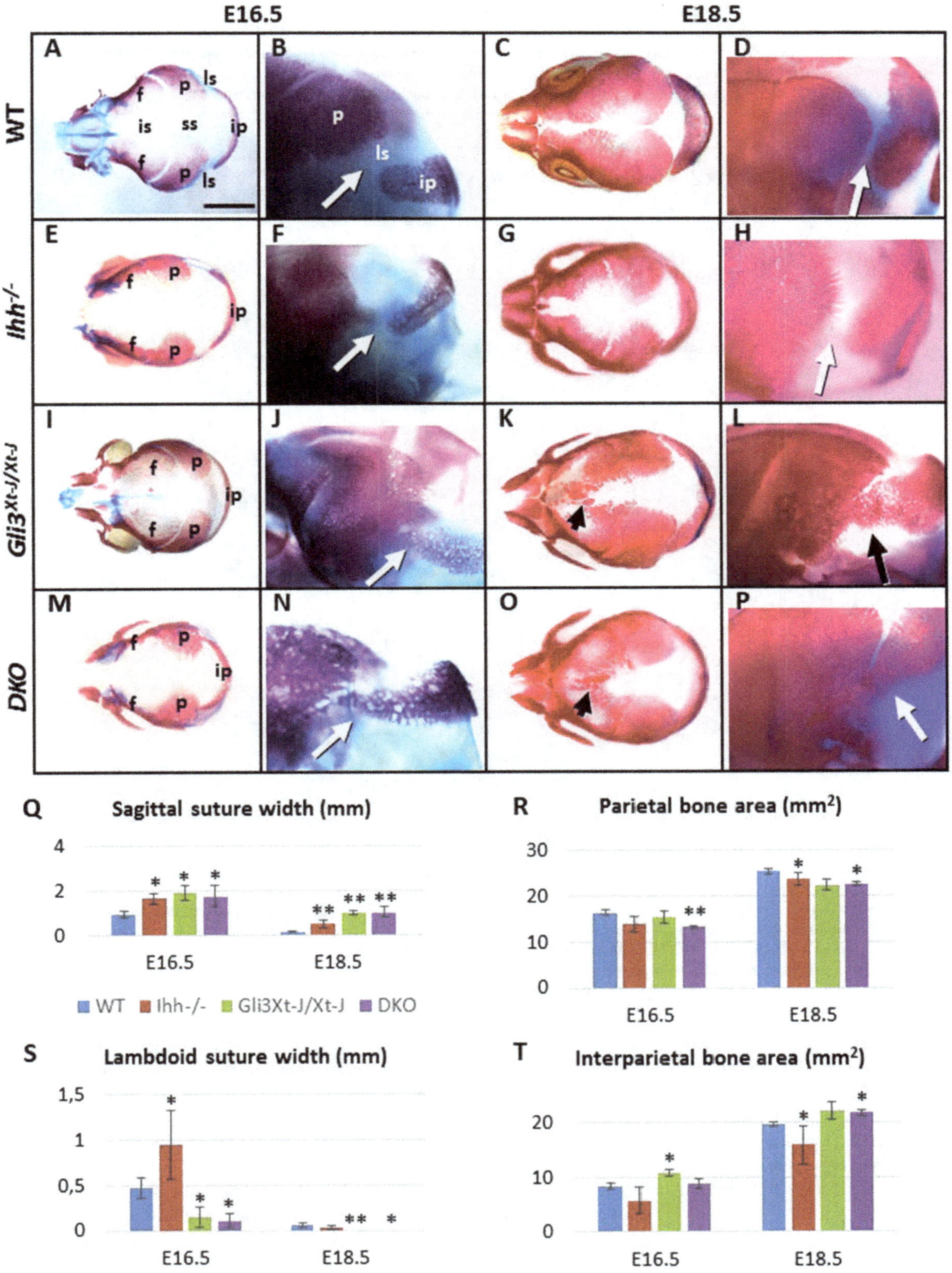

FIGURE 3 | Craniosynostosis of $Gli3^{Xt-J/Xt-J}$ mice is IHH ligand independent. **(A–P)** Alizarin Red-S and Alcian blue stained WT and mutant embryos. **(Q–T)** Selected suture width and bone area measurements. Compared to WT the calvarial bones of $Ihh^{-/-}$ mice ($n = 8$) are smaller and sutures are wider compared

(Continued)

FIGURE 3 | (to the WT $n = 20$). *Gli3*$^{Xt-J/Xt-J}$ mice ($n = 24$) have heterotopic ossifications in the interfrontal suture. The interparietal bone is larger and the lambdoid sutures are narrower with some samples already fused at E16.5. In contrast the sagittal suture is wider compared WT. Although the calvarial bone areas are reduced at E16.5, deletion of *Ihh* in *Ihh*$^{-/-}$;*Gli3*$^{Xt-J/Xt-J}$ (DKO) ($n = 6$) mice does not prevent the lambdoid sutures fusing (arrows) and heterotopic bones forming in the interfrontal suture (arrowheads) by E18.5. f, frontal bone; ip, interparietal bone; is, interfrontal suture; ls, lambdoid suture; p, parietal bone; ss, sagittal suture; DKO, double knockout (*Ihh*$^{-/-}$;*Gli3*$^{Xt-J/Xt-J}$). (*, $p < 0.1$, **, $p < 0.01$ compared to WT). Error bars standard deviation. Scale bar 2 mm.

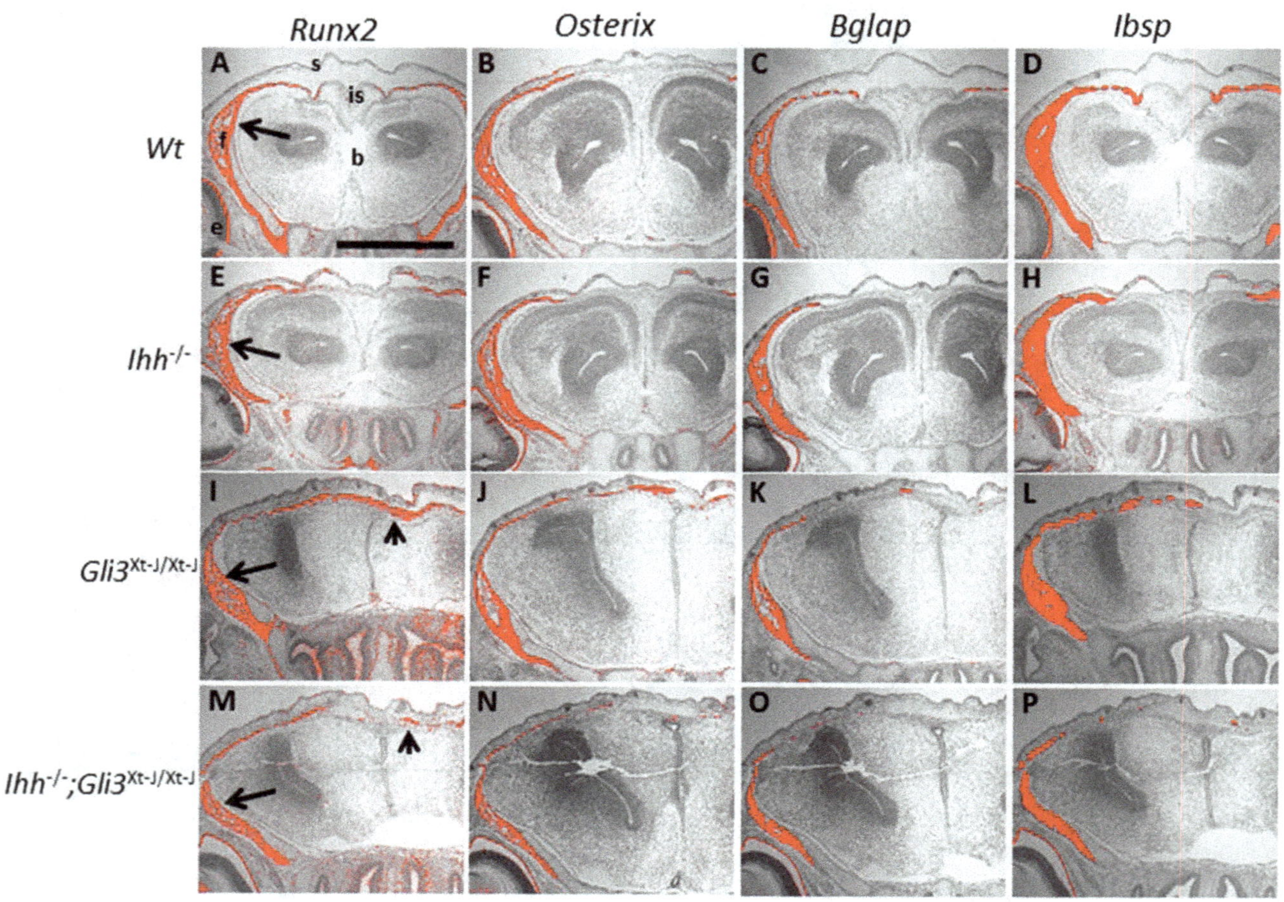

FIGURE 4 | Osteoblasts differentiate in the absence of *Ihh* and *Gli3*. **(A–P)** E15.5 Frontal sections. *Runx2*, *Osterix* (*Osx*), *Bglap* (*Osteocalcin*) and *Integrin binding sialoprotein* (*Ibsp*) are all expressed in the WT frontal bones, shown by *in situ* hybridization **(A–D** arrows). All markers are also expressed in the *Ihh*$^{-/-}$ frontal bones, but the interfrontal suture is wider **(E–H)**. In *Gli3*$^{Xt-J/Xt-J}$ **(I–L)** and *Ihh*$^{-/-}$;*Gli3*$^{Xt-J/Xt-J}$ **(M–P)** calvaria *Runx2*, *Osx*, *Bglap* and *Ibsp* are expressed in the frontal bones, but expression also extends to the interfrontal suture (arrowheads). b, brain; e, eye; f, frontal bone; is, interfrontal suture; s, skin. Scale bar 500 μm.

that Runx2 protein was downregulated (**Figures 6A,B**). Ihh protein levels were significantly ($p < 0.001$) downregulated with *Runx2* siRNA, when compared to negative controls (**Figures 6A,B**). The regulation of *Ihh* by *Runx2* was then tested in embryonic calvarial organ culture with reduced expression of *Ihh* observed adjacent to beads coated in *Runx2* siRNA, assayed by whole mount *in situ* hybridization (**Figure 6C**).

DISCUSSION

Suture biogenesis involves the balance between the promotion and suppression of osteogenesis. The correct location specificity of the positive and negative osteo-inductive signals is important so that aberrant bone formation does not take place. It is not only important that the size and shape of the bones are controlled and that ectopic bones do not form but also that sutures stay patent to allow for continued brain and craniofacial growth.

Here, we show how skull bone size and shape are tightly controlled by hedgehog signaling in maintaining the required balance of progenitor cells and functioning osteoblasts, with Gli3 having a pivotal role. Gli3R acts as an inhibitor of osteogenesis in a location specific manner by repressing the osteo-inductive key players, RUNX2-II and IHH. GLI3R can act to negatively regulate RUNX2 or the function of RUNX2 via a least three possible mechanisms: GLI3 inhibits RUNX2 by competitively

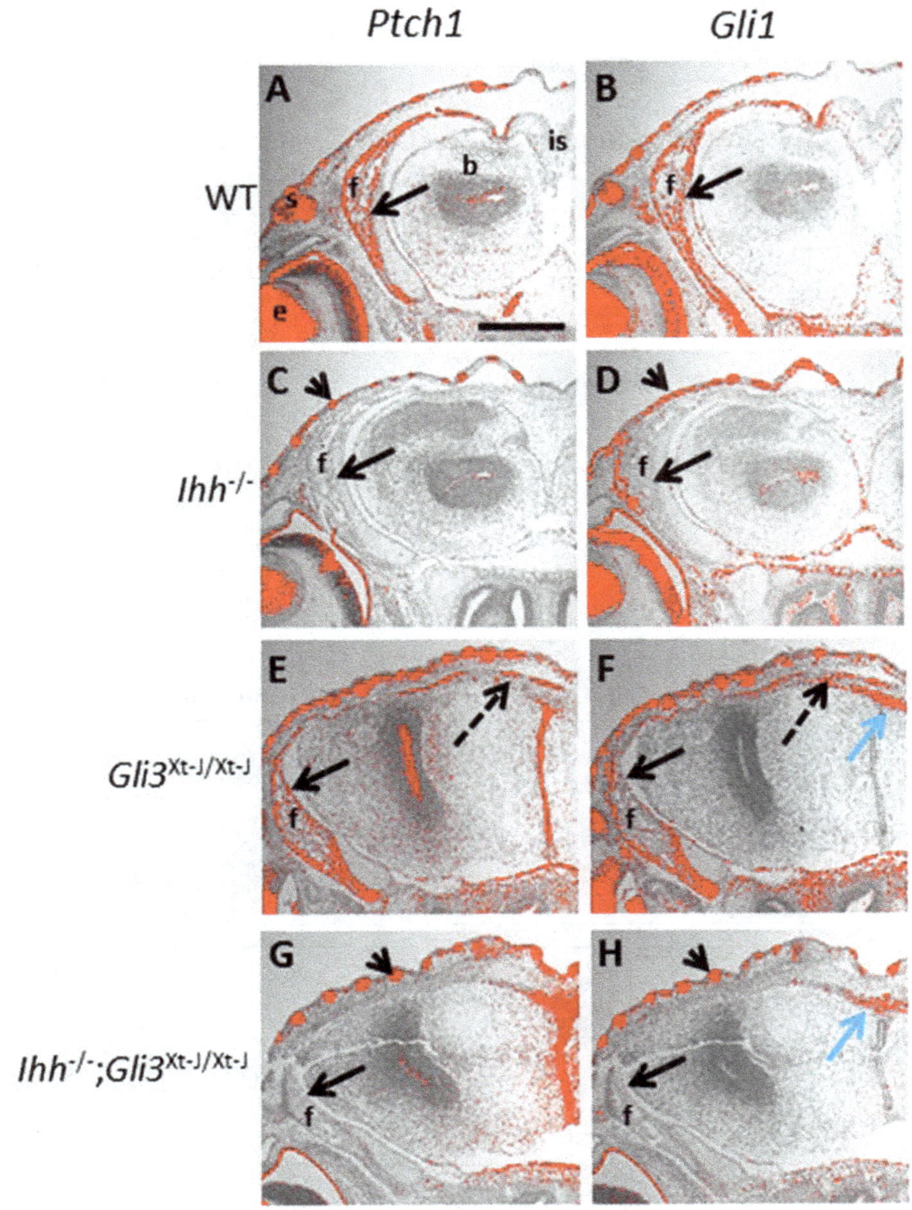

FIGURE 5 | *Ptch1* and *Gli1* expression are not restored in $Gli3^{Xt-J/Xt-J}$ calvaria by deletion of *Ihh*. **(A–H)** Hh target genes *Ptch1* and *Gli1* are upregulated by Hh ligand, E15.5 frontal sections are expressed in the developing WT frontal bone, shown by *in situ* hybridization (**A,B,** black arrows). However, in $Ihh^{-/-}$ frontal bones *Ptch1* and *Gli1* are not expressed confirming that Ihh is the only Hh ligand expressed at this stage and that it activates *Ptch1* and *Gli1* (**C,D,** black arrows). In $Gli3^{Xt-J/Xt-J}$ mice *Ptch1* and *Gli1* are expressed in the frontal bone (**E,F** black arrows), and in the interfrontal bones in the suture (**E,F** dotted black arrows). But in $Ihh^{-/-};Gli3^{Xt-J/Xt-J}$ calvaria expression of both *Ptch1* and *Gli1* is absent (**G,H** black arrows). In $Ihh^{-/-}$ and $Ihh^{-/-};Gli3^{Xt-J/Xt-J}$ mice *Ptch1* and *Gli1* are expressed in the skin where they are activated by Shh (**C,D,G,H** arrowheads). In $Gli3^{Xt-J/Xt-J}$ and $Ihh^{-/-};Gli3^{Xt-J/Xt-J}$ mice *Gli1* is ectopically expressed in the apical midline of the malformed cerebrum, intracranial to the interfrontal suture where it is activated by Shh (**F,H** blue arrow). b, brain; e, eye; f, frontal bone; is, interfrontal suture; s, skin. Scale bar 1mm.

binding to the BGLAP (osteocalcin) promoter (Ohba et al., 2008; Lopez-Rios et al., 2012); GLI3 inhibits BMP2-DLX5 activation of RUNX2; and GLI3 upregulates *Twist1* which directly represses *Runx2* (Bialek et al., 2004; Tanimoto et al., 2012). RUNX2-I is down regulated in $Gli3^{Xt-J/Xt-J}$ sutures and RUNX2-II upregulated. This is consistent with the expression of *Runx2-I* by a more immature osteoprogenitor population than those cells that express *Runx2-II* (Park et al., 2001; Tanimoto et al., 2012).

The effects of *Ihh* deletion on endochondral ossification are dramatic with long bones lacking osteoblasts (St-Jacques et al., 1999). IHH promotes osteogenesis in the orthotopic bone collar of endochondral bones through simultaneous GLI3 suppression and GLI2 activation (Hilton et al., 2005; Joeng

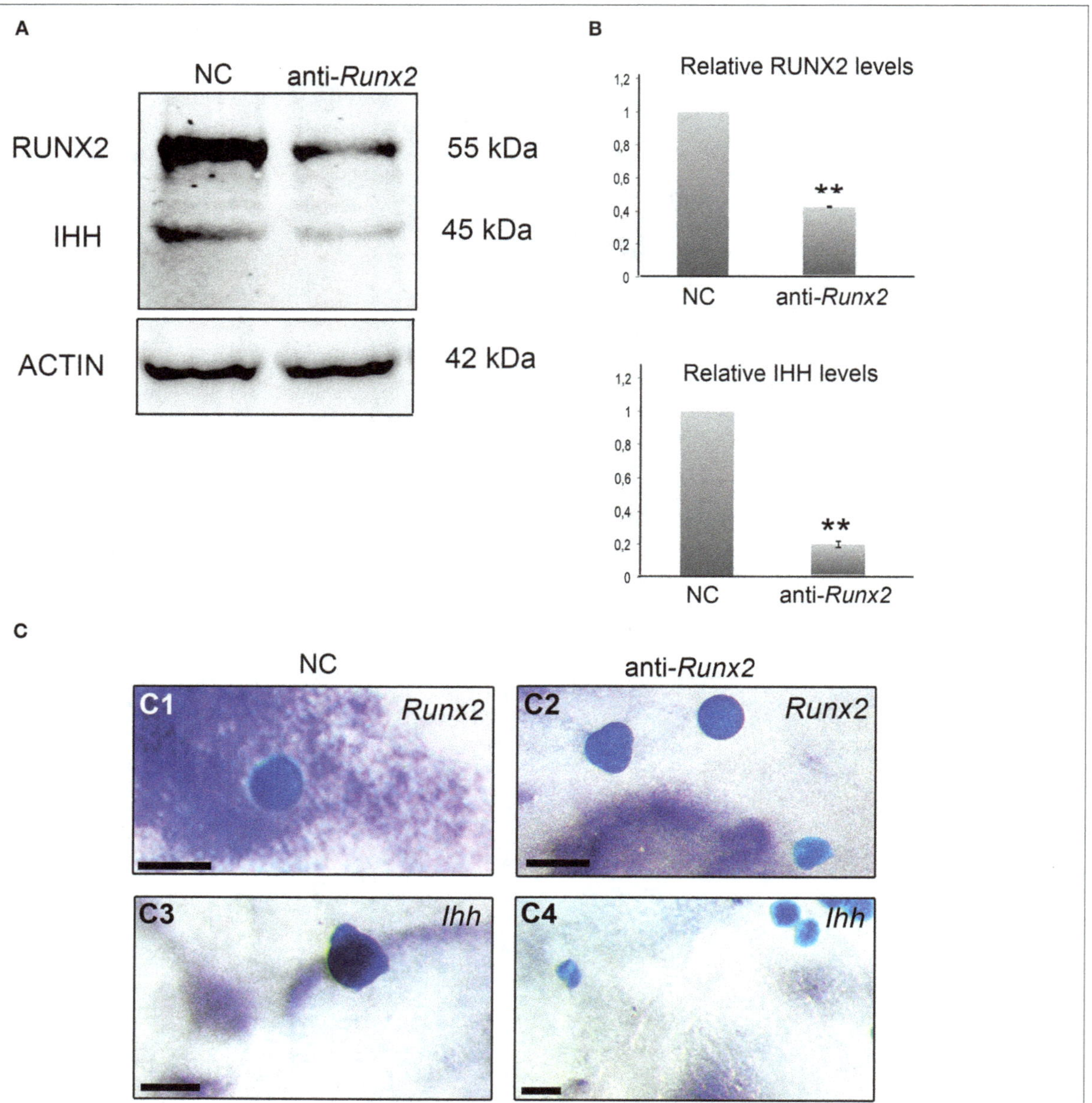

FIGURE 6 | RUNX2 regulates the expression of IHH. **(A)** Protein lysates from negative control siRNA (NC) and *Runx2* siRNA treated calvarial osteoblasts analyzed by western blotting with anti-RUNX2 and anti-IHH antibodies (triplicate). *Runx2* siRNA downregulates RUNX2 and IHH. **(B)** Results are normalized against Actin antibody staining, and normalized values are compared and shown as columns with standard error, with 1 representing the WT osteoblasts. Statistical values calculated using Student's *t*-test, with $p < 0.001$ considered highly significant (**, $p < 0.001$). **(C)** Mouse E15.5 calvaria cultured with Affi-gel blue agarose beads soaked in negative control siRNA (NC) ($n = 6$) and anti-*Runx2* siRNA ($n = 32$), and subsequently analyzed by *Runx2* **(C1, C2)** and *Ihh* **(C3, C4)** *in situ* hybridization, with 28 out of 32 beads showing a reduction of *Ihh* **(C4)**. Note *Runx2* and *Ihh* expression adjacent to the negative control (NC) beads **(C1, C3)** but no *Runx2* and *Ihh* expression adjacent to the anti-*Runx2* siRNA beads **(C2, C4)**. scale bar 100 μm.

and Long, 2009). Genetic expression of a constitutive *Gli2* activator is insufficient to rescue the defective osteoblastic differentiation in $Ihh^{-/-}$ mice. However, the additional removal of *Gli3* restores *Runx2* and *Osx* expression (Joeng and Long, 2009). The regulation of osteogenesis in the calvaria differs from that in long bones as $Ihh^{-/-}$ calvaria express *Runx2* and *Osx* (**Figures 4E,F**). That said, IHH positively regulates intramembranous osteogenesis with *IHH* duplications resulting in an overexpression of IHH being associated with craniosynostosis, and $Ihh^{-/-}$ mice exhibiting small calvarial bones with expanded sutures (**Figures 3E–H**) (Klopocki et al., 2011; Lenton et al., 2011). Despite us demonstrating that IHH is the functional ligand for HH regulated osteogenesis in the calvaria (**Figures 5C,D**), deletion of *Ihh* in $Gli3^{Xt-J/Xt-J}$ calvaria was not sufficient to rescue the craniosynostosis (**Figures 3M–P**). Despite the lack of IHH targets (*Ptch1* and *Gli1*) in $Ihh^{-/-};Gli3^{Xt-J/Xt-J}$ mice (**Figures 5G,H**). This highlights the repressive role of GLI3 and also that

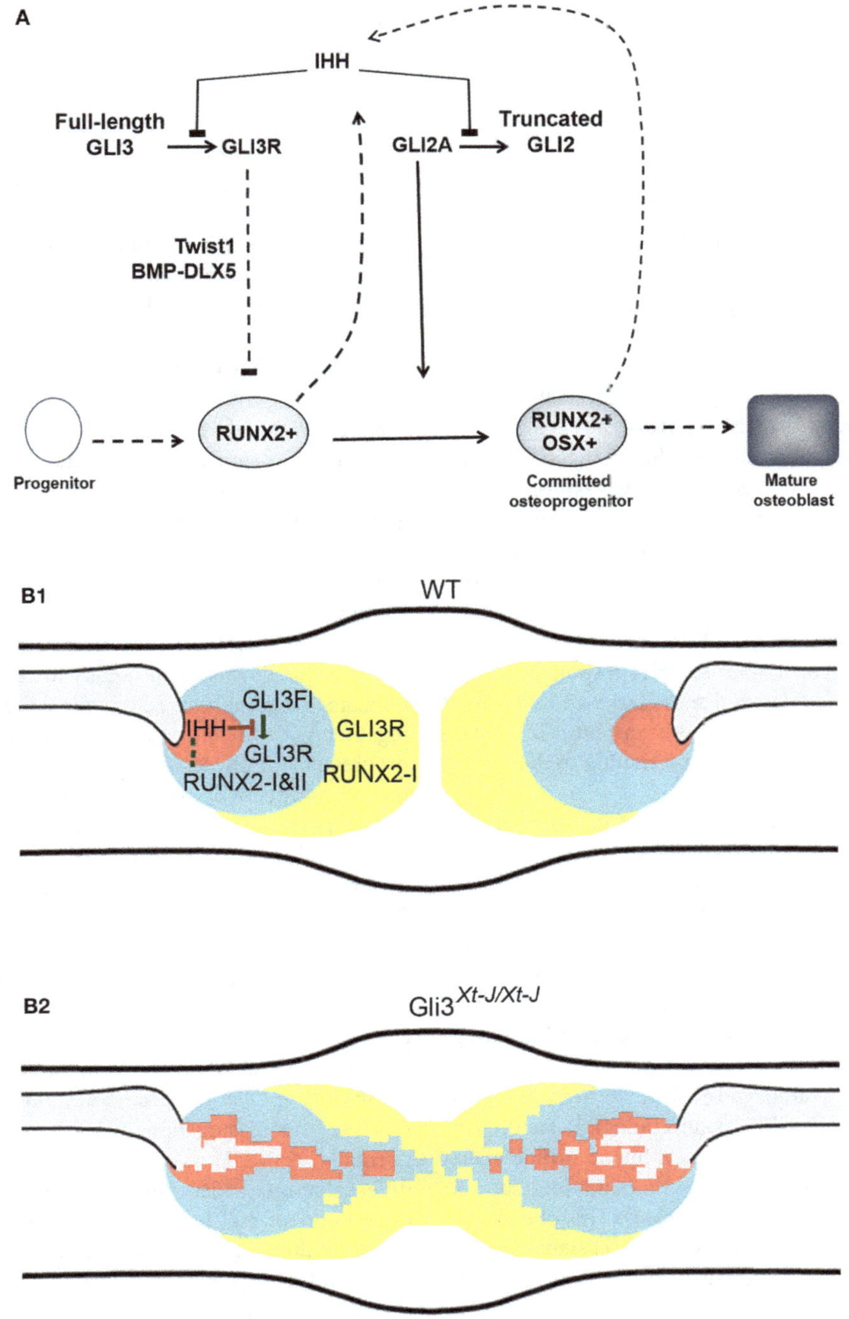

FIGURE 7 | Tight regulation of calvarial osteogenesis by GLI3. **(A)** IHH inhibits the proteolytic truncation of GLI3 into its repressor form (Wang et al., 2000). GLI3R inhibits RUNX2 by competitively binding to the BGLAP (osteocalcin) promoter (Ohba et al., 2008; Lopez-Rios et al., 2012); GLI3R inhibits BMP2-DLX5 activation of RUNX2; and GLI3R upregulates *Twist1* which directly represses *Runx2* (Bialek et al., 2004; Tanimoto et al., 2012). IHH promotes GLI2A which permits the progression of osteoblast differentiation from RUNX2-positive to RUNX2-positive/OSX-positive progenitors (Shimoyama et al., 2007). Our data suggests that RUNX2 may also participate in the regulation IHH. Figure is adapted from (Joeng and Long, 2009), and (Long and Ornitz, 2013) (Joeng and Long, 2009; Long and Ornitz, 2013). **(B1)** Osteogenesis in the normal suture. GLI3 primarily acts as an inhibitor of intramembranous ossification at the periphery of the bones calvarial bones. The truncated repressor form of GLI3 (GLI3R) is the predominant isoform in the undifferentiated sutural mesenchyme (yellow) and at the peripheral edge of the osteogenic condensation (blue). GLI3R restricts ossification and limits the proliferation rate of the mesenchymal osteoprogenitor cells by upregulating *Twist1* **(1)**. In midsutural mesenchyme *Runx2-I* expression by relatively undifferentiated progenitors is high, while in the osteogenic condensation the *Runx2* promoter is activated and both *Runx2* isoforms are upregulated. *Ihh* expression is highly localized within the osteogenic condensation possibly resulting in a short range activation of target genes, including GLI2A. GLI3 repressor limits bone formation at the edge of the osteogenic condensation. In the osteogenic condensation RUNX2-I and RUNX2-II act in a feedback loop by upregulating IHH (dashed line). Within the Ihh signaling domain (red) the truncation of GLI3FL to GLI3R does not occur and osteogenesis is

(Continued)

FIGURE 7 | activated. Outside the IHH signaling domain, GLI3R is generated which inhibits osteogenesis and maintains suture patency. **(B2)** In *Gli3*$^{Xt-J/Xt-J}$ calvaria, as GLI3R does not function, the tight regulation of osteogenesis is lost. This permits the expression domains of IHH and RUNX2 to expand and bone to form across the suture. Key: GLI3 Full length (GLI3FL), GLI3 repressor (GLI3R), undifferentiated sutural mesenchyme (yellow), osteogenic condensation periphery (blue), osteogenic condensation center (red), bone matrix (gray).

craniosynostosis is not just excessive osteogenesis but a patterning defect.

Analysis of *Ihh* zebrafish mutants suggests that Ihh is involved in osteoprogenitor recruitment and proliferation and ultimately the regulation of dermal bone outgrowth and shape (Huycke et al., 2012). Also, following local retroviral mis-expression of *Ihh* in the developing chick frontal bone a developmentally later role for Ihh has been suggested where it regulates the transition from preosteoblastic progenitors to osteoblasts (Abzhanov et al., 2007).

Our results do not exclude the possibility that GLI3 has other roles during calvarial development even prior to the establishment of sutures. Inactivation of the BMP responsive transcription factors *Msx1* and *Msx2* from neural crest cells from E9.5–E10.5 causes heterotopic ossification in the interfrontal suture due to an alteration in the fate of the early migrating neural crest cells (Roybal et al., 2010). A population of calvarial mesenchymal cells arise from HH-responsive *Gli1*-positive cells in the cephalic paraxial mesoderm and although this transcriptional activation of *Gli1* is transient, GLI3 may have a role in controlling migration and patterning of these cells (Deckelbaum et al., 2012).

During calvarial osteoblast differentiation *Gli3* is expressed prior to *Ihh* expression and then it functions as a repressor of HH target genes. During limb patterning the situation is similar, as GLI3 and dHand prepattern the limb bud before dHand activates SHH signaling (te Welscher et al., 2002). Evidence also shows that mouse limbs expressing only GLI3R have only one digit and thus resemble *Shh* null allele mice. The primary mechanism by which SHH patterns the anteriorposterior limb is by inhibiting the GLI3R formation (Cao et al., 2013).

Two mouse models of craniosynostosis have been reported with abnormal processing of GLI3 as an etiological factor. An ENU-induced mouse model representing a hypomorphic allele of *Ptch1* has bilateral craniosynostosis of the lambdoid suture, similar to *Gli3*$^{Xt-J/Xt-J}$ mice (Feng et al., 2013). This phenotype is caused by a ligand-independent activation of HH signaling and a decrease in GLI3R. Fuzzy is a regulator of cilia trafficking and consequently HH signaling. Despite, *Fuzzy* null allele mice have increased repression of GLI3R they also exhibit craniosynostosis, all be it a different suture from that fused in *Gli3*$^{Xt-J/Xt-J}$ and *Ptch1* mutant mice. The coronal suture fusion seen in *Fuz*$^{-/-}$ mice is associated with elevated fibroblast growth factor signaling which is known to play a role in regulating suture patency (Tabler et al., 2013).

We found that in *Gli3*$^{Xt-J/Xt-J}$ cells, RUNX2 and IHH are elevated and silencing *Runx2* decreases *Ihh* expression (**Figures 6A,B**). This suggests that RUNX2 may control *Ihh* expression during calvarial osteoblast differentiation, which would be analogous to its role during chondrogenesis (Yoshida et al., 2004). *Ihh* is expressed by progenitors in the osteogenic fronts (**Figures 1A,B**) and it signals to the cells within the osteogenic condensation to differentiate via a GLI2-driven mechanism. Proteolytic processing of GLI3 into the repressor isoform is inhibited in these cells allowing osteoblast differentiation to proceed. *Runx2* is upregulated and in turn activates *Ihh* expression (**Figures 2A–C**).

CONCLUSIONS

The stepwise differentiation of osteoblasts from mesenchymal progenitors through developmental stages characterized by the expression of SOX9, RUNX2, and OSX is well described (Long and Ornitz, 2013) (**Figure 7A**). IHH acts at 2 stages prior to and post Runx2 positive cells (Joeng and Long, 2009). IHH inhibits the post translational cleavage of GLI transcription factors into truncated repressor forms (Wang et al., 2000). Thus, when IHH is expressed GLI1 and −2 function as activators of downstream targets to regulate osteogenesis. GLI1 regulates calvarial stem cells while GLI2 acts an activator which, together with the simultaneous removal of GLI3R, allows the progression of uncommitted RUNX2-positive osteoprogenitors into committed RUNX2-positive/OSX-positive osteoprogenitors (Shimoyama et al., 2007; Joeng and Long, 2009; Zhao et al., 2015).

We and others have previously shown that GLI3R regulates calvarial osteogenesis by negatively regulating the action of RUNX2. With RUNX2, GLI3R competitively binds to the BGLAP (osteocalcin) promoter (Ohba et al., 2008; Lopez-Rios et al., 2012). GLI3R inhibits the Bmp2-Dlx5 activation of Runx2 and upregulates TWIST1 which directly represses RUNX2 (Bialek et al., 2004; Tanimoto et al., 2012).

We show that IHH is the functional HH ligand in the late embryonic mouse calvaria. But unlike Ihh$^{-/-}$ endochondral bones, osteoblastogenesis in Ihh$^{-/-}$ calvaria progresses normally. So IHH is not essential for calvarial osteoblastic differentiation (St-Jacques et al., 1999). As IHH regulates the conversion of full-length GLI3 into GLI3R, within the IHH signaling domain the truncation of GLI3FL to GLI3R does not occur and osteogenesis is activated. Outside the IHH signaling domain, in immature mesenchymal progenitor cells, GLI3R is generated which inhibits osteogenesis (**Figure 7B**). Here we demonstrate a location specific regulatory role for GLI3R within the suture which is independent of *Ihh* expression, as *IHH* deletion does not rescue craniosynostosis exhibited by Gli3$^{Xt-J/Xt-J}$ mice. We show that GLI3 represses the expression of *Runx2-II* and *Ihh*, and elevates *Runx2-I*. And that IHH is regulated by RUNX2 in calvarial osteoblasts and calvarial explants. This raises the possibility of a regulatory feedback circuit to control calvarial osteogenesis and suture patency.

While we have found some interesting results with regard to intra-suture regulation of, particularly, the interfrontal suture, we have not made extensive analyses of different sutures and at multiple developmental stages. With these limitations in mind, caution is emphasized when extrapolating conclusions we make from data mainly from the interfrontal suture to other sutures.

Taken together, we have presented evidence how GLI3R, RUNX2 and IHH regulate the stage and location of osteoblast differentiation in the calvarial sutures, which ultimately controls skull bone patterning, shape and size.

AUTHOR CONTRIBUTIONS

Study design: LV, TM, MH, MT, AV, and DR, Data collection, analysis, and interpretation: LV, TM, MH, MT, YK, DK, AV, and DR, Drafting manuscript and final version approval: LV, TM, MH, MT, YK, DK, AV, and DR, Responsibility for the integrity of the data analysis: LV, TM, MH, MT, YK, DK, AV, and DR.

Jusélius Foundation (4702957), Academy of Finland (257472) and FINDOS.

ACKNOWLEDGMENTS

We are grateful to Airi Sinkko and Marjatta Kivekäs for excellent technical assistance.

SUPPLEMENTARY MATERIAL

Supplementary Figure 1 | IHH does not affect the expression of *Gli3* mRNA. **(A–D)** *Gli1*, −2 and −3 expression levels in WT primary calvaria derived cells analyzed by RT-qPCR at 1, 2, 6, and 24 h in response to application of 50, 100 and 250 ng/ml of recombinant mouse IHH. Exogenous IHH did not alter the mRNA levels of *Gli2* or *Gli3*. At 24 h, IHH exposure resulted in a gradual up-regulation of *Gli1* expression in a dose-dependent manner (not statistically significant). As *Gli1* is a known target of hedgehog signaling activation this response was seen as a positive control.

REFERENCES

Abzhanov, A., Rodda, S. J., McMahon, A. P., and Tabin, C. J. (2007). Regulation of skeletogenic differentiation in cranial dermal bone. *Development* 134, 3133–3144. doi: 10.1242/dev.002709

Bialek, P., Kern, B., Yang, X., Schrock, M., Sosic, D., Hong, N., et al. (2004). A twist code determines the onset of osteoblast differentiation. *Dev. Cell* 6, 423–435. doi: 10.1016/S1534-5807(04)00058-9

Bourgeois, P., Bolcato-Bellemin, A. L., Danse, J. M., Bloch-Zupan, A., Yoshiba, K., Stoetzel, C., et al. (1998). The variable expressivity and incomplete penetrance of the twist-null heterozygous mouse phenotype resemble those of human Saethre-Chotzen syndrome. *Hum. Mol. Genet.* 7, 945–957. doi: 10.1093/hmg/7.6.945

Cao, T., Wang, C., Yang, M., Wu, C., and Wang, B. (2013). Mouse limbs expressing only the Gli3 repressor resemble those of Sonic hedgehog mutants. *Dev. Biol.* 379, 221–228. doi: 10.1016/j.ydbio.2013.04.025

Deckelbaum, R. A., Holmes, G., Zhao, Z., Tong, C., Basilico, C., and Loomis, C. A. (2012). Regulation of cranial morphogenesis and cell fate at the neural crest-mesoderm boundary by engrailed 1. *Development* 139, 1346–1358. doi: 10.1242/dev.076729

Feng, W., Choi, I., Clouthier, D. E., Niswander, L., and Williams, T. (2013). The Ptch1(DL) mouse: a new model to study lambdoid craniosynostosis and basal cell nevus syndrome-associated skeletal defects. *Genesis* 51, 677–689. doi: 10.1002/dvg.22416

Fujiwara, M., Tagashira, S., Harada, H., Ogawa, S., Katsumata, T., Nakatsuka, M., et al. (1999). Isolation and characterization of the distal promoter region of mouse Cbfa1. *Biochim. Biophys. Acta* 1446, 265–272. doi: 10.1016/S0167-4781(99)00113-X

Handorf, A. M., Chamberlain, C. S., and Li, W. J. (2015). Endogenously produced Indian hedgehog regulates TGFbeta-driven chondrogenesis of human bone marrow stromal/stem cells. *Stem Cells Dev.* 24, 995–1007. doi: 10.1089/scd.2014.0266

Hilton, M. J., Tu, X., Cook, J., Hu, H., and Long, F. (2005). Ihh controls cartilage development by antagonizing Gli3, but requires additional effectors to regulate osteoblast and vascular development. *Development* 132, 4339–4351. doi: 10.1242/dev.02025

Hurst, J. A., Jenkins, D., Vasudevan, P. C., Kirchhoff, M., Skovby, F., Rieubland, C., et al. (2011). Metopic and sagittal synostosis in greig cephalopolysyndactyly syndrome: five cases with intragenic mutations or complete deletions of GLI3. *Eur. J. Hum. Genet.* 19, 757–762. doi: 10.1038/ejhg.2011.13

Huycke, T. R., Eames, B. F., and Kimmel, C. B. (2012). Hedgehog-dependent proliferation drives modular growth during morphogenesis of a dermal bone. *Development* 139, 2371–2380. doi: 10.1242/dev.079806

Joeng, K. S., and Long, F. (2009). The Gli2 transcriptional activator is a crucial effector for Ihh signaling in osteoblast development and cartilage vascularization. *Development* 136, 4177–4185. doi: 10.1242/dev.041624

Kim, H. J., Rice, D. P., Kettunen, P. J., and Thesleff, I. (1998). FGF-, BMP- and Shh-mediated signalling pathways in the regulation of cranial suture morphogenesis and calvarial bone development. *Development* 125, 1241–1251.

Klopocki, E., Lohan, S., Brancati, F., Koll, R., Brehm, A., Seemann, P., et al. (2011). Copy-number variations involving the IHH locus are associated with syndactyly and craniosynostosis. *Am. J. Hum. Genet.* 88, 70–75. doi: 10.1016/j.ajhg.2010.11.006

Koziel, L., Wuelling, M., Schneider, S., and Vortkamp, A. (2005). Gli3 acts as a repressor downstream of Ihh in regulating two distinct steps of chondrocyte differentiation. *Development* 132, 5249–5260. doi: 10.1242/dev.02097

Lana-Elola, E., Rice, R., Grigoriadis, A. E., and Rice, D. P. (2007). Cell fate specification during calvarial bone and suture development. *Dev. Biol.* 311, 335–346. doi: 10.1016/j.ydbio.2007.08.028

Lee, R. T., Zhao, Z., and Ingham, P. W. (2016). Hedgehog signalling. *Development* 143, 367–372. doi: 10.1242/dev.120154

Lenton, K., James, A. W., Manu, A., Brugmann, S. A., Birker, D., Nelson, E. R., et al. (2011). Indian hedgehog positively regulates calvarial ossification and modulates bone morphogenetic protein signaling. *Genesis* 49, 784–796. doi: 10.1002/dvg.20768

Litingtung, Y., Dahn, R. D., Li, Y., Fallon, J. F., and Chiang, C. (2002). Shh and Gli3 are dispensable for limb skeleton formation but regulate digit number and identity. *Nature* 418, 979–983. doi: 10.1038/nature01033

Long, F., and Ornitz, D. M. (2013). Development of the endochondral skeleton. *Cold Spring Harb. Perspect. Biol.* 5:a008334. doi: 10.1101/cshperspect.a008334

Lopez-Rios, J., Speziale, D., Robay, D., Scotti, M., Osterwalder, M., Nusspaumer, G., et al. (2012). GLI3 constrains digit number by controlling both progenitor proliferation and BMP-dependent exit to chondrogenesis. *Dev. Cell* 22, 837–848. doi: 10.1016/j.devcel.2012.01.006

Maeno, T., Moriishi, T., Yoshida, C. A., Komori, H., Kanatani, N., Izumi, S., et al. (2011). Early onset of Runx2 expression caused craniosynostosis, ectopic bone formation, and limb defects. *Bone* 49, 673–682. doi: 10.1016/j.bone.2011.07.023

Marigo, V., Johnson, R. L., Vortkamp, A., and Tabin, C. J. (1996). Sonic hedgehog differentially regulates expression of GLI and GLI3 during limb development. *Dev. Biol.* 180, 273–283. doi: 10.1006/dbio.1996.0300

Maruyama, T., Jeong, J., Sheu, T. J., and Hsu, W. (2016). Stem cells of the suture mesenchyme in craniofacial bone development, repair and regeneration. *Nat. Commun.* 7:10526. doi: 10.1038/ncomms10526

McDonald-McGinn, D. M., Feret, H., Nah, H. D., Bartlett, S. P., Whitaker, L. A., and Zackai, E. H. (2010). Metopic craniosynostosis due to mutations in GLI3: a novel association. *Am. J. Med. Genet.* 152A, 1654–1660. doi: 10.1002/ajmg.a.33495

Ohba, S., Kawaguchi, H., Kugimiya, F., Ogasawara, T., Kawamura, N., Saito, T., et al. (2008). Patched1 haploinsufficiency increases adult bone mass and modulates Gli3 repressor activity. *Dev. Cell* 14, 689–699. doi: 10.1016/j.devcel.2008.03.007

Park, M. H., Shin, H. I., Choi, J. Y., Nam, S. H., Kim, Y. J., Kim, H. J., et al. (2001). Differential expression patterns of Runx2 isoforms in cranial suture morphogenesis. *J. Bone Miner. Res.* 16, 885–892. doi: 10.1359/jbmr.2001.16.5.885

Rice, D. P., Aberg, T., Chan, Y., Tang, Z., Kettunen, P. J., Pakarinen, L., et al. (2000). Integration of FGF and TWIST in calvarial bone and suture development. *Development* 127, 1845–1855.

Rice, D. P., Connor, E. C., Veltmaat, J. M., Lana-Elola, E., Veistinen, L., Tanimoto, Y., et al. (2010). Gli3Xt-J/Xt-J mice exhibit lambdoid suture craniosynostosis which results from altered osteoprogenitor proliferation and differentiation. *Hum. Mol. Genet.* 19, 3457–3467. doi: 10.1093/hmg/ddq258

Rice, D. P., and Rice, R. (2008). Locate, condense, differentiate, grow and confront: developmental mechanisms controlling intramembranous bone and suture formation and function. *Front. Oral Biol.* 12, 22–40. doi: 10.1159/0000115030

Rice, R., Connor, E., and Rice, D. P. (2006). Expression patterns of hedgehog signalling pathway members during mouse palate development. *Gene Expr. Patterns* 6, 206–212. doi: 10.1016/j.modgep.2005.06.005

Rice, R., Kallonen, A., Cebra-Thomas, J., and Gilbert, S. F. (2016). Development of the turtle plastron, the order-defining skeletal structure. *Proc. Natl. Acad. Sci. U.S.A.* 113, 5317–5322. doi: 10.1073/pnas.1600958113

Rice, R., Rice, D. P., Olsen, B. R., and Thesleff, I. (2003). Progression of calvarial bone development requires Foxc1 regulation of Msx2 and Alx4. *Dev. Biol.* 262, 75–87. doi: 10.1016/S0012-1606(03)00355-5

Roybal, P. G., Wu, N. L., Sun, J., Ting, M. C., Schafer, C. A., and Maxson, R. E. (2010). Inactivation of Msx1 and Msx2 in neural crest reveals an unexpected role in suppressing heterotopic bone formation in the head. *Dev. Biol.* 343, 28–39. doi: 10.1016/j.ydbio.2010.04.007

Shimoyama, A., Wada, M., Ikeda, F., Hata, K., Matsubara, T., Nifuji, A., et al. (2007). Ihh/Gli2 signaling promotes osteoblast differentiation by regulating Runx2 expression and function. *Mol. Biol. Cell* 18, 2411–2418. doi: 10.1091/mbc.E06-08-0743

St-Jacques, B., Hammerschmidt, M., and McMahon, A. P. (1999). Indian hedgehog signaling regulates proliferation and differentiation of chondrocytes and is essential for bone formation. *Genes Dev.* 13, 2072–2086.

Tabler, J. M., Barrell, W. B., Szabo-Rogers, H. L., Healy, C., Yeung, Y., Perdiguero, E. G., et al. (2013). Fuz mutant mice reveal shared mechanisms between ciliopathies and FGF-related syndromes. *Dev. Cell* 25, 623–635. doi: 10.1016/j.devcel.2013.05.021

Tanimoto, Y., Veistinen, L., Alakurtti, K., Takatalo, M., and Rice, D. P. (2012). Prevention of premature fusion of calvarial suture in GLI-Kruppel family member 3 (Gli3)-deficient mice by removing one allele of Runt-related transcription factor 2 (Runx2). *J. Biol. Chem.* 287, 21429–21438. doi: 10.1074/jbc.M112.362145

te Welscher, P., Fernandez-Teran, M., Ros, M. A., and Zeller, R. (2002). Mutual genetic antagonism involving GLI3 and dHAND prepatterns the vertebrate limb bud mesenchyme prior to SHH signaling. *Genes Dev.* 16, 421–426. doi: 10.1101/gad.219202

Veistinen, L., Takatalo, M., Tanimoto, Y., Kesper, D. A., Vortkamp, A., and Rice, D. P. (2012). Loss-of-Function of Gli3 in mice causes abnormal frontal bone morphology and premature synostosis of the interfrontal suture. *Front. Physiol.* 3:121. doi: 10.3389/fphys.2012.00121

Wang, B., Fallon, J. F., and Beachy, P. A. (2000). Hedgehog-regulated processing of Gli3 produces an anterior/posterior repressor gradient in the developing vertebrate limb. *Cell* 100, 423–434. doi: 10.1016/S0092-8674(00)80678-9

Yoshida, C. A., Yamamoto, H., Fujita, T., Furuichi, T., Ito, K., Inoue, K., et al. (2004). Runx2 and Runx3 are essential for chondrocyte maturation, and Runx2 regulates limb growth through induction of Indian hedgehog. *Genes Dev.* 18, 952–963. doi: 10.1101/gad.1174704

Zhang, S., Xiao, Z., Luo, J., He, N., Mahlios, J., and Quarles, L. D. (2009). Dose-dependent effects of Runx2 on bone development. *J. Bone Miner. Res.* 24, 1889–1904. doi: 10.1359/jbmr.090502

Zhao, H., Feng, J., Ho, T. V., Grimes, W., Urata, M., and Chai, Y. (2015). The suture provides a niche for mesenchymal stem cells of craniofacial bones. *Nat. Cell Biol.* 17, 386–396. doi: 10.1038/ncb3139

10

Early Determination of the Periodontal Domain by the Wnt-Antagonist Frzb/Sfrp3

Thimios A. Mitsiadis[1], Pierfrancesco Pagella[1] and Claudio Cantù[2]*

[1] *Orofacial Development and Regeneration, Institute of Oral Biology, Centre for Dental Medicine, Medical Faculty, University of Zurich, Zurich, Switzerland,* [2] *Institute of Molecular Life Sciences, University of Zurich, Zurich, Switzerland*

Correspondence:
Thimios A. Mitsiadis
thimios.mitsiadis@zzm.uzh.ch

Odontogenesis results from the continuous and reciprocal interaction between cells of the oral epithelium and cranial neural crest-derived mesenchyme. The canonical Wnt signaling pathway plays a fundamental role in mediating these interactions from the earliest stages of tooth development. Here we analyze by *in situ* hybridization the expression patterns of the extracellular Wnt antagonist *Frzb/Sfrp3*. Although *Frzb* is expressed in dental mesenchymal cells from the earliest stages of odontogenesis, its expression is absent from a tiny population of mesenchymal cells immediately adjacent to the invaginating dental epithelium. Cell proliferation studies using BrdU showed that the *Frzb* expressing and *Frzb* non-expressing cell populations display different proliferative behavior during the initial stages of odontogenesis. DiI-mediated cell-fate tracing studies demonstrated that the *Frzb* expressing cells contribute to the formation of the dental follicle, the future periodontium. In contrast the *Frzb* non-expressing cells give rise to the dental pulp. The present results indicate that Frzb is discriminating the presumptive periodontal territory from the rest of the dental mesenchyme from the very beginning of odontogenesis, where it might act as a barrier for the diffusion of Wnt molecules, thus regulating the activation of Wnt-dependent transcription within dental tissues.

Keywords: Frzb/Srfp3, Wnt signaling, tooth development, cell fate, dental pulp, dental follicle, periodontium

INTRODUCTION

Odontogenesis is characterized by the sequential and reciprocal interactions between cells of the oral epithelium and the cranial neural crest-derived mesenchyme and proceeds through a series of well-defined morphological steps, namely bud, cap, bell, and cytodifferentiation/mineralization stages (Mitsiadis and Graf, 2009). Ectomesenchymal cells form two distinct and specialized tooth components, the dental papilla that gives rise to the pulp and the dentin-producing odontoblasts, and the dental follicle, which surrounds the developing dental epithelium and forms the periodontium (Mitsiadis and Graf, 2009; Krivanek et al., 2017).

All stages of tooth development are mediated by the exchange of a big variety of signaling molecules between homotypic and heterotypic cell populations (Mitsiadis and Graf, 2009; Mitsiadis and Luder, 2011; Jussila and Thesleff, 2012; Balic and Thesleff, 2015). Among these molecules, the secreted lipid-modified Wnt glycoproteins trigger the evolutionarily conserved Wnt signaling pathway, a molecular cascade important for the development of virtually all organs (Clevers, 2006). One previous study has shown that several extracellular Wnt ligands and Wnt inhibitors are expressed in specific stages and compartments during odontogenesis (Sarkar and Sharpe, 1999).

Although many reports addressed the role of the canonical Wnt/β-catenin-mediated signaling in the formation and regeneration of dental tissues (Aurrekoetxea et al., 2012, 2016; Liu et al., 2014; Zhang et al., 2016; Babb et al., 2017) a unifying picture of its activity during odontogenesis is still missing (Tamura and Nemoto, 2016). The critical requirement of Wnt signaling during tooth development has been already evidenced, since the genetic loss of β-catenin, or the specific abrogation of β-catenin-dependent transcription, leads to arrested tooth formation at early stages (Liu et al., 2008; Cantù et al., 2017).

The action of the Wnt ligands in the extracellular matrix is regulated by physiologically secreted Wnt antagonists (or negative regulators) such as the ones belonging to the family of Secreted Frizzled Related Proteins (SFRPs), which possess a cysteine-rich domain homologous to the Wnt-binding domain of Frizzled (Frzb) receptors (Cruciat and Niehrs, 2013) and are implicated as tumor suppressors in several forms of cancer (Zimmerli et al., 2017).

Frzb (known as Frzb1 or Sfrp3, Secreted Frizzled Related Protein 3) was initially identified as a chondrogenic factor during bone morphogenesis (Hoang et al., 1996). It was subsequently shown to modulate the activity of XWnt8 during *Xenopus* dorsoventral axis development (Leyns et al., 1997) and to repress canonical Wnt signaling in other contexts (Person et al., 2005). Here we identify *Frzb* as a novel marker of the neural crest-derived mesenchymal cells that contribute to dental follicle formation, the future periodontium. *Frzb* expression at the earliest stages of odontogenesis allows distinguishing two dental mesenchymal cell populations with clearly defined developmental fates.

MATERIALS AND METHODS

Cell Proliferation Analysis

All animals were maintained and handled according to the Swiss Animal Welfare Law and in compliance with the regulations of the Cantonal Veterinary Office, Zurich (License 11/2014). *In vivo* cell proliferation in dental tissues was analyzed by immunohistochemistry for phosphorylated Histone 3 (pH3; rabbit Ab, 1:200; Upstate, Charlottesville, VA) and bromodeoxyuridine (BrdU). For the latter, a BrdU cell proliferation kit (Boehringer Mannheim, Germany) was used. Foster mothers were injected intraperitoneally with 5 mg/ml of BrdU in PBS at a concentration of 50 mg/kg body-weight, 60 min before embryos were sacrificed. BrdU-positive cells in developing teeth of E13–E15 embryos were analyzed on 14 μm cryosections after staining with an anti-BrdU antibody. Immunohistochemistry was performed as described earlier (Mitsiadis et al., 2008). Cells were counted with the CellCounter Plugin, ImageJ. Statistical Analysis was performed with GraphPad Prism 7 (*t*-test).

Lineage Tracing Using DiI Labeling

DiI (1, 10, di-octadecyl-3, 3, 30,-tetramethylindo-carbocyanine perchlorate; Molecular probes cell tracker CM-DiI, C-7000) injection was performed to various locations of mesenchymal cells surrounding the dental epithelial ingrowths of cultured mandible slices to monitor cell kinetics. Briefly, E13 mouse mandibles were carefully dissected out from the head, placed upon a chopping plate of a McIlwain tissue chopper (Mickle Laboratory Engineering Co., Ltd., Guilford, UK), orientated to obtain frontal sections and finally cut into 250 μm thick slices. Slices containing the molar tooth buds were selected and cultured. DiI, which is highly lipophilic dye intercalating into the cell membranes, was dissolved in ethanol (EtOH) at 2.5 μg/μl (stock solution) and then diluted 1–9 in 0.2 M sucrose. Thereafter, small amounts of DiI were injected using a mouth-controlled micropipette made from a 50 mm borosilicate glass into different areas of the condensing dental mesenchyme, either in mesenchymal cells contacting the molar bud epithelium or in condensing cells located at a more distant area from the tooth epithelium (Mitsiadis et al., 2008; Gruenbaum-Cohen et al., 2009).

Slice Cultures and Imaging

DiI labeled slices were placed upon Millipore filters coated with growth factor reduced Matrigel basement membrane matrix (BD Biosciences). The slices were completely encapsulated by an additional layer of Matrigel that served to structurally support the morphology of the explants during their development. The filters were supported above the culture medium by metal grids within Petri dishes. The culture medium was composed of Dulbecco's Minimum Essential Medium (DMEM) supplemented with 1% penicillin/streptomycin, 2 mM L-glutamine and 15% fetal calf serum (FCS). Slices were cultured up to 4 days in a 37°C/5% CO2 air-jacketed incubator. After culturing, samples were fixed in 4% paraformaldehyde (PFA) for 30 min, washed with PBS and then embedded in wax and sectioned at 8 μm.

The initial positions of the DiI injection and the subsequent location of the DiI-labeled cells were monitored throughout the culture period using a Leica dissecting microscope equipped with UV light (Leica Microsystems Ltd., Germany).

In Situ Hybridization

Frzb in situ hybridization probe was kindly provided by Prof. De Robertis (Leyns et al., 1997). The labeled probe was ethanol-precipitated, resuspended in 100 mM DTT, diluted in hybridization solution (60% deionized formamide, 20 mM Tris-HCl, 5 mM EDTA, pH 8, 0.3 M NaCl, 0.5 mg/ml yeast RNA, 5% dextran sulfate). *In situ* hybridization was performed according to standard procedures (Mitsiadis et al., 1995). Briefly, slides were incubated with the probe at 60°C. After intense washing, the slides were incubated in blocking solution (20% Normal Goat Serum) and anti-digoxigenin (DIG)-AP (alkaline phosphatase conjugate) Fab-fragment (Boehringer Mannheim, 1093 274) diluted 1:1,000 in blocking solution. The color reaction was developed using Nitro Blue Tetrazolium (NBT, Sigma N-6876) and 5-Bromo-4-Chloro-3-Indolyl Phosphate (BCIP, Sigma B-8503) in staining solution 2% NaCl, 5% MgCl2, 10% Tris-HCl pH 9.5, 1% Tween-20. *In situ* hybridization immediately followed by BrdU immunohistochemistry was performed in cryosectioned slides of E13–E15 mouse embryos to show the correlation between *Frzb* expression and cell proliferation (Mitsiadis et al.,

2008). No hybridization signal was detected with the sense probe at these developmental stages.

RESULTS

Frzb Is Expressed in a Subpopulation of Dental Mesenchymal Cells

To determine the potential role of Frzb in odontogenesis, we analyzed its expression pattern during the early stages of mouse tooth development (**Figure 1A**). We monitored the expression of *Frzb* in the developing mouse tooth germs from embryonic day 11 (E11; initiation stage) to E15 (cap stage). Intense hybridization signal was observed in the mesenchyme of the mandible during the tooth initiation period (E11) (**Figure 1B**). During the dental epithelial invagination to the underlying mesenchyme (early bud stage, E12), *Frzb* mRNA was restricted in mesenchymal cells located at the areas of molar (**Figures 1C,D**) and incisor (**Figure 1E**) formation. At this stage, the hybridization signal was strikingly absent from a layer of mesenchymal cells nearby the epithelium (**Figures 1C–E**, red asterisk). However, *Frzb* was strongly expressed in mesenchymal cells that are not in close contact with the dental epithelium (**Figures 1C–E**). This observation was confirmed by transcript localization at E13 (late bud stage) (**Figures 1F,G**). At the cap stage (E14–E15), *Frzb* hybridization signal was absent from the cells composing the dental papilla, while *Frzb* expression was strong in the peripheral regions of the developing tooth germ (**Figures 1H,I**).

Differential Proliferation of Presumptive Dental Papilla and Follicle Cells

We then wondered whether this distinct *Frzb* expression pattern in the developing dental mesenchyme could correlate with dissimilar proliferative behavior between these two cell populations (*Frzb* expressing and *Frzb* non-expressing cells). To test this hypothesis, pregnant females were injected with BrdU and tooth germs of E13–E15 embryos were analyzed for cell proliferation. At E13 (bud stage), two territories could be observed according to BrdU immunoreactivity. Cell proliferation was significantly lower in the mesenchyme nearby the epithelium (**Figure 2A**, red asterisk), which does not express *Frzb* (Frzb$^-$, **Figure 2G**), when compared to the mesenchyme that is most distant from the epithelium (**Figure 2A**; green arrowheads) and expresses *Frzb* (*Frzb*$^+$, **Figures 2G,J**). At the subsequent cap stage (E14–E15), the proliferation status of the two cell populations switched: abundant mitotic activity was observed in mesenchymal cells forming the dental papilla (**Figures 2B,C**; green arrowheads) outside the Frzb expression domain (*Frzb*$^-$, **Figures 2H,I**). In contrast, proliferative activity was sporadically detected in the forming dental follicle (**Figures 2B,C**; green arrowheads) that expresses *Frzb* (*Frzb*$^+$, **Figures 2H–J**). To confirm the differential proliferation status between cells of the dental follicle (*Frzb*$^+$ cells) and dental papilla (*Frzb*$^-$ cells), we stained E13–E15 tooth germs for phospho-Histone H3 (pH3), which marks cells in active mitosis (M phase) (**Figures 2D–F**). pH3 immunohistochemistry showed that *Frzb*$^+$ cells of the dental follicle proliferate significantly more than *Frzb*$^-$ cells of the presumptive dental papilla at E13 (**Figures 2D,K**). A proliferative switch occurred at E14–E15, when *Frzb*$^+$ cells of the follicle display a significantly lower mitotic activity than *Frzb*$^-$ cells of the papilla (**Figures 2F,I,K**).

Frzb Expressing Cells Mark the Presumptive Dental Follicle

To test if the *Frzb* expressing cells selectively contribute to the formation of dental follicle, we labeled subsets of the *Frzb* expressing (**Figure 3A**) and non-expressing (**Figure 3E**) mesenchymal domains with DiI at the bud stage and followed the fate of DiI-positive cells (**Figures 3B–D,F–H**). DiI-positive cells that were located in the territory of *Frzb* expression participated in the formation of the dental follicle of the cap (2 days of culture) and early bell (4 days of culture) staged teeth (**Figures 3B–D**). As DiI does not allow simultaneous labeling of the entire *Frzb* expression domain, we marked different sub-regions in a significant number of experiments ($n > 10$). In all experiments realized, DiI staining was never observed neither in the dental papilla compartment of these developing teeth, nor in other tissues formed far away from the tooth germ (**Figures 3C,D,I,J**). Conversely, DiI labeled cells in direct contact with the dental epithelium (*Frzb*$^-$ cells) contributed to dental papilla formation at the cap (2 days of culture) and early bell (4 days of culture) stages ($n > 10$; **Figures 3F–H**). Sections of the tooth germs of the early bell stage indicated dental papilla cells stained with DiI (**Figures 3G,H,K,L**). Since DiI injection was performed in both tooth mesenchymal cell populations in this experiment, DiI labeled cells were present in both dental follicle and dental papilla cells. Due to the intrinsic limitations of this technique we rarely obtained DiI labeling in dental epithelial cells when injection was performed in mesenchymal cells immediately adjacent to dental epithelial bud (**Figures 3E,F,I**).

DISCUSSION

Cranial neural crest-derived mesenchymal cells play a crucial role in tooth formation and are recognizable since the earliest stages of odontogenesis due to their positivity to classical neural crest or dental mesenchyme-specific markers such as *Pax9* (Bonczek et al., 2017), *Barx1* (Mitsiadis et al., 1998), and *midkine (MK)* (Mitsiadis et al., 1995). These cells have been historically considered as a homogeneous population of cells; nevertheless, the dental mesenchyme generates highly specialized adult soft tissues, such as the pulp and the periodontium (Jiménez-Rojo et al., 2014; Otsu et al., 2014; Mitsiadis et al., 2015). It is therefore of great interest the discovery of new markers that would allow distinguishing the subsets of mesenchymal cells possessing different differentiation commitments. Here we identify *Frzb* as a novel dental mesenchymal marker. Importantly, *Frzb* is specifically expressed from the earliest tooth developmental stages in mesenchymal cells that are not in direct contact with the dental epithelium. This specific expression pattern only partially overlaps with the expression domain of other well-established dental mesenchymal markers, such as *Pax9* (**Figure 4A**). One previous report described the expression of

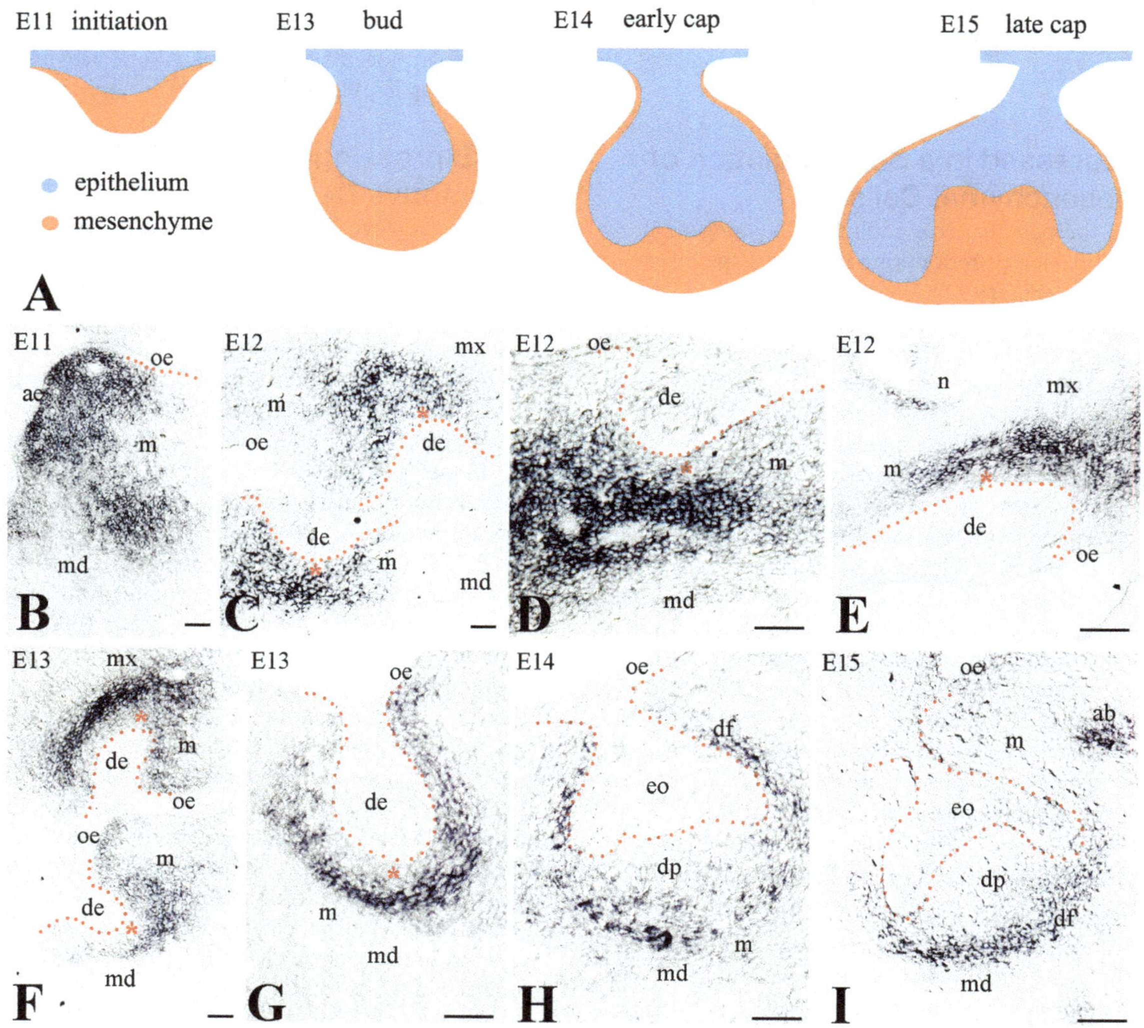

FIGURE 1 | Expression of *Frzb* transcript in developing tooth germs by digoxigenin *in situ* hybridization on cryosections **(A)** Schematic representation of the early developmental tooth stages (E11–E15). **(B)** At E11, *Frzb* is expressed in the mandibular and maxillary mesenchyme, while it is excluded from the tooth germ. **(C–G)** At the bud stage (E12–E13), *Frzb* is expressed in the dental mesenchyme, but excluded from the 1–3 cell layers immediately adjacent to the dental epithelium (red asterisks), both in molars **(C,D,G)** and incisors **(E,F)**. **(H,I)** At the cap stage (E14–E15), *Frzb* expression consistently marks the dental follicle, while it is absent from the dental papilla. ab, alveolar bone; ae, aboral epithelium; de, dental epithelium; df, dental follicle; dp, dental papilla; eo, enamel organ; m, mesenchyme; md, mandible; mx, maxilla; oe, oral epithelium; n, nose. Scale bars: 100 μm.

Frzb in the dental mesenchyme (Sarkar and Sharpe, 1999). However, the radioactive *in situ* hybridization technique that was used for the detection of the transcripts did not offer sufficient resolution to distinguish the absence of *Frzb* mRNA expression in the cell layers immediately adjacent to the dental epithelium. Based on *Frzb* expression we could identify two functionally distinct cell domains: one expressing *Frzb* that will give rise to the dental follicle, and another non-expressing *Frzb* that will form the dental papilla. This important finding shows for the first time the presence of two functionally distinct cell populations in the tooth mesenchyme and their commitment for generating specialized dental structures of the tooth at very early developmental stages (**Figure 4B**). During early odontogenesis (E11–E12), the thickened dental epithelium is surrounded by mesenchymal cells that condense and actively proliferate (Mitsiadis et al., 2003; Mitsiadis and Graf, 2009). These combined activities of cell migration, adhesion and proliferation within the mesenchyme are controlled by signaling and cell adhesion molecules such as fibroblast growth factors, midkine, syndecan. Dental mesenchyme is important for the tooth shape determination that involves alternated and well-orchestrated proliferations of distinct cell populations throughout odontogenesis. Initially, active proliferative events in the territory that will give rise to dental follicle/periodontium correlate with *Frzb* expression. This initial process of active cell proliferation within the *Frzb* expression domain determines the size of the periodontal domain that is important for proper tooth germ development and its integration in the growing

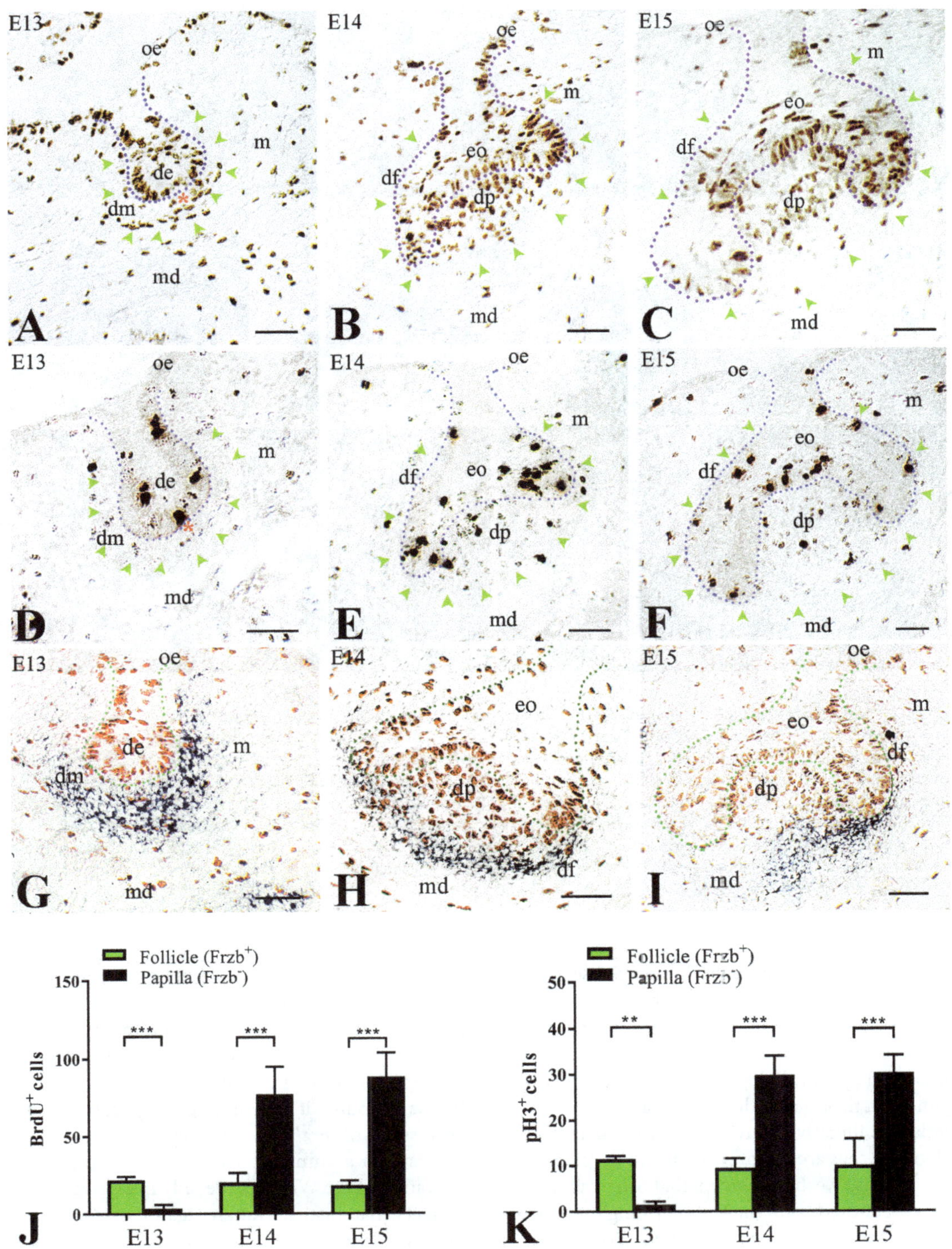

FIGURE 2 | Differential proliferative behavior of dental mesenchymal populations. **(A)** BrdU immunostaining showing intense proliferation in the presumptive dental follicle region (green arrowheads), and little proliferation in the presumptive dental papilla (red asterisk). **(B,C)** At E14–E15, cell proliferation is concentrated in the dental papilla, while it is very limited in the dental follicle (green arrowheads). **(D)** At E13, phosphorylated Histone H3 (pH3) immunostaining indicates cell mitosis in the presumptive dental follicle region (green arrowheads), and little mitotic activity in the presumptive dental papilla (red asterisk). **(E,F)** At E14 and E15, pH3 immunolabelling shows intense mitotic activity in dental papilla and moderate in dental follicle. **(G–I)** Combined BrdU immunostaining (red) and *Frzb in situ* hybridization (blue) shows the correlation between cell proliferation and *Frzb* expression within the dental follicle and papilla at E13 **(G)**, E14 **(H)** and E15 **(I)**. **(J)** Quantification of $BrdU^+$ cells in dental follicle and dental papilla at E13, E14, and E15. $n = 5$ vs. 5. **(K)** Quantification of $pH3^+$ cells in the dental follicle and dental papilla at E13, E14, and E15 ($n = 5$ vs. 5). de, dental epithelium; df, dental follicle; dm, dental mesenchyme; dp, dental papilla; eo, enamel organ; m, mesenchyme; md, mandible; oe, oral epithelium. Scale bars: 100 μm. $^{**}p < 0.001$; $^{***}p < 0.0001$.

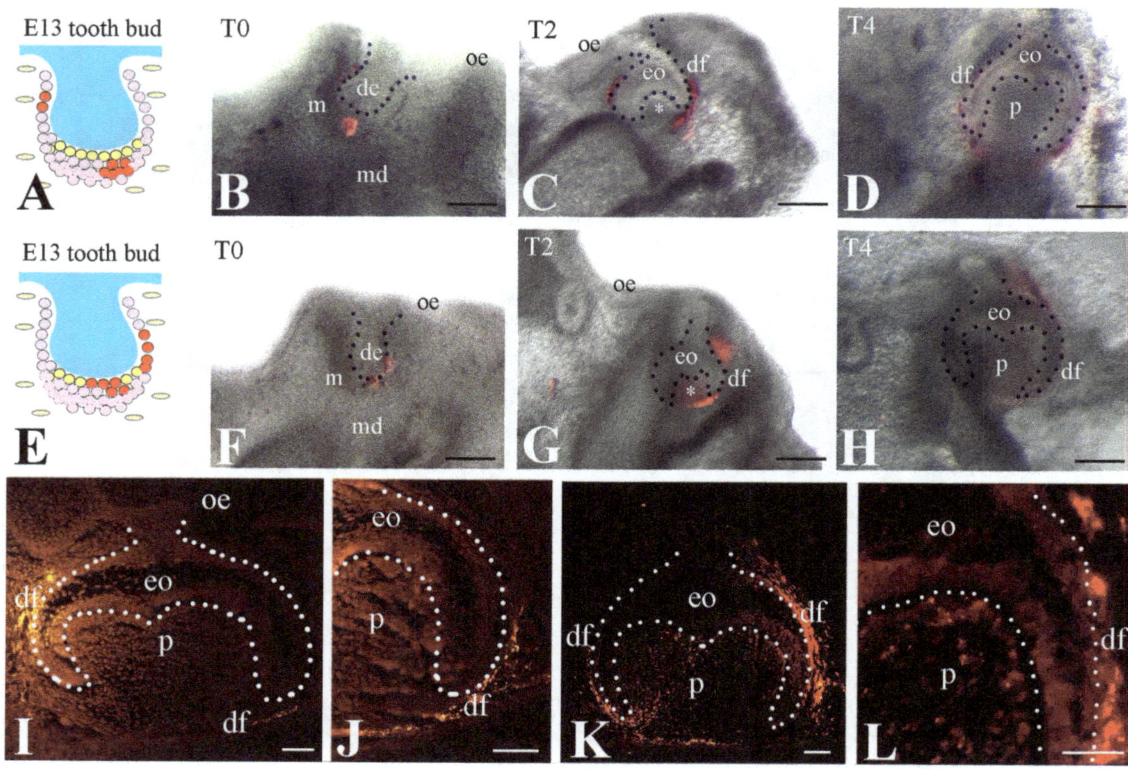

FIGURE 3 | Tracing of DiI-labeled cells from the *Frzb*$^+$ and the *Frzb*$^-$ mesenchymal territories. **(A–D)** DiI-tracing of presumptive follicular cells (n > 10 per location of injection). DiI was injected in the dental mesenchymal region distant from the dental epithelium **(A,B)**. After 2 **(C)** and 4 **(D)** days, the marked cells and their progeny gave rise uniquely to the dental follicle, as no fluorescence could be detected within the dental papilla (white asterisk in **C**). **(E–H)** DiI-tracing of mesenchymal cells both distant and adjacent to the dental epithelium. DiI was injected in close proximity to the dental epithelium **(E,F)**. After 2 **(G)** and 4 **(H)** days, DiI labeling could be observed in the papilla (white asterisk in **(G)** and in the dental follicle domain. **(I–L)** Dark field pictures showing DiI-tracing of distant mesenchymal cells (see **A**) at day 4. When DiI was injected at a distance from the dental epithelium, DiI$^+$-cells (bright yellow color) were observed only in the dental follicle **(I,J)**. Worth note that some epithelial cells next to the dental follicle were also injected with DiI during the procedure. In contrast, when both distant and adjacent mesenchymal cells were injected with DiI, fluorescence was observed in the dental pulp and dental follicle **(K,L)**. de, dental epithelium; df, dental follicle; eo, enamel organ; m, mesenchyme; md, mandible; oe, oral epithelium; p, pulp. Scale bars: **(B–D/F–H)** 200 μm; **(I–L)**: 100 μm.

surrounding environment (e.g., alveolar bone). Subsequently, once *Frzb* expressing cells have delimited the dental papilla domain, cells from this tiny *Frzb*-negative territory start to actively proliferate in order to increase the tissue size. This process is accompanied by morphological rearrangements within the growing epithelium that dictate the tooth shape.

The differential proliferative activities between dental pulp cells and dental follicle cells are not only limited to development. In our previous studies, we have shown that when pulp and follicle cells are co-cultured, they never intermingle and they assume an organization reminiscent of the *in vivo* situation, with follicle cells surrounding and engulfing pulp cells (Schiraldi et al., 2012). These cell populations appear to have a clear genetic memory and compete for their own territory even *in vitro*. Our results indicate that these two cell populations are functionally and molecularly discriminated from the earliest stages of odontogenesis, thus providing a developmental basis to their clear and persistent peculiarity. Future studies are required to understand the molecular mechanisms underlying the early specification and fate of these cell populations. In this regard, *Frzb*-based genetic lineage tracing fluorescent analysis on transgenic mouse models might be instrumental to understand the exact contribution of *Frzb*-expressing cells to tooth development as well as to the formation and the regeneration of the periodontium. Since Frzb is an extracellular Wnt antagonist, it is tempting to speculate that the restricted expression of *Frzb* to a subset of mesenchymal cells could generate an asymmetric barrier whose function is to limit the activation of the Wnt cascade only in certain cells. It is plausible, in fact, that distinct differentiation fates require cells to be Wnt-responsive, while others necessitate the inhibition of this pathway, as it occurs for the early development of the mouse heart (Marvin et al., 2001) and the eye lens (Cantù et al., 2014; Cvekl and Ashery-Padan, 2014). In this scenario, Frzb might restrict the activity of the secreted Wnt ligands to the oral epithelium and to the presumptive dental papilla. Consistently, many genes encoding for Wnt ligands are specifically expressed from the oral epithelium throughout tooth development (Sarkar and Sharpe, 1999) and genetic and molecular evidence indicates that the epithelium must remain responsive to canonical Wnt

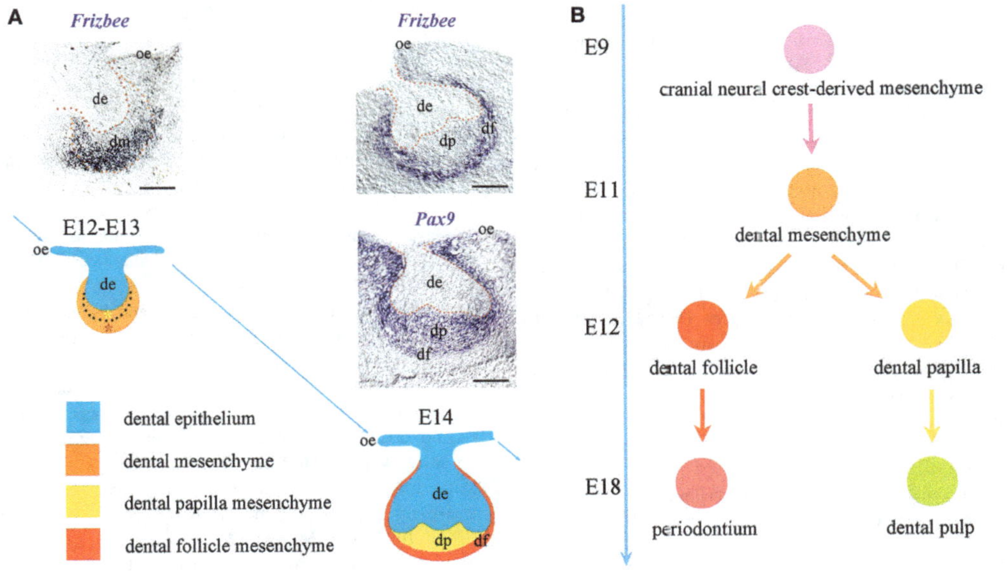

FIGURE 4 | *Frzb* expression determinates the presumptive periodontal territory from the earliest stages of odontogenesis. **(A)** Differently from well-established dental mesenchymal markers (e.g., *Pax9*), *Frzb* is expressed solely in the territory that will give rise to the periodontium from the very beginning of odontogenesis. **(B)** *Frzb* expression pattern suggests that the commitment of dental mesenchymal cells toward either follicle/periodontium or papilla/pulp formation occurs already from the bud stage of tooth development (E12–E13). Scale bars: 200 μm.

signaling. When a mutated, transcriptionally silent, version of β-catenin is exclusively expressed in the epithelium (i.e., epithelial cells become unresponsive to canonical Wnt signaling), tooth development stops abruptly (Cantù et al., 2017). Intriguingly, *Frzb* expression coincides with the dental mesenchymal territory that receives the growing neurons (Pagella et al., 2014). Indeed, from the earliest stages of odontogenesis, nerve fibers grow toward the tooth germ and progressively innervate the dental follicle. On the contrary, these nerves do not penetrate the dental papilla mesenchyme until the late stage of tooth mineralization (Pagella et al., 2014). It is thus possible that *Frzb* expression could regulate tooth innervation and probably morphogenesis. Indeed, increasing evidence indicates that innervation plays an active role in organ morphogenesis and development (Kumar and Brockes, 2012; Pagella et al., 2014). Taken together the present results suggest that the developing dental follicle necessitates a specific inhibition of the activity of the Wnt ligands. Conditional knockout and overexpression studies will constitute fundamental approaches to determine the exact role of Frzb in odontogenesis.

Both the dental pulp (formed by the *Frzb* non-expressing dental papilla cells) and the periodontal ligament (formed by the *Frzb* expressing dental follicle) contain stem cells, the dental pulp and the periodontal ligament stem cell populations, which hold the promise of regenerative approaches (Huang et al., 2009; Mitsiadis et al., 2011; Jiménez-Rojo et al., 2014). The present findings increase the arsenal of markers that permits the specific isolation of mesenchymal cells with desired differentiation potential by the combined use of mesenchymal markers. An increased knowledge of the regulation of mesenchymal dental cells will allow the future development of novel treatments for dental tissue repair and regeneration.

AUTHOR CONTRIBUTIONS

TM designed the project, performed the experiments, interpreted the data, and wrote the manuscript; PP and CC contributed to the interpretation of the data and wrote the manuscript.

ACKNOWLEDGMENTS

We thank Prof. E. De Robertis (UCLA, USA) for kindly providing the plasmid used for the generation of the *Frzb* probe. This work was supported by funds of the University of Zurich.

REFERENCES

Aurrekoetxea, M., Irastorza, I., García-Gallastegui, P., Jiménez-Rojo, L., Nakamura, T., Yamada, Y., et al. (2016). Wnt/β-catenin regulates the activity of epiprofin/Sp6, SHH, FGF, and BMP to coordinate the stages of odontogenesis. *Front. Cell Dev. Biol.* 4:25. doi: 10.3389/fcell.2016.00025

Aurrekoetxea, M., Lopez, J., García, P., Ibarretxe, G., and Unda, F. (2012). Enhanced Wnt/β-catenin signalling during tooth morphogenesis impedes cell differentiation and leads to alterations in the structure and mineralisation of the adult tooth. *Biol. Cell* 104, 603–617. doi: 10.1111/boc.201100075

Babb, R., Chandrasekaran, D., Carvalho Moreno Neves, V., and Sharpe, P. T. (2017). Axin2-expressing cells differentiate into reparative odontoblasts via autocrine Wnt/β-catenin signaling in response to tooth damage. *Sci. Rep.* 7:3102. doi: 10.1038/s41598-017-03145-6

Balic, A., and Thesleff, I. (2015). Tissue interactions regulating tooth development and renewal. *Curr. Top. Dev. Biol.* 115, 157–186. doi: 10.1016/bs.ctdb.2015.07.006

Bonczek, O., Balcar, V. J., and Sery, O. (2017). PAX9 gene mutations and tooth agenesis: a review. *Clin. Genet.* 92, 467–476. doi: 10.1111/cge.12986

Cantù, C., Pagella, P., Shajiei, T. D., Zimmerli, D., Valenta, T., Hausmann, G., et al. (2017). A cytoplasmic role of Wnt/β-catenin transcriptional cofactors Bcl9, Bcl9l, and Pygopus in tooth enamel formation. *Sci. Signal.* 10, 1–11. doi: 10.1126/scisignal.aah4598

Cantù, C., Zimmerli, D., Hausmann, G., Valenta, T., Moor, A., Aguet, M., et al. (2014). Pax6-dependent, but β-catenin-independent, function of Bcl9 proteins in mouse lens development. *Genes Dev.* 28, 1879–1884. doi: 10.1101/gad.246140.114

Clevers, H. (2006). Wnt/β-catenin signaling in development and disease. *Cell* 127, 469–480. doi: 10.1016/j.cell.2006.10.018

Cruciat, C. M., and Niehrs, C. (2013). Secreted and transmembrane wnt inhibitors and activators. *Cold Spring Harb. Perspect. Biol.* 5, 1–26. doi: 10.1101/cshperspect.a015081

Cvekl, A., and Ashery-Padan, R. (2014). The cellular and molecular mechanisms of vertebrate lens development. *Development* 141, 4432–4447. doi: 10.1242/dev.107953

Gruenbaum-Cohen, Y., Tucker, A. S., Haze, A., Shilo, D., Taylor, A. L., Shay, B., et al. (2009). Amelogenin in cranio-facial development: the tooth as a model to study the role of amelogenin during embryogenesis. *J. Exp. Zool. B Mol. Dev. Evol.* 312, 445–457. doi: 10.1002/jez.b.21255

Hoang, B., Moos, M., Vukicevic, S., and Luyten, F. P. (1996). Primary structure and tissue distribution of *frzb*, a novel protein related to Drosophila frizzled, suggest a role in skeletal morphogenesis. *J. Biol. Chem.* 271, 26131–26137. doi: 10.1074/jbc.271.42.26131

Huang, G. T.-J., Gronthos, S., and Shi, S. (2009). Mesenchymal stem cells derived from dental tissues vs. those from other sources: their biology and role in regenerative medicine. *J. Dent. Res.* 88, 792–806. doi: 10.1177/0022034509340867

Jiménez-Rojo, L., Granchi, Z., Woloszyk, A., Filatova, A., Pagella, P., and Mitsiadis, T. A. (2014). "Regenerative dentistry: stem cells meet nanotechnology," in *Horizons in Clinical Nanomedicine, 1st Edn.*, eds V. Karagkiozaki and S. Logothetidis (Singapore: Pan Standford Publishing), 255–288.

Jussila, M., and Thesleff, I. (2012). Signaling networks regulating tooth organogenesis and regeneration, and the specification of dental mesenchymal and epithelial cell lineages. *Cold Spring Harb. Perspect. Biol.* 4:a008425. doi: 10.1101/cshperspect.a008425

Krivanek, J., Adameyko, I., and Fried, K. (2017). Heterogeneity and developmental connections between cell types inhabiting teeth. *Front. Physiol.* 8:386. doi: 10.3389/fphys.2017.00376

Kumar, A., and Brockes, J. P. (2012). Nerve dependence in tissue, organ, and appendage regeneration. *Trends Neurosci.* 35, 691–699. doi: 10.1016/j.tins.2012.08.003

Leyns, L., Bouwmeester, T., Kim, S. H., Piccolo, S., and De Robertis, E. M. (1997). Frzb-1 is a secreted antagonist of Wnt signaling expressed in the Spemann organizer. *Cell* 88, 747–756. doi: 10.1016/S0092-8674(00)81921-2

Liu, F., Chu, E. Y., Watt, B., Zhang, Y., Gallant, N. M., Andl, T., et al. (2008). Wnt/beta-catenin signaling directs multiple stages of tooth morphogenesis. *Dev. Biol.* 313, 210–224. doi: 10.1016/j.ydbio.2007.10.016

Liu, W., Konermann, A., Guo, T., Jäger, A., Zhang, L., and Jin, Y. (2014). Canonical Wnt signaling differently modulates osteogenic differentiation of mesenchymal stem cells derived from bone marrow and from periodontal ligament under in fl ammatory conditions. *Biochim. Biophys. Acta* 1840, 1125–1134. doi: 10.1016/j.bbagen.2013.11.003

Marvin, M. J., Di Rocco, G., Gardiner, A., Bush, S. M., and Lassar, A. B. (2001). Inhibition of Wnt activity induces heart formation from posterior mesoderm. *Genes Dev.* 15, 316–327. doi: 10.1101/gad.855501

Mitsiadis, T. A., and Graf, D. (2009). Cell fate determination during tooth development and regeneration. *Birth Defects Res. C Embryo Today* 87, 199–211. doi: 10.1002/bdrc.20160

Mitsiadis, T. A., and Luder, H. U. (2011). Genetic basis for tooth malformations: from mice to men and back again. *Clin. Genet.* 80, 319–329. doi: 10.1111/j.1399-0004.2011.01762.x

Mitsiadis, T. A., Chéraud, Y., Sharpe, P., and Fontaine-Pérus, J. (2003). Development of teeth in chick embryos after mouse neural crest transplantations. *Proc. Natl. Acad. Sci. U.S.A.* 100, 6541–6545. doi: 10.1073/pnas.1137104100

Mitsiadis, T. A., Feki, A., Papaccio, G., and Catón, J. (2011). Dental pulp stem cells, niches, and notch signaling in tooth injury. *Adv. Dent. Res.* 23, 275–279. doi: 10.1177/0022034511405386

Mitsiadis, T. A., Mucchielli, M. L., Raffo, S., Proust, J. P., Koopman, P., and Goridis, C. (1998). Expression of the transcription factors Otlx2, Barx1 and Sox9 during mouse odontogenesis. *Eur. J. Oral Sci.* 106, 112–116. doi: 10.1111/j.1600-0722.1998.tb02161.x

Mitsiadis, T. A., Orsini, G., and Jimenez-Rojo, L. (2015). Stem cell-based approaches in dentistry. *Eur. Cells Mater.* 30, 248–257. doi: 10.22203/eCM.v030a17

Mitsiadis, T. A., Salmivirta, M., Muramatsu, T., Muramatsu, H., Rauvala, H., Lehtonen, E., et al. (1995). Expression of the heparin-binding cytokines, midkine (MK) and HB-GAM (pleiotrophin) is associated with epithelial-mesenchymal interactions during fetal development and organogenesis. *Development* 121, 37–51.

Mitsiadis, T. A., Tucker, A. S., De Bari, C., Cobourne, M. T., and Rice, D. P. C. (2008). A regulatory relationship between Tbx1 and FGF signaling during tooth morphogenesis and ameloblast lineage determination. *Dev. Biol.* 320, 39–48. doi: 10.1016/j.ydbio.2008.04.006

Otsu, K., Kumakami-Sakano, M., Fujiwara, N., Kikuchi, K., Keller, L., Lesot, H., et al. (2014). Stem cell sources for tooth regeneration: current status and future prospects. *Front. Physiol.* 5:36. doi: 10.3389/fphys.2014.00036

Pagella, P., Jiménez-Rojo, L., and Mitsiadis, T. A. (2014). Roles of innervation in developing and regenerating orofacial tissues. *Cell. Mol. Life Sci.* 71, 2241–2251. doi: 10.1007/s00018-013-1549-0

Person, A. D., Garriock, R. J., Krieg, P. A., Runyan, R. B., and Klewer, S. E. (2005). Frzb modulates Wnt-9a-mediated β-catenin signaling during avian atrioventricular cardiac cushion development. *Dev. Biol.* 278, 35–48. doi: 10.1016/j.ydbio.2004.10.013

Sarkar, L., and Sharpe, P. T. (1999). Expression of Wnt signalling pathway genes during tooth development. *Mech. Dev.* 85, 197–200. doi: 10.1016/S0925-4773(99)00095-7

Schiraldi, C., Stellavato, A., D'Agostino, A., Tirino, V., D'Aquino, R., Woloszyk, A., et al. (2012). Fighting for territories: time-lapse analysis of dental pulp and dental follicle stem cells in co-culture reveals specific migratory capabilities. *Eur. Cell. Mater.* 24, 426–440. doi: 10.22203/eCM.v024a30

Tamura, M., and Nemoto, E. (2016). Role of the Wnt signaling molecules in the tooth. *Jpn. Dent. Sci. Rev.* 52, 75–83. doi: 10.1016/j.jdsr.2016.04.001

Zhang, L., Liu, W., Zhao, J., Ma, X., Shen, L., Zhang, Y., et al. (2016). Mechanical stress regulates osteogenic differentiation and RANKL / OPG ratio in periodontal ligament stem cells by the Wnt/β-catenin pathway. *Biochim. Biophys. Acta* 1860, 2211–2219. doi: 10.1016/j.bbagen.2016.05.003

Zimmerli, D., Hausmann, G., Cantù, C., and Basler, K. (2017). Pharmacological interventions in the Wnt pathway: inhibition of Wnt secretion versus disrupting the protein-protein interfaces of nuclear factors. *Br. J. Pharmacol.* doi: 10.1111/bph.13864. [Epub ahead of print].

11

The Role of Na:K:2Cl Cotransporter 1 (NKCC1/SLC12A2) in Dental Epithelium during Enamel Formation in Mice

Rozita Jalali[1,2]*, Johannes C. Lodder[3], Behrouz Zandieh-Doulabi[1], Dimitra Micha[4], James E. Melvin[5], Marcelo A. Catalan[5,6], Huibert D. Mansvelder[3], Pamela DenBesten[7] and Antonius Bronckers[1†]

[1] Department of Oral Cell Biology, Academic Centre for Dentistry Amsterdam (ACTA), Amsterdam Movement Sciences, University of Amsterdam, VU University Amsterdam, Amsterdam, Netherlands, [2] Department of Functional Anatomy, Academic Centre for Dentistry Amsterdam (ACTA), MOVE Research Institute Amsterdam, University of Amsterdam, VU University Amsterdam, Amsterdam, Netherlands, [3] Department Integrative Neurophysiology, Center for Neurogenomics and Cognitive Research, VU University, Amsterdam, Netherlands, [4] Department of Clinical Genetics, VU University Medical Center, Amsterdam Movement Sciences, Netherlands, [5] Secretory Mechanisms and Dysfunction Section, NIDCR/NIH, Bethesda, MD, United States, [6] Departamento de Ciencias Químicas y Farmacéuticas, Facultad de Ciencias de la Salud, Universidad Arturo Prat, Iquique, Chile, [7] Department of Orofacial Sciences, School of Dentistry, University of California, San Francisco, San Francisco, CA, United States

Correspondence:
Rozita Jalali
r.jalali@acta.nl

†Retired.

Na^+:K^+:2Cl^- cotransporters (NKCCs) belong to the *SLC12A* family of cation-coupled Cl^- transporters. We investigated whether enamel-producing mouse ameloblasts express NKCCs. Transcripts for *Nkcc1* were identified in the mouse dental epithelium by RT-qPCR and NKCC1 protein was immunolocalized in outer enamel epithelium and in the papillary layer but not the ameloblast layer. In incisors of *Nkcc1*-null mice late maturation ameloblasts were disorganized, shorter and the mineral density of the enamel was reduced by 10% compared to wild-type controls. Protein levels of gap junction protein connexin 43, Na^+-dependent bicarbonate cotransporter e1 (NBCe1), and the Cl^--dependent bicarbonate exchangers SLC26A3 and SLC26A6 were *upregulated* in *Nkcc1*-null enamel organs while the level of NCKX4/SLC24A4, the major K^+, Na^+ dependent Ca^{2+} transporter in maturation ameloblasts, was slightly downregulated. Whole-cell voltage clamp studies on rat ameloblast-like HAT-7 cells indicated that bumetanide increased ion-channel activity conducting outward currents. Bumetanide also reduced cell volume of HAT-7 cells. We concluded that non-ameloblast dental epithelium expresses NKCC1 to regulate cell volume in enamel organ and provide ameloblasts with Na^+, K^+ and Cl^- ions required for the transport of mineral- and bicarbonate-ions into enamel. Absence of functional *Nkcc1* likely is compensated by other types of ion channels and ion transporters. The increased amount of Cx43 in enamel organ cells in *Nkcc1*-null mice suggests that these cells display a higher number of gap junctions to increase intercellular communication.

Keywords: mineralization, ion transport, pH regulation, SLC26A, gap junctions

INTRODUCTION

Ion transport by ameloblasts is critical for the formation of fully mineralized dental enamel. Disturbance in transport of mineral and/or bicarbonate ions (either local and/or systemic) during enamel development can lead to permanent enamel abnormalities (Lacruz et al., 2010a, 2012).

To form and mature apatite crystals, maturation ameloblasts transport mineral ions as calcium and phosphate into the forming enamel using apical plasma membrane transporter(s) such as Na^+-Ca^{2+}exchangers (NXC1,3) (Okumura et al., 2010) and Na^+-K^+-Ca^{2+} exchangers (NCKX4/SLC24A family) (Hu et al., 2012; Parry et al., 2013; Bronckers et al., 2015a). However, formation of each unit cell of the hydroxyapatite crystal also releases ~8 protons (Ryu et al., 1998) that need to be buffered to prevent acidification and arrest of mineral accretion. In order to buffer protons, ameloblasts have been proposed to secrete bicarbonate ions into the enamel space that neutralize H^+ (Smith, 1998). Bicarbonate is taken up by ameloblasts basolaterally from the extracellular fluid by bicarbonate-transporting proteins such as electrogenic (NBCe) and electroneutral (NBCn) Na^+-dependent bicarbonate cotransporters expressed in the ameloblasts during secretion- and maturation phase of amelogenesis (Josephsen et al., 2010; Lacruz et al., 2013; Jalali et al., 2014; Bori et al., 2016). During maturation phase ameloblasts also generate bicarbonates by producing carbonic acid (H_2CO_3) from CO_2 and H_2O via cytosolic carbonic anhydrase 2 (Car2) (Bori et al., 2016). During the maturation phase the bicarbonate ions are secreted by ameloblasts into the enamel space by coordinated activity of basolateral AE2, and apically by CFTR and members of the SLC26A family: SLC26A1, SLC26A3/Dra, SLC26A4/Pendrin, SLC26A6/Pat1 and SLC26A7 (Lyaruu et al., 2008; Lacruz et al., 2010b, 2012, 2013; Bronckers et al., 2011, 2015a; Jalali et al., 2015; Yin et al., 2015).

Recent studies suggested that non-ameloblast epithelial cells connected to the basal side of the ameloblasts are also involved in transepithelial transport, based on the expression of NBCe1 (Josephsen et al., 2010; Lacruz et al., 2010b; Jalali et al., 2014) and Na^+-K^+-ATPase and ATPase activity in papillary layer (Garant and Sasaki, 1986; Glynn, 2002; Josephsen et al., 2010). Accumulation of Na^+ and K^+ and reduction of Cl^- in hypomineralizing enamel of *Cftr*- null and *Ae2*- null mice suggested that in wild type mice Na^+ and K^+ are removed but that Cl^- is taken up from the forming maturation enamel (Bronckers et al., 2015a). It was speculated that maturation ameloblasts remove Na^+ and K^+ from the enamel space by a yet unknown mechanism which is impaired in *Cftr*-null and *Ae2*-null mice. Potential transporters for potassium and sodium reabsorption in ameloblasts may correspond to Na^+:K^+:$2Cl^-$ (NKCC) cotransporters, which are sensitive to loop diuretics such as bumetanide and furosemide (Gagnon et al., 1998).

Na^+-K^+-Cl^- cotransporters (NKCCs) aid in the active transport of sodium, potassium and chloride in or out of the cells (Haas, 1994). The SLC12A family contains two Na^+:K^+:$2Cl^-$ cotransporters, NKCC1 and NKCC2, encoded by two different genes (*SLC12A2* and *SLC12A1*, respectively). NKCC1 is widely distributed throughout the body. In salivary glands, basolateral NKCC1 mediates the transport of sodium, potassium and chloride from blood into the acinar cells. Lack of functional NKCC1 results in dramatic reduction of the volume of secreted saliva (Evans et al., 2000). NKCC1 is also necessary for establishing the potassium-rich endolymph that bathes part of the cochlea, the organ necessary for hearing. Inhibition of NKCC1, as with furosemide or bumetamide, can result in deafness (Delpire et al., 1999). NKCC2 has a more restricted distribution and is specifically found in the apical membrane of cells in the thick ascending limb of the loop of Henle and the macula densa in nephrons where it serves both in sodium absorption and tubuloglomerular feedback (Lytle et al., 1995). Expression of *Slc12a2/Nkcc1* messenger RNA was reported in mouse enamel epithelium in bud to bell stage teeth (embryonic stage E15–postnatal day 3), suggesting a possible involvement of NKCC1 in enamel organ development (Hübner et al., 2001).

In this study, we tested the hypothesis that NKCC1 plays a role in the ion transport by dental epithelium during enamel formation. The enamel organs of mice and HAT-7 cells, a rat ameloblast-like cell line derived from the cervical loop of a rat incisor (Kawano et al., 2002), were analyzed for expression of NKCC1 at the protein level. The effect of the null mutation of *Nkcc1* on enamel development, cell-size and enamel mineralization was studied by histology, immunohistochemistry, micro-computed tomography and Western blotting. To understand the role of NKCC1 cell volume regulation, we exposed *in vitro* HAT-7 cells to bumetanide and measured cell volume using the calcein-quenching method (Ye et al., 2015). The effect of bumetamide was also tested on electrophysiology of HAT-7 membranes by patch clamp.

MATERIALS AND METHODS

Tissues

Nkcc1-null mutant mice used for this study were generated and genotyped as previously described (Flagella et al., 1999). One hemi-maxillary incisor of each mouse was used for immunohistological studies and the other one was freeze-dried for micro-CT analysis and western blotting. For each genotypic mouse strain, at least three wild-type mice and three null mutant mice were analyzed.

All experiments were approved by the Committee for Animal Care (Vrije Universiteit Amsterdam; ACTA-12-01) and by the Animal Care and Use Committee of the National Institute of Dental and Craniofacial Research, National Institutes of Health (ASP 13–686). The methods were carried out in accordance with the approved guidelines.

Cell Culture

HAT-7 cells were grown in DMEM/F12 (Sigma-Aldrich, St. Louis, MO, USA) with 10% HyClone fetal bovine serum, 100 U/mL of penicillin, 10 μg/mL of streptomycin (Sigma-Aldrich) and 10^{-5} mM dexamethasone in humidified atmosphere containing 5% CO_2 at 37°C (Bori et al., 2016).

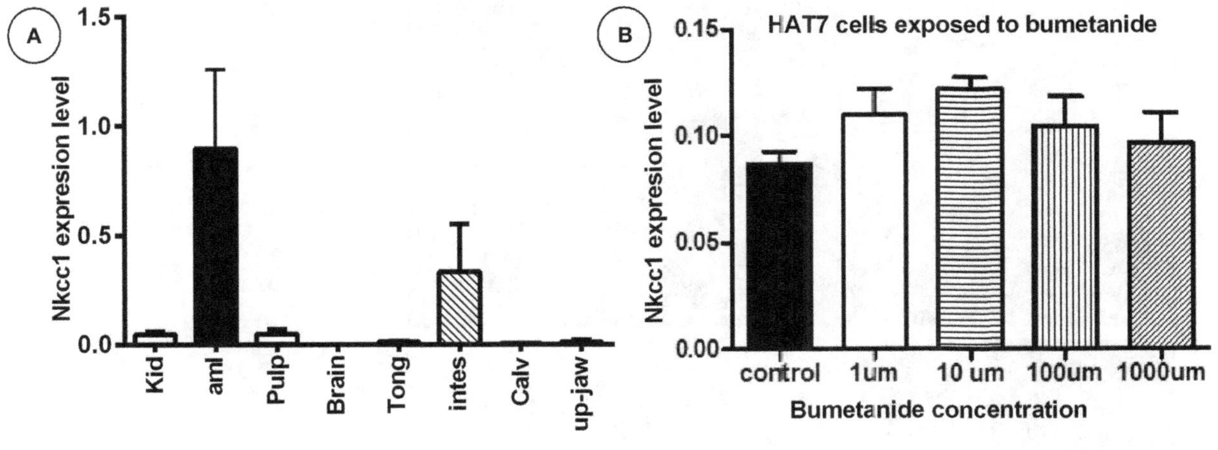

FIGURE 1 | High mRNA expression of *Nkcc1* in mouse enamel organ **(A)** and HAT-7 cells **(B)** and effect of bumetanide on *Nkcc1* expression in HAT-7 cells **(B)**. In **(A)** total RNA was extracted from different tissues and *Nkcc1* expression values normalized for ywhaz. Tissues are listed along X-axis (average for $n = 3$ mice). **(B)** Total RNA was isolated from HAT-7 cells treated with zero (control) and different concentrations of bumetanide (1, 10, 100, and 1,000 µM). kid: kidney; amlb, ameloblasts/enamel organ; pulpa, pulp; tong: tongue; stom, stomac; m3calv, MC3T3 mouse calvarial cell line; intes intestine; calv, calvaria.

Histology

Mouse jaws were fixed by immersion in 5% paraformaldehyde in 0.1 M phosphate buffer pH 7.3 and embedded in paraffin. Calcified tissues from mice older than 2 weeks were first decalcified in 4% EDTA, pH 7.3 for 2–3 weeks at 4°C. Salivary glands were fixed in Bouin's fixative (75 ml of saturated picric acid, 25 ml of 40% formaldehyde, and 5 ml of glacial acetic acid) at room temperature for 48 h and processed into 5–7 µm thick paraffin sections. Dewaxed sections were stained with 1% hematoxylin (1 min) and eosin (5 min) (HE) or used for immunohistochemicals staining.

Quantifications in Cells of the Enamel Organ

At 40x objective pictures of secretory and maturation stage of enamel organ were made and images selected based on the anatomical position in the tooth. The length of the long axis of secretory and maturation ameloblasts was measured in sagittal sections using imaging software (image J).

Real Time Quantitative Polymerase Chain Reaction (RT-qPCR)

Total RNA was extracted from HAT-7 cells and various fresh mouse tissues using the NucleoSpin RNA/protein kit (Macherey-Nagel, Düren, Germany) according to the manufacturer's instructions. First strand cDNA synthesis was performed in a 20 µl reverse transcription reaction containing 200 ng of total RNA using VILO kit (Invitrogen) according to the manufacturer's instructions. Real-time PCR analysis was performed to analyze expression of *Slc12a2* (*Nkcc1*) with the primer sequences (FW:5' GAAGAAAGTACTCCAACCAGAGATG 3'; REV: 5' CTGAAGTAGACAATCCTGTGATA 3'; size: 232 bps) and the housekeeping protein tyrosine 3-monooxygenase (*Ywhaz*) with sequences (FW:5'GATGAAGCCATTGCTGAACTTG3'; REV:5'CTATTTGTGGGACAGCATGGA3'; size:229 bps) shown by using the LightCycler 480 system based on SYBR Green I dye (Roche Applied Science, Indianapolis, IN, USA). The LightCycler reactions were prepared in 20 µl total volume with 7 µl PCR-H_2O, 0.5 µl forward primer (0.2 µM), 0.5 µl reverse primer (0.2 µM), 10 µl LightCycler Mastermix (LightCycler 480 SYBR Green I Master; Roche Applied Science, IN, USA), to which 2 µl of 5 times diluted cDNA was added as PCR template. Controls in the real-time RT-PCR reaction included RT reactions without the reverse transcriptase (control for DNA carry over) and RT reactions without template (control for reagent contamination). With the Light Cycler software, the crossing points were assessed based on a standard curve of five serial dilutions ranging from 10 ng to 1.6 pg of cDNA. PCR efficiency (E) was automatically calculated using the fit point method ($E = 10^{-1}$/slope). Gene expression data were used only if the PCR efficiency was within a 1.85–2.0 range. For each gene the amount of measured DNA was normalized to that of YWHAZ housekeeping gene to calculate relative gene expression. The relative gene expression in different tissues was normalized to kidney levels for each gene in the graphs.

Immunohistochemistry

Dewaxed paraffin sections were rinsed in phosphate buffered saline (PBS) and subjected to antigen retrieval in 10 mM citrate buffer (pH 6.0) either at 60°C overnight or for 20 min in microwave at 95°C. Endogenous peroxidase was blocked with a peroxidase block solution (Envision kit, Dakocytomation) for 5 min. Sections were washed 3x in tris-buffered saline (TBS). Non-specific staining was blocked for 30 min with 2% BSA after which sections were incubated overnight at 4°C with primary antibodies. These were (1) goat anti-NKCC1 (Santa Cruz, affinity purified, catalog number SC-21545), raised against the N-terminal end of human NKCC1. (2) Mouse anti-NCKX4 monoclonal antibodies (IgG2b isotype) from NeuroMab

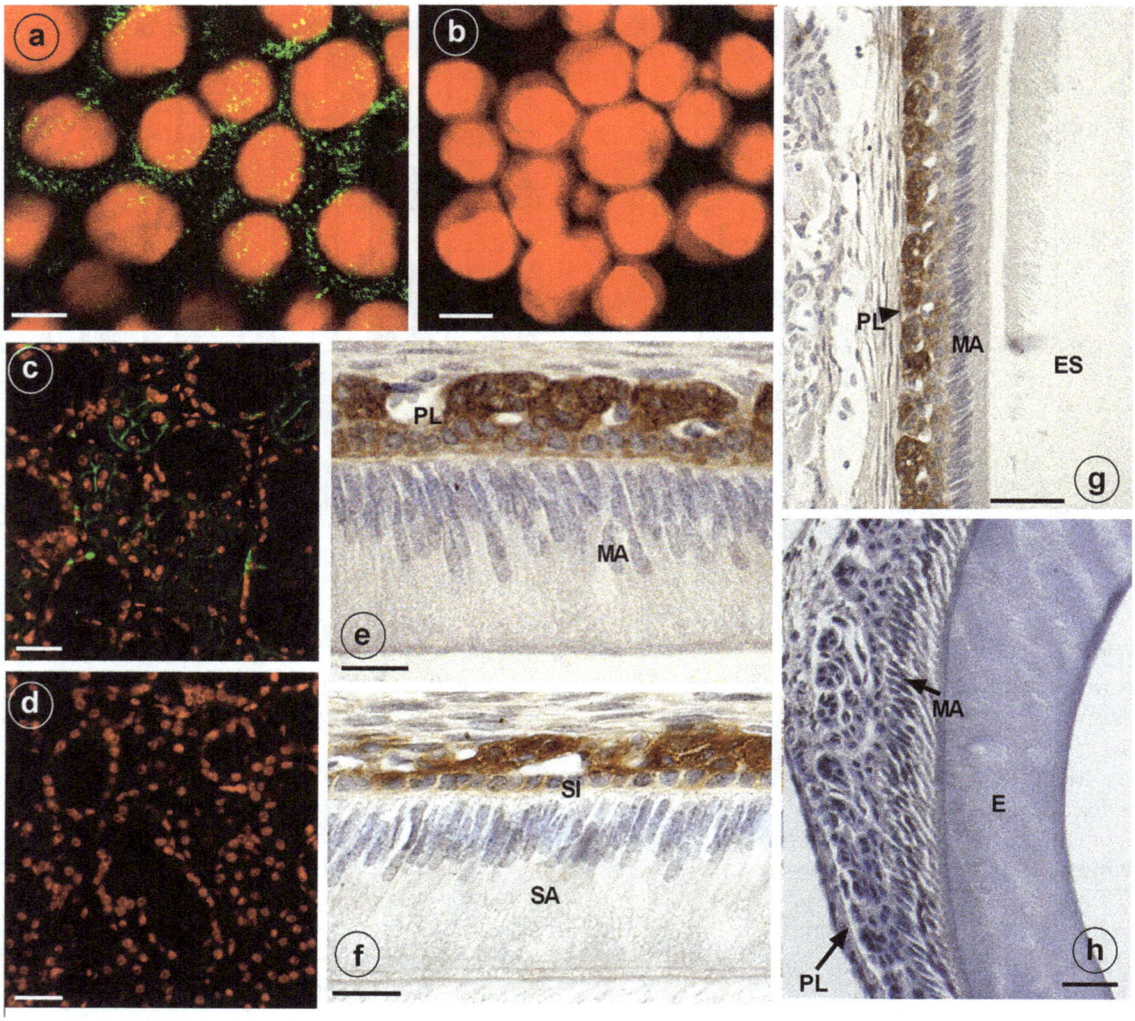

FIGURE 2 | Immunostaining of NKCC1 protein in HAT-7 cells, developing mouse dental epithelium and mouse salivary glands. NKCC1 expression as green punctuate grains near the plasma membranes of cultured HAT-7 cells stained with anti-NKCC1 **(A)** or with non-immune IgG (**B**, control) and visualized using Alexa488-coupled secondary antibody. Panels **(C,D)** show salivary glands of a wild type **(C)** and *Nkcc1* null mouse **(G)** stained with anti-NKCC1. NKCC1 staining in mouse dental epithelium at secretory stage **(F)** and in maturation stage **(E,G)** in papillary layer. Absence of staining with anti-NKCC1 in salivary gland **(D)** and incisor **(H)** of a *Nkcc1*-null mouse confirms the specificity of primary antibody. Note: all the stainings have been tested in triplicate in three mice. E, enamel; ES, enamel space; SA, ameloblasts secretory stage; MA, ameloblasts maturation stage; P, pulp; PL, papillary layer; SI, stratum intermedium.

(UC Davis/NIH NeuroMab Facility, catalog # N414/25). (3) Matched non-immune IgG (1:200–1:300) or normal serum (same concentration as primary antibodies) served as controls. After overnight incubation at 4°C with primary antibodies, sections were washed three times in TBS and incubated with rabbit anti-goat secondary antibody conjugated to peroxidase (Thermo Scientific) for 1 h at room temperature. After washing staining was visualized using DAB (EnVision kit), counterstained with hematoxylin. For immunofluorescent staining, goat anti mouse-IgG conjugated to Alexa Fluor 488 (5 μg/mL; Invitrogen) was used and counterstained with propidium iodine (Vector Laboratories, Burlingame, CA, USA). Immunohistochemistry images were acquired with a Leica EL6000 or Axio Zoom V16 microscope.

Microcomputed Tomography (microCT)

To determine the degree of mineral content, hemi-maxillae were scanned at a resolution of 8 μm voxels in a microCT-40 high-resolution scanner (Scanco Medical, AG, Bassersdorf, Switzerland) to measure mineral density in enamel. An internal standard made of solid-sintered apatite (5-mm diameter, 1.5–2.0 mm thick, solid sintered) with density of 2.9 ± 0.2 g/mL (a gift from Himed; http://www.himed.com) was used as high-density standard. Beginning at the apical part of the incisor and moving toward the tip, cross-sectioned images through the incisors were collected at sequential intervals of 300 μm in maturation-stage and 60 μm in secretory-stage enamel. In each slice, the mineral density of enamel was measured halfway through the enamel layer at three sites within a circular area, with a diameter of 7 μm

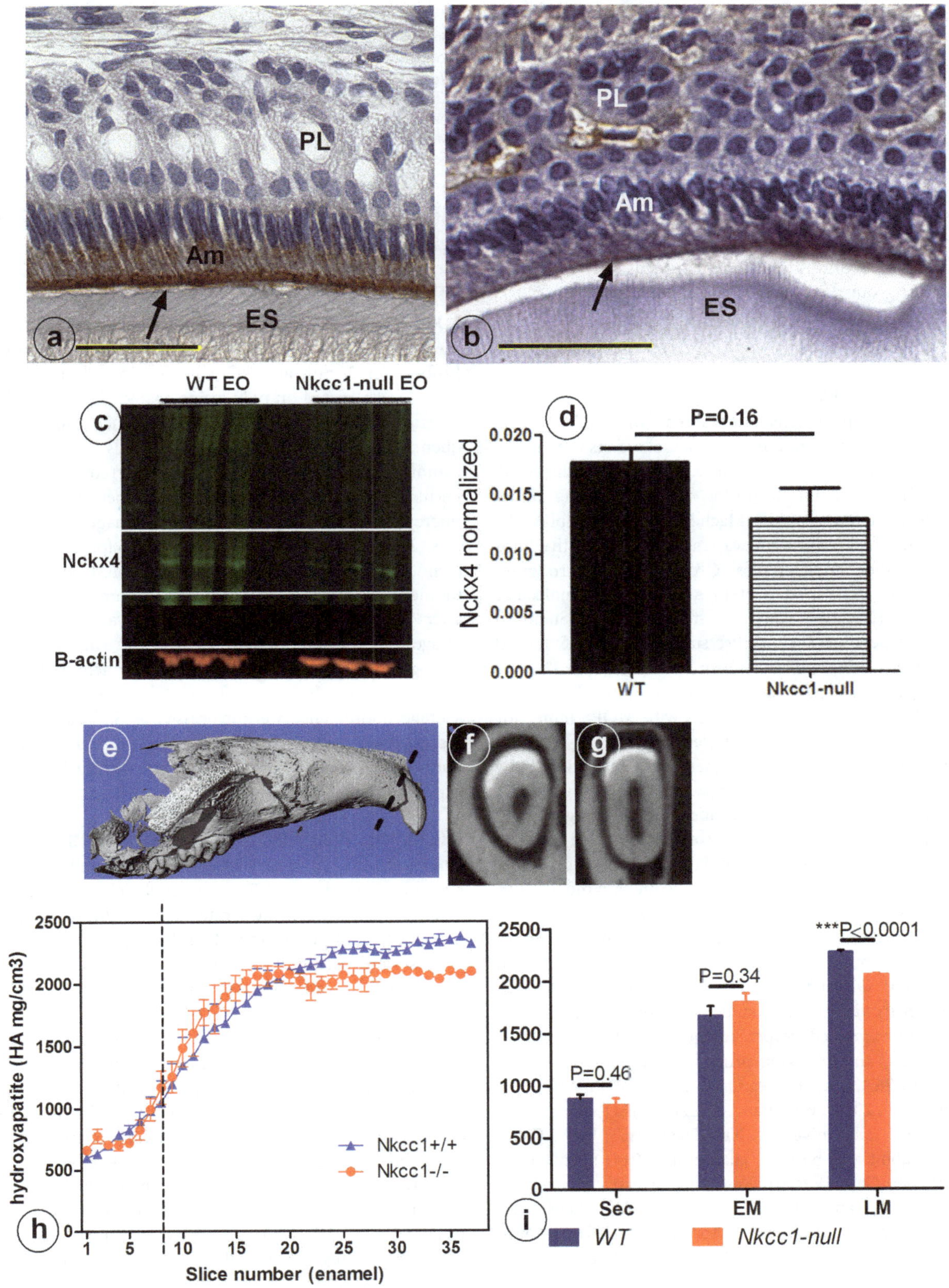

FIGURE 3 | Reduced NCKX4 protein expression in enamel organ **(A–D)** and lower mineral density **(E–I)** of advanced maturation stage maxillary incisor enamel of *Nkcc1* null mice upper incisors ($n = 3$) **(A–D)** and decrease in maturation mineral density in mouse upper incisor ($n = 3$). Panels **(E–I)** shows the importance of NKCC1 *(Continued)*

FIGURE 3 | Continued
for enamel mineralization. Nckx4 expression (arrows) in WT **(A)** and *Nkcc1*-null maturation ameloblast **(B)**. Total protein was extracted from WT and *Nkcc1*-null enamel organs ($n = 3$ mice) and NCKX4 expression analyzed by western blot **(C)**. Graph bar shows semi-quantitative NCKX4 band density normalized to that of ß-actin **(D)**. Mineral density measured by micro-CT plotted against slice numbers **(H)**. Blue color represents WT and red *Nkcc1*-null upper incisor; maturation stage starts at the dotted line. In **(I)** the bar graphs with the same color (blue and red) represent measurements of mineral density in different stages of amelogenesis (sec, secretory; EM, early maturation; LM, late maturation). Panels **(E–G)** show 3D reconstruction, virtual cross section of WT and *Nkcc1*-null upper incisor respectively. Circles in **(F)** indicate sites of measurement per slice.

at the mesial, lateral, and central sides. Mean values and standard error of mean (SEM) of the mineral density were calculated and presented as mean ±SEM. Independent Student's *t*-test was used to compare the groups. Statistical significance was set at $p < 0.05$ level.

Western Blotting

From freeze-dried upper incisors obtained from wild-type and $Nkcc1^{-/-}$ mice early maturation stage enamel organs were micro dissected. The apical half of the enamel organ was dissected, dissolved in non-reducing condition in SDS loading buffer (from Nucleospin Triprep kit, Macherey-Nagel, supplied by Bioke, Leiden, NL) and protein was measured using the BCA protein assay (Bio-Rad, Hercules, CA). Twenty micro gram of enamel organ denatured protein and 10 µg of molecular weight markers [Novex® Sharp Pre-stained Protein Standard (# LC5800) or SeeBlue® Plus2 Pre-stained Protein Standard (#LC5925)] were subjected to electrophoresis in a 3–8% Tris acetate Nupage gel with Tris acetate running buffer for 60 min at 150 V or 4–12% Bis-Tris Protein Gels with MOPS buffer for 35 min at 200 V. and subsequently electroblotted by an iBlot device (Invitrogen) on nitrocellulose membrane according to the manufacturer's instructions. Membranes were blocked with BSA 2% for 1 h at room temperature and incubated overnight (4°C) with the primary antibodies. Blots were washed three times in PBS and incubated with IRDye secondary antibodies (LI-COR). Visualization and quantification was carried out with the LI-COR Odyssey scanner and software (LI-COR Biosciences). Actin was detected at 680 nm wavelength (shown as red) and other primary antibodies and tubulin were detected at 800 nm wavelength (shown as green). Quantification was performed using Odyssey software. Intensity values of the bands were normalized for actin or tubulin and expressed as percentage of wild type (100%). For western blots the following primary antibodies were used: rabbit anti-SLC26A3/Dra (Research Genetics, Huntsville, AL, USA) (Jalali et al., 2015), rabbit anti-SLC26A6/Pat1 (donated by Dr. P. Aronson, Yale University, New Haven, CT, USA) (Jalali et al., 2015), rabbit anti-NBCe1 (Jalali et al., 2014) (donated by Dr. W.F. Boron, Case Western Reserve University, Cleveland, Ohio, USA), rabbit anti-NCKX4 (NeuroMab, UC Davis/NIH, # N414/25), rabbit anti-connexin (Abcam, #ab11370), mouse anti-β-actin antibody (Sigma, A2228) and rabbit anti-tubulin antibody (Abcam, ab59680). Secondary antibodies: IRDye 800CW conjugated goat anti-rabbit IgG (H+L) highly cross-adsorbed (LI-COR; Product number: 926–32,211) and IRDye 680CW conjugated goat anti-mouse IgG (H+L) highly-cross adsorbed (LI-COR; Product number: 926–32,220). Dilutions: anti-β-actin and anti-tubulin (1:1,000); other primary antibodies (1:250); secondary antibodies (1:10,000).

Imaging of Volume Decrease after Exposure to Bumetanide

HAT-7 cells were loaded with 5 µM Calcein-AM (Molecular Probes) for 20 min at 37°C. Changes in cell volume of single HAT-7 cells, plated on poly-lysine coated glass cover slips, were assessed by measuring calcein fluorescence using the calcein-quenching method (Ye et al., 2015). Cells were bathed in iso-osmotic solution (20–22°C) and transferred to a continuously perfused (5 ml/min) recording chamber, equipped with a microscope with 10X objective. An image was taken every 30 s. At the start images were obtained for 5 min in the iso-osmotic solution to establish the baseline. Cells were exposed to media supplemented with 10 µM bumetanide for 30 min, after which the iso-osmotic solution was re-introduced and images were taken for another 10 min. The cell surface and average fluorescence of each cell in the acquired images was calculated using Image-J software. Changes in cell surface and average fluorescence were expressed as S_t/S_0 and F_t/F_0 ratios, respectively, where S_0 and F_0 are the average cell surface area and fluorescence under iso-osmotic treatment at the beginning of the experiment.

Electrophysiological Recordings

Cover slips bearing HAT-7 cells were transferred to the recording chamber, containing 1.5 ml external solution. The external solution was changed at a rate of 1.5 ml/min using a gravity driven constant perfusion system. During the recordings, HAT-7 cells were perfused with standard artificial Cerebral Spinal Fluid (aCSF) containing (in mM): 126 NaCl, 3KCl, 10 D-glucose, 26 $NaHCO_3$, 1.2 NaH_2PO_4, 2 $CaCl_2$ and 1 $MgSO_4$, carboxygenated with 95% O_2 and 5% CO_2 to obtain pH 7.4 and an osmolality of 300 mOsm. For electrophysiological recordings, we used a EPC-8 amplifier and a Instrutech ICT-18 (all from Heka, D-67466 Lambrecht, Germany). Cells were identified and patched using an Olympus IX51 inverted microscope equipped with a LCAcn 40x 0.55nA ph2 objective (all Olympus corporation, Tokyo, Japan). Glass pipettes for whole-cell and cell attached recordings were made from borosilicate capillaries (OD 1.5 mm, ID 0.86 mm; Harvard Apparatus, Holliston, MA, USA) using a Sutter P-87 micro-electrode puller (Sutter instruments, USA) and displayed a resistance of 2.5–5 MΩ. Glass microelectrodes were filled with intracellular solution containing (in mM): 110 K-Gluconate, 10 KCl, 10 HEPES, 0.4 NaGTP, 4 Mg_2ATP and 10 K-Phosphocreatine (pH 7.3 adjusted with KOH, 290 mOsm). HAT-7 cells were gently

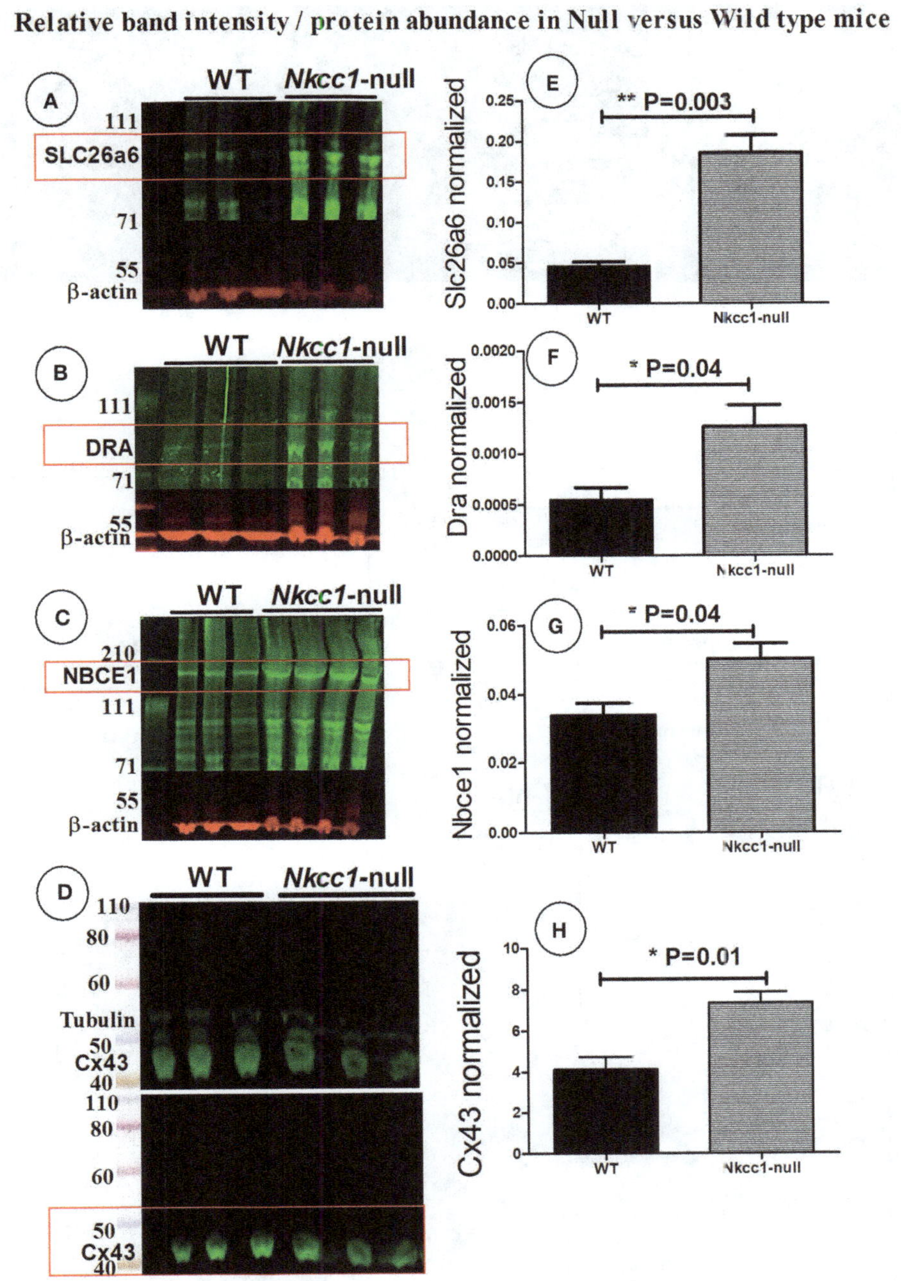

I Enamel Organ Genotype	Western blot probed with			
	Anti-SLC26A6	Anti-DRA	Anti-NBCE1	Anti-CX43
Nkcc1-null	+303 %**	+143.4 %*	+47.4 %*	+78 %*

FIGURE 4 | SLC26a6, DRA, NBCe1 and CX43 proteins possibly compensate during lost *Nkcc1* gene expression. Expression of SLC26a6 **(A)**, DRA **(B)**, NBCe1 **(C)**, and Cx43 **(D)** protein extracts of enamel organs of WT and *Nkcc1* null mice by western blotting. Graph bars **(E–G)** show semi-quantitative SLC26a6, DRA, NBCe1 bands normalized to ß-actin. The CX43 bands were normalized to tubulin **(H)**. Table **(I)** presents a summary of the quantification.

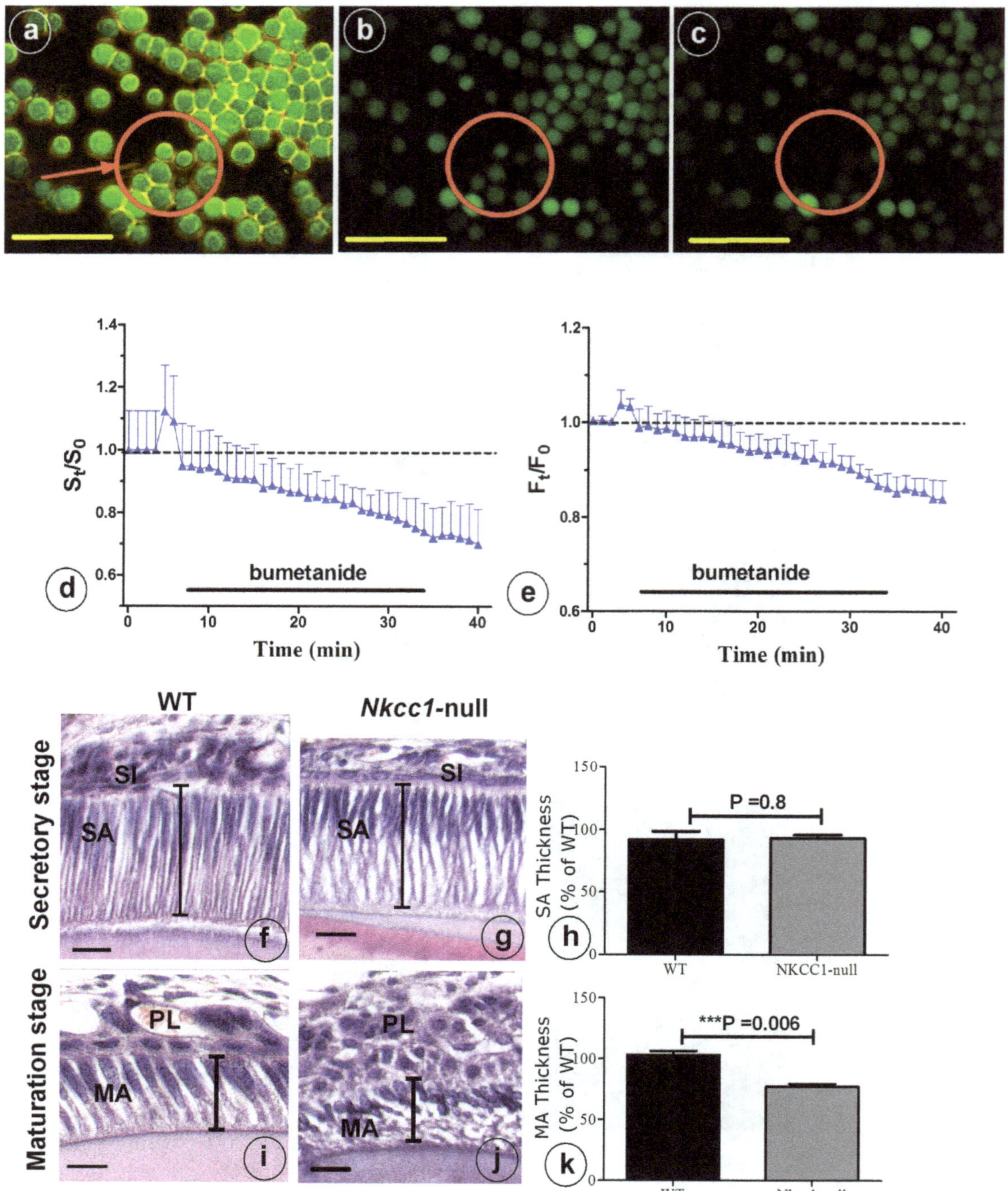

FIGURE 5 | NKCC1-dependent regulatory volume decrease. **(A)** HAT-7 cells were loaded with 5 μM Calcein-AM for 20 min. Cells were bathed in a iso-osmotic solution that was switched to 10 μM bumetanide solution for 30 min as indicated by black bars in **(D,E)**. Changes in cell volume of single HAT-7 cells (arrow in **A**). **(B)** 2 min after bumetanide exposure; **(C)** 7 min after bumetanide exposure. **(D)** Average relative cell surface and **(E)** fluorescence, obtained under iso-osmotic with and without 10 μM bumetanide ($n = 10$). Length of ameloblast cells in *Nkcc1*-null **(G–J)** and WT mice stained with hematoxylen-eosin was measured using Image-J software ($n = 3$). Bar diagrams show the difference between ameloblasts length in the secretion stage **(H)** and maturation stage **(K)** of amelogenesis in WT and *Nkcc1*-null mice. SA, secretory ameloblasts; MA, advanced maturation ameloblasts; SI, stratum intermedium; PL, papillary layer. Lines indicate length of the cells in **(F,G,I,J)**; results for **(F,G)** summarized in **(H)**, while results for **(I,J)** are summarized in **(K)**. Bars = 50 μm.

lifted from the cover slip and placed in front of a piezo-driven theta-barrel electrode (TGC 200; Harvard Apparatus, Holliston, MA, USA), filled with standard aCSF on one side and standard aCSF supplemented with 10 μM bumetanide (B1158000 Sigma-Aldrich) on the other side. By changing the position of the barrel bumetanide was applied during the whole-cell recording. Voltage ramps from −70 to 80 mV (500 ms) were applied under control and in the presence of 10 μM bumetanide.

The cell attached recordings were made by filling the recording pipet with aCSF for the control recordings and with aCSF supplemented 10 μM bumetanide for experimental recordings. All data was acquired using an internal 7-pole Bessel filter (5 kHz) and a sample frequency of 20 kHz. Recordings with an access resistance above 12 mΩ were excluded form analysis.

RESULTS

Slc12a2 mRNA Expression in Mouse Tissues and Rat HAT-7 Cells

Transcripts for *Nkcc1/Slc12a2* normalized for *Ywhaz* housekeeping gene were detectable in enamel organ and intestine (high), pulp and kidney moderate-(low); in the remaining tissues tested expression was very low or below detection limit (**Figure 1A**; Supplementary Figure 1). HAT-7 cells also expressed *Nkcc1* transcripts (**Figure 1B**).

Bumetanide blocks activity of the NKCC's. To test whether this blocking agent also could affect *Nkcc1* expression level in enamel epithelium, HAT-7 cells were exposed to various concentrations of this inhibitor for 45 min, washed, and incubated for 9 h in medium without inhibitor. Then total RNA was isolated and the amount of *Nkcc1* transcripts measured by RT-qPCR (**Figure 1B**). Bumetanide did not change the number of transcripts of *Nkcc1*.

NKCC1 Expression in HAT-7 Cells, Mouse Enamel Organ, and Salivary Glands

Anti-NKCC1 antibodies stained plasma membranes in HAT-7 cells as fine granular material (**Figure 2A**). Replacing primary (mouse) antibodies for normal non-immune mouse IgG failed to stain these membranes in HAT-7 cells (**Figure 2B**).

Strong immunostaining was detected in the basolateral plasma membranes of the acinar cells of salivary glands, a well-established site of NKCC1 expression (Evans et al., 2000) (**Figure 2C**).

In upper incisors, in presecretory stage and during the secretory and maturation stage, the plasma membrane of outer enamel epithelium cells was immunopositive for NKCC1 (**Figures 2E,F**; Supplementary Figure 2). No staining was seen in ameloblasts. Weaker staining was seen in dental epithelium between ameloblasts and outer enamel epithelium. Strong staining was apparent in the papillary layer (intracellular and membranes) during maturation (**Figures 2E,G**).

Sections from salivary glands (**Figure 2D**) and enamel organ from *Nkcc1*-null mice (**Figure 2H**) incubated with anti-NKCC1 failed to immunostain the tissues, validating the specificity of the antibodies.. In developing molar tooth germs similar stainings were obtained: a strong staining for NKCC1 in outer enamel but no staining in ameloblasts (Supplementary Figure 3).

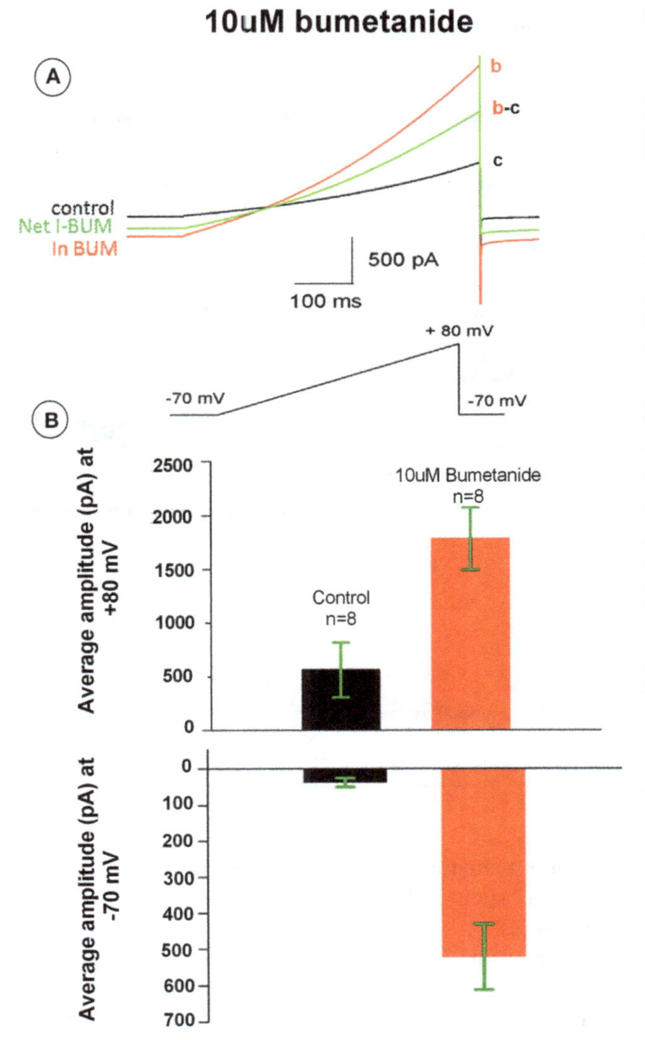

FIGURE 6 | (A) Bumetanide 10 μM increased whole-cell membrane currents across the voltage range from −70 to +80 mV. The black tracing curve c is the control and the red aCSF tracing curve b is the current in the presence of 10 μM bumetanide. The green tracing curve b-c is the net current induced by 10 μM bumetanide. **(B)** Outward currents measured at +80 mV (upper) and inward current at −70 mV (lower). Bars show the average amplitude of control and 10 μM bumetanide ($n = 8$).

NKCC1 Expression is Important for Enamel Organ Function and Enamel Mineralization

Slc12a2 (or *Nkcc1*) knockout mice exhibit growth retardation with a 30% incidence of death by the time of weaning. They are deaf, have less body fat, reduced mean arterial blood pressure, exhibit reduced cAMP-induced short circuit currents in jejunum, cecum, and trachea, unusual head postures, and engage in circling behaviors and rapid spinning, but have difficulty maintaining their balance (Flagella et al., 1999). Incisors of *Nkcc1*-null mice showed no obvious gross changes. Analysis of upper incisor enamel of *Nkcc1*-null mice showed no significant change in mineral density in enamel during secretory stage but

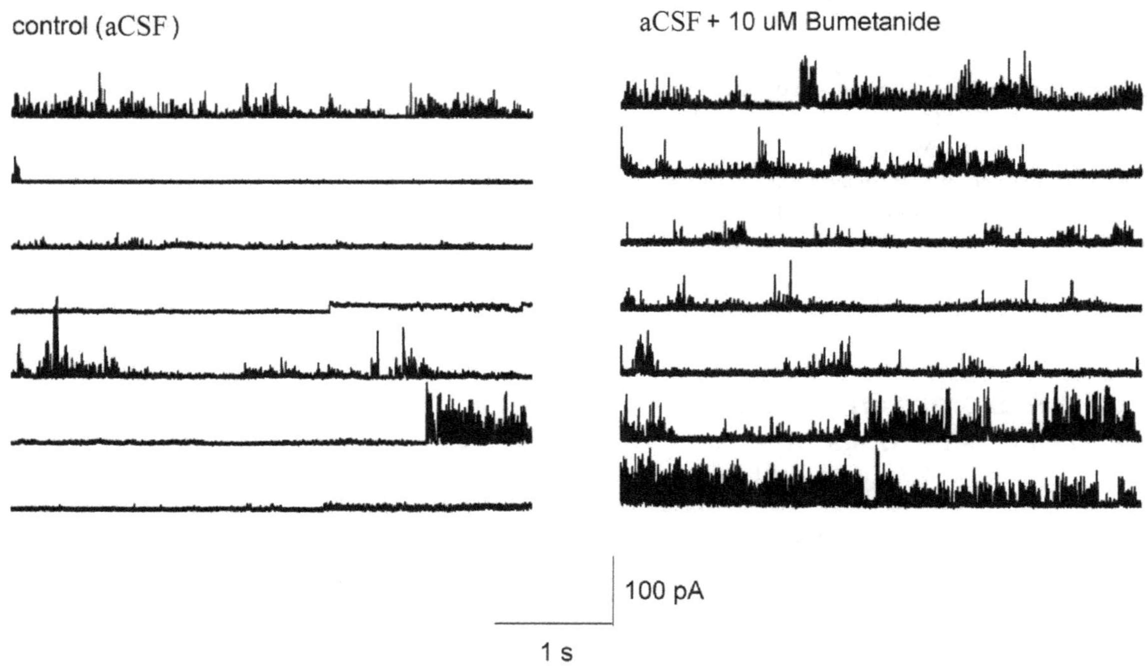

FIGURE 7 | Representative tracings showing the effect of 10 μM bumetanide on the channel activity in HAT-7 cells. Left figure shows the channel activity obtained from cell-attached patch with aCSF in the recording pipet at 0 mV. Right figure shows the channel activity obtained when the recording pipet was filled with aCSF + 10 μM bumetanide and clamped at 0 mV.

a reduction at maturation stage, reaching a final density that was reduced about 10% compared to controls ($P < 0.0001$) (**Figures 3E–I**).

Next we examined expression of NCKX4 (sodium/calcium-potassium exchanger-4) a major transcellular calcium transporter in maturation ameloblasts, to determine whether calcium transport is affected in *Nkcc1*-null incisors. Nckx4 protein was strongly expressed in the apical membrane of maturation ameloblasts of wild type mice (**Figure 3A**), but its antibody-associated staining was weaker in *Nkcc1*-null mice (**Figure 3B**). Western blot analysis (**Figure 3C**) of protein extracts from wild type and *Nkcc1*-null maturation enamel organ, showed a small (but not significant) reduction of NCKX4 protein in *Nkcc1*-null enamel organ (**Figure 3D**).

Upregulation of SLC26A6, DRA, NBCe1 and Gap Junction (Cx43) Protein Expression in *Nkcc1*-Null Enamel Organ by Western Blotting

To examine if the expression of other Na^+ and Cl^- ion transporters or/ and gap junction channels could compensate for the absence of NKCC1, we tested maturation stage enamel organs of *Nkcc1*-null mice for changes in protein levels of SLC26A6, DRA, NBCel and Cx43 by Western blotting (**Figures 4A–H**). Total protein extracted from *Nkcc1* -null enamel organs showed a 303% increase of SLC26A6/PAT1 ($P = 0.003$) (**Figures 4A,E**) compared with wild type a, 143% increase for SLC26A3/DRA ($P = 0.04$) (**Figures 4B,F**), 47% increase for NBCel ($P = 0.04$) (**Figures 4C,G**) and 78% increase for Cx43 ($P = 0.01$) (**Figures 4D,H**). The results are summarized in **Figure 4I**.

Regulation of Cell Volume Is Impaired in *Nkcc1*-Null Enamel Organ and HAT-7 Cells Exposed to Bumetanide

NKCC1 is one of the proteins involved in cell volume recovery after cell shrinkage in kidney (Walker et al., 2002). Analysis of histological sections of *Nkcc1*-null upper mouse incisors showed that late maturation ameloblasts lost their polarization and that the cells of the papillary layer were shorter compared to that seen in wild type controls. However, secretory stage ameloblasts and stratum intermedium seemed hardly or not affected in the null mutants in comparison to wild type mice (**Figures 5F,G,I,J**). To examine a possible role of NKCC1 in regulating cell volume in ameloblasts, we measured cell volume changes of single HAT-7 cells *in vitro* by measuring cell size (surface area measurements) and by using the calcein-quenching method before and after bumetanide (10 uM) treatment, (**Figures 5A–E**). Bumetanide decreased cell volume as measured directly (**Figure 5D**) and by loss of fluorescence (**Figure 5E**). In incisors of *Nkcc1*-null mice the values of the long axes of secretory ameloblasts were not different from those in wild types (**Figures 5F–H**) but were significantly shorter (~25%; $P < 0.0001$; **Figures 5I–K**) in maturation ameloblasts.

Bumetanide Increases Membrane Conductance in HAT-7 Cells

Bumetanide has been previously shown to induce potassium currents in canine kidney cells. To test whether bumetanide affects the membrane ionic conductance in HAT-7 cells, electrophysiological whole-cell voltage-clamp recordings were made from these cells. The membrane potential was ramped from −70 to +80 mV. In control conditions, the voltage ramp induced a small membrane current that reversed at −30 mV. Application of bumetanide (10 μM) increased membrane currents across the entire membrane potential range (**Figure 6A**). The outward current measured at +80 mV increased about 3-fold, whereas the inward current measured at −70 mV was 20-fold enlarged (**Figures 6A,B**). The increase of membrane currents induced by bumetanide hardly reversed upon washout (not shown). To our surprise, the bumetanide-induced currents reversed at −30 mV. Given that for the recording solutions used in these experiments the equilibrium potential for potassium was −95 mV, for chloride −65 mV and for sodium and calcium above +60 mV, this suggests that most likely a mixed ionic current was activated by bumetanide-block of NKCC transporters.

Bumetanide Increases Ion Channel Activity in HAT-7 Cells

It is not known whether the effect of bumetanide on the membrane conductance required block of NKCC transporters across the entire cell membrane, or whether this effect could also be induced locally. To determine this, we made cell-attached recordings from HAT-7 cells and applied bumetanide only to the membrane patch inside the patch pipette. The pipette potential was kept at 0 mV. In control recordings, ion channel activity and occasional discrete single channel openings were observed that were alternated by silent periods ($n = 10$, **Figure 7**). At this pipette potential, only outward currents were observed. During recordings in which bumetanide (10 uM) was included in the recording pipette, ion channel activity conducting outward currents increased ($n = 10$, **Figure 7**). No discrete amplitude levels could be distinguished, which suggests that blocking NKCC transporters with bumetanide augments the activity of multiple ion channels in the membrane patch. These results suggest that the effects of bumetanide on membrane ionic conductance could be induced locally in a patch of the cell membrane.

DISCUSSION

The present study demonstrates that in mice enamel organ epithelium in secretory and maturation stage expresses NKCC1 at the mRNA and protein level. Without NKCC1 enamel was slightly less mineralized, at visual inspection without gross change in enamel structure. The upregulation of NBCe1, DRA and PAT1 in enamel organs of *Nkcc1* null mice suggest that NKCC1 can be at least in part compensated by typical pH regulators as reported for salivary glands and duodenum epithelium in *Nkcc1* null mice (Evans et al., 2000; Walker et al., 2002). This suggests that NKCC1 is involved in enamel mineralization possibly by providing amloblasts Cl^- crucial for bicarbonate secretion but its role is limited. However, it cannot be excluded that some of the defects in enamel mineralization are secondary due to systemic changes brought about by changes in other tissues in *Nckk1*- null mice.

The reduction in mineral density of enamel in *Nkcc1* null mice was relatively small (10%) in comparison with the reduction in *Cftr*-null mice (47%, Bronckers et al., 2015b) and in *Ae2*- null mice (57% Lyaruu et al., 2014), two transporters critical for pH regulation by maturation ameloblasts. The reduction in mineral density in *Nkcc1* null mice could be due to: (1) a slightly increased acidification associated with reduced intracellular Cl^- levels in ameloblasts resulting from less NKCC1-mediated Cl^- transport in the papillary layer. The rather normal gross appearance of incisor enamel and the fact the mineral density changes appear quite late in comparison to the severe mineral reduction and porotic changes in enamel of *Cftr*-null and *Ae2*- null mice seen early in maturation make this option less likely. (2) Reduction of the cytosolic levels of K^+ or a reduced number of apical NCKX4 in maturation ameloblasts needed for NCKX4-mediated Ca^{2+} transport by maturation ameloblasts. (3). Reduction in the levels of Na^+ in ameloblasts required for Na-Pi2b mediated phosphate transport (Bronckers et al., 2015a).

Ameloblast did not express NKCC1 but papillary layer cells highly expressed the cotransporter. To reach forming enamel ions transported by NKCC1 into the papillary layer need to pass from papillary layer into ameloblasts. The enhanced expression of connex43 points to a mechanism for such transport. Ameloblasts and papillary layer have been suggested to act as a functional unit in passing ions from outer enamel epithelium to ameloblasts through gap junctions (Josephsen et al., 2010). Gap junctions are structures passing through the plasma membranes of two adjacent cells forming small pores that enable direct intracellular transport of ions and small molecules/peptides (Toth et al., 2010). The significance of communication between enamel organ cells is exemplified in $Gja1Jrt^{-/+}$ mice in which enamel formation was severely affected by a decrease in the number of gap junctions in the enamel organ (Toth et al., 2010). Upregulation of connexin43 in enamel organ of *Nkcc1*-null mice may occur to increase the number of gap junctions to compensate for changes in ion transport due to absence of NKCC1.

Our histological and electrophysiological results suggest that NKCC1 is involved in amelogenesis. The distribution of NKCC1 in enamel organs, and the reduction in cell height of ameloblast layer in *Nkcc1*-null mice suggests that during amelogenesis the symporter NKCC1 serves to import Na^+, K^+, and Cl^- from blood vessels, regulates cell volume of dental epithelium and likely water transport across the ameloblast layer. Transport of large amounts of Cl^- and Na^+ across epithelial cells, for example by Cl^- channels and cotransporters such as CFTR, NKCC2 and NKCC1, is required for fluid transport (e.g., in kidney) and maintenance or changes in cell volume. Volume changes in ameloblasts during normal amelogenesis are substantial indicated by the changes in the long axes of ameloblasts when moving from differentiation into secretion stage, reaching maximal values at full secretion stage, followed by a 50% reduction during transitional and early maturation stage. In *Nkcc1*-null mice the maturation ameloblasts were shorter than in wild type controls. Exposing HAT-7 cells to 10 μM bumetanide caused cell volume decrease without altering the number of *Nkcc1*-mRNA transcripts suggesting that iso-osmotically shrinkage accrued after adding bumetanide. These data are in line with a function of NKCC1 in cell volume regulation and ion transport.

In short, NKCC1 is highly expressed in non-ameloblast enamel organ epithelium. A reduction in mineral density of enamel, shortening of ameloblast cell body and upregulation of other ion transporters when NKCC1 is absent suggests that NKCC1 regulates cell volume and ion transport but can be partly compensated by enhanced activity of other ion transporters.

AUTHOR CONTRIBUTIONS

Conceived and designed the experiments: RJ, AB, PD, and JL; Performed the experiments: RJ, JL, BZ-D, DM, JM, and MC; Wrote the manuscript: RJ, AB; Edited the manuscript: JL, DM, JM, MC, HM, PD, and AB.

ACKNOWLEDGMENTS

The authors thank Dr. P. Aronson (Yale University New Haven CT, USA) for providing anti-SLC26A6, Dr. W. F. Boron (Case Western, Cleveland, OH, USA) for anti-NBCE1. Ben K. A. Nelemans and Manuel Schmitz Orthopedic Surgery (VU Medical Center, MOVE Research Institute Amsterdam, the Netherlands) for their help in microscopic examination of the samples. The authors thank Dr. H. Harada (Department of Anatomy, Developmental Biology Division, Iwata Medical University Iwate, Japan) for donating HAT07 cells. This study was supported in part by the Intramural Research Program of the National Institute of Dental and Craniofacial Research (NIDCR), NIH (JEM, DE000738) and the NIDCR Veterinary Research Core (DE000740).

REFERENCES

Bori, E., Guo, J., Rácz, R., Burghardt, B., Földes, A., Kerémi, B., et al. (2016). Evidence for bicarbonate secretion by ameloblasts in a novel cellular model. *J. Dent. Res.* 95, 588–596. doi: 10.1177/0022034515625939

Bronckers, A. L., Guo, J., Zandieh-Doulabi, B., Bervoets, T. J., Lyaruu, D. M., Li, X., et al. (2011). Developmental expression of solute carrier family 26A member 4 (SLC26A4/pendrin) during amelogenesis in developing rodent teeth. *Eur. J. Oral Sci.* 119, 185–192. doi: 10.1111/j.1600-0722.2011.00901.x

Bronckers, A. L., Lyaruu, D., Jalali, R., Medina, J., Zandieh-Doulabi, B., and Denbesten, P. (2015a). Ameloblast modulation and transport of Cl−, Na+, and K+ during amelogenesis. *J. Dent. Res.* 94, 1740–1747. doi: 10.1177/0022034515606900

Bronckers, A. L., Lyaruu, D. M., Guo, J., Bijvelds, M. J., Bervoets, T. J., Zandieh-Doulabi, B., et al. (2015b). Composition of mineralizing incisor enamel in cystic fibrosis transmembrane conductance regulator-deficient mice. *Eur. J. Oral Sci.* 123, 9–16. doi: 10.1111/eos.12163

Delpire, E., Lu, J., England, R., Dull, C., and Thorne, T. (1999). Deafness and imbalance associated with inactivation of the secretory Na-K-2Cl co-transporter. *Nat. Genet.* 22, 192–195. doi: 10.1038/9713

Evans, R. L., Park, K., Turner, R. J., Watson, G. E., Nguyen, H.-V., Dennett, M. R., et al. (2000). Severe impairment of salivation in Na+/K+/2Cl− cotransporter (NKCC1)-deficient mice. *J. Biol. Chem.* 275, 26720–26726. doi: 10.1074/jbc.M003753200

Flagella, M., Clarke, L. L., Miller, M. L., Erway, L. C., Giannella, R. A., Andringa, A., et al. (1999). Mice lacking the basolateral Na-K-2Cl cotransporter have impaired epithelial chloride secretion and are profoundly deaf. *J. Biol. Chem.* 274, 26946–26955. doi: 10.1074/jbc.274.38.26946

Gagnon, F., Orlov, S. N., Tremblay, J., and Hamet, P. (1998). Complete inhibition of Na+, K+, Cl− cotransport in Madin-Darby canine kidney cells by PMA-sensitive protein kinase. *Biochimica et Biophysica Acta* 1369, 233–239. doi: 10.1016/S0005-2736(97)00225-3

Garant, P. R., and Sasaki, T. (1986). Ultracytochemistry of ouabain-sensitive K+-dependent p-nitrophenyl phosphatase in rat incisor enamel organ. *Anat. Rec.* 216, 1–9. doi: 10.1002/ar.1092160102

Glynn, I. M. (2002). A hundred years of sodium pumping. *Ann. Rev. Physiol.* 64, 1–18. doi: 10.1146/annurev.physiol.64.081501.130716

Haas, M. (1994). The Na-K-Cl cotransporters. *Am. J. Physiol. Cell Physiol.* 267, C869–C885.

Hu, P., Lacruz, R. S., Smith, C. E., Smith, S. M., Kurtz, I., and Paine, M. L. (2012). Expression of the sodium/calcium/potassium exchanger, NCKX4, in ameloblasts. *Cells Tissues Organs* 196, 501–509. doi: 10.1159/000337493

Hübner, C. A., Lorke, D. E., and Hermans-Borgmeyer, I. (2001). Expression of the Na-K-2Cl-cotransporter NKCC1 during mouse development. *Mech. Dev.* 102, 267–269. doi: 10.1016/S0925-4773(01)00309-4

Jalali, R., Guo, J., Zandieh-Doulabi, B., Bervoets, T., Paine, M., Boron, W., et al. (2014). NBCe1 (SLC4A4) a potential pH regulator in enamel organ cells during enamel development in the mouse. *Cell Tissue Res.* 358, 433–442. doi: 10.1007/s00441-014-1935-4

Jalali, R., Zandieh-Doulabi, B., Denbesten, P., Seidler, U., Riederer, B., Wedenoja, S., et al. (2015). Slc26a3/Dra and Slc26a6 in murine ameloblasts. *J. Dent. Res.* 94, 1732–1739. doi: 10.1177/0022034515606873

Josephsen, K., Takano, Y., Frische, S., Praetorius, J., Nielsen, S., Aoba, T., et al. (2010). Ion transporters in secretory and cyclically modulating ameloblasts: a new hypothesis for cellular control of preeruptive enamel maturation. *Am. J. Physiol. Cell Physiol.* 299, C1299–C1307. doi: 10.1152/ajpcell.00218.2010

Kawano, S., Morotomi, T., Toyono, T., Nakamura, N., Uchida, T., Ohishi, M., et al. (2002). Establishment of dental epithelial cell line (HAT-7) and the cell differentiation dependent on Notch signaling pathway. *Connect. Tissue Res.* 43, 409–412. doi: 10.1080/03008200290000637

Lacruz, R. S., Nanci, A., Kurtz, I., Wright, J. T., and Paine, M. L. (2010a). Regulation of pH during amelogenesis. *Calcif. Tissue Int.* 86, 91–103. doi: 10.1007/s00223-009-9326-7

Lacruz, R. S., Nanci, A., White, S. N., Wen, X., Wang, H., Zalzal, S. F., et al. (2010b). The sodium bicarbonate cotransporter (NBCe1) is essential for normal development of mouse dentition. *J. Biol. Chem.* 285, 24432–24438. doi: 10.1074/jbc.M110.115188

Lacruz, R. S., Smith, C. E., Moffatt, P., Chang, E. H., Bromage, T. G., Bringas, P., et al. (2012). Requirements for ion and solute transport, and pH regulation during enamel maturation. *J. Cell. Physiol.* 227, 1776–1785. doi: 10.1002/jcp.22911

Lacruz, R., Smith, C., Kurtz, I., Hubbard, M., and Paine, M. (2013). New paradigms on the transport functions of maturation-stage ameloblasts. *J. Dent. Res.* 92, 122–129. doi: 10.1177/0022034512470954

Lyaruu, D. M., Bronckers, A. L., Mulder, L., Mardones, P., Medina, J. F., Kellokumpu, S., et al. (2008). The anion exchanger Ae2 is required for enamel maturation in mouse teeth. *Matrix Biol.* 27, 119–127. doi: 10.1016/j.matbio.2007.09.006

Lyaruu, D. M., Medina, J. F., Sarvide, S., Bervoets, T. J., Everts, V., Denbesten, P., et al. (2014). Barrier formation: potential molecular mechanism of enamel fluorosis. *J. Dent. Res.* 93, 96–102. doi: 10.1177/00220345135 10944

Lytle, C., Xu, J.-C., Biemesderfer, D., and Forbush, B. (1995). Distribution and diversity of Na-K-Cl cotransport proteins: a study with monoclonal antibodies. *Am. J. Physiol. Cell Physiol.* 269, C1496–C1505.

Okumura, R., Shibukawa, Y., Muramatsu, T., Hashimoto, S., Nakagawa, K.-I., Tazaki, M., et al. (2010). Sodium-calcium exchangers in rat ameloblasts. *J. Pharmacol. Sci.* 112, 223–230. doi: 10.1254/jphs.09267FP

Parry, D. A., Poulter, J. A., Logan, C. V., Brookes, S. J., Jafri, H., Ferguson, C. H., et al. (2013). Identification of mutations in SLC24A4, encoding a potassium-dependent sodium/calcium exchanger, as a cause of amelogenesis imperfecta. *Am. J. Hum. Genet.* 92, 307–312. doi: 10.1016/j.ajhg.2013. 01.003

Ryu, O., Hu, C.-C., and Simmer, J. (1998). Biochemical characterization of recombinant mouse amelogenins: protein quantitation, proton absorption, and relative affinity for enamel crystals. *Connect. Tissue Res.* 38, 207–214. doi: 10.3109/03008209809017038

Smith, C. (1998). Cellular and chemical events during enamel maturation. *Crit. Rev. Oral Biol. Med.* 9, 128–161. doi: 10.1177/10454411980090020101

Toth, K., Shao, Q., Lorentz, R., and Laird, D. (2010). Decreased levels of Cx43 gap junctions result in ameloblast dysregulation and enamel hypoplasia in Gja1Jrt/+ mice. *J. Cell. Physiol.* 223, 601–609. doi: 10.1002/jcp.22046

Walker, N. M., Flagella, M., Gawenis, L. R., Shull, G. E., and Clarke, L. L. (2002). An alternate pathway of cAMP-stimulated Cl– secretion across the NKCC1-null murine duodenum. *Gastroenterology* 123, 531–541. doi: 10.1053/gast.2002.34757

Ye, S., Armah, S., Xu, Q., and Reddy, M. (2015). Calcein's quenching *in vitro* method for assessing dietary iron bioavailability. *FASEB J.* 29:LB336. doi: 10.1096/fj.1530-6860

Yin, K., Lei, Y., Wen, X., Lacruz, R. S., Soleimani, M., Kurtz, I., et al. (2015). SLC26A gene family participate in pH regulation during enamel maturation. *PLoS ONE* 10:e0144703. doi: 10.1371/journal.pone.0144703

12

Stemodia maritima L. Extract Decreases Inflammation, Oxidative Stress and Alveolar Bone Loss in an Experimental Periodontitis Rat Model

*Alrieta H. Teixeira[1,2], Jordânia M. de Oliveira Freire[1], Luzia H. T. de Sousa[1], Antônia T. Parente[3], Nayara A. de Sousa[3], Angela M. C. Arriaga[4], Francisca R. Lopes da Silva[4], Iracema M. Melo[2], Igor I. Castro da Silva[2], Karuza M. A. Pereira[5], Paula Goes[6], José J. do Nascimento Costa[7], Gerardo Cristino-Filho[3], Vicente de Paulo T. Pinto[3], Hellíada V. Chaves[2] and Mirna M. Bezerra[1,3]**

[1] RENORBIO, Federal University of Ceará, Fortaleza, Brazil, [2] Dentistry School, Federal University of Ceará, Sobral, Brazil, [3] Medical School, Federal University of Ceará, Sobral, Brazil, [4] Department of Organic and Inorganic Chemistry, Federal University of Ceará, Fortaleza, Brazil, [5] Department of Morphology, Medical School, Federal University of Ceará, Fortaleza, Brazil, [6] Department of Pathology and Legal Medicine, Medical School, Federal University of Ceará, Fortaleza, Brazil, [7] UNINTA University Center, Sobral, Brazil

***Correspondence:**
Mirna M. Bezerra
mirnabrayner@gmail.com

Periodontitis is very prevalent worldwide and is one of the major causes of tooth loss in adults. About 80% of the worldwide population use medicinal plants for their health care. *Stemodia maritima* L. (*S. maritima*) antioxidant and antimicrobial effects *in vitro* as well as anti-inflammatory properties. Herein, the potential therapeutic effect of *S. maritima* was assessed in rats subjected to experimental periodontitis (EP). EP was induced in female Wistar rats by nylon thread ligature around 2nd upper left molars for 11 days. Animals received (*per os*) *S. maritima* (0.2; 1 or 5 mg/kg) or vehicle (saline + DMSO) 1 h before ligature and then once daily for 11 days. The naive group had no manipulation. After this time-point, the animals were terminally anesthetized, and the maxillae were removed for morphometric and histological analyzes (HE). Gingival tissues were dissected to cytokine levels detection (TNF-α, IL1-β, CINC-1, and IL-10), enzymes superoxide dismutase (SOD), and catalase (CAT) analysis, as well as gene expression (TNF-α, IL-1β, RANK, and iNOS) by qRT-PCR. Systemic parameters (weight variation, plasma levels of hepatic enzymes aspartate aminotransferase (AST) and alanine aminotransferase (ALT), creatinine, total alkaline phosphatase (TALP), and bone alkaline phosphatase (BALP) were performed. Histological analysis of the stomach, liver, kidney, and heart was also performed. *S. maritima* (5 mg/kg) decreased alveolar bone loss, TNF-α and CINC-1 gingival levels, oxidative stress, and transcription of TNF-α, IL1-β, RANK, and iNOS genes. It elevated both BALP activity and IL-10 gingival levels. The animals showed no any signs of toxicity. In conclusion, *S. maritima* reduced pro-inflammatory cytokine production, oxidative stress, and alveolar bone loss in a pre-clinical trial of periodontitis. *S. maritima* is a potential tool for controlling the development of periodontitis.

Keywords: *Stemodia maritima* L., periodontitis, inflammation, oxidative stress, bone loss

INTRODUCTION

Current concepts define periodontitis as a chronic inflammatory disease that compromises the integrity of the tooth-supporting tissues. It is an imbalance between the polymicrobial biofilm and the immune-inflammatory response and includes genetic and environmental risk factors (Genco and Borgnakke, 2013; Hajishengallis, 2014). The periodontal tissue breakdown is mainly mediated by the release of pro inflammatory cytokines (TNF-α, IL-1, and IL-8/CXCL8 (in humans) or CINC-1/CXCL1 (in rats) as well as the production of reactive oxygen species (ROS) (Liao et al., 2014; Hienz et al., 2015; Silva et al., 2015; Gomes et al., 2016).

Mechanical therapy and surgical procedures have been used to treat periodontitis (Wang et al., 2014). Nevertheless, these procedures are not always satisfactory. Thus, adjunctive therapies may be necessary including antibiotics and non-steroidal anti-inflammatory drugs. The major disadvantage of these agents is the development of bacterial resistance and gastric/renal toxicity. Thus, the search for newer and safer therapeutic agents continues to overcome these limitations. Phytochemicals isolated from plants are considered good alternatives to synthetic chemicals. In recent years, the use of plant extracts has gained popularity (Alviano and Alviano, 2009; Chandra Shekar et al., 2015; Kala et al., 2015; Ramesh et al., 2016) and some of these extracts have been used to treat periodontitis or repair bone defects (Guimarães et al., 2016; Lima et al., 2017; Oliveira et al., 2017).

In this regard, earlier chemical studies on *Stemodia maritima* L. (Plantaginaceae family, formely Scrophulariaceae), which is used in traditional medicine to treat inflammatory disorders, reported the isolation of flavonoids, diterpenes, and other compounds associated with larvicidal and antiviral activities (Rodrigues et al., 2010; Russell et al., 2011). Our group studied the phytochemicals in *S. maritima* L., and described the isolation of the natural compound, stemodinol along with seven known compounds (da Silva et al., 2014). Antioxidant and antimicrobial activities were observed on crenatoside, stemodinoside B, and stemodin. These are natural compounds also derived from *S. maritima* L. (da Silva et al., 2014).

Despite these data, there is no study in the literature focusing on inflammatory bone resorption using *S. maritima* L. extract or its bioactive phytochemicals. Thus, considering the involvement of both polymicrobial biofilm (Genco and Borgnakke, 2013; Hajishengallis, 2014) and oxidative stress (Tóthová et al., 2015; Lima et al., 2017) in periodontitis, and the potential therapeutic effect of *S. maritima* L., the goal of this study was to investigate the efficacy of *S. maritima* L. extract in a rat periodontitis model.

Abbreviations: cDNA, Complementary Deoxyribonucleic Acid; CINC-1, Rat cytokine-induced neutrophil chemoattractant - 1; DMSO, Dimethyl sulfoxide; dNTP, Deoxynucleotide; DTT, Dithiothreitol; EDTA, Ethylenediaminetetraacetic acid; HE, Hematoxylin and eosin; IL-10, Interleukin 10; IL1-β, Interleukin 1 beta; NBT, Nitro-blue tetrazolium; qRT-PCR, Reverse Transcription Polymerase Chain Reaction; RANK, Receptor activator of nuclear factor-kappaB; RNA, Ribonucleic Acid; TNF-α, Tumor Necrosis Factor-alpha.

MATERIALS AND METHODS

Plant Material

S. maritima L. (*S. maritima* or Sm) is a common shrub that grows widely in the northeast region of Brazil, near the seacoasts. It belongs to Plantaginaceae family, tribe Gratioleae Benth (Albach et al., 2005). Dr. F. S. Cavalcanti and Prof. E. P. Nunes identified the plant and a voucher specimen (# 38483) was registered at Frisco Bezerra Herbarium, Federal University of Ceará, Fortaleza, Brazil. For this study, the extract was obtained from fresh leaves of Sm collected during the flowering stage along Fleixeiras Beach, Ceará, Brazil (da Silva et al., 2014).

Animals

The experimental procedures and treatments performed on animals were approved by the Animal Research Ethics Committee of Federal University of Ceará (Permit number: 08/2013) in accordance with the guidelines from the Brazilian Society of Laboratory Animal Science - SBCAL/COBEA). Female Wistar rats, 10-weeks-old and weighting 200 ± 20 g were housed in appropriated cages of polypropylene and maintained on a 12 h-12 h light-dark cycles with a constant room temperature of 25°C and received water and food *ad libitum*.

Experimental Design

For the initial experiment, 30 animals were randomly divided into five specific groups ($n = 6$ in each group): unchallenged group (naive), three experimental periodontitis-challenged groups (EP) receiving oral gavage (*per os*) in different concentrations of *S. maritima* (0.2, 1, or 5 mg/kg) or 0.9% saline solution + DMSO (vehicle). Experimental Periodonttis (EP) was performed as previously described (Bezerra et al., 2002). Briefly, the animals were anesthetized with ketamine and xylazine (90:10 mg/kg, i.p.) and a sterilized nylon suture thread (3.0 Nylpoint, Ceará, Brazil) was placed around the second left maxillary molar. To facilitate suture placement, a guide through the medial and distal interproximal spaces was made using a 5.0 suture needle (Point Suture, Ceará, Brazil). Groups received vehicle and *S. maritima* (*per os*) 1 h before periodontitis induction and once daily, during 11 days. After this time, blood samples were obtained and an overdose of ketamine and xylazine (300:30 mg/kg; i.p.) were used to euthanize the animals. The maxillae were removed to analyze the total bone resorption area. Hystopathological analyses was performed with another animals following the same above designed groups ($n = 30$).

Sm at a dose of 5 mg/kg was found to be the most effective dose against alveolar bone loss (ABL), and therefore this dose was selected for the experiments. Subsequent series of experiments were conducted with the following groups: non-ligated (naive - animals not subjected to EP); ligature only (vehicle), and ligature plus treatment with *S. maritima* 5 mg/kg diluted in 0.9% saline solution + DMSO (*S. maritima* 5) to quantification of gingival levels of cytokines TNF-α, IL-1β, CINC-1 and IL-10 ($n = 18$), antioxidant enzymes superoxide dismutase (SOD) and catalase (CAT) ($n = 18$) and qRT-PCR analysis of TNF-α, IL-1β, RANK, and iNOS ($n = 18$). All these assays were performed using the gingival tissues from surrounding maxillary left molars (the half of the maxillae with ligature).

Measurement of Alveolar Bone Loss

After the period of EP the maxillae were removed, divided in half and fixed in buffered formalin (10%) for 24 h. Following, the maxillae were defleshed and kept in 8% sodium hypochlorite for 4 h (Pimentel et al., 2012). After that, the specimens were washed in running water and stained with methylene blue (1%) to differentiate bone from teeth. Then, hemi-maxillae were fixed in a piece of wax with their occlusal planes parallel to the ground and long axes perpendicular to the camera and photographed with a 6.1-megapixel digital camera (Canon® 60D). ImageJ® software (National Institute of Health, Bethesda, MD, USA) were used for measurement of ABL, as described previously (Kuhr et al., 2004). The buccal area (mm^2) corresponding to the exposed roots and coronary surface of the molars was calculated and obtained and subtracted from the correspondent area (mm^2) of the normal right hemi-maxillae.

After definition of the most effective dose, one sample of each group was scanned using a high resolution microcomputed tomography (micro-CT) system (SkyScan 1174; Bruker-microCT, Kontich, Belgic, 50 kV and 800 μA) with a 0.5 mm aluminium filter and 15% beam hardening correction and ring artifacts reduction. We used 180 degrees of rotation and exposure range of 1 degree, time of scanning 38 min. Each specimen was scanned with acquisition of images every 0.7°, filed in TIFF format, with resolution of 19.7 μm and saved on a hard disk. After reconstruction of the images (NRecon v1.6.9; Bruker-microCT) 3D models were created with help of CTAn software v.1.12 program (Bruker-microCT) in accordance with the recommended guidelines.

Histopathological Analysis

The maxillae with ligature were fixed in 10% neutral-buffer formalin (10%) and demineralized in formic acid (10%). The specimens went through the process of dehydration, paraffin embedment, and after were sectioned in a mesio-distal plane for hematoxylin and eosin (HE) staining. The area between the first and second molars where ligatures had been placed was sectioned in 4 μm thickness sections and evaluated under light microscopy considering the inflammatoryparameters such as cell influx and alveolar bone and cementum integrity. Previously standardized scores ranging from 0 to 3 were used (Lima et al., 2000; Leitão et al., 2005). Score 0 indicates absence of or only discrete presence of inflammatory cell infiltration cellular infiltration (restricted to the marginal gingiva, preserved alveolar process and cementum; score 1 represents moderate inflammatory cellular infiltration all over the insert gingiva, some minor alveolar process resorption and intact cementum; score 2 represents accentuated cellular infiltration in both gingiva and periodontal ligament, accentuated degradation of the alveolar process, and partial destruction of cementum; score 3 indicates accentuated cellular infiltration with complete resorption of the alveolar process and intense destruction of cementum. Two examiners who were masked to the identity of samples performed histologic evaluation.

Plasma Bone Alkaline Phosphatase (BALP)

The plasma concentration of bone alkaline phosphatase was obtained from blood samples collected from the retro-orbital plexus on the 11th day using the thermo-activation method, as previously described (Whitby and Moss, 1975). The samples were heated up to 56°C for 10 min. Serum levels of BALP were calculated by subtracting the concentration of the heated alkaline phosphatase in serum from the concentration of the total alkaline phosphatase (TALP) in serum. The analysis was performed according to the manufacturer's instructions (Labest, Lagoa Santa, MG, Brazil).

Quantification of Cytokine Levels in Gingival Tissue

The stored gingival tissues were used to determine the concentrations of TNF-α, IL-1β, CINC-1 and IL-10 using specific commercially available kits (DuoSet Elisa kit, R&D Systems Inc., MN, USA). The inflammatory mediators' levels were determined by enzyme-linked immunosorbent assay (ELISA) using respective standard curves. Results were shown as picogram/ml (pg/ml). All kits were used according manufacturer's instructions.

Superoxide Dismutase (SOD) and Catalase (CAT) Levels in Gingival Tissue

The gingivae removed on 11th day were used to evaluate the effect of *S. maritima* 5 mg/kg on the oxidative stress. The SOD activity was assayed according the protocol previously described (Beauchamp and Fridovich, 1971). In a dark room, the gingival samples were homogenized in 20 μl of ice-cold phosphate buffer at 15,000 G for 20 min. The supernatants were mixed with a solution comprised of phosphate buffer (50 nM), EDTA (100 nM) and L-methionine (19.5 mM) in a pH of 7.8. Then, 150 ml of a solution of riboflavin (10 nM) and nitro NBT (750 nM) was added and the mixture was exposed to light (20 W) for 15 min. The absorbance of the samples was measured at 560 nm. The results are expressed as grams of SOD per ml.

The measurement of O_2 production rate and H_2O in proportion of H_2O_2 was calculated to obtain CAT activity. Briefly, 20 μl of gingival homogenate was mixed with a solution comprised of 3% H_2O_2 and Tris-HCl EDTA buffer (5 nM, pH 8.0). The absorbance was measure immediately and 6 min after preparing the samples at a 230 nm wavelength (Maehly and Chance, 1954).

qRT-PCR Analysis of TNF-α, IL-1β, RANK, and iNOS Levels

Total RNA was extracted from gingivae tissues using the TRIzol reagent (Invitrogen, São Paulo, Brazil). The RNA concentration was estimated by reading the absorbance at 260 nm and was checked for purity at 280 nm in a spectrophotometer (Amersham Biosciences, Cambridge, England). For each sample, the RNA concentrations used to synthesize cDNA were adjusted to 1,000 ng/mL. Before the reverse transcription reaction, samples of RNA were incubated for 5 min at 70°C and then cooled in ice. The reverse transcription was performed in a total volume of 20 μL composed of 10 μL of sample RNA, 4 μL reverse transcriptase buffer (Invitrogen), 8 units RNAsin, 150 units of reverse transcriptase Superscript III, 0.036U random primers, 10 mM DTT and 0.5 mM of each dNTP (Invitrogen). The mixture was incubated at 42°C for 1 h, subsequently at 80°C for 5 min and finally stored at −20°C. The negative control was prepared under the same conditions but without addition of reverse transcriptase.

Quantitative real-time polymerase chain reaction (qRT-PCR) was performed in triplicate to determine the gingival levels of mRNA for TNF-α, IL1-β, RANK and iNOS. Each reaction contained 10 μL of SYBR® Green Master Mix (Applied Biosystems, Warrington, UK), 7,3 μL of ultra-pure water, 1 μL of cDNA and 0.5 μM of each primer and was performed in StepOne Real-Time PCR (Applied Biosystems, Warrington, UK) thermocycler. The thermal cycling profile for the first round of qRT-PCR was initial denaturation and activation of the polymerase for 10 min at 95°C, followed by 40 cycles of 15 s at 95°C, 30 s at 58°C, and 30 s at 72°C. The final extension was for 10 min at 72°C. The primers were designed by using the PrimerQuest® Tool https://www.idtdna.com/Primerquest/Home/Index. The primers used in this study are shown in **Table 1**. The glyceraldehyde 3-phosphate dehydrogenase (GAPDH) was used as endogenous control for normalization of messenger RNA expression. The specificity of each primer pair was confirmed by melting curve analysis of qRT-PCR products. Relative quantifications of mRNA were carried out using the comparative threshold (CT) cycle method. The delta-delta-Ct method was used to transform the Ct values into normalized relative expression levels (Livak and Schmittgen, 2001).

Subchronic Toxicity Evaluation

Variation of body mass, organ weight alteration and biochemical and histopathological parameters were evaluated in animals treated daily during 11 consecutive days with a single dose of *S. maritima* 5 mg/kg and saline + DMSO. Peripheral blood samples were collected in order to obtain biochemical analysis of aspartate aminotransferase (AST) and alanine aminotransferase (ALT) levels and creatinine (Labtest, Lagoa Santa, MG, Brazil).

After sacrificing the animals, the liver, kidney and heart were removed and weighed. The stomach was also removed for histological analysis. The organs were fixed with formalin and then dehydrated with increasing concentrations of ethanol and embedded in paraffin. The blocs were sliced in 5 μm thick sections, stained with hematoxylin-eosin (HE) and observed at light microscope (Leica DM 2000, Wetzlar, Germany).

TABLE 1 | Description of biomarkers, gene, primer sequences and NCBI accession numbers.

Biomarkers	Gene	Primer sequence (5′-3′)	NCBI
Inflammatory modulators	TNF-α	**S-**CGGGGTGATCGGTCCCAACAAG	NM_012675.3
		A-GTGGTTTGCTACGACGTGGGC	
	IL-1β	**S-**TGCTGTCTGACCCATGTGAG	NM_031512.2
		A-CCAAGGCCACAGGGATTTTG	
	iNOS	**S-**AGGCACAAGACTCTGACACC	NM_012611.3
		A-GGTAGGGTAGAGGAGGGGAG	
Bone makers	RANK	**S-**AGGGAAAACGCTGACAGCTAA	NM_001271235.1
		A-CCAACACAATGGTCCCCTGA	
Reference gene	GAPDH	**S-**GGACCAGGTTGTCTCCTGTG	NM_017008.4
		A-CATTGAGAGCAATGCCAGCC	

Statistical Analysis

Shapiro-Wilk normality test was performed to analyze the data. Results are presented as means ± standard error (SEM) or as medians when appropriate. ANOVA followed by Tukey test or Games-Howell test were used to compare means and Kruskal–Wallis and Dunn tests were used to compare medians. $P < 0.05$ was considered significant. Analyses were performed using IBM SPSS Statistics for Windows, Version 20.0. Armonk, NY or GraphPad Prism 6 software, San Diego, CA, USA.

RESULTS

Alveolar Bone Loss and Histopathological Analysis

No significant ABL was observed in the naive group (**Figures 1a,b**). Data indicated that *S. maritima* 5 mg/kg was the most effective dose protecting against ABL. Gavage (*per os*) administration of *S. maritima* 5 mg/kg 1 h before the placement of the ligature and once daily for 11 days resulted in a significant ($P < 0.05$) inhibition of ABL (2.37 ± 0.53) (**Figures 1a,bG,H**), compared to the group that received the vehicle only (4.47 ± 0.22) (**Figures 1a,bD,E**).

Histopathologic analysis of animals subjected to EP (vehicle group) demonstrated accentuated inflammatory cell infiltration, breakdown of alveolar bone, collagen fiber derangement within the periodontal ligament, and resorption of cementum, receiving a median score of 3 (range 2 to 3) (**Table 2**). The periodontium of animals treated with *S. maritima* 5 mg/kg showed preservation of the alveolar process and cementum, reduction of the inflammatory cell infiltration, and partial preservation of collagen fibers of the periodontal ligament (**Figures 1bC,F,I**), receiving a median score of 1 (range 1 to 2) (**Table 2**). These values were statistically different ($P < 0.05$), compared with the vehicle group.

Plasma Bone-Specific Alkaline Phosphatase (BALP)

Experimental periodontitis decreased BALP serum levels and the treatment with *S. maritima* 5 mg/kg resulted in a significant increase in the BALP serum levels ($P < 0.05$), when compared with the vehicle group (**Figure 2**).

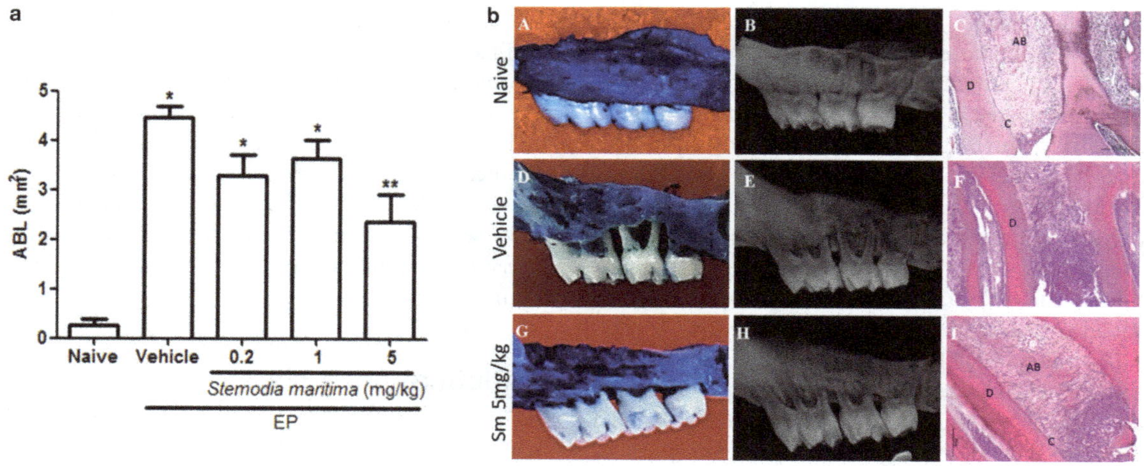

FIGURE 1 | (a) Effect of oral gavage of vehicle (saline + DMSO) and Sm extracts concentrations on alveolar bone loss (0.2, 1, and 5 mg/kg) in experimental periodontitis. Data represent the mean ± SEM of six animals/group. $^*P < 0.05$ was considered significantly different compared to the naïve control group; $^{**}P < 0.05$ was considered significantly different compared to vehicle group (saline + DMSO). (ANOVA and Games-Howell *post-hoc* test). **(b)** Macroscopic view (first column), microCT images (second column) and histological aspects (third column) of Naive, Vehicle and Sm 5 mg/kg. Data represent the mean ± SEM of six animals/group. **(A–C)** Indicates normal maxilla (naive), showing integrity of its components (c, Cementum; d, Dentine and ab, Alveolar bone). **(D–F)** Shows maxilla subjected to experimental periodontitis that received only the vehicle (saline + DMSO), showing severe bone resorption, inflammatory infiltrate in gingiva and periodontal ligament, extensive cementum destruction and total resorption of the alveolar process. **(G–I)** Indicate maxilla after 11 days of experimental periodontitis treated with Sm 5 mg/kg showing discrete cell influx and preservation of the alveolar process and cementum. Magnification x100.

TABLE 2 | Effect of oral gavage of Sm extracts and vehicle (saline + DMSO) on histopathologic score of rat maxillae.

			***Stemodia maritima* (Sm) mg/kg**		
	Naive	**Vehicle**	**0.2**	**1**	**5**
Escores (median values and range)	0 (0–0)	3 (2–3)*	2 (1–2)	2 (2–2)	1 (1–2)**

$^*P < 0.05$ vs. naive group (CONTROL); $^{**}P < 0.05$ vs. vehicle group (animals submitted to experimental periodontitis and treated with saline + DMSO) (Kruskal-Wallis followed by Dunn's test).

Effects of *S. maritima* on Cytokine Levels in Gingival Tissue

Periodontitis challenge was associated with significant ($P < 0.05$) increase of pro-inflammatory cytokines (TNF-α, IL-1β, and CINC-1) in gingival tissue; at the same time it was observed a significant ($P < 0.05$) decrease in gingival levels of IL-10, an anti-inflammatory cytokine, when compared to naive group. Treatment with Sm 5 mg/kg significantly ($P < 0.05$) decreased TNF-α and CINC-1 but no significant difference was observed in IL-1β gingival levels; also, *S. maritima* 5 mg/kg increased IL-10 levels, when compared to vehicle treated group (**Figures 3A–D**).

Superoxide Dismutase and Catalase Levels in Gingival Tissue

In the present study periodontitis induction resulted in a significant ($P < 0.05$) reduction of SOD and CAT levels in gingival tissue, when compared with naive group. *S. maritima* 5 mg/kg significantly ($P < 0.05$) increased both markers for oxidative stress in gingival tissue, when compared with vehicle group (**Figures 4A,B**).

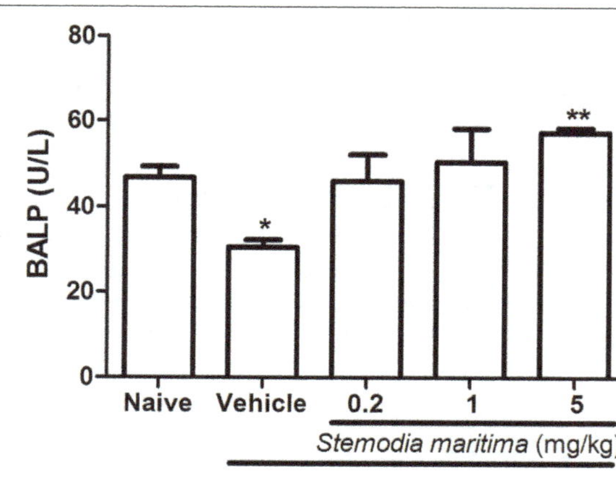

FIGURE 2 | Effects of Sm 5 mg/kg and saline + DMSO (vehicle) on the plasma bone alkaline phosphatase (BALP) in experimental periodontitis in rats. Data represent the mean ± SEM of six animals/group. $^*P < 0.05$ compared with naïve group (control); $^{**}P < 0.05$ compared with vehicle group (animals submitted to experimental periodontitis and treated with saline + DMSO) (ANOVA and Games-Howell *post-hoc* test).

qRT-PCR Analysis of TNF-α, IL-1β, RANK and iNOS Levels

The vehicle groups showed significant increase in TNF-α (**Figure 5A**), IL-1β (**Figure 5B**), RANK (**Figure 5C**) and iNOS (**Figure 5D**) mRNA expression, when compared with

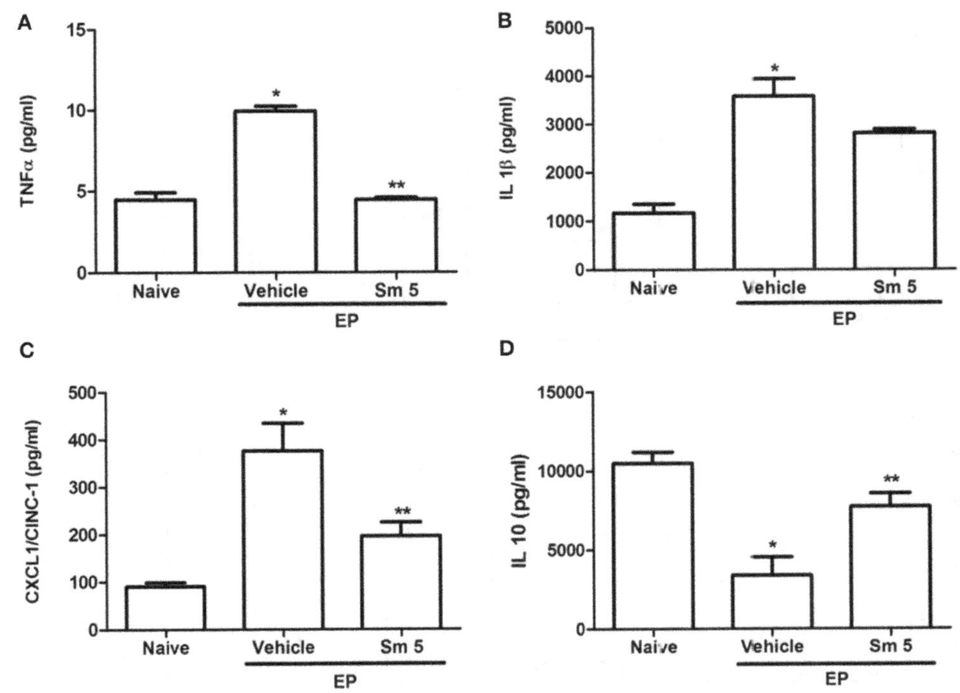

FIGURE 3 | Effects of Sm 5 mg/kg and saline + DMSO (vehicle) on TNF-α **(A)**, IL-1β **(B)**, CINC-1 **(C)** and IL-10 **(D)** in gingival tissues levels. Data represent the mean ± SEM of six animals/group. *$P < 0.05$ compared with naïve group (control); **$P < 0.05$ compared with vehicle group (animals submitted to experimental periodontitis and treated with saline + DMSO) (ANOVA and Tukey's *post-hoc* test).

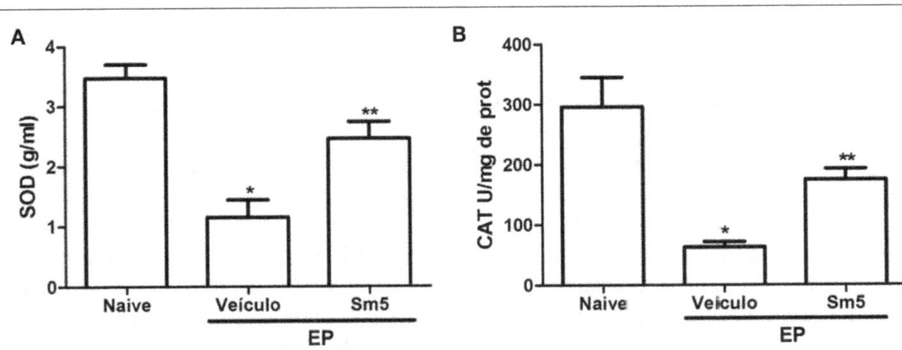

FIGURE 4 | Effects of Sm 5 mg/kg on superoxide dismutase **(A)** and catalase **(B)** concentrations in gingival tissues. Data represent the mean ± SEM of six animals/group. *$P < 0.05$ compared with naïve group (control); **$P < 0.05$ compared with vehicle group (animals submitted to experimental periodontitis and treated with saline + DMSO) (ANOVA and Tukey's *post-hoc* test).

the naive control group. Administration of *S. maritima* 5 mg/kg significantly reduced mRNA expression in all parameters evaluated compared to vehicle group (**Figure 5**).

Analysis of Toxicity

No signs of systemic illness, adverse pharmacological events or changes in behavior were observed throughout the experimental period. *S. maritima* 5 mg/kg or vehicle did not affect the animals' body mass or the wet weight of the livers, kidneys or hearts compared to the naive control throughout the study period. Gross necropsy findings did not show any abnormalities. A single-dose of *S. maritima* (5 mg/kg) or vehicle (saline + DMSO) over 11 consecutive days had no significant histological alterations in the hepatic, renal parenchyma, and cardiac tissue. The values obtained for ALT/AST and creatinine did not differ from the control group.

DISCUSSION

Ligature-induced periodontitis is a well-established animal model. While it has some limitations, the structure and organization of the periodontal tissues are similar to those of

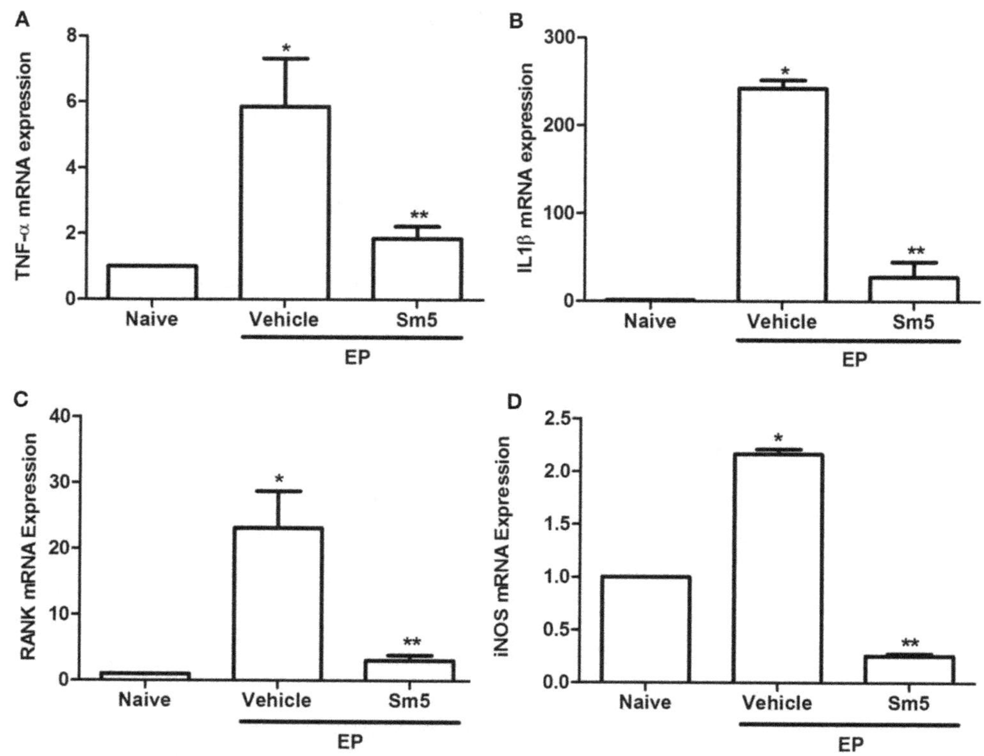

FIGURE 5 | Effects of Sm 5 mg/kg on tumor necrosis factor alpha (TNF-α) **(A)**, interleukin 1β (IL-1β) **(B)**, RANK **(C)**, and inducible nitric oxide synthase (iNOS) **(D)** mRNA levels in experimental periodontitis in rats. Data represent the mean ± SEM. *$P < 0.05$ compared with naïve group (control); **$P < 0.05$ compared with vehicle group (animals submitted to experimental periodontitis and treated with saline + DMSO) (ANOVA and Tukey's *post-hoc* test).

humans. Further, rat models have fewer limitations than *in vitro* models that cannot reproduce the complexity of interactions among the oral microbiome, environmental factors, and the immune/inflammatory host response (Struillou et al., 2010; Oz and Puleo, 2011; Hajishengallis et al., 2015). In this model, ligature causes mechanical trauma, and affects tissue integrity to induce an inflammatory response, increase oxidative stress, and destroy the periodontal ligament leading to significant bone loss (Bezerra et al., 2000; Guimarães et al., 2016; Lima et al., 2017; Oliveira et al., 2017). Alternative and preventive treatment options are essential to overcome the adverse effects of both antimicrobial and anti-inflammatory agents as an adjunct to conventional mechanical and surgical treatments (Chandra Shekar et al., 2015; Ramesh et al., 2016).

Chemical studies on *S. maritima* reported the isolation of diterpenes and flavonoids showing antiviral, cytotoxic, and larvicidal activities (Hufford et al., 1991; Rodrigues et al., 2010). Further, it was showed that *S. maritima* compounds have *in vitro* inhibitory activity of both lipids peroxidation and cyclooxygenase 1 and 2 (Hufford et al., 1992; Russell et al., 2011). Besides, our research group demonstrated that *S. maritima* has antioxidant activity *in vitro* and it also has activity against some bacterial strains (da Silva et al., 2014). However, it is important to mention that there is no study in the literature using *S. maritima* extract or its identified compounds on bone resorption models. These data encouraged us to investigate whether *S. maritima* extract could be useful to ameliorate the bone loss during periodontitis.

The protective effect of *S. maritima* on alveolar bone loss was associated with an increase in plasma bone-specific alkaline phosphatase (BALP) suggesting that 5 mg/kg *S. maritima* prevents bone resorption and stimulates bone formation. Many studies have verified the effects of medicinal plants on ABL using a similar periodontitis model (Sezer et al., 2013; Hatipoglu et al., 2015; Saglam et al., 2015; Guimarães et al., 2016). Sezer et al. (2013) showed that the systemic use of *Ginko biloba* extract on reducing ABL. Hatipoglu et al. (2015) assessed ABL from microcomputed tomography (micro CT) images, and verified less bone resorption in animals treated with *Crataegus orientalis* extracts. Recently, Guimarães et al. (2016) observed the ability of the *Matricaria recutita* extract to inhibit TNF-α and IL-1β cytokines. These treatments prevented the osteoclast activation via RANKL-OPG. Lima et al. (2017) demonstrated anti-inflammatory and anti-oxidant activities with *Calendula officinalis*.

Cytokines play a significant role in periodontitis. Here, we showed that *S. maritima* (5 mg/kg) significantly increased IL-10 gingival levels, an anti-inflammatory cytokine, while decreasing the pro-inflammatory cytokines TNF-α and CINC-1. Alternative therapeutic approaches based that inhibit TNF-α production have been successfully used for the pre-clinical and clinical treatment of chronic inflammatory diseases, particularly rheumatoid arthritis and temporomandibular joint disorders (Feldmann, 2002; Araújo et al., 2013; Freitas et al., 2016; Alves et al., 2017). Further, when mRNA expression for TNF-α, IL-1β, iNOS, and RANK were evaluated, *S. maritima* 5 mg/kg significantly reduced mRNA expression for all these genes compared to the vehicle group. Cytokines amplify the inflammatory response in periodontitis (Duarte et al., 2015). It seems contradictory that *S. maritima* 5 mg/kg reduced mRNA expression for IL-1β without affecting IL-1β gingival levels. Here, we hypothesized that the IL1-β levels detected by ELISA in gingival samples might derive from a pre-formed pool because the increase in IL-1β levels after periodontitis challenge precedes the increase in mRNA. Studies analyzing the effects of resveratrol, a naturally occurring product found in numerous plants showed similar results (Casati et al., 2013; Tamaki et al., 2014).

The release of large amounts of NO by iNOS plays a major role in immune-inflammatory events including periodontitis (Leitão et al., 2005; Tamaki et al., 2014; Martins et al., 2016). TNF-α and IL-1 trigger the transcription of the iNOS resulting in the increase production of NO. On the other hand, the significant increase of IL-10 levels in gingival tissues could also decrease iNOS gene expression (Gadek-Michalska et al., 2013). Some components of medicinal plants might inhibit nuclear transcription factor-kB binding activity and downregulate the expression of iNOS (Kim et al., 2005; Cai et al., 2008). These results are in accordance with our present data since the extract of *S. maritima* decreased transcription of iNOS genes.

Oxidative stress plays a central role in periodontitis (Tóthová et al., 2015; Lima et al., 2017). This study demonstrated that experimental periodontitis in rats leads to oxidative stress as indicated by a significant reduction in SOD and CAT levels in gingival tissue. This effect was reduced in animals treated with *S. maritima* (5 mg/kg), which suggests that the beneficial effects of *S. maritima* are at least partially related to its antioxidative properties. *Calendula offinalis* extract also presents ability to reduce oxidative stress by increasing superoxide dismutase (SOD), catalase (CAT) and reduced gluthatione (GSH) enzymes and decreasing malonaldeyde (MDA) levels in gingival tissue (Lima et al., 2017).

The regulation of the critical cytokine macrophage colony-stimulating factor, RANK ligand is essential to the differentiation of osteoclasts. Our results indicated that ligature-induced periodontitis in rats is associated with an increase in the RANK mRNA levels in periodontal tissues, and the treatment with *S. maritima* (5 m/kg) could reduce RANK expression.

Medicinal plants have been historically used for treatment of numerous human diseases (Varela-López et al., 2015; de Oliveira et al., 2016; Ramesh et al., 2016). The leaves and stem of *S. maritima* can treat stomach pain and fluid retention, although the literature still lacks studies that confirm the safety of this plant. Thus, in this study we used biochemical and histopathological analysis to show that the administration of *S. maritima* (5 mg/kg) did not promote any signs of toxicity when administered for 11 consecutive days.

This study observed that 5 mg/kg *S. maritima* extract reduced alveolar bone loss, inflammation, and oxidative stress in a ligature-induced model of periodontitis in rats without causing any systemic changes. These data are in accordance with previous results from our group, which demonstrated via *in vitro* assays that *S. maritima* has anti-inflammatory, antioxidant and antibacterial properties (da Silva et al., 2014). We also found evidence that, at least in part, the effectiveness of *S. maritima* depends upon a positive balance between pro and anti-inflammatory cytokines that decrease TNF-α, IL-1β, and CINC-1 gingival levels while increasing IL-10. This effect might also modulate both iNOS activity and RANK levels, to improve antioxidative events.

To the best of our knowledge, there are no existing reports evaluating the efficacy of *S. maritima* extract in a preclinical trial of rat periodontitis. Although additional studies are needed, these data suggest that *S. maritima* is a potential tool for controlling the development of periodontitis.

AUTHOR CONTRIBUTIONS

AT and JF treated the animals, performed all assays, analysis and interpretation of data. LdS induced periodontitis. AA and FL performed the collection and extraction of plant material. NdS performed cytokines analysis. IM, KP, and IC performed histolopathogical analysis. AP assisted in laboratory experiments. JC performed quantitative qRT-PCR analysis. GC-F and VP performed and analyzed the *S. maritima* Linn toxicity profile. MB, HC, and PG designed and supervised the study. AT and MB wrote the paper. All authors critically reviewed and approved the manuscript.

ACKNOWLEDGMENTS

This work was supported by Brazilian grants from Conselho Nacional de Pesquisa (CNPq) (grant #471974/2013-7), and Coordenação de Aperfeiçoamento de Pessoal de Nível Superior (Capes) / Fundação Cearense de Apoio ao Desenvolvimento Científico e Tecnológico (Funcap) (grant # AE1-0052-000180100/2011). The authors are grateful to Bruno C. Vasconcelos from the School of Dentistry, Federal University of Ceará, Sobral, Ceará, Brazil for the microCT images.

REFERENCES

Albach, D. C., Meudt, H. M., and Oxelman, B. (2005). Piecing together the "new" Plantaginaceae. *Am. J. Bot.* 92, 297–315. doi: 10.3732/ajb.92.2.297

Alves, S. M., Abreu, S. C., Lemos, J. C., Gomes, F. I. F., Alves, S. M., do Val, D. R., et al. (2017). Anti-inflammatory and anti-nociceptive effects of strontium ranelate on the zymosan-induced temporomandibular joint inflammatory hypernociception in rats depend on TNF-α inhibition. *Pharmacol. Rep.* 69, 764–772. doi: 10.1016/j.pharep.2017.03.007

Alviano, D. S., and Alviano, C. S. (2009). Plant extracts: search for new alternatives to treat microbial diseases. *Curr. Pharm. Biotechnol.* 10, 106–121. doi: 10.2174/138920109787048607

Araújo, A. A., Souza, T. O., Moura, L. M., Brito, G. A., Aragão, K. S., Araújo, L. S., et al. (2013). Effect of telmisartan on levels of IL-1, TNF-α, down-regulated COX-2, MMP-2, MMP-9 and RANKL/RANK in an experimental periodontitis model. *J. Clin. Periodontol.* 40, 1104–1111. doi: 10.1111/jcpe.12160

Beauchamp, C., and Fridovich, I. (1971). Superoxide dismutase: improved assays and an assay applicable to acrylamide gels. *Anal. Biochem.* 44, 276–287. doi: 10.1016/0003-2697(71)90370-8

Bezerra, M. M., Brito, G. A., Ribeiro, R. A., and Rocha, F. A. (2002). Low-dose doxycycline prevents inflammatory bone resorption in rats. *Braz. J. Med. Biol. Res.* 35, 613–616. doi: 10.1590/S0100-879X2002000500015

Bezerra, M. M., de Lima, V., Alencar, V. B., Vieira, I. B., Brito, G. A., and Ribeiro, R. (2000). Selective cyclooxygenase-2 inhibition prevents alveolar bone loss in experimental periodontitis in rats. *J. Periodontol.* 71, 1009–1014. doi: 10.1902/jop.2000.71.6.1009

Cai, X., Li, C., Du, G., and Cao, Z. (2008). Protective effects of baicalin on ligature-induced periodontitis in rats. *J. Periodontal Res.* 43, 14–21. doi: 10.1111/j.1600-0765.2007.00989.x

Casati, M. Z., Algayer, C., Cardoso da Cruz, G., Ribeiro, F. V., Casarin, R. C., Pimentel, S. P., et al. (2013). Resveratrol decreases periodontal breakdown and modulates local levels of cytokines during periodontitis in rats. *J. Periodontol.* 84, e58–e64. doi: 10.1902/jop.2013.120746

Chandra Shekar, B. R., Nagarajappa, R., Suma, S., and Thakur, R. (2015). Herbal extracts in oral health care - a review of the current scenario and its future needs. *Pharmacogn. Rev.* 9, 87–92. doi: 10.4103/0973-7847.162101

da Silva, F., Rodrigues, F., Gomes, A., Arriaga, A., Mafezoli, J., Lemos, T., et al. (2014). Phytochemical study, antioxidant and antibacterial activities of *Stemodia maritima*. *Quim Nov.* 37, 1474–1478. doi: 10.5935/0100-4042.20140255

de Oliveira, J. S., Pinto, M. S. C., Santana, L. A. B., Pinto, A. S. B., di Lenardo, D., and Vasconcelos, D. F. P. (2016). Biological effects of medicinal plants on induced periodontitis: a systematic review. *Int. J. Dent.* 2016:3719879. doi: 10.1155/2016/3719879

Duarte, P. M., Bastos, M. F., Fermiano, D., Rabelo, C. C., Perez-Chaparro, P. J., Figueiredo, L. C., et al. (2015). Do subjects with aggressive and chronic periodontitis exhibit a different cytokine/chemokine profile in the gingival crevicular fluid? A systematic review. *J. Periodontal Res.* 50, 18–27. doi: 10.1111/jre.12180

Feldmann, M. (2002). Development of anti-TNF therapy for rheumatoid arthritis. *Nat. Rev. Immunol.* 2, 364–371. doi: 10.1038/nri802

Freitas, R. S., do Val, D. R., Fernandes, M. E., Gomes, F. I., de Lacerda, J. T., SantiGadelha, T., et al. (2016). Lectin from *Abelmoschus esculentus* reduces zymosan-induced temporomandibular joint inflammatory hypernociception in rats via heme oxygenase-1 pathway integrity and tnf-alpha and il-1β suppression. *Int. Immunopharmacol.* 38, 313–323. doi: 10.1016/j.intimp.2016.06.012

Gadek-Michalska, A., Tadeusz, J., Rachwalska, P., and Bugajski, J. (2013). Cytokines, prostaglandins and nitric oxide in the regulation of stress-response systems. *Pharmacol. Rep.* 65, 1655–1662. doi: 10.1016/S1734-1140(13)71527-5

Genco, R. J., and Borgnakke, W. S. (2013). Risk factors for periodontal disease. *Periodontology 2000* 62, 59–94. doi: 10.1111/j.1600-0757.2012.00457.x

Gomes, F. I., Aragao, M. G., Barbosa, F. C., Bezerra, M. M., de Paulo Teixeira Pinto, V., and Chaves, H. V. (2016). Inflammatory cytokines interleukin-1β and tumour necrosis factor-α- novel biomarkers for the detection of periodontal diseases: a literature review. *J. Oral Maxillofac. Res.* 7:e2. doi: 10.5037/jomr.2016.7202

Guimarães, M. V., Melo, I. M., Adriano Araújo, V. M., Tenazoa Wong, D. V., Roriz Fonteles, C. S., Moreira Leal, L. K., et al. (2016). Dry extract of *Matricaria recutita* L. (Chamomile) prevents ligature-induced alveolar bone resorption in rats via inhibition of tumor necrosis factor-α and interleukin-1β. *J. Periodontol.* 87, 706–715. doi: 10.1902/jop.2016.150411

Hajishengallis, G. (2014). Immunomicrobial pathogenesis of periodontitis: keystones, pathobionts, and host response. *Trends Immunol.* 35, 3–11. doi: 10.1016/j.it.2013.09.001

Hajishengallis, G., Lamont, R. J., and Graves, D. T. (2015). The enduring importance of animal models in understanding periodontal disease. *Virulence* 6, 229–235. doi: 10.4161/21505594.2014.990806

Hatipoglu, M., Saglam, M., Köseoglu, S., Köksal, E., Keleş, A., and Esen, H. H. (2015). The effectiveness of *Crataegus orientalis* M Bieber. (Hawthorn) extract administration in preventing alveolar bone loss in rats with experimental periodontitis. *PLoS ONE* 10:e0128134. doi: 10.1371/journal.pone.0128134

Hienz, S. A., Paliwal, S., and Ivanovski, S. (2015). Mechanisms of bone resorption in periodontitis. *J. Immunol. Res.* 2015:615486. doi: 10.1155/2015/615486

Hufford, C. D., Badria, F. A., Abou-Karam, M., Shier, W. T., and Rogers, R. D. (1991). Preparation, characterization, and antiviral activity of microbial metabolites of stemodin. *J. Nat. Prod.* 54, 1543–1552. doi: 10.1021/np50078a008

Hufford, C. D., Oguntimein, B. O., and Muhammad, I. (1992). New stemodane diterpenes from *Stemodia maritima*. *J. Nat. Prod.* 55, 48–52. doi: 10.1021/np50079a007

Kala, B. S., Gunjan, C., Disha, N., and Shobha, P. (2015). Treatment of periodontal disease - a herbal approach. *Int. J. Pharm. Sci. Rev. Res.* 33, 126–136.

Kim, D. H., Cho, K. H., Moon, S. K., Kim, Y. S., Kim, D. H., Choi, J. S., et al. (2005). Cytoprotective mechanism of baicalin against endothelial cell damage by peroxynitrite. *J. Pharm. Pharmacol.* 57, 1581–1590. doi: 10.1211/jpp.57.12.0008

Kuhr, A., Popa-Wagner, A., Schmoll, H., Schwahn, C., and Kocher, T. (2004). Observations on experimental marginal periodontitis in rats. *J. Periodontal Res.* 39, 101–106. doi: 10.1111/j.1600-0765.2004.00710.x

Leitão, R. F., Ribeiro, R. A., Chaves, H. V., Rocha, F. A., Lima, V., and Brito, G. A. (2005). Nitric oxide synthase inhibition prevents alveolar bone resorption in experimental periodontitis in rats. *J. Periodontol.* 76, 956–963. doi: 10.1902/jop.2005.76.6.956

Liao, C. H., Fei, W., Shen, Z. H., Yin, M. P., and Lu, C. (2014). Expression and distribution of TNF-α and PGE_2 of periodontal tissues in rat periodontitis model. *Asian Pac. J. Trop. Med.* 7, 412–416. doi: 10.1016/S1995-7645(14)60067-5

Lima, M. d. R., Lopes, A. P., Martins, C., Brito, G. A. C., Carneiro, V. C., and Goes, P. (2017). The effect of *Calendula officinalis* on oxidative stress and bone loss in experimental periodontitis. *Front. Physiol.* 8:440. doi: 10.3389/fphys.2017.00440

Lima, V., Bezerra, M. M., de Menezes Alencar, V. B., Vidal, F. D., da Rocha, F. A., de Castro Brito, G. A., et al. (2000). Effects of chlorpromazine on alveolar bone loss in experimental periodontal disease in rats. *Eur. J. Oral Sci.* 108, 123–129. doi: 10.1034/j.1600-0722.2000.00766.x

Livak, K. J., and Schmittgen, T. D. (2001). Analysis of Relative Gene Expression Data Using Real-Time Quantitative, PCR and the $2^{-\Delta\Delta C}T$ Method. *Methods* 25, 402–408. doi: 10.1006/meth.2001.1262

Maehly, A. C., and Chance, B. (1954). The assay of catalases and peroxidases. *Methods Biochem. Anal.* 1, 357–424. doi: 10.1002/9780470110171.ch14

Martins, C. S., Leitão, R. F. C., Costa, D. V., Melo, I. M., Santos, G. S., Lima, V., et al. (2016). Topical HPMC/S-nitrosoglutathione solution decreases inflammation and bone resorption in experimental periodontal disease in rats. *PLoS ONE* 11:e0153716. doi: 10.1371/journal.pone.0153716

Oliveira, G. J., Paula, L. G., Souza, J. A., Spin-Neto, R., Stavropoulos, A., and Marcantonio, R. A. (2017). Effects of avocado/soybean unsaponifiables (ASU) on the treatment of ligature-induced periodontitis in rats. *Braz. Oral Res.* 31, 1–11. doi: 10.1590/1807-3107bor-2017.vol31.0028

Oz, H. S., and Puleo, D. A. (2011). Animal models for periodontal disease. *J. Biomed. Biotechnol.* 2011:754857. doi: 10.1155/2011/754857

Pimentel, S. P., Barrella, G. E., Casarin, R. C. V., Cirano, F. R., Casati, M. Z., Foglio, M. A., et al. (2012). Protective effect of topical *Cordia verbenacea* in a rat periodontitis model: immune-inflammatory, antibacterial and morphometric assays. *BMC Complement. Altern. Med.* 12:224. doi: 10.1186/1472-6882-12-224

Ramesh, A., Varghese, S. S., Doraiswamy, J. N., and Malaiappan, S. (2016). Herbs as an antioxidant arsenal for periodontal diseases. *J. Intercult. Ethnopharmacol.* 5, 92–96. doi: 10.5455/jice.20160122065556

Rodrigues, F. E. A., Lima, J. Q., Santiago, G. M. P., Mafezoli, J., Braz-filho, R., and Arriaga, A. M. C. (2010). Diterpene and other constituents from *Stemodia maritima* (Scrophulariaceae). *J. Braz. Chem. Soc.* 21, 1581–1586. doi: 10.1590/S0103-50532010000800025

Russell, F. A., Mulabagal, V., Thompson, D. R., Singh-Wilmot, M. A., Reynolds, W. F., Nair, M. G., et al. (2011). Stemodin-derived analogues with lipid peroxidation, cyclooxygenase enzymes and human tumour cell proliferation inhibitory activities. *Phytochemistry* 72, 2361–2368. doi: 10.1016/j.phytochem.2011.08.024

Saglam, M., Köseoglu, S., Hatipoglu, M., Esen, H. H., and Köksal, E. (2015). Effect of sumac extract on serum oxidative status, RANKL/OPG system and alveolar bone loss in experimental periodontitis in rats. *J. Appl. Oral Sci.* 23, 33–41. doi: 10.1590/1678-775720140288

Sezer, U., Kara, M. I., ErcIyas, K., Özdemir, H., Üstün, K., Özer, H., et al. (2013). Protective effects of ginkgo biloba extract on ligature-induced periodontitis in rats. *Acta Odontol. Scand.* 71, 38–44. doi: 10.3109/00016357.2011.650195

Silva, N., Abusleme, L., Bravo, D., Dutzan, N., Garcia-Sesnich, J., Vernal, R., et al. (2015). Host response mechanisms in periodontal diseases. *J. Appl. Oral Sci.* 23, 329–355. doi: 10.1590/1678-775720140259

Struillou, X., Boutigny, H., Soueidan, A., and Layrolle, P. (2010). Experimental animal models in periodontology: a review. *Open Dent. J.* 4, 37–47. doi: 10.2174/1874210601004010037

Tamaki, N., Cristina Orihuela-Campos, R., Inagaki, Y., Fukui, M., Nagata, T., and Ito, H. O. (2014). Resveratrol improves oxidative stress and prevents the progression of periodontitis via the activation of the Sirt1/AMPK and the Nrf2/antioxidant defense pathways in a rat periodontitis model. *Free Radic. Biol. Med.* 75, 222–229. doi 10.1016/j.freeradbiomed.2014.07.034

Tóthová, L., Kamodyová, N., Cervenka, T., and Celec, P. (2015). Salivary markers of oxidative stress in oral diseases. *Front. Cell. Infect. Microbiol.* 5:73. doi: 10.3389/fcimb.2015.00073

Varela-López, A., Bullón, P., Giampieri, F., and Quiles, J. (2015). Non-nutrient, naturally occurring phenolic compounds with antioxidant activity for the prevention and treatment of periodontal diseases. *Antioxidants* 4, 447–481. doi: 10.3390/antiox4030447

Wang, T.-F., Jen, I.-A., Chou, C., and Lei, Y.-P. (2014). Effects of periodontal therapy on metabolic control in patients with type 2 diabetes mellitus and periodontal disease. *Medicine* 93:e292. doi: 10.1097/MD.0000000000000292

Whitby, L. G., and Moss, D. W. (1975). Analysis of heat inactivation curves of alkaline phosphatase isoenzymes in serum. *Clin. Chim. Acta* 59, 361–367. doi: 10.1016/0009-8981(75)90012-1

13

Expression of Nerve Growth Factor (NGF), TrkA and $p75^{NTR}$ in Developing Human Fetal Teeth

Thimios A. Mitsiadis* and Pierfrancesco Pagella

Orofacial Development and Regeneration, Institute of Oral Biology, Center for Dentistry (ZZM), University of Zurich, Zurich, Switzerland

***Correspondence:**
Thimios A. Mitsiadis
thimios.mitsiadis@zzm.uzh.ch

Nerve growth factor (NGF) is important for the development and the differentiation of neuronal and non-neuronal cells. NGF binds to specific low- and high-affinity cell surface receptors, respectively, $p75^{NTR}$ and TrkA. In the present study, we examined by immunohistochemistry the expression patterns of the NGF, $p75^{NTR}$, and TrkA proteins during human fetal tooth development, in order to better understand the mode of NGF signaling action in dental tissues. The results obtained show that these molecules are expressed in a wide range of dental cells of both epithelial and mesenchymal origin during early stages of odontogenesis, as well as in nerve fibers that surround the developing tooth germs. At more advanced developmental stages, NGF and TrkA are localized in differentiated cells with secretory capacities such as preameloblasts/ameloblasts secreting enamel matrix and odontoblasts secreting dentine matrix. In contrast, $p75^{NTR}$ expression is absent from these secretory cells and restricted in proliferating cells of the dental epithelium. The temporospatial distribution of NGF and $p75^{NTR}$ in fetal human teeth is similar, but not identical, with that observed previously in the developing rodent teeth, thus indicating that the genetic information is well-conserved during evolution. The expression patterns of NGF, $p75^{NTR}$, and TrkA during odontogenesis suggest regulatory roles for NGF signaling in proliferation and differentiation of epithelial and mesenchymal cells, as well as in attraction and sprouting of nerve fibers within dental tissues.

Keywords: human, tooth, development, nerve growth factor, odontoblast, ameloblast, TrkA, $p75^{NTR}$

INTRODUCTION

The roles of nerve growth factor (NGF) in the development, survival and maintenance of selected group of neurons of the peripheral and central nervous system have been thoroughly evaluated in the last few decades (Chao, 2003; Lu et al., 2005; Reichardt, 2006; Ichim et al., 2012; Lewis and Carter, 2014). Dependence of neurons on NGF varies as a function of the stage of development. Additional members of the NGF-related family of neurotrophic molecules include brain-derived neurotrophic factor (BDNF), neurotrophin-3 (NT-3), neurotrophin-4 (NT-4; also known as NT-4/5 or NT-5), and neurotrophin-6 (NT-6; Chao, 2003; Lu et al., 2005; Reichardt, 2006; Lewis and Carter, 2014). NGF-related neurotrophins (NTFs) support the survival and outgrowth of various neuronal populations (Reichardt, 2006; Ichim et al., 2012). Target cells for NTFs bear specific cell-surface receptors and their presence is indicative of a potentially responsive cell (Chao, 2003; Reichardt, 2006). Two binding affinities of NTFs to their receptors, one high, the other low, have

been described. A transmembrane glycoprotein called low-affinity NGF receptor ($p75^{NTR}$) binds all NTFs with low-affinity (Radeke et al., 1987; Chao, 1992; Reichardt, 2006). However, it is still unclear whether the low-affinity form is capable of mediating all biological responses of NTFs. The products of the tyrosine kinase *trk* family of proto-oncogenes bind also NTFs, and are components of the high-affinity receptor. The *trk* gene family is formed of three characterized genes, *trkA, trkB, trkC* (Chao, 1992; Barbacid, 1994; Reichardt, 2006; Lewis and Carter, 2014). The *trkA* gene encodes a 140 kDa glycoprotein with a tyrosine kinase activity, which functions as a NGF receptor (Klein et al., 1991). Functional high-affinity NGF binding requires either co-expression and binding to both $p75^{NTR}$ and TrkA (Kaplan et al., 1991) or binding to dimers of TrkA (Chao, 2003; Reichardt, 2006).

Novel roles for NTFs in embryonic development are proposed by the presence of $p75^{NTR}$ and Trk receptors during organ morphogenesis and differentiation of non-neuronal cells (Chesa et al., 1988; Yan and Johnson, 1988; Represa and Bernd, 1989; von Bartheld et al., 1991; Nakamura et al., 2007; Di Girolamo et al., 2008; Truzzi et al., 2011; Tomellini et al., 2015). Indeed, expression of both $p75^{NTR}$ and NGF in the developing rodent teeth (Yan and Johnson, 1988; Byers et al., 1990; Mitsiadis et al., 1992, 1993; Mitsiadis and Luukko, 1995) suggests that NTFs play multiple roles in odontogenesis, dental cell function, and tooth homeostasis. The tooth develops as a result of sequential and reciprocal interactions between the oral ectoderm and the cephalic neural crest-derived mesenchyme (Mitsiadis and Graf, 2009). Differentiation of tooth-specific cells gives rise to the mesenchymal-derived odontoblasts that produce the organic matrix of dentine, and the epithelial-derived ameloblasts that elaborate the enamel matrix proteins. In rodents, concomitant expression of $p75^{NTR}$ and NGF in dental mesenchyme is correlated with odontoblast differentiation, whereas in dental epithelium their co-expression corresponds mostly to proliferative phenomena (Mitsiadis et al., 1992, 1993; Mitsiadis and Luukko, 1995). These findings indicate that NGF may be implicated in morphogenetic and mineralization events by affecting either proliferation or differentiation of dental cells (Mitsiadis et al., 1993).

Although numerous studies are undertaken in rodents to understand the role of NGF signaling in tooth development and regeneration, only limited studies exist in humans. Previous data have focused only on the localization of $p75^{NTR}$ in both embryonic and adult teeth. These reports have shown that in the developing fetal teeth $p75^{NTR}$ is expressed transiently in both dental papilla mesenchyme and inner dental epithelium (Christensen et al., 1993), whereas in adult teeth the receptor is present only in unmyelinated axons and Schwann cells of the pulp (Maeda et al., 1992). To date, there is no available data on the distribution of both NGF and TrkA proteins in the developing human teeth. The present study was conducted to localize areas and specific dental cells that express NGF, $p75^{NTR}$, and TrkA in developing human teeth, in order to better understand the mode of NGF action in dental tissues.

MATERIALS AND METHODS

Embryonic Tissues

Tissues

Human fetal tissues were obtained from legal abortions. The material comprised teeth from 19 fetuses (5–23 gestational weeks). The gestation age was estimated from the fetal foot length and from the last menstruation of the mother. Embryos were non-infected, and all tissues were both macroscopically and microscopically normal. The fetuses were immediately fixed in 10% buffered formalin for 48 h to 5 days according to the fetus size. Maxillary and mandibular jaws from 5 to 15 weeks old embryos and fetuses were embedded in Paraplast at 56°C, while the samples ranged in age from 19 to 23 gestational weeks (g.w.) were decalcified for 3 weeks in formic acid/10% formalin prior to embedding in Paraplast. Four to six micrometer thick sections were used for immunohistochemistry. This study was carried out in compliance with the French legislation, after approval of the Regional Ethics Committee of Development and Reproduction of the U.F.R. of Medicine of Reims-France (INSERM 314 Reims).

Materials

Antibodies

Preparation, purification and characterization of polyclonal anti-NGF antibodies have been described (Mitsiadis et al., 1992, 1993). Affinity purified mouse anti-human $p75^{NTR}$ monoclonal antibody was the kind gift of Dr. E. M. Johnson Jr. and Dr. C. Osborn (St. Louis, USA). The purification and characterization of the 20.4 antibody, which recognizes the human $p75^{NTR}$, has been already described (Ross et al., 1984; Grob et al., 1985; Chesa et al., 1988). Polyclonal TrkA antibody was purchased from Abcam (ab76291).

Chemicals

Vector Vectastain ABC kit was purchased from Biosys (Compiègne, France). Other chemicals were obtained from Sigma (St. Louis, MO, USA).

Immunohistochemistry

Immunoperoxidase staining was performed as previously described (Mitsiadis et al., 1992, 1993, 2003). Briefly, the sections were deparaffinized, treated with 0.4% pepsin, exposed to a 0.3% solution of hydrogen peroxide in methanol, and then incubated overnight at 4°C in a humid atmosphere either with polyclonal anti-NGF and anti-TrkA antibodies diluted 1:300 in PBS containing 0.2% BSA, or with the monoclonal anti-$p75^{NTR}$ antibody 20.4 (1:1000 dilution). Positive peroxidase staining produces red/brown color on light microscopy. After staining the sections were mounted with Eukit. In control sections the antibodies were omitted.

RESULTS

Tooth development proceeds in three well-characterized morphological stages: the bud, cap, and bell stages. At the 5–7th gestational week (g.w.), the epithelial dental buds represent the first epithelial ingrowth into the neural crest-derived mesenchyme at sites corresponding to the position of the future fetal teeth. At that stage, weak NGF immunostaining was evident only in the dental mesenchyme (**Figures 1A, 2A**), a pattern similar to that observed for TrkA (**Figure 1C**). While p75^{NTR} labeling was absent from both epithelial and mesenchymal components at the 5th g.w., intense immunoreactivity was seen only in nerve fibers next to the developing tooth germ (**Figures 1B, 3A**).

Three epithelial cell populations compose the dental epithelium at the cap stage of development (8–15th g.w.): the outer dental epithelium, the inner dental epithelium and the stellate reticulum. The mesenchyme surrounded by the inner dental epithelium gives rise to the dental papilla (future dental pulp), whereas the mesenchyme limiting the dental papilla and encapsulating the enamel organ forms the dental follicle, which gives rise to the supporting tissues of the tooth (future

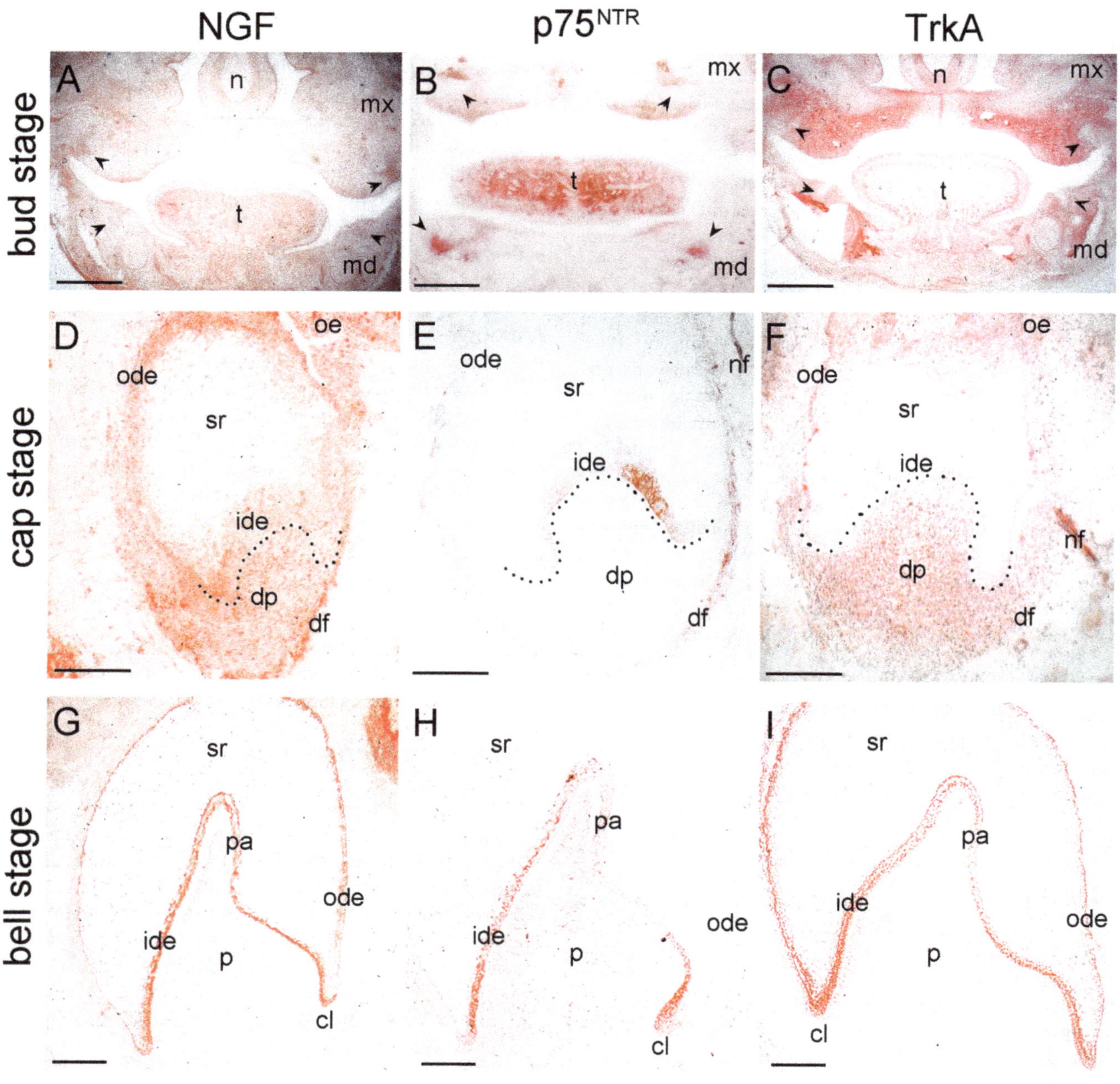

FIGURE 1 | Distribution of NGF, p75^{NTR}, and TrkA proteins in developing human teeth. (A–C) Frontal sections of human fetal head with tooth germs at bud/early cap stage (arrowheads). Immunostaining is seen in red color. **(D–F)** Tooth germs at the late cap stage. NGF **(D)**, p75^{NTR} **(E)**, and TrkA **(F)** immunoreactivities. Note the staining in the nerve fibers (nf) in the dental follicle (df). **(G–I)** Tooth germs at the early bell stage. NGF **(G)**, p75^{NTR} **(H)**, and TrkA **(I)** immunostainings. Dotted lines represent the border between the dental epithelial and mesenchymal components. Abbreviations: cl, cervical loop; dp, dental papilla; ide, inner dental epithelium; md, mandible; mx, maxilla; n, nose; nf, nerve fibers; ode, outer dental epithelium; oe, oral epithelium; p, dental pulp; pa, preameloblasts; sr, stellate reticulum; t, tongue. Scale bars: **(A–C)** 1 mm, **(D–I)** 100 μm.

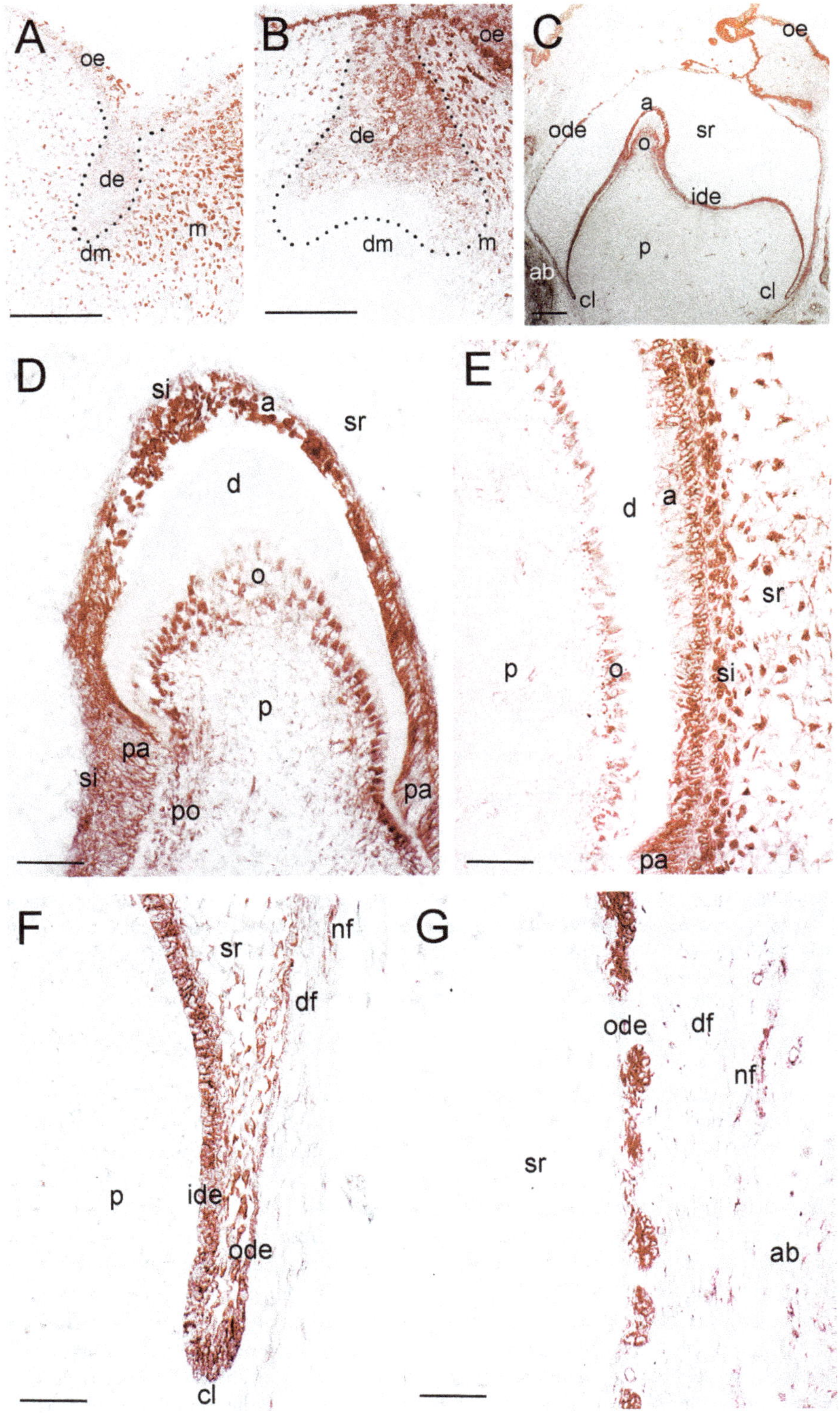

FIGURE 2 | Distribution of the NGF protein in developing human teeth. (A) NGF immunoreactivity (red color) in a tooth germ at the bud stage. **(B)** NGF expression in a tooth germ at the early cap stage. **(C–G)** NGF staining in a tooth germ at the late bell stage. **(D–G)** Higher magnifications of **(C)**, representing the tip of the cusp area **(D)**, an area of the flanks of the forming tooth crown **(E)**, the cervical loop territory **(F)**, and the dental follicle territory **(G)**. Dotted lines represent the border between the dental epithelial and mesenchymal components. Abbreviations: a, ameloblasts; ab, alveolar bone; cl, cervical loop; d, dentinee; de, dental epithelium; df, dental follicle; dm, dental mesenchyme; ide, inner dental epithelium; m, mesenchyme; nf, nerve fibers; o, odontoblasts; ode, outer dental epithelium; oe, oral epithelium; p, dental pulp; pa, preameloblasts; po, preodontoblasts; si, stratum intermedium; sr, stellate reticulum. Scale bars: **(A–C)** 100 μm, **(D–G)** 25 μm.

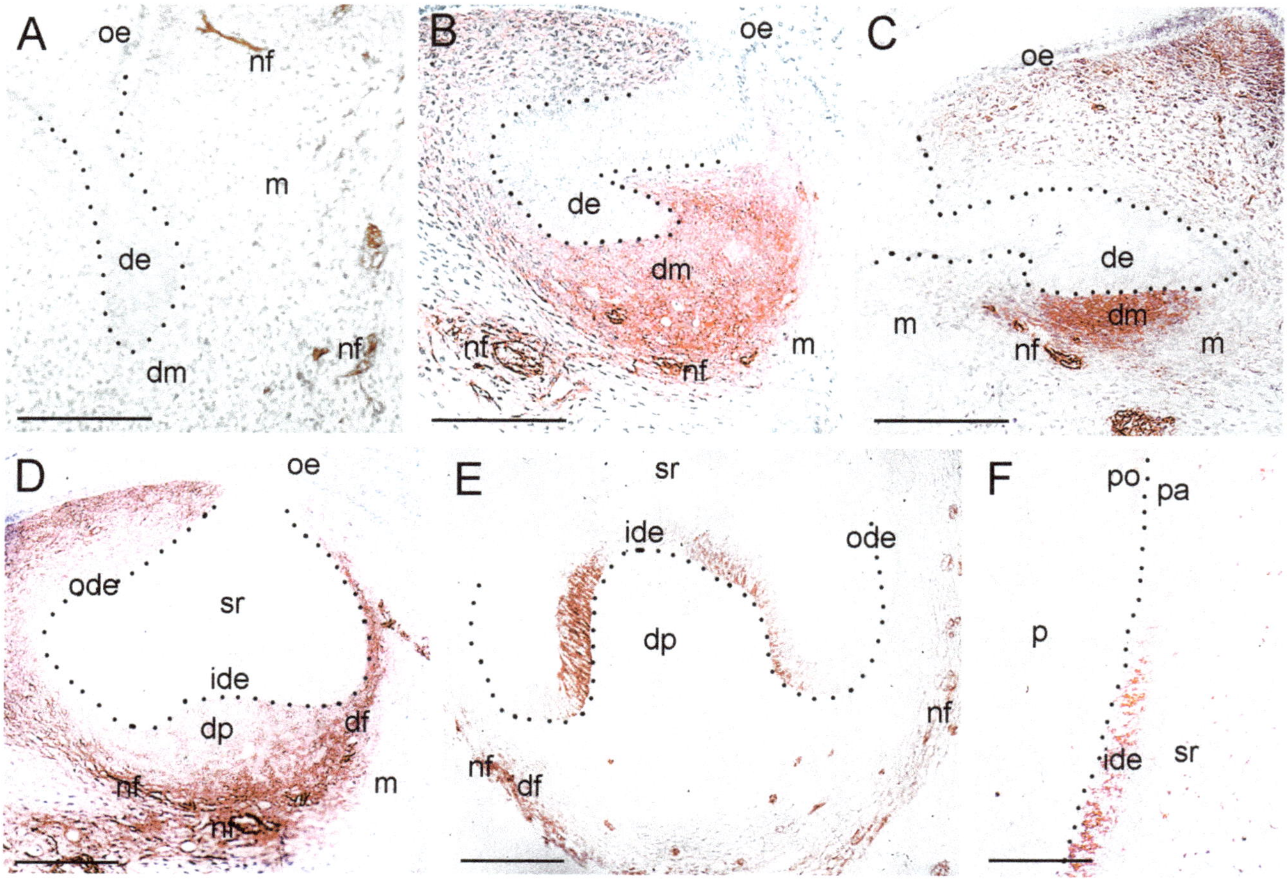

FIGURE 3 | Expression of p75^{NTR} during tooth development. (A) A tooth germ at the bud stage. Note the p75^{NTR} immunoreactivity (red color) in the nerve fibers (nf) approaching the tooth germ. **(B–E)** Tooth germs at the cap stage of development. Note that p75^{NTR} staining in mesenchyme is localized in the dental mesenchyme (dm) at the early cap stage **(B,C)**, while the staining is mostly seen in the dental follicle (df) at the late cap stage **(D,E)**. Cells from the inner dental epithelium (ide) start to express p75^{NTR}, while no staining is detected in the dental papilla (dp) at this late stage **(E)**. Note that nerve fibers (nf) surrounding the dental follicle are strongly stained. **(F)** Higher magnification of the flank area of a tooth germ at the early bell stage of development (**Figure 1H**). Restricted p75^{NTR} reactivity in undifferentiated cells of the inner dental epithelium. Note that the staining is absent in dental pulp (p). Dotted lines represent the border between the dental epithelial and mesenchymal components. Additional abbreviations: de, dental epithelium; m, mesenchyme; ode, outer dental epithelium; oe, oral epithelium; pa, preameloblasts; po, preodontoblasts; sr, stellate reticulum. Scale bars: 100 μm.

periodontium). During the cap stage, NGF expression was highly dynamic. At early cap stage NGF immunoreactivity was absent from the dental mesenchyme and the adjacent dental epithelium, while it was present in the dental epithelium located far from the mesenchyme (**Figure 2B**). At the late cap stage, however, NGF was clearly expressed in the inner and outer dental epithelia, in the dental papilla and dental follicle, while expression was very weak in the stellate reticulum (**Figure 1D**). p75^{NTR} expression was also extremely dynamic at this stage. At the 8th g.w. (early cap stage), intense p75^{NTR} staining was seen in the condensed dental mesenchyme as well as growing nerve axons, while p75^{NTR} staining was absent from all cells of the dental epithelium (**Figures 3B,C**). At the late cap stage (12th g.w.), p75^{NTR} expression decreased in the dental papilla, while the staining was concentrated in the dental follicle surrounding the dental epithelium (**Figure 3D**). At 15th g.w., p75^{NTR} labeling was restricted in proliferating cells of the inner dental epithelium, in cell of the dental follicle, as well as in nerve fibers (**Figures 1E, 3E**). At the early cap stage (8th g.w.), TrkA immunoreactivity was absent from both the dental epithelium and dental mesenchyme, while staining was observed in the mesenchyme surrounding the developing tooth germ (**Figure 4A**). At the late cap stage (15th g.w.), TrkA staining was localized in the dental papilla, as well as in nerve fibers surrounding the tooth germ (**Figures 2F, 4B**).

Continuous growth of the tooth germ leads to the bell stage of development (18th–23rd g.w.). The cells of the inner dental epithelium and outer dental epithelium rapidly proliferate in an apical direction and the tooth shape (i.e., crown morphology) is now observable. Dentinogenesis is initiated at the tips of the cusps at the late bell stage (23rd g.w.). Changes occur in peripheral undifferentiated dental pulp cells, which are separated from the inner dental epithelium by a cell-free zone. Mesenchymal cells adjoining this zone polarize, differentiate into odontoblasts and start to secrete the organic matrix of predentinee/dentinee. Changes also occur in the adjacent inner

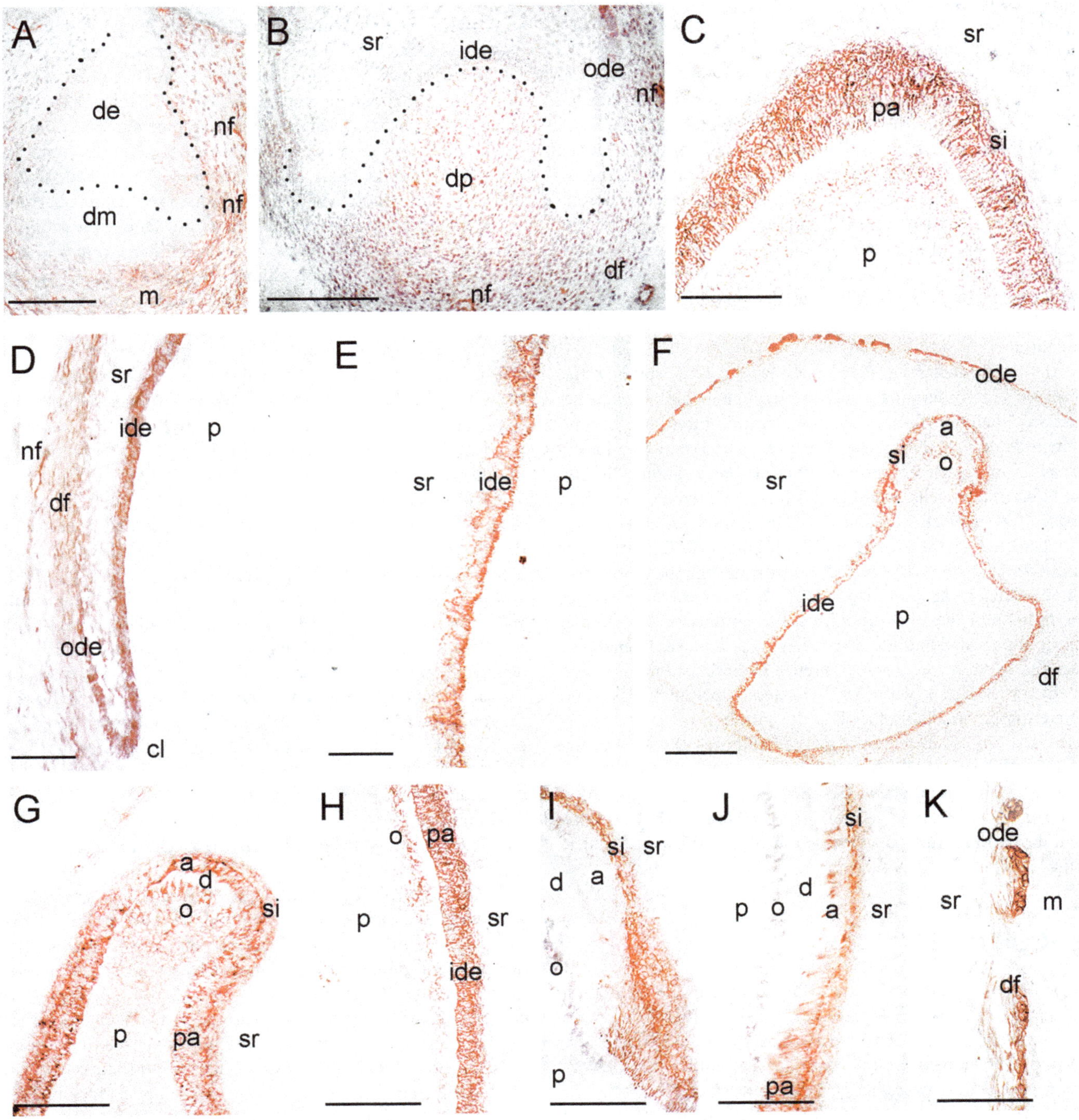

FIGURE 4 | Expression of TrkA during tooth development. (A) A tooth germ at the early cap stage of development. TrkA immunoreactivity in red color. **(B)** Higher magnification of a tooth germ at the late cap stage of development (**Figure 1F**). **(C–E)** Higher magnifications of a tooth germ at the early bell stage of development (**Figure 1I**), representing the tip of the cusp area **(C)**, the cervical loop and dental follicle territories **(D)**, and an area of the flanks of the forming tooth crown **(E)**. **(F–K)** TrkA staining in tooth germs at the late bell stage of development. **(G–K)** Higher magnifications representing the tip of the cusp areas **(G,I)**, areas of the flanks of the forming tooth crown **(H,J)**, and the dental follicle territory **(K)**. Dotted lines represent the border between the dental epithelial and mesenchymal components. Abbreviations: a, ameloblasts; cl, cervical loop; d, dentinee; de, dental epithelium; df, dental follicle; dm, dental mesenchyme; dp, dental papilla; ide, inner dental epithelium; m, mesenchyme; nf, nerve fibers; o, odontoblasts; ode, outer dental epithelium; p, dental pulp; pa, preameloblasts; si, stratum intermedium; sr, stellate reticulum. Scale bars: **(A,B,F)** 100 μm, **(C–E, G–J)** 25 μm.

dental epithelial cells that change their shape, stop dividing, polarize, and differentiate into preameloblasts/ameloblasts that assume their enamel-forming function. During the early bell stage (18th g.w.), NGF immunoreactivity was observed in all dental epithelial cells, whereas the labeling was absent from the dental pulp (**Figure 1G**). $p75^{NTR}$ staining was evident in proliferating cells of the inner dental epithelium but the staining was considerably decreased in preameloblasts at the tip of the cusp (**Figures 1H, 3F**). Strong TrkA labeling was detected in cells of the inner dental epithelium, preameloblasts, stratum intermedium, and cells of the outer dental epithelium (**Figures 1I, 4C–E**), while a very weak staining was detected in pulp fibroblasts at the cusp area (**Figure 4C**). No TrkA immunoreactivity was detected in the stellate reticulum.

At the late bell stage (23rd g.w.) strong NGF staining was observed in undifferentiated (i.e., inner dental epithelium, outer dental epithelium, stellate reticulum, stratum intermedium) and differentiated dental epithelial (i.e., preameloblasts, ameloblasts) as well as in preodontoblasts, and odontoblasts (**Figures 2C–E**). Undifferentiated cells exhibited a strong NGF labeling on their surface (**Figures 2E–G**). Weak NGF immunoreactivity was also detected in the dental follicle (**Figures 2E–G**), while the staining was stronger in nerve fibers surrounding the tooth germ (**Figures 2F,G**). At this stage, $p75^{NTR}$ immunoreactivity was absent in ameloblasts, odontoblasts, and fibroblasts of the dental pulp, but persisted in undifferentiated inner dental epithelial cells near the cervical loop region (**Figure 3F** and data not shown). In contrast, TrkA labeling was detected in preameloblasts and differentiating ameloblasts, while the staining was considerably decreased in mature ameloblasts (**Figures 4F–J**). In the dental pulp, strong TrkA immunoreactivity was observed in differentiating odontoblasts, but this reactivity was significantly reduced in secreting odontoblasts (**Figures 4F–J**). TrkA immunostaining was also expressed in cells of the dental follicle (**Figure 4K**).

DISCUSSION

Sequential and reciprocal interactions between oral epithelium and cranial neural crest-derived mesenchyme result in tooth formation and generation of specific hard tissues, the enamel and dentine (Mitsiadis and Graf, 2009; Jussila and Thesleff, 2012). The present study describes the distribution of NGF, $p75^{NTR}$, and TrkA proteins in the developing human fetal teeth, and confirms that their temporospatial distribution in human dental tissues is very similar with that observed previously in rodents (Yan and Johnson, 1988; Byers et al., 1990; Mitsiadis et al., 1992, 1993; Mitsiadis and Luukko, 1995). NGF is expressed in the epithelium during the early stages of tooth development, while $p75^{NTR}$ and TrkA are first expressed in the mesenchyme. The expression of NGF, TrkA, and $p75^{NTR}$ in the tooth germ significantly precedes the onset of tooth innervation. This pattern of expression suggests a paracrine mode of action of NGF during this stage of odontogenesis and also indicates a role of this molecule in epithelial-mesenchymal interactions. Our present data in humans and previous findings in rodents show $p75^{NTR}$ expression in the condensed mesenchyme of the cap staged molars (Mitsiadis et al., 1992; Mitsiadis and Luukko, 1995). Adhesive functions have been proposed for $p75^{NTR}$ during neuronal development (Chao, 1992; Mirnics et al., 2005), suggesting that this low affinity NGF receptor may be implicated in the condensation of the neural crest-derived mesenchyme and its specification in dental mesenchyme. $p75^{NTR}$ expression in dental follicle coincides with the outgrowths of the maxillary and mandibular nerves around the tooth germs. One of the proposed functions of $p75^{NTR}$ is to increase the local concentrations of NGF (Chao, 1992), thus providing a tropic and trophic support for specific neurons that follow the concentration gradients of NGF.

At later stages of tooth formation, when cytodifferentiation starts, NGF and TrkA are distributed in proliferating cells of the inner dental epithelium, as well as in preameloblasts and the enamel secreting ameloblasts. However, $p75^{NTR}$ expression in dental epithelium is more restricted and confined to undifferentiated, still proliferating, inner dental epithelial cells. The same pattern of $p75^{NTR}$ distribution has been previously detected in human fetal teeth (Christensen et al., 1993) and in the developing rat molars (Byers et al., 1990; Mitsiadis et al., 1992, 1993; Mitsiadis and Luukko, 1995). Concomitant NGF, TrkA, and $p75^{NTR}$ expression in proliferating cells of the inner dental epithelium suggests that NGF may act as a mitogenic factor. In fact, this function of NGF has been already evidenced in the developing human skin (Yaar et al., 1991), human airway smooth muscles (Freund-Michel et al., 2006), and the whisker follicles of the mouse (Davies et al., 1987). During cytodifferentiation, NGF and TrkA are localized around the nucleus and in the apical part of differentiating and functional ameloblasts, whereas $p75^{NTR}$ is not expressed in these cells, thus indicating that NGF can accomplish its biological activities (i.e., differentiation, enamel matrix synthesis, and deposition) in these cells through the TrkA receptor.

In the dental pulp NGF and TrkA are co-expressed in polarizing and differentiated odontoblasts, also indicating that NGF, upon binding to the TrkA receptor, could regulate the function and differentiation of mesenchymal cells, as suggested by previous *in vitro* studies (Arany et al., 2009). The expression pattern of NGF in the pulp of developing human teeth is identical to that previously observed in the pulp of developing rodent teeth (Mitsiadis et al., 1992, 1993; Mitsiadis and Luukko, 1995), illustrating a close correlation between the appearance of NGF and the process of odontoblast differentiation. The present results also confirm prior studies on $p75^{NTR}$ expression in embryonic human teeth, where this low-affinity NGF receptor was absent from dental pulp cells at the bell stage (Christensen et al., 1993). However, in contrast to our previous findings in developing rodent teeth showing $p75^{NTR}$ expression in preodontoblasts and cells of the sub-odontoblastic layer (Mitsiadis et al., 1992, 1993), in human teeth these two cell populations lack $p75^{NTR}$, thus indicating that the mode of NGF action could be variable according to the species.

In the developing human tooth germs, NGF, $p75^{NTR}$, and TrkA are also expressed in the dental follicle (i.e., future

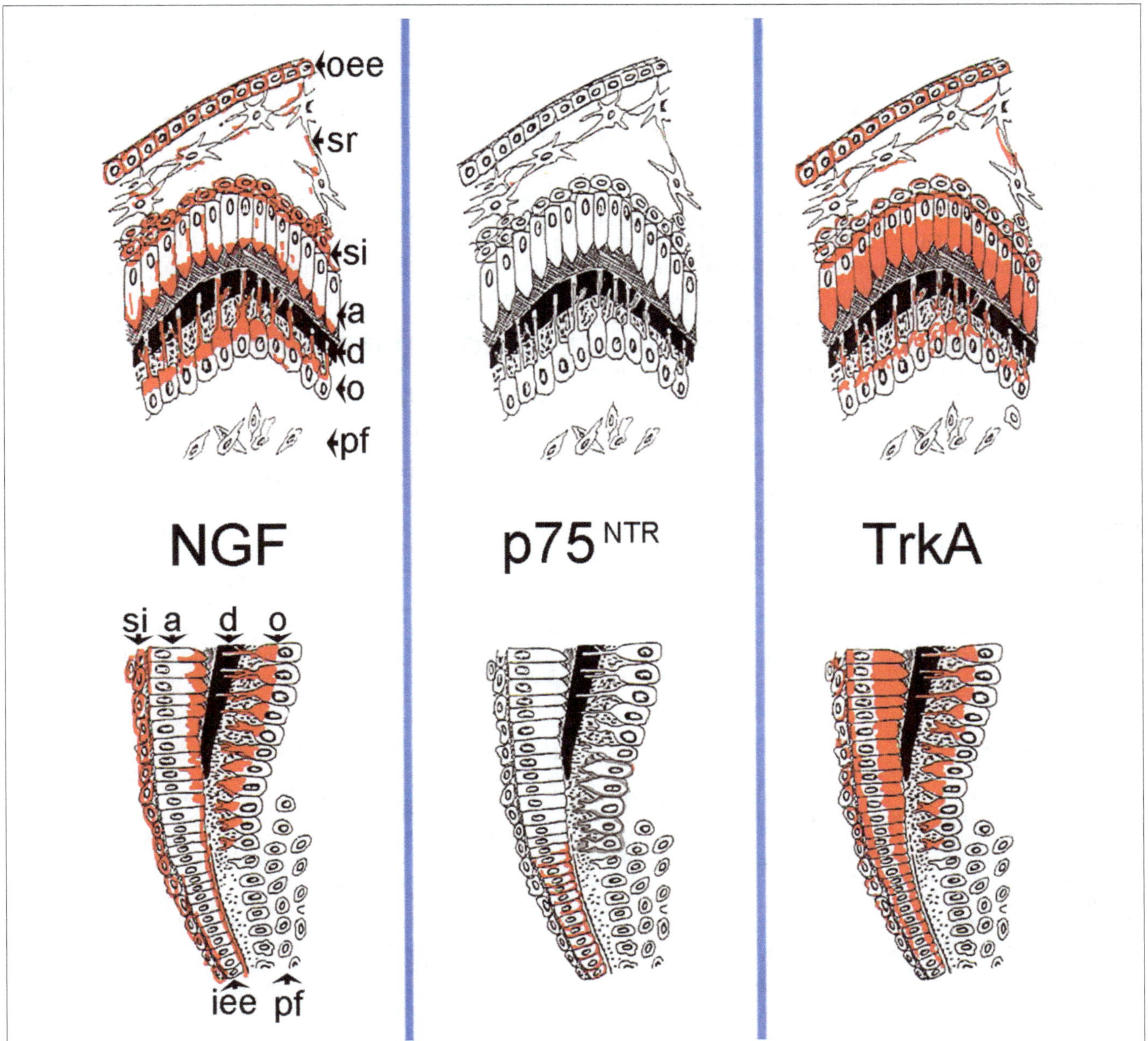

FIGURE 5 | Schematic illustration of the expression patterns of the NGF, p75^{NTR}, TrkA proteins in developing human teeth during the differentiation/mineralization events. On the top is represented the tip of the cusp territory, on the bottom the flank of the tooth crown territory. Abbreviations: oee, outer enamel epithelium; sr, stellate reticulum; si, stratum intermedium; a, ameloblasts; d, dentinee; o, odontoblasts; pf, pulp fibroblasts; iee, inner enamel epithelium.

periodontium), where mark mainly the nerve fibers. It has been shown that NGF and TrkA play a fundamental role in the innervation and nociception of dental tissues, since mutations in the gene coding for TrkA (i.e., *NTRK1*) leads to pain insensitivity and in some cases to tooth agenesis (Bonkowsky et al., 2003; Gao et al., 2013). In rodents, tooth movement up-regulates NGF, p75^{NTR}, and TrkA expression in the periodontal ligament, which is associated with increased sensory nerve fibers sprouting and pain perception (O'Hara et al., 2009). NGF and TrkA expression in the dental follicle indicates that these molecules might modulate nerve growth and sprouting in the periodontal ligament of human teeth in both physiological and pathological conditions. Similarly, NGF expression is up-regulated upon injury in the pulp of mouse molars, leading to massive sprouting of TrkA expressing nerve fibers toward the site of injury (Sarram et al., 1997). The above mentioned findings suggest that innovative strategies could be applied in dental clinics for patients pain relief, since TrkA-positive nerve fibers are important mediators of pain perception in dental tissues (Sullins et al., 2000; Gao et al.,

2013; Kyrkanides et al., 2015). Inhibition of NGF/TrkA signaling could be an effective approach to eliminate or reduce pain associated with dental pathologies and clinical interventions. In this context, NGF/TrkA/p75^{NTR} gained enormous attention as potential targets for treatments against cancer-associated pain, leading to the development and trial of several classes of small-molecule-inhibitors and antibodies targeting this signaling axis (Demir et al., 2016).

Apart from its implication in pain perception, the neuro-attractive effect of NGF signaling could be an important modulator of tooth development and regeneration. Innervation plays a key role in the development and the regeneration of orofacial organs (Pagella et al., 2014), and consists one of the fundamental component of stem cell niches (Katayama et al., 2006; Méndez-Ferrer et al., 2008; Knox et al., 2013; Pagella et al., 2015). Both the periodontium and the dental pulp host various stem cell populations that guarantee their repair and regeneration. It has been evidenced on mouse models that tooth injury leads to the activation of NGF signaling and the concomitant attraction of nerve fibers (Sarram et al., 1997; Yamashiro et al., 2000; Kaukua et al., 2014), which might provide necessary but so far unidentified cues for proper formation and regeneration of dental tissues.

In conclusion, the present findings suggest a regulatory role for NGF in both mesenchymal and epithelial components of the developing human teeth. NGF, p75^{NTR}, and TrkA expression in dental tissues (**Figure 5**) indicates a function for NGF signaling in cell proliferation, differentiation and mineralization events during odontogenesis, paralleling its role in the development of the nervous system. More precisely, expression of all these three molecules in inner dental epithelial cells correlates with their proliferation status, while co-expression of NGF and TrkA alone in dental epithelial and mesenchymal cells is associated with their differentiation into ameloblasts and odontoblasts. Moreover, expression of the NGF, p75^{NTR}, and TrkA proteins in nerve fibers of the developing human teeth indicates that NGF signaling is also involved in their sprouting and attraction toward dental tissues.

AUTHOR CONTRIBUTIONS

TM and PP equally contributed to the collection of data, analysis of results, writing, and editing of the manuscript.

ACKNOWLEDGMENTS

We are grateful to Professor Dr. D. Laurent-Maquin and Dr. D. Gaillard (INSERM UMR-S 926 "Interfaces Biomatériaux/Tissus Hôtes," U.F.R. d'Odontologie de Reims, France) for kindly providing us with human tissues. This work was supported by funds of the University of Zurich. The authors confirm that there are no conflicts of interest associated with this work.

REFERENCES

Arany, S., Koyota, S., and Sugiyama, T. (2009). Nerve growth factor promotes differentiation of odontoblast-like cells. *J. Cell. Biochem.* 106, 539–545. doi: 10.1002/jcb.22006

Barbacid, M. (1994). The Trk family of neurotrophin receptors. *J. Neurobiol.* 25, 1386–1403. doi: 10.1002/neu.480251107

Bonkowsky, J. L., Johnson, J., Carey, J. C., Smith, A. G., and Swoboda, K. J. (2003). An infant with primary tooth loss and palmar hyperkeratosis: a novel mutation in the NTRK1 gene causing congenital insensitivity to pain with anhidrosis. *Pediatrics* 112, e237–e241. doi: 10.1542/peds.112.3.e237

Byers, M. R., Schatteman, G. C., and Bothwell, M. (1990). Multiple functions for NGF receptor in developing, aging and injured rat teeth are suggested by epithelial, mesenchymal and neural immunoreactivity. *Development* 109, 461–471.

Chao, M. V. (1992). Neurotrophin receptors: a window into neuronal differentiation. *Neuron* 9, 583–593. doi: 10.1016/0896-6273(92)90023-7

Chao, M. V. (2003). Neurotrophins and their receptors: a convergence point for many signalling pathways. *Nat. Rev. Neurosci.* 4, 299–309. doi: 10.1038/nrn1078

Chesa, P. G., Rettig, W. J., Thomson, T. M., Old, L. J., and Melamed, M. R. (1988). Immunohistochemical analysis of nerve growth factor receptor expression in normal and malignant human tissues. *J. Histochem. Cytochem.* 36, 383–389. doi: 10.1177/36.4.2831267

Christensen, L. R., Møllgård, K., Kjaer, I., and Janas, M. S. (1993). Immunocytochemical demonstration of nerve growth factor receptor (NGF-R) in developing human fetal teeth. *Anat. Embryol.* 188, 247–255. doi: 10.1007/BF00188216

Davies, A., Bandtlow, C., and Heumann, R. (1987). Timing and site of NGF synthesis in developing skin in relation to innnervation and expression of the receptor. *Nature* 326, 353–357. doi: 10.1038/326353a0

Demir, I. E., Tieftrunk, E., Schorn, S., Friess, H., and Ceyhan, G. O. (2016). Nerve growth factor & TrkA as novel therapeutic targets in cancer. *Biochim. Biophys. Acta Rev. Cancer* 1866, 37–50. doi: 10.1016/j.bbcan.2016.05.003

Di Girolamo, N., Sarris, M., Chui, J., Cheema, H., Coroneo, M. T., and Wakefield, D. (2008). Localization of the low-affinity nerve growth factor receptor p75 in human limbal epithelial cells. *J. Cell. Mol. Med.* 12, 2799–2811. doi: 10.1111/j.1582-4934.2008.00290.x

Freund-Michel, V., Bertrand, C., and Frossard, N. (2006). TrkA signalling pathways in human airway smooth muscle cell proliferation. *Cell. Signal.* 18, 621–627. doi: 10.1016/j.cellsig.2005.06.007

Gao, L., Guo, H., Ye, N., Bai, Y., Liu, X., Yu, P., et al. (2013). Oral and craniofacial manifestations and two novel missense mutations of the NTRK1 gene identified in the patient with congenital insensitivity to pain with anhidrosis. *PLoS ONE* 8:e66863. doi: 10.1371/journal.pone.0066863

Grob, P. M., Ross, A. H., Koprowski, H., and Bothwell, M. (1985). Characterization of the human melanoma nerve growth factor receptor. *J. Biol. Chem.* 260, 8044–8049.

Ichim, G., Tauszig-Delamasure, S., and Mehlen, P. (2012). Neurotrophins and cell death. *Exp. Cell Res.* 318, 1221–1228. doi: 10.1016/j.yexcr.2012.03.006

Jussila, M., and Thesleff, I. (2012). Signaling networks regulating tooth organogenesis and regeneration, and the specification of dental mesenchymal and epithelial cell lineages. *Cold Spring Harb. Perspect. Biol.* 4:a008425. doi: 10.1101/cshperspect.a008425

Kaplan, D. R., Hempstead, B. L., Martin-zanca, D., Chao, M. V., and Paradat, L. F. (1991). The trk proto-oncogene product : a signal transducing receptor for nerve growth factor. *Science* 252, 554–558. doi: 10.1126/science.1850549

Katayama, Y., Battista, M., Kao, W.-M., Hidalgo, A., Peired, A. J., Thomas, S., et al. (2006). Signals from the sympathetic nervous system regulate hematopoietic stem cell egress from bone marrow. *Cell* 124, 407–421. doi: 10.1016/j.cell.2005.10.041

Kaukua, N., Shahidi, M. K., Konstantinidou, C., Dyachuk, V., Kaucka, M., Furlan, A., et al. (2014). Glial origin of mesenchymal stem cells in a tooth model system. *Nature* 513, 551–554. doi: 10.1038/nature13536

Klein, R., Nanduri, V., Jing, S., Lamballe, F., Tapley, P., Bryant, S., et al. (1991). The trkB tyrosine protein kinase is a receptor for brain-derived neurotrophic factor and neurotrophin-3. *Cell* 66, 395–403. doi: 10.1016/0092-8674(91)90628-C

Knox, S. M., Lombaert, I. M. A., Haddox, C. L., Abrams, S. R., Cotrim, A., Wilson, A. J., et al. (2013). Parasympathetic stimulation improves epithelial organ regeneration. *Nat. Commun.* 4:1494. doi: 10.1038/ncomms2493

Kyrkanides, S., Huang, H., and Faber, R. D. (2015). Neurologic regulation and orthodontic tooth movement. *Front. Oral Biol.* 18, 64–74. doi: 10.1159/000351900

Lewis, G. R., and Carter, B. D. (2014). *Neurotrophic Factors*. Heidelberg; New York, NY; Dordrecht; London: Springer. doi: 10.1007/978-3-642-45106-5

Lu, B., Pang, P. T., and Woo, N. H. (2005). The yin and yang of neurotrophin action. *Nat. Rev. Neurosci.* 6, 603–614. doi: 10.1038/nrn1726

Maeda, T., Sato, O., Iwanaga, T., and Takano, Y. (1992). Immunocytochemical localization of nerve growth factor receptor (NGFR) in human teeth. *Proc. Finnish Dent. Soc. Suom. Hammaslääkäriseuran Toim.* 88(Suppl. 1), 557–562.

Méndez-Ferrer, S., Lucas, D., Battista, M., and Frenette, P. S. (2008). Haematopoietic stem cell release is regulated by circadian oscillations. *Nature* 452, 442–447. doi: 10.1038/nature06685

Mirnics, Z. K., Yan, C., Portugal, C., Kim, T.-W., Saragovi, H. U., Sisodia, S. S., et al. (2005). P75 neurotrophin receptor regulates expression of neural cell adhesion molecule 1. *Neurobiol. Dis.* 20, 969–985. doi: 10.1016/j.nbd.2005.06.004

Mitsiadis, T. A., Couble, P., Dicou, E., Rudkin, B. B., and Magloire, H. (1993). Patterns of nerve growth factor (NGF), proNGF, and p75 NGF receptor expression in the rat incisor: comparison with expression in the molar. *Differentiation* 54, 161–175. doi: 10.1111/j.1432-0436.1993.tb01599.x

Mitsiadis, T. A., Dicou, E., Joffre, A., and Magloire, H. (1992). Immunohistochemical localization of nerve growth factor (NGF) and NGF receptor (NGF-R) in the developing first molar tooth of the rat. *Differentiation* 49, 47–61. doi: 10.1111/j.1432-0436.1992.tb00768.x

Mitsiadis, T. A., and Graf, D. (2009). Cell fate determination during tooth development and regeneration. *Birth Defects Res. C Embryo Today* 87, 199–211. doi: 10.1002/bdrc.20160

Mitsiadis, T. A., and Luukko, K. (1995). Neurotrophins in odontogenesis. *Int. J. Dev. Biol.* 39, 195–202.

Mitsiadis, T. A., Rome, A., Lendahl, U., Sharpe, P. T., and Christophe, J. (2003). Notch2 protein distribution in human teeth under normal and pathological conditions. *Exp. Cell Res.* 282, 101–109. doi: 10.1016/s0014-4827(02)00012-5

Nakamura, T., Endo, K., and Kinoshita, S. (2007). Identification of human oral keratinocyte stem/progenitor cells by neurotrophin receptor p75 and the role of neurotrophin/p75 signaling. *Stem Cells* 25, 628–638. doi: 10.1634/stemcells.2006-0494

O'Hara, A. H., Sampson, W. J., Dreyer, C. W., Pierce, A. M., and Ferguson, I. A. (2009). Immunohistochemical detection of nerve growth factor and its receptors in the rat periodontal ligament during tooth movement. *Arch. Oral Biol.* 54, 871–878. doi: 10.1016/j.archoralbio.2009.06.003

Pagella, P., Jiménez-Rojo, L., and Mitsiadis, T. A. (2014). Roles of innervation in developing and regenerating orofacial tissues. *Cell. Mol. Life Sci.* 71, 2241–2251. doi: 10.1007/s00018-013-1549-0

Pagella, P., Neto, E., Lamghari, M., and Mitsiadis, T. A. (2015). Investigation of orofacial stem cell niches and their innervation through microfluidic devices. *Eur. Cells Mater.* 29, 213–223.

Radeke, M., Misko, T., and Hsu, C. (1987). Gene transfer and molecular cloning of the rat nerve growth factor receptor. *Nature* 325, 593–597. doi: 10.1038/325593a0

Reichardt, L. F. (2006). Neurotrophin-regulated signalling pathways. *Philos. Trans. R. Soc. Lond. B Biol. Sci.* 361, 1545–1564. doi: 10.1098/rstb.2006.1894

Represa, J., and Bernd, P. (1989). Nerve growth factor and serum differentially regulate development of the embryonic otic vesicle and cochleovestibular ganglion *in vitro*. *Dev. Biol.* 134, 21–29. doi: 10.1016/0012-1606(89)90074-2

Ross, A. H., Grobt, P., Bothwellt, M., Elders, D. E., Ernstt, C. S., Maranot, N., et al. (1984). Characterization of nerve growth factor receptor in neural crest tumors using monoclonal antibodies. *Biochemistry* 81, 6681–6685.

Sarram, S., Lee, K. F., and Byers, M. R. (1997). Dental innervation and CGRP in adult p75-deficient mice. *J. Comp. Neurol.* 385, 297–308.

Sullins, J. S., Carnes, D. L., Kaldestad, R. N., and Wheeler, E. F. (2000). Time course of the increase in trk A expression in trigeminal neurons after tooth injury. *J. Endod.* 26, 88–91. doi: 10.1097/00004770-200002000-00007

Tomellini, E., Touil, Y., Lagadec, C., Julien, S., Ostyn, P., Ziental-Gelus, N., et al. (2015). Nerve growth factor and prongf simultaneously promote symmetric self-renewal, quiescence, and epithelial to mesenchymal transition to enlarge the breast cancer stem cell compartment. *Stem Cells* 33, 342–353. doi: 10.1002/stem.1849

Truzzi, F., Marconi, A., Atzei, P., Panza, M. C., Lotti, R., Dallaglio, K., et al. (2011). P75 neurotrophin receptor mediates apoptosis in transit-amplifying cells and its overexpression restores cell death in psoriatic keratinocytes. *Cell Death Differ.* 18, 948–958. doi: 10.1038/cdd.2010.162

von Bartheld, C. S., Patterson, S. L., Heuer, J. G., Wheeler, E. F., Bothwell, M., and Rubel, E. W. (1991). Expression of nerve growth factor (NGF) receptors in the developing inner ear of chick and rat. *Development* 113, 455–470.

Yaar, M., Grossman, K., Eller, M., and Gilchrest, B. A. (1991). Evidence for nerve growth factor-mediated paracrine effects in human epidermis. *J. Cell Biol.* 115, 821–828. doi: 10.1083/jcb.115.3.821

Yamashiro, T., Fujiyama, K., Fukunaga, T., Wang, Y., and Takano-Yamamoto, T. (2000). Epithelial rests of Malassez express immunoreactivity of TrkA and its distribution is regulated by sensory nerve innervation. *J. Histochem. Cytochem.* 48, 979–984. doi: 10.1177/002215540004800711

Yan, Q., and Johnson, E. M. (1988). An immunohistochemical study of the nerve growth factor receptor in developing rats. *J. Neurosci.* 8, 3481–3498.

14

Multiple Cranial Organ Defects after Conditionally Knocking Out *Fgf10* in the Neural Crest

Tathyane H. N. Teshima*[1], *Silvia V. Lourenco*[1] *and Abigail S. Tucker*[2]

[1] *Department of Stomatology, School of Dentistry, University of Sao Paulo, São Paulo, Brazil,*

[2] *Department of Craniofacial Development and Stem Cell Biology, King's College London, London, UK*

Correspondence:
Abigail S. Tucker
abigail.tucker@kcl.ac.uk

Fgf10 is necessary for the development of a number of organs that fail to develop or are reduced in size in the null mutant. Here we have knocked out *Fgf10* specifically in the neural crest driven by *Wnt1cre*. The *Wnt1creFgf10fl/fl* mouse phenocopies many of the null mutant defects, including cleft palate, loss of salivary glands, and ocular glands, highlighting the neural crest origin of the *Fgf10* expressing mesenchyme surrounding these organs. In contrast tissues such as the limbs and lungs, where *Fgf10* is expressed by the surrounding mesoderm, were unaffected, as was the pituitary gland where *Fgf10* is expressed by the neuroepithelium. The circumvallate papilla of the tongue formed but was hypoplastic in the conditional and *Fgf10* null embryos, suggesting that other sources of FGF can compensate in development of this structure. The tracheal cartilage rings showed normal patterning in the conditional knockout, indicating that the source of *Fgf10* for this tissue is mesodermal, which was confirmed using *Wnt1cre-dtTom* to lineage trace the boundary of the neural crest in this region. The thyroid, thymus, and parathyroid glands surrounding the trachea were present but hypoplastic in the conditional mutant, indicating that a neighboring source of mesodermal *Fgf10* might be able to partially compensate for loss of neural crest derived *Fgf10*.

Keywords: *Fgf10*, ocular glands, thyroid, palate, cranial glands, CVP

INTRODUCTION

Fgf10 is an essential signaling molecule from the fibroblast growth factor family and is involved in the development of many organs, signaling through *Fgfr2b* in the epithelium (Ohuchi et al., 2000). Patients with mutations in one copy of the *Fgf10* ligand or its receptor have Lacrimo Acoustic Dental Digital (LADD) syndrome (OMIM 149730) or the related Aplasia of Salivary and Lacrimal Gland (ASLG) syndrome (OMIM 180920), characterized by defects in a variety of cranial glands (Rohmann et al., 2006). Mice with a complete knockout of *Fgf10* die at birth due to a complete lack of lungs and limbs and formation of a cleft palate (Min et al., 1998; Sekine et al., 1999; Rice et al., 2004). As in patients, loss of *Fgf10* also impacts on the development of a number of cranial glands, with null mutants showing complete loss of the salivary glands, thyroid gland, pituitary gland (Ohuchi et al., 2000), ocular glands (Govindarajan et al., 2000; Makarenkova et al., 2000) and the circumvallate papilla (CVP) housing the Von Ebner's glands in the tongue (Petersen et al., 2011). The salivary glands have been shown to arrest at the prebud stage, with heterozygous mice showing a delay in development that leads to later gland hypofunction (Jaskoll et al., 2005; May et al., 2015). The pituitary gland starts to initiate in the *Fgf10* null with an infolding of the oral epithelium to form Rathke's pouch at the back of the mouth, but the ectoderm is associated with high levels of apoptosis and the pouch disappears by E13.5 (Ohuchi et al., 2000). Other glands form but are reduced in size, such as the thymus glands (Ohuchi et al., 2000; Revest et al., 2001), and more subtle defects are also observed in the inner ear, in the patterning of the trachea cartilage rings, in the teeth and in the skin and hair follicles (Ohuchi et al., 2000; Pauley et al., 2003; Sala et al., 2011). In these organs loss of *Fgf10* may be compensated for by the presence of *Fgf7* or *Fgf3*, which can both bind to the same receptor (Zhang et al., 2006). In keeping with this loss of both *Fgf10* and *Fgf3* leads to a more severe defect in the inner ear (Wright and Mansour, 2003), and knockout of the receptor *Fgfr2b* leads to additional defects not observed in *Fgf10* knockouts, such as arrest of tooth development at the bud stage (De Moerlooze et al., 2000).

During development *Fgf10* is expressed in the mesenchyme that surrounds many developing organs (lungs, limbs, ocular glands, palatal shelves, salivary glands (Bellusci et al., 1997; Moustakas et al., 2011; Wells et al., 2013). In contrast its receptor, Fgfr2b, is expressed in epithelial structures overlying these regions, emphasizing the importance of epithelial-mesenchymal interactions (Peters et al., 1992; Orr-Urtreger et al., 1993; Rice et al., 2004). In the developing brain *Fgf10* is expressed in the infundibulum, which signals to the developing oral epithelium during pituitary gland development (Takuma et al., 1998). Early on during facial development *Fgf10* is expressed in the oral epithelium of the first pharyngeal arch (Kettunen et al., 2000; Wells et al., 2013), with expression also observed in the tooth germ epithelium in some species (Moustakas et al., 2011). In the otic region *Fgf10* is first expressed in the mesoderm derived mesenchyme around the otic epithelium at E8.75 and then in the otic cup and otic vesicle at E9 and E9.5 (Wright and Mansour, 2003). *Fgf10* is therefore expressed in a range of tissues during development.

In this paper we have conditionally knocked out *Fgf10* specifically in neural crest derived tissue using the *Wnt1*cre transgenic line (Chai et al., 2000). Previously a conditional knockout of *Fgf10* has been carried out using *Dermo1* cre, which led to specific loss of *Fgf10* in the mesoderm around the developing lungs, resulting in lung branching defects (Abler et al., 2009). By knocking out *Fgf10* in neural crest derived tissues only we aim to investigate which phenotypes in the null mutant are a consequence specifically of *Fgf10* expression in the neural crest. A number of tissues in the head are known to be derived from the neural crest. These include the mesenchyme around the developing salivary glands, thyroid and thymus glands, teeth, and the palatine bone (Chai et al., 2000; Jiang et al., 2000; Jaskoll et al., 2002; Müller et al., 2008; Johansson et al., 2015). The *Fgf10* expressing mesenchyme that underlies the forming CVP in the tongue is also neural crest derived (Hosokawa et al., 2010). The origin of the tissue around the developing ocular glands has not been confirmed as the developing eye is surrounded by neural crest derived mesenchyme and lateral plate mesoderm, which together forms the periocular mesenchyme (Langenberg et al., 2008). In contrast the limbs and lungs are surrounded by mesoderm and so would be predicted to develop normally in the conditional *Wnt1cre Fgf10* mice. The pituitary would also be expected to be normal in these conditional mutants as the source of the *Fgf10* is the neuroectodermal infundibulum (Takuma et al., 1998). In addition we compare the conditional knockout to the phenotype in the null *Fgf10* mouse to clarify the role of neural crest derived *Fgf10* in a variety of craniofacial tissues, and identify a few discrepancies with the published literature.

MATERIALS AND METHODS

Transgenic Mice

Fgf10 floxed (Fgf10A02 tmc1c) mice on a C57Bl6 background were produced by MRC-Harwell as part of the International Mouse Phenotyping Consortium (IMPC; Pettitt et al., 2009; Skarnes et al., 2011; Bradley et al., 2012). *Fgf10fl/fl* females were crossed to *Wnt1cre/Fgf10 fl/+* males to generate *Wnt1creFgf10fl/fl* embryos (3 litters), collected at E14.5, E15.5, and E19.5 (E14.5 $n = 3$; E15.5 $n = 3$; E19.5 $n = 2$). These conditional mutants were compared to *Fgf10fl/fl* littermates that did not carry the cre and were therefore phenotypically wildtype. A total of 6 *Fgf10* null embryos generated on a mixed C57Bl6/CD1 background (E14.5, E15.5, E18.5) were used to compare the conditional phenotype with that of the complete null.

Wnt1cre males were mated to *tdTomato* reporter females (Gt(ROSA)26 Sor tm14(CAG-tdTomato)Hze JAX labs) to lineage trace the neural crest and were viewed with a Nikon SMZ25 fluorescence microscope.

The *Wnt1cre* mouse is widely used for neural crest specific knockout studies, however, it has been linked to elevated levels of Wnt signaling in the midbrain, particularly in *Wnt1cre* Tg/Tg embryos (Lewis et al., 2013). We used *Wnt1cre* Tg/+ mice for our crosses to reduce this effect. In addition, no facial phenotype was observed in *Wnt1cre* embryos compared to WT littermate controls (data not shown), agreeing with results that show that any midbrain dysmorphologies caused by the *Wnt1cre* line do not cause cranial shape changes (Heuze et al., 2014).

Pregnant mice were culled using schedule 1 culling methods at E14.5 to E19.5, just prior to giving birth. All procedures were carried out as agreed by the UK Home Office and King's College London. Animals were housed in approved non-specific-pathogen-free conditions. Animal experiments conform to ARRIVE (animal research: reporting of *in vivo* experiments) guidelines.

Embryos were photographed using a Leica dissecting microscope.

Skeletal Preps

E19.5 embryos were skinned and eviscerated before fixing in 95% Ethanol. Samples were then stained in alcian blue and alizarin red to stain cartilages and bones, respectively. Embryos were cleared in 0.5% KOH and stored in glycerol and photographed using a Leica dissecting microscope.

Histology

Embryos were fixed in 4% paraformaldehyde and dehydrated through an ethanol or methanol series before embedding in wax. Sections were cut on a microtome at 8 μm and slides were stained with a trichrome stain (Haematoxylin, alcian blue and sirrus red). Sections were photographed using a Nikon microscope.

Thymus Analysis

To compare the size of the thymus glands in the conditional mutants the thymus glands from 3 *Fgf10fl/fl* mice and 4 *Wnt1cre Fgf10fl/fl* mice were assessed using histology sections at E14.5. The number of sections with a thymus was multiplied by the thickness of the sections (8 μm) to give the total extent of the gland. This was then compared using a student *t*-test where significance was $P < 0.05$.

Radioactive *In situ* Hybridisation

CD1 mice were used for expression of *Fgf10*. *Fgf10* probe was a gift from Ivor Mason. *In situ* hybridisation on wax sections was carried out according to previously published protocols (Kettunen et al., 2000). *Fgf10* antisense probe was synthesized using 35S labeled UTP and signal was identified using sliver emulsion, which when developed showed positive signal as white grains under darkfield. The magic wand tool in photoshop was used to pseudocolour the white grains red and this layer was overlain on top of the light field image to produce a final compound image.

RESULTS

Normal Lung, Limb and Pituitary Development but Defective Palate Formation in *Wnt1cre Fgf10* Conditional Mutants

In agreement with previous studies we observed expression of *Fgf10* in the developing lung, limb, ocular glands, palate, salivary glands, and epithelium of the developing maxilla and mandible (**Figure 1**). As expected conditional mutants (*Wnt1creFgf10fl/fl*) had normally developing lungs at E19.5 (**Figures 2A,B**; $N = 2/2$). Histology of the lungs matched that of littermate controls (*Fgf10fl/fl*; **Figures 2C,D**), as although there are *Wnt1cre* positive cells located within the developing lungs these are associated with the intrinsic nervous system, which does not express *Fgf10* (Freem et al., 2010). The limbs also formed normally ($N = 8/8$), in contrast to complete loss of these structure in *Fgf10* null mutants (**Figures 2E,F**; $N = 6/6$).

In the palate *Fgf10* is expressed in the mesenchyme adjacent to the oral epithelium (**Figure 1D**). Palate development was disrupted in the conditional mutants with a failure in development of the palatal shelves at E15.5 (**Figures 3A,B**; $N = 3/3$), suggesting problems in shelf development similar to those observed in the null (Rice et al., 2004). Just before birth (E19.5) defects in formation of the palatine processes of the maxilla and palatine bone were clear, leaving the vomer visible when viewed from the oral side (**Figures 3C,D**; $N = 2/2$). Due to the cleft palate the conditional mutant would not be predicted to survive past birth, and, in agreement with this, no mutants were discovered at P1 (postnatal day 1) in one litter where the mother was left to litter down.

In the *Fgf10* null the ectoderm part of the pituitary (Rathke's pouch), which forms the anterior lobe, is completely lost due to high apoptosis at early stages of development (Ohuchi et al., 2000). In contrast the posterior lobe, which is derived from the neuroectoderm, is apparent at E13.5 but regresses in the absence of the anterior lobe and has been reported to be lost by E15.5 (Ohuchi et al., 2000). In agreement with the published data, we observed a complete loss of the ectodermally derived portion of the pituitary at E15.5 in the *Fgf10* null mice, but the posterior lobe was still present at this stage (**Figure 3G**). It was also still evident at E18.5 (**Figure 3H**), suggesting that this part of the pituitary is not dependent on the presence of the anterior lobe as previously proposed. The conditional mutant showed normal development of both the anterior and posterior lobe of the pituitary at E15.5 (**Figures 3E,F**), indicating no requirement for neural crest derived Fgf10 in its formation.

Development of a Hypoplastic CVP and Loss of Salivary and Ocular Glands in *Wnt1cre Fgf10* Conditionals

Salivary glands are absent in *Fgf10* nulls. In keeping with this result the salivary glands were completely absent in the conditional mutant (**Figures 4A–C,E–G**; $N = 8/8$), although a mesenchymal capsule still formed despite the lack of any branching epithelium (**Figure 4G**), phenocopying the null phenotype (Wells et al., 2013). These results are in agreement with the neural crest origin of the salivary gland mesenchyme (Jaskoll et al., 2002).

Slightly unexpectedly, the conditional mutants also formed a circumvallate papilla (CVP) at the back of the tongue (**Figures 4D,H**; $N = 3/3$). The CVP was smaller in size compared to littermate controls and the two fingers of invaginating epithelium were reduced, similar to the phenotype observed in *Eda* pathway mutants (Wells et al., 2011). We checked the development of the CVP in *Fgf10* null embryos, where the CVP has been recorded as missing, and found that the CVP was present but reduced in size in the *Fgf10* null embryos at E15.5 ($N = 3/3$), similar to the phenotype in the conditional knockout, indicating that the CVP can initiate in the absence of *Fgf10* (**Figure 4K**).

Fgf10 is expressed at high levels in the mesenchyme around the developing eye during the stages of ocular gland development (**Figure 1C**). At E15.5 the Harderian gland had initiated in littermate controls at the back of the eye, while this gland was missing in the conditional mutant, despite the presence of a mesenchymal capsule (**Figures 4I,J**; $N = 3/3$). This is in agreement with previous research that *Fgf10* expression is essential for the formation of ocular glands, and confirms that the source of *Fgf10* is the neural crest around the eye.

Hypoplasia of Neck Glands but Normal Tracheal Cartilage Patterning in Conditional Mutants

The thyroid gland was present, but reduced in size in the conditional mutants (**Figures 5A,B**; $N = 3/3$). This suggests either that not all *Fgf10* signaling required for formation of this gland is neural crest derived, or that in fact this gland can develop in the absence of *Fgf10*. To confirm this we looked at development of the thyroid in *Fgf10* null mutants. A small

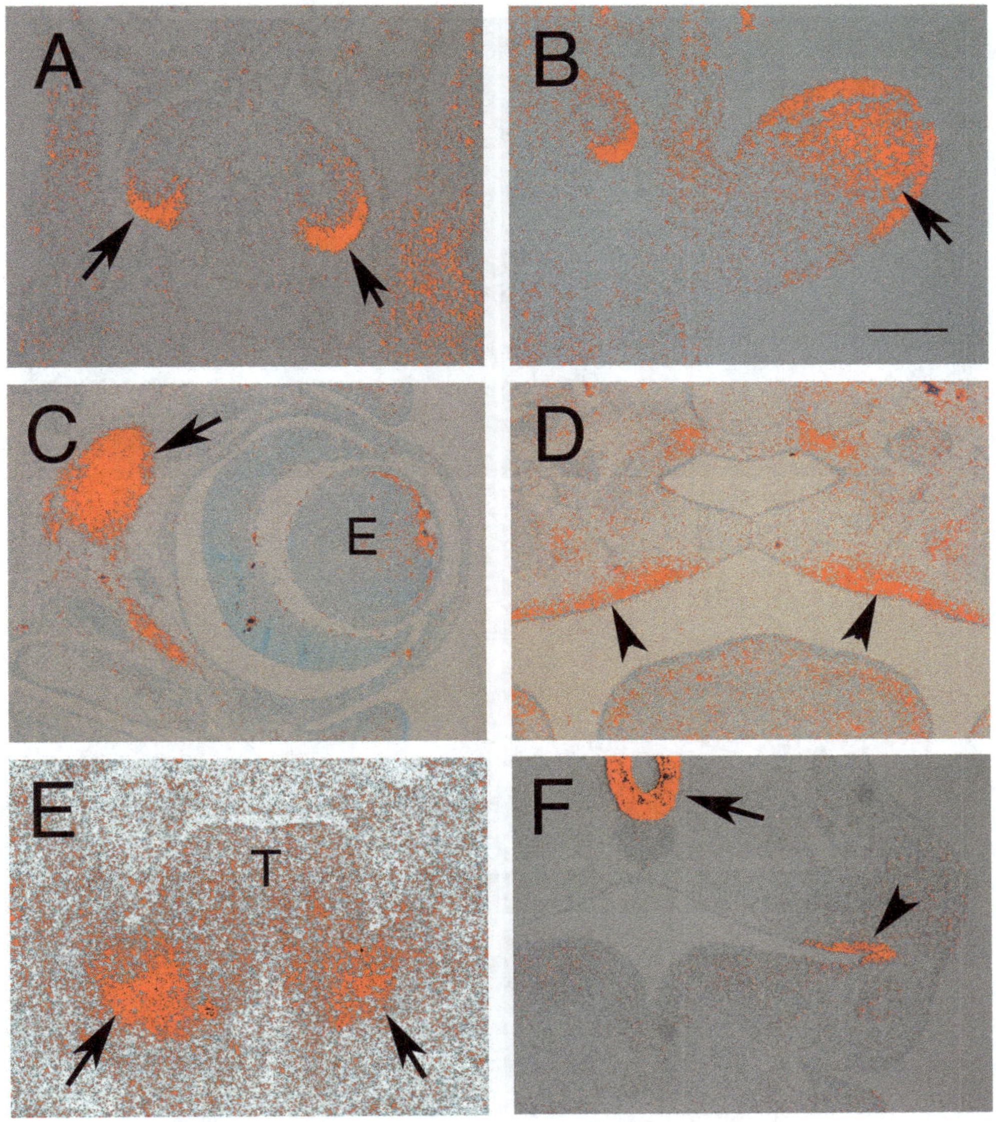

FIGURE 1 | Expression of *Fgf10* in the developing embryo. (A,B,F) E10.5 Frontal sections. **(C,D)** E15.5 frontal sections. **(E)** E12.5 Frontal section. Red grains indicate signal. **(A)** Developing lungs. *Fgf10* is expressed around the tips of the epithelial lung buds (arrows). **(B)** Developing Limb. *Fgf10* is expressed in the mesenchyme in the distal part of the limb (arrows). **(C)** Developing eye (e). *Fgf10* is expressed in the mesenchyme at the back of the eye (arrow). **(D)** Developing palate. *Fgf10* is expressed in the mesenchyme adjacent to the palatal epithelium (arrowsheads). **(E)** Developing salivary gland. *Fgf10* is expressed in the mesenchyme (arrows) underlying the epithelial buds on either side of the tongue (T). **(F)** Developing pituitary and molars. *Fgf10* is expressed at the base of the brain (arrow) underlying rathke's pouch and in the oral epithelium (arrowhead). Scale bars in **(B)** = 200 μm, same scale **(A,C–F)**.

thyroid was observed in 2/3 cases, and in both cases was unilateral, indicating that the thyroid is able to initiate in the absence of *Fgf10* (**Figure 5C**). The gland tissue was located in the correct place, under the cricoid cartilage, indicating that migration cues were unaffected in the mutant, however the gland did not extend as far anteriorly toward the thyroid cartilage. The null gland when present was smaller than that observed in the conditional mutant suggesting another source of Fgf10 might be available for development of this gland in the conditional mutant. Alternatively development of this gland might depend on interaction with other tissues, not affected in the conditional. As the parathyroids migrate to the thyroid we checked for the presence of these glands in our samples. The parathyroids were normally positioned next to the thyroid in the conditional mutant, but as with the thyroid were slightly hypoplastic (**Figures 5D,E**). No evidence of parathyroids were observed in the *Fgf10* null mutant mice ($N = 3$; **Figures 5F**), suggesting again an alternative non-neural crest source for parathyroid gland development in our conditional mutants. The thymus glands in the *Fgf10* null mutants have been shown to be hypoplastic (Ohuchi et al., 2000; Revest et al., 2001). In the conditional mutants the thymus glands were present (**Figures 5G,H**) but appeared slightly reduced in size in the conditional mutant at E15.5, although analysis at E14.5 showed

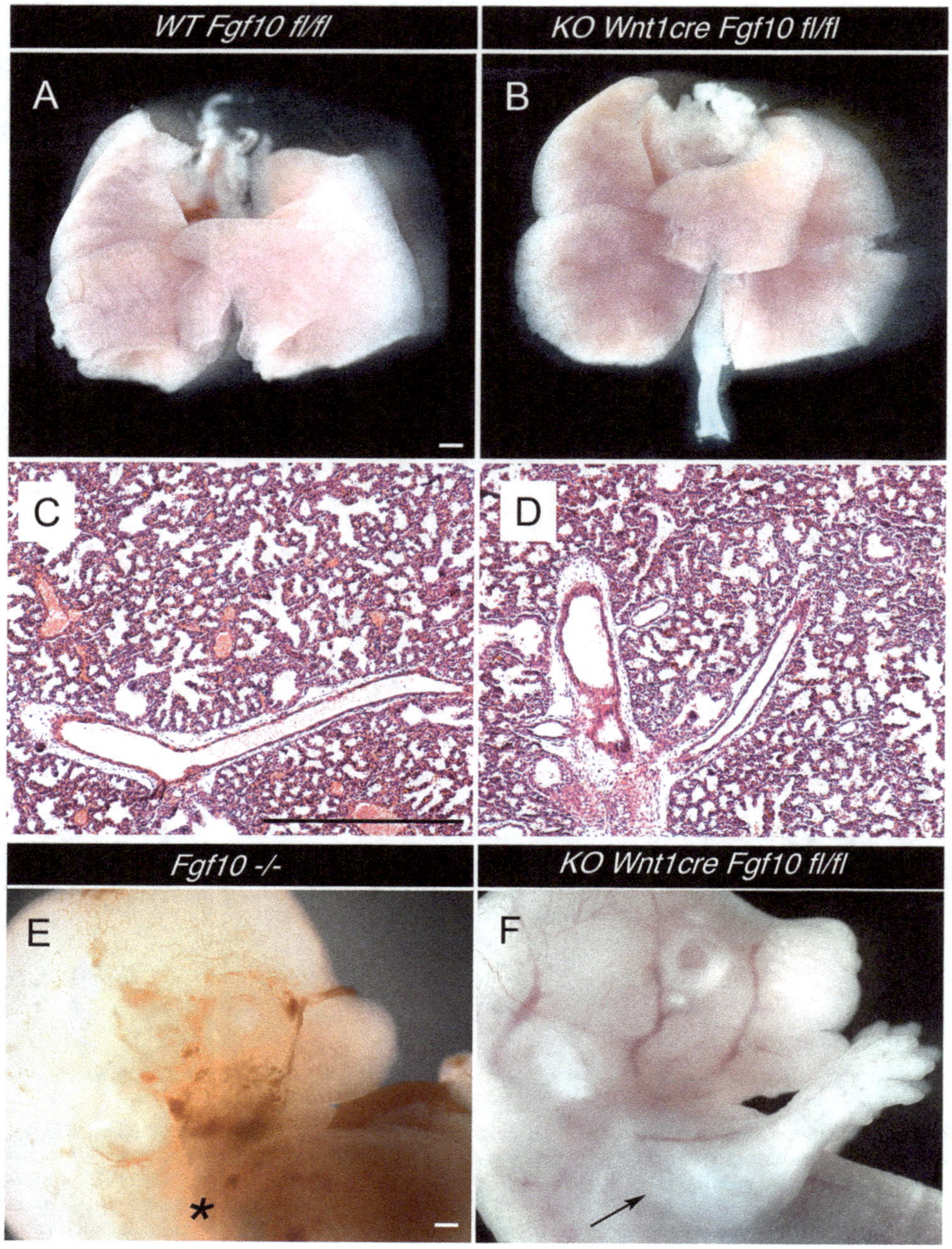

FIGURE 2 | Normal development of lungs and limbs in *Wnt1creFgf10* mutant mice. (A,C) *Fgf10 fl/fl* Control. **(B,D,F)** *Wnt1creFgf10 fl/fl* mutant. **(E)** Fgf10 null mutant. **(A,B)** Dissected lungs E19.5. **(C,D)** Lung histology at E19.5. **(E)** Absence of limbs in null *Fgf10* mutant at E14.5 (*). **(F)** Normal limb development in the conditional mutant (arrow). Scale bars: 500 μm.

no statistically significant difference ($P = 0.684$). This is in contrast to the null where the thymus glands are much smaller by this stage (Revest et al., 2001). In each case, therefore, the neck glands were less severely affected in the conditional compared to the null mutant.

We therefore decided to confirm the position of the boundary between the neural crest and mesoderm in this region of the neck. Tracheas from *Wnt1cre-tdTom* reporter mice were dissected out with the glands removed at P0 to identify the limit of the neural crest, which was found to lie between the thyroid (*Wnt1* positive) and cricoid (*Wnt1* negative) cartilages, with the tracheal rings being mesodermal (**Figure 5K**). This therefore places the thymus, thyroid and parathyroids within the mesoderm, despite the glands themselves having a neural crest origin. In the *Fgf10* null the trachea cartilages are severely mispatterned (Sala et al., 2011). We therefore investigated tracheal cartilage formation at

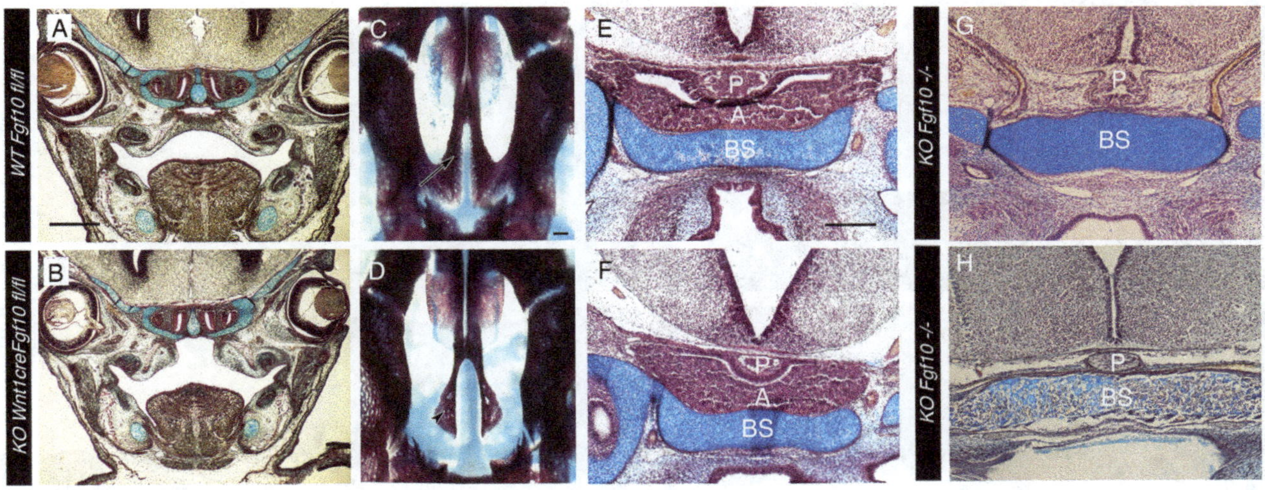

FIGURE 3 | Cleft palate but normal pituitary formation in *Wnt1creFgf10* mutant mice. (A,C,E) *Fgf10 fl/fl* Control. **(B,D,F)** *Wnt1creFgf10* mutant. **(G,H)** *Fgf10 −/−*. **(A,B)** Frontal histology sections through the palate at the level of the molars at E15.5. The palatal shelves have not formed correctly in the conditional mutant. **(C,D)** Skeletal preps of the palate at E19.5. Arrow in C points to the WT palatal processes of the maxilla that have met in the midline. These processes are missing in the conditional mutant and the underlying vomer (arrowhead) is visible. **(E–H)** Developing pituitary gland. **(E,F)** The anterior and posterior lobes form as normal in the conditional mutant at E15.5. **(G,H)** The anterior lobe is missing but the posterior lobe is still evident in the *Fgf10* null at E15.5 **(G)** and E18.5 **(H)**. A = anterior lobe derived from oral ectoderm. P = Posterior lobe derived from neuroepithelium. BS = Basisphenoid. Scale bars in **(A,B)** = 500 μm. Scale bars **(C,D)** = 200 μm. Scale bars **(E–H)** = 200 μm.

E19.5 by skeletal prep in the conditional mutants. As expected, given the limit of the neural crest in this region, the cartilage rings were unaffected in the conditional mutants ($N = 2/2$), matching the pattern in littermate controls (**Figures 5I,J**).

DISCUSSION

The development of the ocular and submandibular and sublingual salivary glands was completely dependent on *Fgf10* signaling from the neural crest derived mesenchyme, with development arresting at early initiation stages as in the null. This paper therefore confirms that the *Fgf10* expressing ocular and salivary gland mesenchyme is derived from the neural crest. As expected, palate development was also disrupted after loss of *Fgf10* in the neural crest derived mesenchyme of the developing palatal shelves, and the conditional mutation is likely to cause lethality.

In contrast to these cranial glands other more posterior glands, such as the thyroid, thymus, and parathyroids did not phenocopy the complete loss of *Fgf10*. The thymus, parathyroids and thyroid initiate within neural crest derived mesenchyme (Müller et al., 2008; Johansson et al., 2015) and then migrate more posteriorly to sit within mesodermally derived mesenchyme, as supported by our neural crest lineage analysis of the trachea, and previous lineage tracing that mentions the tracheal rings are not neural crest derived (Matsuoka et al., 2005). All of these glands are severely affected in the *Fgf10* null but the conditional mutants had a milder phenotype. In all three glands it is possible that other Fgfs and alternative signaling pathways are able to compensate for the initial loss of *Fgf10* in this tissue, allowing their initiation, while mesodermal *Fgf10* may be able to act once the glands have reached their final positions in the neck. In agreement with this *Fgf10* is expressed in the mesenchyme around the thymus at E13.5, a stage after the glands have reached their final position (Revest et al., 2001), and is strongly expressed in the ventral mesenchyme of the developing trachea from E14.5 (Sala et al., 2011). Mesodermal Fgf10 is therefore in the right place to be able to signal to the more posterior glands. It is also possible that signals between these tissues and other neighboring structures are important for their development, and that their presence is interdependent.

Early on in development *Fgf10* is strongly expressed in the oral epithelium. It was therefore possible that some of the orally derived structures would have a reduced phenotype when compared to the *Fgf10* null. The glands of the oral cavity, however, appeared to mimic the null phenotype indicating that only the loss of *Fgf10* in the neural crest was critical. Moreover the epithelial expression appeared to have no influence on the developing teeth, the molars having only a very minor defect in relative size similar to the null (Ohuchi et al., 2000). It would therefore be interesting to see whether knocking out *Fgf10* in the early epithelium has any effect on development of these key structures. As expected development of the pituitary, limbs and lungs was normal in the conditional knockout, in which *Fgf10* was provided by the neuroepithelium and mesoderm rather than neural crest. The tracheal rings were also normal highlighting the fact that the *Fgf10* expressing mesenchyme that forms the cartilage rings is not neural crest derived.

Our comparison of the conditional mutants with the *Fgf10* null mutants revealed a few differences between the phenotype observed in our null mice and in previously published data. For example, although it has been reported that the thyroid fails

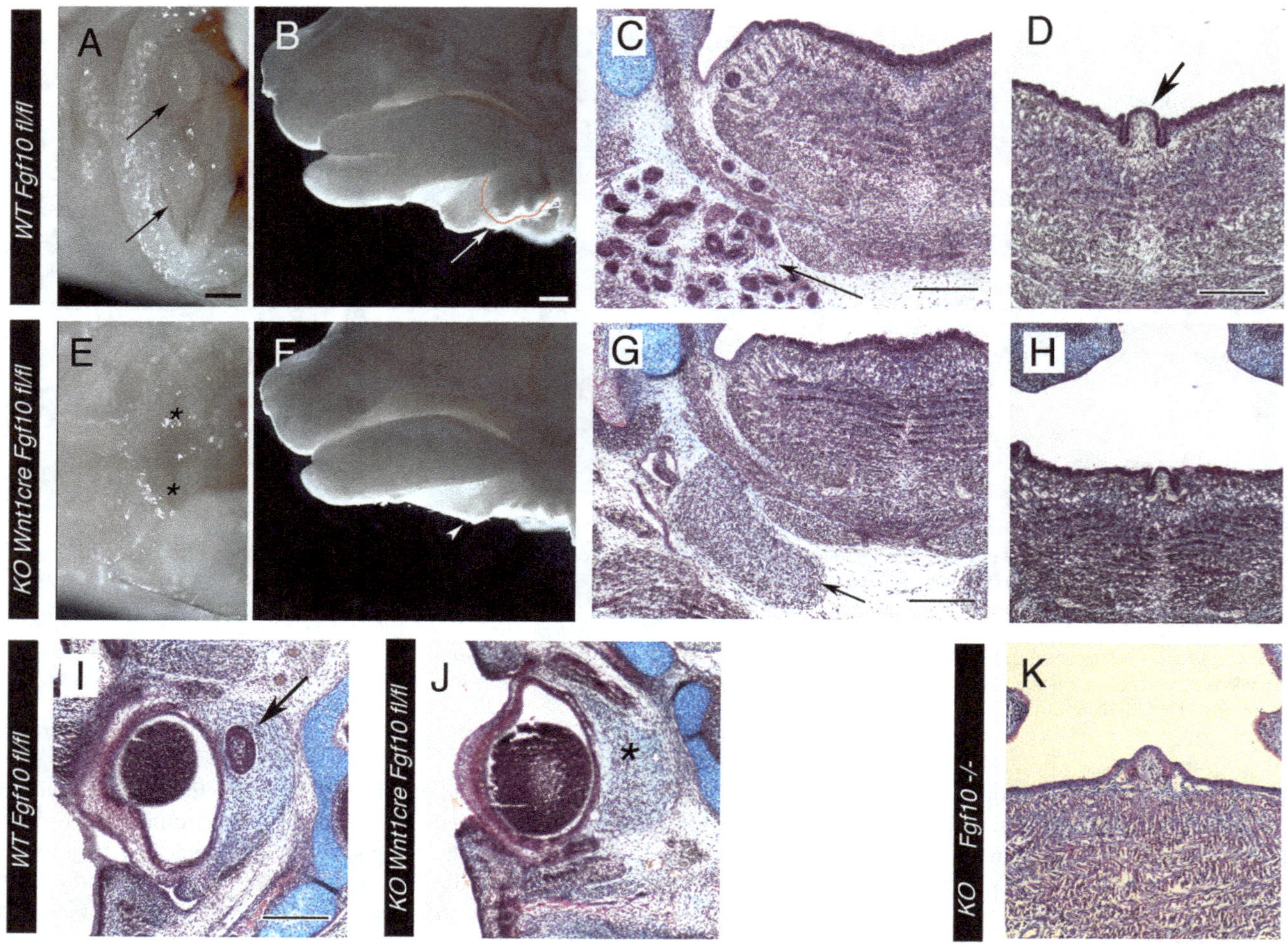

FIGURE 4 | Loss of Salivary and ocular glands in *Wnt1creFgf10* mutant mice. (A–D,I) *Fgf10 fl/fl* Control. **(E–H,J)** *Wnt1creFgf10 fl/fl* mutant. **(K)** *Fgf10 −/−*. **(A,E)** E15.5 head ventral view looking up at the paired submandibular and sublingual glands (arrow). The glands are missing in the mutant (asterix). **(B,F)** E15.5 head dissected down the middle to reveal the glands at the base of the tongue, outlined in red and arrowed. The glands are missing in the conditional mutant (arrowhead). **(C,D,G,H,K)** Frontal sections at the level of the tongue at E15.5. **(C,G)** The branching epithelial tissue of the salivary gland is observed in the control (arrow) but are missing in the mutant. The mesenchymal capsule, however, is still evident (arrow). **(D,H,K)** Posterior tongue showing the single circumvallate papilla (CVP) in the center (arrow in **D**). **(H,K)** A CVP formed in the null and conditional but was smaller than in the WT. **(I,J)** Frontal sections of the eye at E15.5. The harderian gland at the back of the eye failed to form in the conditional mutant (asterix in **J**). Scale bars **(A,B)** = 500 μm, same scale in **(E,F)**. Scale bars **(C,D,G,I)** = 200 μm, same scale in **(H,J,K)**.

to form in *Fgf10* null mice (Ohuchi et al., 2000) in our null mice a small amount of glandular tissue was present around the trachea in the region of the thyroid but this was only observed unilaterally. Interestingly, in the Ohuchi paper although the text states no gland forms the figures highlight a rudimentary thyroid. The thyroid therefore does appear to be able to form in the complete absence of *Fgf10* but is severely hypoplastic, while we saw no evidence of a parathyroid.

We also observed development of a hypoplastic CVP in the tongue, which had previously been reported as missing in the *Fgf10* mutant (Petersen et al., 2011). *Fgf7* is also expressed in the mesenchyme of the developing tongue and may compensate for the loss of *Fgf10* in this structure (Sohn et al., 2011). These differences with the published data may indicate variation due to genetic background. For our studies we investigated *Fgf10* nulls on a mixed C57Bl6/CD1 background, while other papers have used a mixed C57bl6/CBA or C57Bl6/129SVJ or not reported the background used (Min et al., 1998; Sekine et al., 1999; Ohuchi et al., 2000; Rice et al., 2004; Petersen et al., 2011). In fact the arrest in limb development was reported to occur at slightly different time-points when the *Fgf10* knockout was originally reported by two groups, with the difference being suggested to be due to genetic background (Min et al., 1998; Sekine et al., 1999). Our findings have therefore shed light on the structures affected by neural crest expressing *Fgf10* but have also revealed some differences in the published literature which merit further investigation.

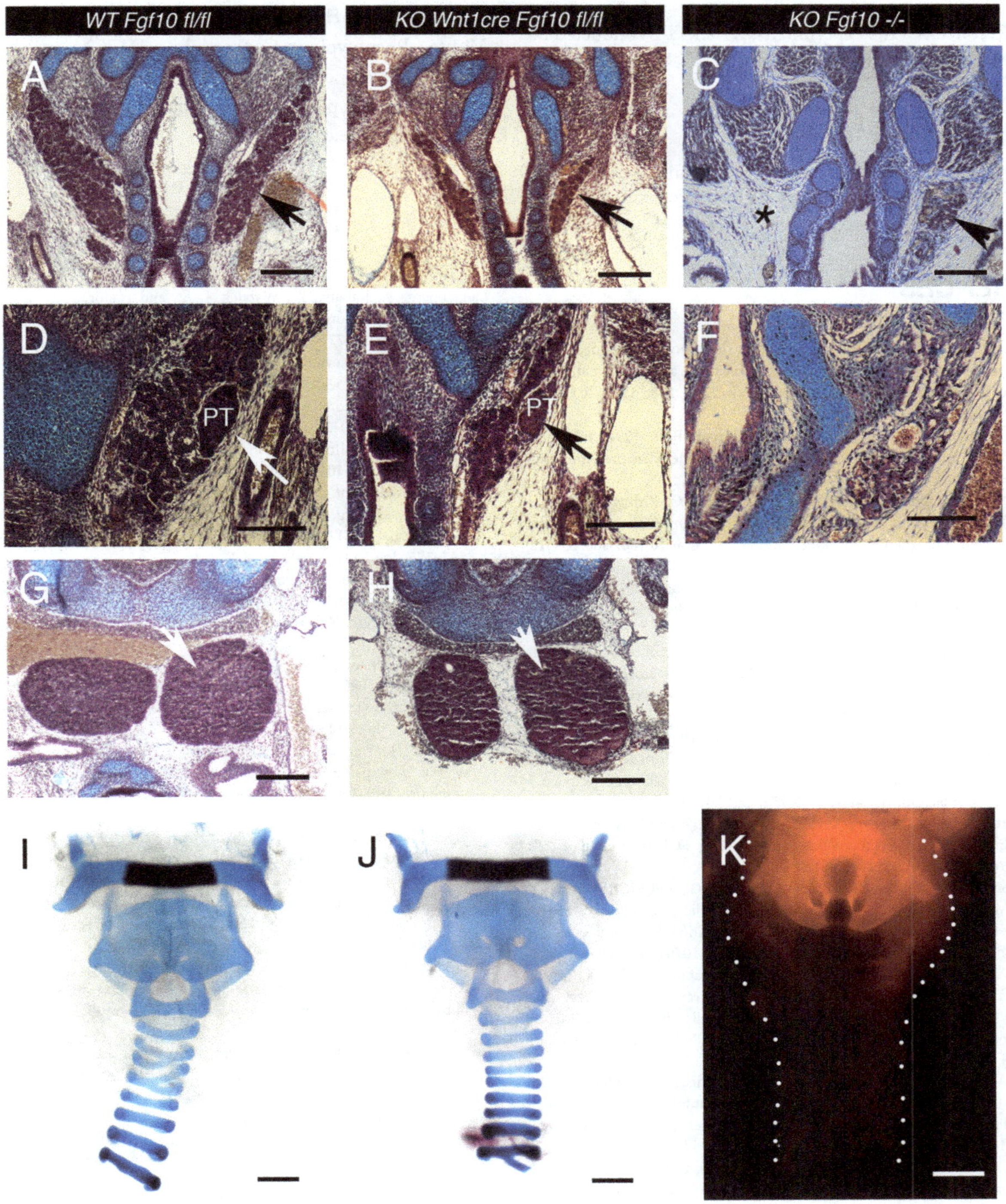

FIGURE 5 | Cranial gland and trachea development in the *Wnt1creFgf10* mutant mice. (A,D,G,I) *Fgf10 fl/fl* Control. **(B,E,H,J)** *Wnt1creFgf10* mutant. **(C,F)** *Fgf10 −/−* null mice. Frontal sections E15.5. **(A,B,C)** Developing thyroid glands (arrowed) A severely hypoplastic gland was observed in the null mutant but was missing on one side (asterix). **(D,E,F)** Developing parathyroid glands (arrows). No parathyroid was observed in the Fgf10 null. **(G,H)** Developing Thymus glands (arrow). **(I,J)** Alcian blue staining for tracheal cartilages at E19.5. Dissected trachea show normal morphology with formation of cartilage rings. **(K)** The neural crest, as marked by red in *Wnt1cre/tdTom* mice, does not extend down the trachea past the thyroid cartilage as shown at Postnatal day 0. PT = parathyroid. Scale bars **(A–C,G,H)** = 200 μm. Scale bars **(D–F)** = 100 μm. Scale bars **(I–K)**: 500 μm.

AUTHOR CONTRIBUTIONS

AT and SL conceived the experiments, AT and TT conducted the experiments and undertook data acquision, AT, SL, and TT wrote the manuscript.

ACKNOWLEDGMENTS

The Fgf10A02 tmc1c mice were obtained from the MRC-Harwell, which distributes these mice on behalf of the European Mouse Mutant Archive (http://www.emmanet.org). The MRC-Harwell is also a member of the International Mouse Phenotyping Consortium (IMPC), which funded the generation of the Fgf10A02 tmc1c mice. Associated primary phenotypic information may be found at http://www.mousephenotype.org.

REFERENCES

Abler, L. L., Mansour, S. L., and Sun, X. (2009). Conditional gene inactivation reveals roles for Fgf10 and Fgfr2 in establishing a normal pattern of epithelial branching in the mouse lung. *Dev. Dyn.* 238, 1999–2013. doi: 10.1002/dvdy.22032

Bellusci, S., Grindley, J., Emoto, H., Itoh, N., and Hogan, B. L. (1997). Fibroblast growth factor 10 (FGF10) and branching morphogenesis in the embryonic mouse lung. *Development* 124, 4867–4878.

Bradley, A., Anastassiadis, K., Ayadi, A., Battey, J. F., Bell, C., Birling, M. C., et al. (2012). The mammalian gene function resource: the International Knockout Mouse Consortium. *Mamm. Genome* 23, 580–586. doi: 10.1007/s00335-012-9422-2

Chai, Y., Jiang, X., Ito, Y., Bringas, P. Jr., Han, J., Rowitch, D. H., et al. (2000). Fate of the mammalian cranial neural crest during tooth and mandibular morphogenesis. *Development* 127, 1671–1679.

De Moerlooze, L., Spencer-Dene, B., Revest, J. M., Hajihosseini, M., Rosewell, I., and Dickson, C. (2000). An important role for the IIIb isoform of fibroblast growth factor receptor 2 (FGFR2) in mesenchymal-epithelial signalling during mouse organogenesis. *Development* 127, 483–492.

Freem, L. J., Escot, S., Tannahill, D., Druckenbrod, N. R., Thapar, N., and Burns, A. J. (2010). The intrinsic innervation of the lung is derived from neural crest cells as shown by optical projection tomography in Wnt1-Cre;YFP reporter mice. *J. Anat.* 217, 651–664. doi: 10.1111/j.1469-7580.2010.01295.x

Govindarajan, V., Ito, M., Makarenkova, H. P., Lang, R. A., and Overbeek, P. A. (2000). Endogenous and ectopic gland induction by FGF-10. *Dev. Biol.* 225, 188–200. doi: 10.1006/dbio.2000.9812

Heuze, Y., Singh, N., Basilico, C., Jabs, E. W., Holmes, G., and Richtsmeier, J. T. (2014). Morphological comparison of the craniofacial phenotypes of mouse models expressing the Apert FGFR2 S252W mutation in neural crest- or mesoderm-derived tissues. *Bone* 63, 101–109. doi: 10.1016/j.bone.2014.03.003

Hosokawa, R., Oka, K., Yamaza, T., Iwata, J., Urata, M., Xu, X., et al. (2010). TGF-beta mediated FGF10 signaling in cranial neural crest cells controls development of myogenic progenitor cells through tissue-tissue interactions during tongue morphogenesis. *Dev. Biol.* 341, 186–195. doi: 10.1016/j.ydbio.2010.02.030

Jaskoll, T., Abichaker, G., Witcher, D., Sala, F. G., Bellusci, S., Hajihosseini, M. K., et al. (2005). FGF10/FGFR2b signaling plays essential roles during *in vivo* embryonic submandibular salivary gland morphogenesis. *BMC Dev. Biol.* 5:11. doi: 10.1186/1471-213X-5-11

Jaskoll, T., Zhou, Y. M., Chai, Y., Makarenkova, H. P., Collinson, J. M., West, J. D., et al. (2002). Embryonic submandibular gland morphogenesis: stage-specific protein localization of FGFs, BMPs, Pax6 and Pax9 in normal mice and abnormal SMG phenotypes in FgfR2-IIIc(+/Delta), BMP7(-/-) and Pax6(-/-) mice. *Cells Tissues Organs* 170, 83–98. doi: 10.1159/000046183

Jiang, X., Rowitch, D. H., Soriano, P., McMahon, A. P., and Sucov, H. M. (2000). Fate of the mammalian cardiac neural crest. *Development* 127, 1607–1616.

Johansson, E., Andersson, L., Örnros, J., Carlsson, T., Ingeson-Carlsson, C., Liang, S., et al. (2015). Revising the embryonic origin of thyroid C cells in mice and humans. *Development* 142, 3519–3528. doi: 10.1242/dev.126581

Kettunen, P., Laurikkala, J., Itäranta, P., Vainio, S., Itoh, N., and Thesleff, I. (2000). Associations of FGF-3 and FGF-10 with signaling networks regulating tooth morphogenesis. *Dev. Dyn.* 219, 322–332.

Langenberg, T., Kahana, A., Wszalek, J. A., and Halloran, M. C. (2008). The eye organizes neural crest cell migration. *Dev. Dyn.* 237, 1645–1652. doi: 10.1002/dvdy.21577

Lewis, A. E., Vasudevan, H. N., O'Neill, A. K., Soriano, P., and Bush, J. O. (2013). The widely used Wnt1-Cre transgene causes developmental phenotypes by ectopic activation of Wnt signaling. *Dev. Biol.* 379, 229–234. doi: 10.1016/j.ydbio.2013.04.026

Makarenkova, H. P., Ito, M., Govindarajan, V., Faber, S. C., Sun, L., McMahon, G., et al. (2000). FGF10 is an inducer and Pax6 a competence factor for lacrimal gland development. *Development* 127, 2563–2572.

Matsuoka, T., Ahlberg, P. E., Kessaris, N., Iannarelli, P., Dennehy, U., Richardson, W. D., et al. (2005). Neural Crest origins of the neck and shoulder. *Nature* 436, 347–355. doi: 10.1038/nature03837

May, A. J., Chatzeli, L., Proctor, G. B., and Tucker, A. S. (2015). Salivary gland dysplasia in Fgf10 heterozygous mice: a new mouse model of xerostomia. *Curr. Mol. Med.* 15, 674–682. doi: 10.2174/156652401566615083114 1307

Min, H., Danilenko, D. M., Scully, S. A., Bolon, B., Ring, B. D., Tarpley, J. E. et al. (1998). Fgf-10 is required for both limb and lung development and exhibits striking functional similarity to Drosophila branchless. *Genes Dev.* 12, 3156–3161. doi: 10.1101/gad.12.20.3156

Moustakas, J. E., Smith, K. K., and Hlusko, L. J. (2011). Evolution and development of the mammalian dentition: insights from the marsupial *Monodelphis domestica*. *Dev. Dyn.* 240, 232–239. doi: 10.1002/dvdy.22502

Müller, S. M., Stolt, C. C., Terszowski, G., Blum, C., Amagai, T., Kessaris, N., et al. (2008). Neural crest origin of perivascular mesenchyme in the adult thymus. *J. Immunol.* 180, 5344–5351. doi: 10.4049/jimmunol.180.8.5344

Ohuchi, H., Hori, Y., Yamasaki, M., Harada, H., Sekine, K., Kato, S., et al. (2000). FGF10 acts as a major ligand for FGF receptor 2 IIIb in mouse multi-organ development. *Biochem. Biophys. Res. Commun.* 277, 643–649. doi: 10.1006/bbrc.2000.3721

Orr-Urtreger, A., Bedford, M. T., Burakova, T., Arman, E., Zimmer, Y., Yayon, A., et al. (1993). Developmental localization of the splicing alternatives of fibroblast growth factor receptor-2 (FGFR2). *Dev. Biol.* 158, 475–486. doi: 10.1006/dbio.1993.1205

Pauley, S., Wright, T. J., Pirvola, U., Ornitz, D., Beisel, K., and Fritzsch, B. (2003). Expression and function of FGF10 in mammalian inner ear development. *Dev. Dyn.* 227, 203–215. doi: 10.1002/dvdy.10297

Peters, K. G., Werner, S., Chen, G., and Williams, L. T. (1992). Two FGF receptor genes are differentially expressed in epithelial and mesenchymal tissues during limb formation and organogenesis in the mouse. *Development* 114, 233–243.

Petersen, C. I., Jheon, A. H., Mostowfi, P., Charles, C., Ching, S., Thirumangalathu, S., et al. (2011). FGF signaling regulates the number of posterior taste papillae by controlling progenitor field size. *PLoS Genet.* 7:e1002098. doi: 10.1371/journal.pgen.1002098

Pettitt, S. J., Liang, Q., Rairdan, X. Y., Moran, J. L., Prosser, H. M., Beier, D. R., et al. (2009). Agouti C57BL/6N embryonic stem cells for mouse genetic resources. *Nat. Methods* 6, 493–495. doi: 10.1038/nmeth.1342

Revest, J.-M., Suniara, R. K., Kerr, K., Owen, J. J. T., and Dickson, C. (2001). Development of the thymus requires signalling through the Fibroblast growth factor receptor R2-IIIb. *J. Immunol.* 167, 1954–1961. doi: 10.4049/jimmunol.167.4.1954

Rice, R., Spencer-Dene, B., Connor, E. C., Gritli-Linde, A., McMahon, A. P., Dickson, C., et al. (2004). Disruption of Fgf10/Fgfr2b-coordinated epithelial-mesenchymal interactions causes cleft palate. *J. Clin. Invest.* 113, 1692–1700. doi: 10.1172/JCI20384

Rohmann, E., Brunner, H. G., Kayserili, H., Uyguner, O., Nürnberg, G., Lew, E. D., et al. (2006). Mutations in different components of FGF signaling in LADD syndrome. *Nat. Genet.* 38, 414–417. doi: 10.1038/ng1757

Sala, F. G., Del Moral, P. M., Tiozzo, C., Alam, D. A., Warburton, D., Grikscheit, T., et al. (2011). FGF10 controls the patterning of the tracheal cartilage rings via Shh. *Development* 138, 273–282. doi: 10.1242/dev.051680

Sekine, K., Ohuchi, H., Fujiwara, M., Yamasaki, M., Yoshizawa, T., Sato, T., et al. (1999). Fgf10 is essential for limb and lung formation. *Nat. Genet.* 21, 138–141. doi: 10.1038/5096

Skarnes, W. C., Rosen, B., West, A. P., Koutsourakis, M., Bushell, W., Iyer, V., et al. (2011). A conditional knockout resource for the genome-wide study of mouse gene function. *Nature* 474, 337–342. doi: 10.1038/nature10163

Sohn, W. J., Jung, H. I., Choi, M. A., Han, J. H., Gwon, G. J., Yamamoto, H., et al. (2011). Reciprocal interactions of Fgf10/Fgfr2b modulate the mouse tongue epithelial differentiation. *Cell Tissue Res.* 345, 265–273. doi: 10.1007/s00441-011-1204-8

Takuma, N., Sheng, H. Z., Furuta, Y., Ward, J. M., Sharma, K., Hogan, B. L., et al. (1998). Formation of Rathke's pouch requires dual induction from the diencephalon. *Development* 125, 4835–4840.

Wells, K. L., Gaete, M., Matalova, E., Deutsch, D., Rice, D., and Tucker, A. S. (2013). Dynamic relationship of the epithelium and mesenchyme during salivary gland initiation: the role of Fgf10. *Biol. Open* 2, 981–989. doi: 10.1242/bio.20135306

Wells, K. L., Mou, C., Headon, D. J., and Tucker, A. S. (2011). Defects and rescue of the minor salivary glands in Eda pathway mutants. *Dev. Biol.* 349, 137–146. doi: 10.1016/j.ydbio.2010.10.012

Wright, T. J., and Mansour, S. L. (2003). FGF signaling in ear development and innervation. *Curr. Topics Dev. Biol.* 57, 225–259. doi: 10.1016/S0070-2153(03)57008-9

Zhang, X., Ibrahimi, O. A., Olsen, S. K., Umemori, H., Mohammadi, M., and Ornitz, D. M. (2006). Receptor specificity of the fibroblast growth factor family. The complete mammalian FGF family. *J. Biol. Chem.* 281, 15694–15700. doi: 10.1074/jbc.M601252200

15

Angled Growth of the Dental Lamina is Accompanied by Asymmetrical Expression of the WNT Pathway Receptor Frizzled 6

Iveta Putnová[1, 2], Hana Dosedělová[1, 2], Vitezslav Bryja[3], Marie Landová[1], Marcela Buchtová[1, 3] and Jan Štembírek[1, 4]*

[1] Laboratory of Molecular Morphogenesis, Institute of Animal Physiology and Genetics, Academy of Sciences, Brno, Czechia, [2] Department of Anatomy, Histology and Embryology, University of Veterinary and Pharmaceutical Sciences, Brno, Czechia, [3] Department of Animal Physiology and Immunology, Institute of Experimental Biology, Masaryk University, Brno, Czechia, [4] Department of Maxillofacial Surgery, University Hospital Ostrava, Ostrava, Czechia

Correspondence:
Marcela Buchtova
buchtova@iach.cz

Frizzled 6 (FZD6) belongs to a family of proteins that serve as receptors in the WNT signaling pathway. FZD6 plays an important role in the establishment of planar cell polarity in many embryonic processes such as convergent extension during gastrulation, neural tube closure, or hair patterning. Based on its role during hair development, we hypothesized that FZD6 may have similar expression pattern and function in the dental lamina, which is also a distinct epithelial protrusion growing characteristically angled into the mesenchyme. Diphyodont minipig was selected as a model species because its dentition closely resemble human ones with successional generation of teeth initiated from the dental lamina. We revealed asymmetrical expression of FZD6 in the dental lamina of early as well as late stages during its regression with stronger expression located on the labial side of the dental lamina. During lamina regression, FZD6-positive cells were found in its superficial part and the signal coincided with the upregulation of molecules involved in epithelial-mesenchymal transition and increased migratory potential of epithelial cells. FZD6-expression was also turned on during differentiation of cells producing hard tissues, in which mature odontoblasts, ameloblasts, or surrounding osteoblasts were FZD6-positive. On the other hand, the tip of successional lamina and its lingual part, in which progenitor cells are located, exhibited FZD6-negativity. In conclusion, asymmetrical expression of FZD6 correlates with the growth directionality and side-specific morphological differences in the dental lamina of diphyodont species. Based on observed expression pattern, we propose that the dental lamina is other epithelial tissue, where planar cell polarity signaling is involved during its asymmetrical growth.

Keywords: FZD6, successional dental lamina, WNT signaling, planar cell polarity (PCP), odontoblast, ameloblast, osteoblast, epithelial remnants

INTRODUCTION

Tooth development is a complex process that is dependent on reciprocal and strictly regulated interactions between the ectoderm-derived epithelium and cranial neural crest-derived mesenchyme (Thesleff et al., 1995). Numerous regulatory genes associated with all stages of tooth formation (patterning, morphogenesis, cytodifferentiation, and mineralization) belong to evolutionarily conserved signaling pathways. They are necessary for individual steps of odontogenesis and are regulated by a precise timing mechanism (Thesleff, 2003; Mitsiadis and Luder, 2011). The WNT signaling pathway has previously been demonstrated to play an important role in mouse as well as human tooth development (Sarkar and Sharpe, 1999; Sarkar et al., 2000; Handrigan and Richman, 2010). FZD members belongs to a family of proteins that serve as receptors in WNT signaling pathways (Fischer et al., 2007; Dijksterhuis et al., 2016; Wang et al., 2016). Their functions include activation of the FZD/β-catenin, FZD/Ca^{+2} and FZD/planar cell polarity signaling pathways (Schulte and Bryja, 2007). To date, 10 FZD proteins have been described in mammals (Schulte and Bryja, 2007; Dijksterhuis et al., 2016). While the expression of several ligands of WNT signaling during odontogenesis has been well-described (Cai et al., 2011; Lin et al., 2011; Wang et al., 2014), little attention has been paid to the expression of individual receptors. Here, we focus on FZD6, which is involved in PCP (planar cell polarity) signaling and is required for the transmission of polarity signals across the plasma membrane in epidermal cells (Wang et al., 2006).

Cellular communication mediated by WNT and FZD has been shown to be essential for proper embryonic development of invertebrates as well as vertebrates. FZD induction has been found in several developmental processes such as the polarized cell movements required for convergent extension during gastrulation in frog and fish (Borello et al., 1999), neural induction and patterning, cell proliferation, cell specification, stem cell differentiation, axonal outgrowth and guidance, and synaptogenesis (Logan and Nusse, 2004; Chien et al., 2009; Wang et al., 2010). Besides these early patterning processes, FZD3 and FZD6 have been reported redundantly to control neural tube closure and planar orientation of hair bundles on a subset of auditory and vestibular sensory cells. In the inner ear, these two proteins are located on the lateral faces of sensory and auxiliary cells in a pattern that correlates with the axis of planar polarity (Wang et al., 2006). The polarity of FZD6 localization with respect to the asymmetric position of the kinocilium is reversed between vestibular hair cells in the cristae of the semicircular canals and auditory hair cells in the organ of Corti (Wang et al., 2006). FZD6 controls macroscopic hair patterning in the mouse and is also expressed in the skin and hair follicles (Guo et al., 2004; Wang et al., 2010; Chang et al., 2016).

Mutations in PCP genes lead to a wide range of developmental defects, including a shortened body axis, a widened neural plate, and neural tube defects (NTDs; Simons and Mlodzik, 2008). In the case of targeted deletion of the *Fzd6* gene, stereotyped whorls on the hind feet, variable whorls and tufts on the head and disorientation of hairs on the torso are evident (Guo et al., 2004). In the $Fzd6^{-/-}$ mouse, the orientations of the earliest born hair follicles are uncorrelated, but over time the follicles reorient to create patterns, which are typical for different body regions and are characterized by a high degree of local arrangement (Wang et al., 2010). Fifty percent of male newborns, but not female $Fzd6^{-/-}$ mice, displayed abnormal claw morphology. The claws are easily lost with age or under increased mechanical stress. The claw disappears or become rudimentary on the hind limbs at the age of 2–3 months. The reason for the significant misbalance between sexes is unknown but it could be due to the more aggressive behavior of males (Fröjmark et al., 2011). Similarly in humans, loss-of-function mutations caused recessive nail dysplasia (Fröjmark et al., 2011; Naz et al., 2012). While several ectodermal derivates have been found to be affected in transgenic mouse lines or humans with defective FZD6, to date, no tooth phenotype has been described.

Here, we analyzed the expression of FZD6, a transmembrane protein of the WNT family, that is known to regulate the number of epithelial differentiation-related genes. During human odontogenesis, *Fzd6* was shown to exhibit weak mRNA expression in the dental epithelium of incisors and molars at 8 and 12 weeks of gestation (Wang et al., 2014). Later during 15 week, *Fzd6* was observed in the inner and outer enamel epithelium and in the surrounding mesenchymal cells (Wang et al., 2014). However, the distribution of FZD6 on protein level has not been analyzed yet. We focused on premolar development in diphyodont dentition during early as well as late mineralization stages of odontogenesis to determine the distribution of its expression throughout development. Labio-lingual differences during the initiation and regression of dental lamina were analyzed to uncover signaling involved in asymmetrical morphology and growth of the lamina. Therefore, the main aim of our study was to describe the expression pattern of FZD6 at the protein level during early odontogenesis in the minipig dentition with a special focus on the asymmetric distribution of FZD6 in the dental lamina during its angled growth and regression. Furthermore, changes in FZD6-positivity in odontoblasts and ameloblasts during their differentiation were determined.

MATERIALS AND METHODS

Embryonic Material

Selected developmental stages of the minipig (E29, E30, E36, E56, E67) were used to analyse the expression of FZD6 during odontogenesis. Minipig embryos and fetuses were obtained from Liběchov animal facility (Liběchov, Czech Republic). The day after insemination was established as day 1 of gestation. Staged embryos and fetuses were obtained by hysterectomy. All samples were fixed in 4% neutral formaldehyde and decalcified in 12.5% EDTA in 4% PFA until the mandibular bones of embryos were soft enough for further processing. Sections were stained with Haematoxylin-Eosin and alternative slides were used for immunohistochemical labeling. All procedures were conducted following a protocol approved by the Laboratory Animal Science Committee of the Institute of Animal Physiology and Genetics, Academy of Sciences (approval no. 020/2010, Liběchov, Czech Republic).

Immunohistochemical Analysis

For detection of FZD6-positivity, we performed immunohistochemical labeling. After deparaffinization and rehydration, antigen retrieval was performed in a water bath (97°C) in citrate buffer (pH = 6) for 20 min. Blocking serum was applied to the sections for 20 min and slides were incubated for 1 h at room temperature with primary FZD6 antibody (cat. no. G260, Antibodies online, 1:200 dilution). The secondary antibody was applied for 30 min. Streptavidin-FITC complex (1:250 dilution, cat. no. 554060, BD Pharmigen, Franklin Lakes, USA) was used for visualization of FZD6-positive cells (30 min). DAPI (cat. no. P36935, Invitrogen, Oregon, USA) or DRAQ5 (1:500 dilution, cat. no. 62254, Thermo Scientific, USA) were applied for the counterstaining. The photos taken under a fluorescence microscope Leica DM LB2 (Leica Microsystems, Germany) were merged together in Adobe Photoshop 7.0 (USA). High power images were taken on confocal microscope Leica SP5 using 40x (air) objectives (Leica Microsystems, Germany) with Leica Application Suite software.

RESULTS AND DISCUSSION

Asymmetrical Expression of FZD6 at Early Stages of Odontogenesis

PCP components are often localized asymmetrically in different types of cells. The Frizzled family was found to be required for producing the correct orientation of cuticular bristles and hairs (Guo et al., 2004). This process is referred to as tissue or planar polarity (Gubb and García-Bellido, 1982; Vinson et al., 1989). Such polarization is often precisely coordinated relative to the axes of a tissue or organ, but the mechanisms underlying this regulation are still poorly understood. As exact coordination of tissue polarity in the labio-lingual axis is necessary to direct the angled growth of dental lamina into the mesenchyme, we wondered whether protein expression FZD6 can be associated with morphological side-related differences in the dental lamina. Indeed, we observed significant differences in the level of FZD6-positivity in distinct areas of the dental lamina at all stages of minipig odontogenesis. Already at the epithelial thickening stage, a strong FZD6 signal was apparent on the labial side of the oral epithelium and in the dental epithelium, especially in its basal layer (**Figure 1A**). The signal became weaker toward its lingual side. Distinct expression was also obvious in the mesenchyme surrounding the epithelial thickening, where more FZD6-positivity was noticeable in the labial area (**Figure 1A**). Later, during dental lamina growth into the mesenchyme, stronger expression was observed also on the labial side of the oral dental interface in comparison with the lingual area (**Figures 1B,C,C′**). At the dental bud stage, FZD6 was only weakly expressed inside the tooth anlagen (**Figures 1D,D′**) while FZD6-immunopositivity was detected in the dental lamina connecting the tooth to the oral epithelium, where stronger expression was located on the labial side (**Figures 1D,D′**).

At the cap stage (**Figure 1E**), distinct expression was found throughout all thicknesses of the oral epithelium and in the dental lamina, but was not apparent inside the tooth anlagen. The signal spread into the cervical loop area during the early bell stage (**Figure 1F**). Almost no signal was visible in the stellate reticulum (**Figure 1F**). The dental papilla and surrounding mesenchyme were FZD6-negative. FZD6-signal was abundant in the basal layer of the oral epithelium at all analyzed stages and became localized to the superficial area of membrane in more differentiated superficial layers of the epithelium (**Figure 1**).

It is known that FZD6 is transducing signals in non-canonical WNT pathway and Wnt5a is one of its representative, which signals upstream of PCP pathway in mammals (Moon et al., 1993; Kilian et al., 2003). It was shown that WNT5a regulates tooth growth, cusp patterning and odontoblast differentiation in developing mouse molars and incisors (Lin et al., 2011). Previously, WNT5a expression was found not only in the dental mesenchyme but also in the dental epithelium in mouse during E14–E17 (Cai et al., 2011). However, we detected FZD6 even at very early stages of epithelial thickening and in the surrounding mesenchyme, and therefore another WNT ligand probably activates signaling at these early stages, which will be necessary to further analyse in future.

FZD can also mediate canonical signaling with activation of β-catenin. WNT3a is strongly expressed in the inner enamel epithelium of humans during the bell stage (Wang et al., 2014). In mice, *Wnt3a* is expressed in the enamel knot at the cap stage (Millar et al., 2003). These expression patterns do not seem to correlate with our observations of a strong signal located in the superficial part of the tooth anlagen whereas deeper parts including enamel knots and cervical loops were FZD6-negative (**Figure 1**).

FZD6 was also distributed in distinct areas of the mesenchyme surrounding epithelial thickenings during the early stages of odontogenesis; however, mesenchymal expression was downregulated and only small spots were visible on the mesenchymal cell surface at older stages. On the other hand, FZD6 was mostly expressed in the epithelium with uniform expression throughout the whole thickness of the oral epithelium. This finding is consistent with observations in FZD6 knockout mice, where numerous genes encoding keratins, keratin-associated proteins and transglutaminases and their substrates were significantly downregulated (Cui et al., 2013). Therefore, the mesenchymal expression pattern is dissimilar to the epithelial signal indicating distinct role of FZD signaling in the epithelium in contrast to the mesenchyme.

FZD6 Expression in the Successional Dental Lamina

During later stages of odontogenesis, the dental lamina protruded deeply into the mesenchyme and morphological changes were obvious in its superficial part (**Figure 2**). In the most superficial area, cells connecting the lamina to the oral epithelium were FZD6-positive (**Figures 2A,B, 3A,A′,B,B′**). Expression in superficial cells even increased following disconnection of the lamina from the oral epithelium (**Figures 2C, 3D,D′,E,E′**). Cells on the labial side separating from the lamina were strongly FZD6-positive similar to the stalk of very flat cells connecting the dental lamina to the tooth (**Figures 2A–C**). On the other hand, the apical tip of the successional lamina was FZD6-negative (**Figures 2A–D, 3C,C′,F,F′**). Therefore, there are significant differences in FZD6 expression through the dental lamina with higher expression maintained in its superficial layers.

While, the most distal tip of the successional dental lamina was FZD6-negative, β-catenin was previously described in the tip and lingual side of the dental lamina in snake and alligator (Wu et al., 2013) and transcription factor Lef1 (Wnt/β-catenin pathway target gene) in corn snake and python dental lamina (Handrigan

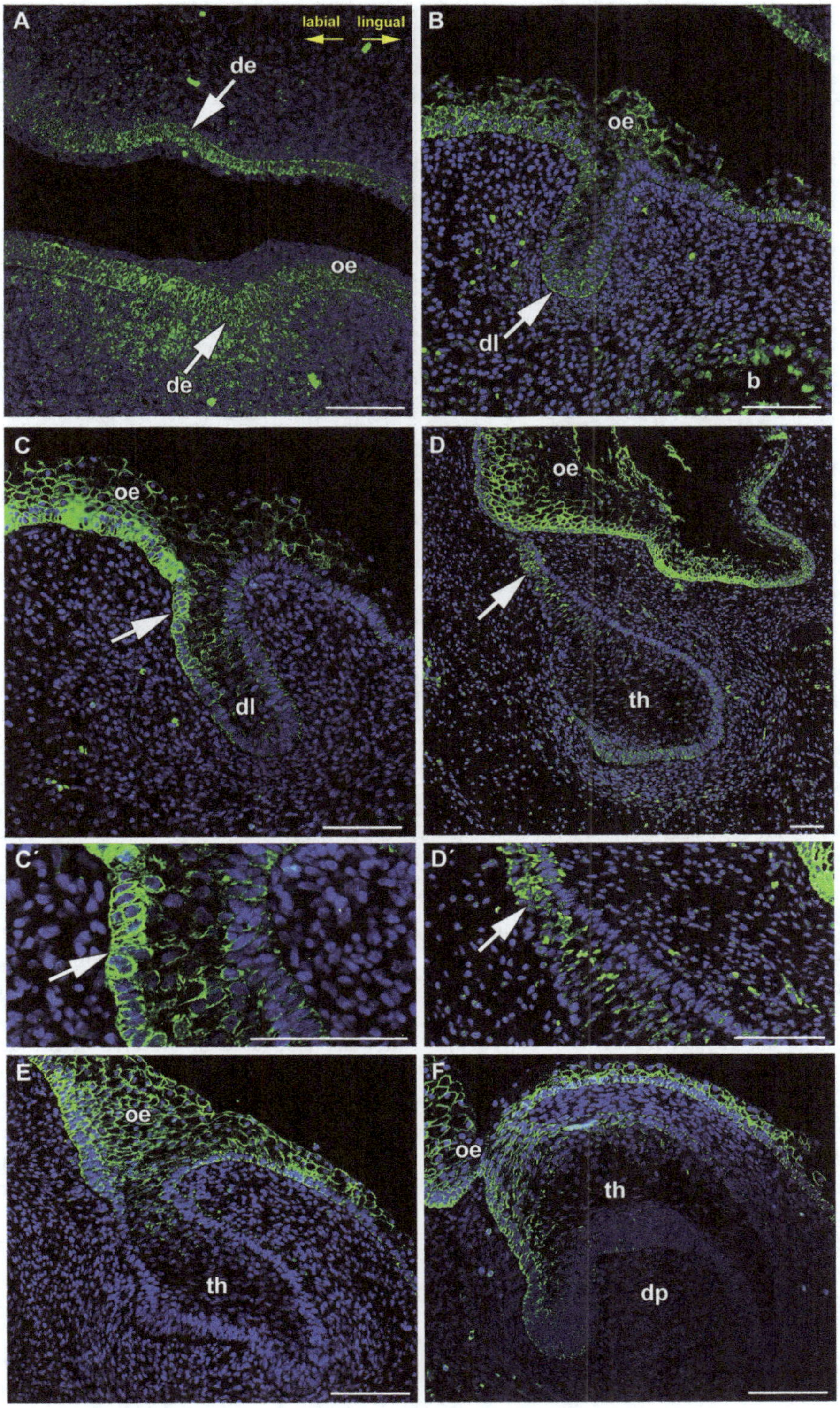

FIGURE 1 | FZD6 expression is asymmetrical in the dental lamina. (A) At epithelial thickening stage, the oral epithelium and surrounding mesenchyme are FZD6-positive. (**B,C,C′** in detail) Later, FZD6-positive signal is located on the labial side (arrow) of the protruding dental lamina. (**D,D′** in detail) At dental bud stage, stronger FZD6-immunopositivity (arrow) was detected on the labial side of dental germ. **(E,F)** At bell stage, the labial cervical loop is more positive that the lingual one. Almost no signal was visible in the stellate reticulum. The dental papilla and surrounding mesenchyme were FZD6-negative. b, bone; de, dental epithelium; dl, dental lamina; dp, dental papilla; oe, oral epithelium; th, tooth. Scale bar = 100 μm.

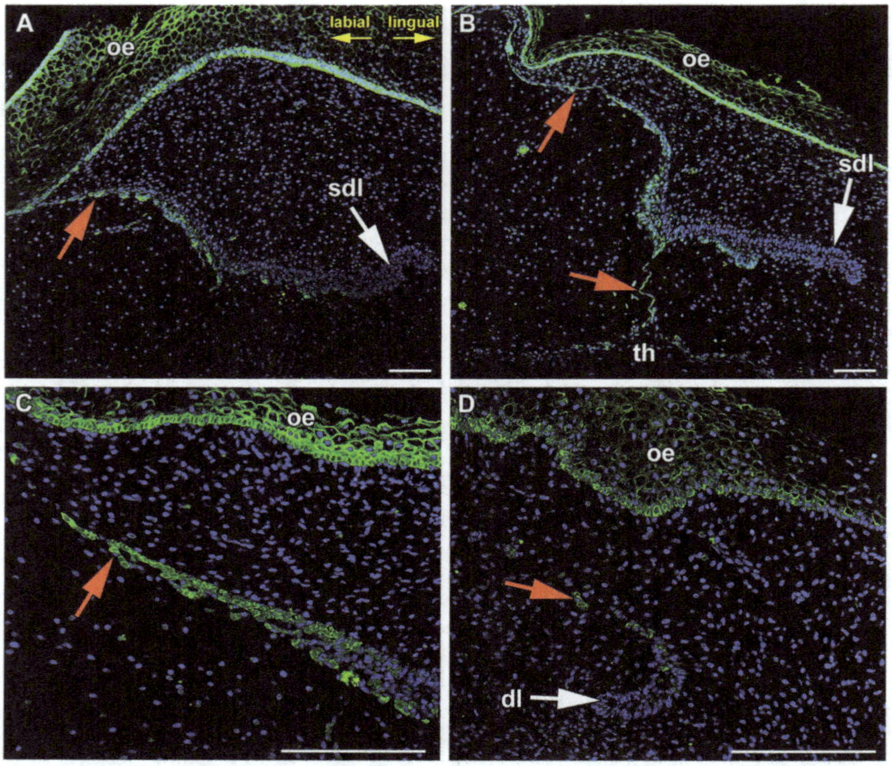

FIGURE 2 | The tip of growing successional dental lamina is FZD6-negative. (A) In the most superficial area, flat cells connecting the lamina to the oral epithelium were FZD6-positive. **(B)** Cells on the labial side separating from the lamina were also FZD-positive similarly to the stalk of very flat cells connecting the dental lamina to the tooth. However, the apical tip of the successional lamina was FZD6-negative. **(C)** When dental lamina disconnected from the oral epithelium, the stronger positivity of Fzd6 was evident in the superficial fragments and epithelial clusters of cells. **(D)** Rudimental interdental lamina exhibited only weak FZD6 expression. dl, dental lamina; oe, oral epithelium; sdl, successional dental lamina; th, tooth; red arrow, epithelial remnants. Scale bar = 100 μm.

and Richman, 2010; Gaete and Tucker, 2013). WNT ligands that signal through β-catenin are involved in stem/progenitor self-renewal and maintenance of cells in a proliferative and undifferentiated state while non-canonical signaling promotes their differentiation (Liu et al., 2009; Grumolato et al., 2010). As non-canonical signaling is known to inhibit WNT/β-catenin canonical signaling (Topol et al., 2003; Mikels and Nusse, 2006), this asymmetrical expression of non-canonical and canonical WNT molecules and the balance among them is critical for the regulation of dental progenitor cell lines similar to that shown in other systems (Grigoryan et al., 2008). Based on our evidence, FZD6 is not expressed in the areas of dental lamina with high cell proliferation or proposed localization of progenitor cells. Therefore, canonical and non-canonical WNT signaling exhibits distinct asymmetrical expression pattern through the lamina, which seems to be aligned with side-specific differences during successional dental lamina formation.

FZD6 Was Strongly Expressed in the Epithelial Remnants and Pearls during Dental Lamina Regression

The minipig similar to human has a diphyodont type of dentition, where only two generation of teeth are initiated. During embryonic period, the dental lamina undergoes major morphological changes and becomes thinner and disconnected from the oral epithelium. Cells are elongated in the superficial area of the dental lamina (Buchtová et al., 2012). Furthermore, they are elongated in the area of the dental stalk connecting the tooth anlagen to the dental lamina. After the dental lamina had disconnected from the oral epithelium, stronger expression of FZD6 was evident in the superficial epithelial cells. In deeper parts of the lamina, the expression of FZD6 was apparent on the side facing the tooth, which undergoes regression (**Figure 2C**). There were also differences in the level of expression along the jaw axis. In the area between teeth, rudimental interdental lamina exhibited only weak FZD6 expression located in the most superficial area (**Figure 2D**).

Later during dental lamina regression, the dental lamina become fragmented, and only occasional epithelial islands remain in the superficial area (**Figure 4A**). Some of these fragments undergo further morphological changes and epithelial pearls become visible along the jaw (Buchtová et al., 2012). Expression was also found in the epithelial clusters during the process of pearl formation (**Figure 4C**) as well as in the basal layer of already formed pearls (**Figure 4B**), while the central area was negative (**Figure 4D**).

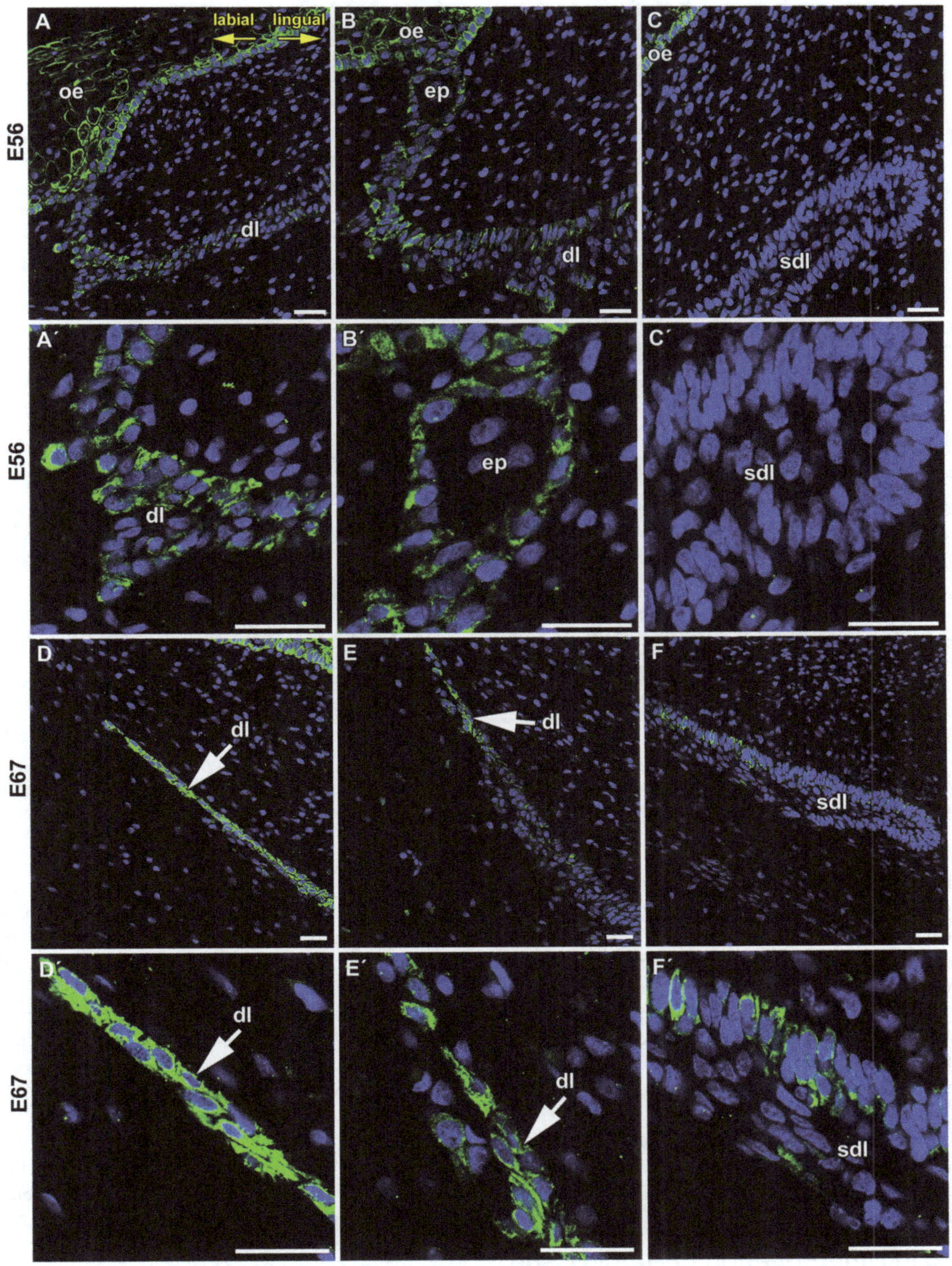

FIGURE 3 | Details of FZD6 expression in the dental lamina. (A,A′,B,B′) Stronger expression of FZD6 was observed in the superficial area of the dental lamina, which was still connected to the oral epithelium. **(C,C′)** No FZD6 expression was found in deeper successional dental lamina while spotted pattern of expression was observed in surrounding mesenchymal cells. **(D,D′)** Later in development, superficial part was disconnected from the oral epithelium and cells exhibited strong FZD6-positivity. **(E,E′)** Expression was gradually lost in the central part of the lamina. **(F,F′)** The tip of the successional lamina was negative similar to younger stage, only few positive cells were found in more superficial position. dl, dental lamina; ep, epithelial pearl; oe, oral epitheliuml; sdl, successional dental lamina. Scale bar = 25 μm.

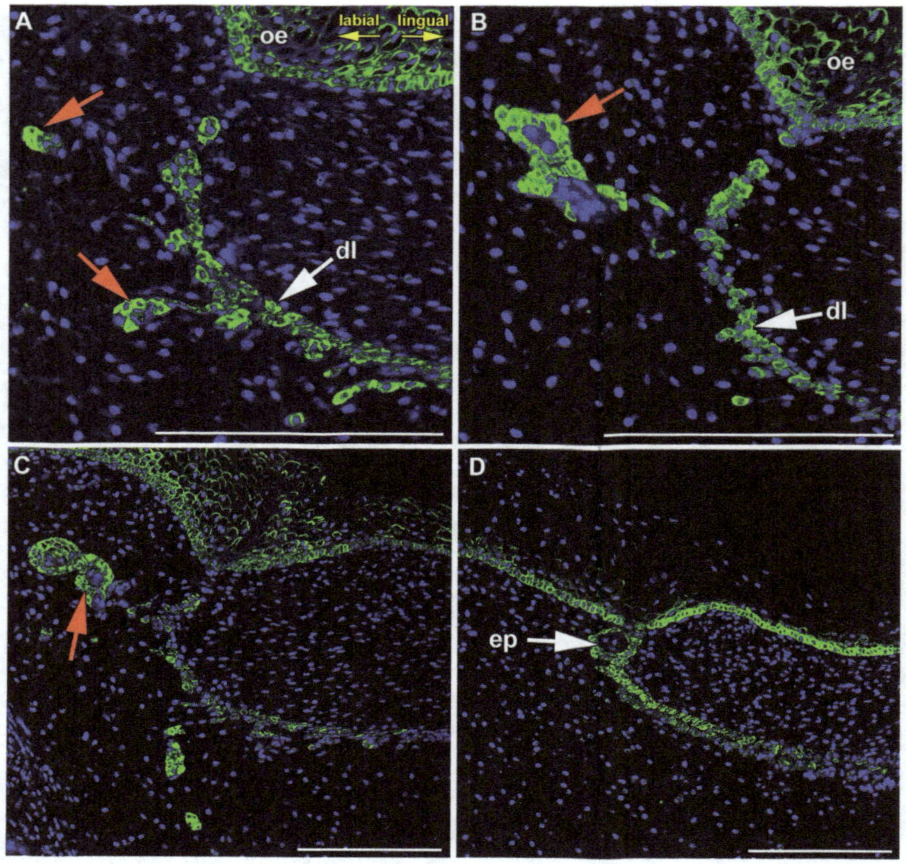

FIGURE 4 | FZD6 expression in epithelial remnants and pearls. (A,B) Localized and cytoplasmatic expression of FZD6 was found in epithelial remnants. **(C)** The expression was found in the epithelial clusters during process of pearl formation as well as in the basal layer of already formed pearls **(D)**, while their central area was negative. ep, epithelial pearl; red arrow, epithelial remnants. Scale bar = 100 μm.

Interestingly, distinct expression was obvious especially in the basal layers of the lamina epithelium facing the tooth where clusters of elongated cells were moving out of the dental lamina. The expression of FZD6 during lamina regression coincides with the upregulation of molecules involved in epithelial-mesenchymal transition of epithelial cells (Buchtová et al., 2012). Our observations that cells moving from the dental lamina are FZD6-positive is consistent with the previously known role of PCP proteins in notochord or somite cell elongation during their convergent extension (Keller et al., 2000; Keller, 2002; Seifert and Mlodzik, 2007) as well as regulation of cell polarity and directed motility during gastrulation in frogs and fish, and neural tube and eyelid closure in mammals (Wang et al., 2006; Seifert and Mlodzik, 2007).

Frizzled 6 in Differentiation of Hard-Tissue Producing Cells

Both canonical and non-canonical WNT pathways were previously shown to be involved in the differentiation of hard-tissue producing cells (Millar et al., 2003; Lin et al., 2011; Sakisaka et al., 2015). WNT signaling was shown to promote the differentiation of dental follicle cells into the cementoblast or osteoblast phenotype (Peng et al., 2010; Du et al., 2012; Sakisaka et al., 2015; Nemoto et al., 2016). Moreover, Wnt5a overexpression promotes the differentiation of dental papilla cells and increased the expression of mineralization-related genes (Peng et al., 2010).

In agreement with these findings, FZD6 expression was switched on during the differentiation of odontoblasts, ameloblasts, and osteoblasts in minipigs (**Figure 5**) at time when the production of hard tissues started. Differentiated and secretory ameloblasts were FZD6-positive while non-differentiated cells of the inner enamel epithelium were negative (**Figures 5A,A′**). A similar pattern was observed in the dental papilla where differentiated odontoblasts exhibiting dentin production were FZD6-positive (**Figures 5A,A′**). Almost no signal was found in the stellate reticulum or stratum intermedium (**Figure 5A**). On the other hand, the outer enamel epithelium was positive, especially the superficial clusters of cells during disruption of the enamel organ by blood vessels. FZD6 signal was also located in the structures surrounding teeth in the jaw such as alveolar bones, in which osteoblasts were positive (**Figures 5B,B′**) along with the secretory area of salivary glands or their ducts (**Figures 5C,C′**).

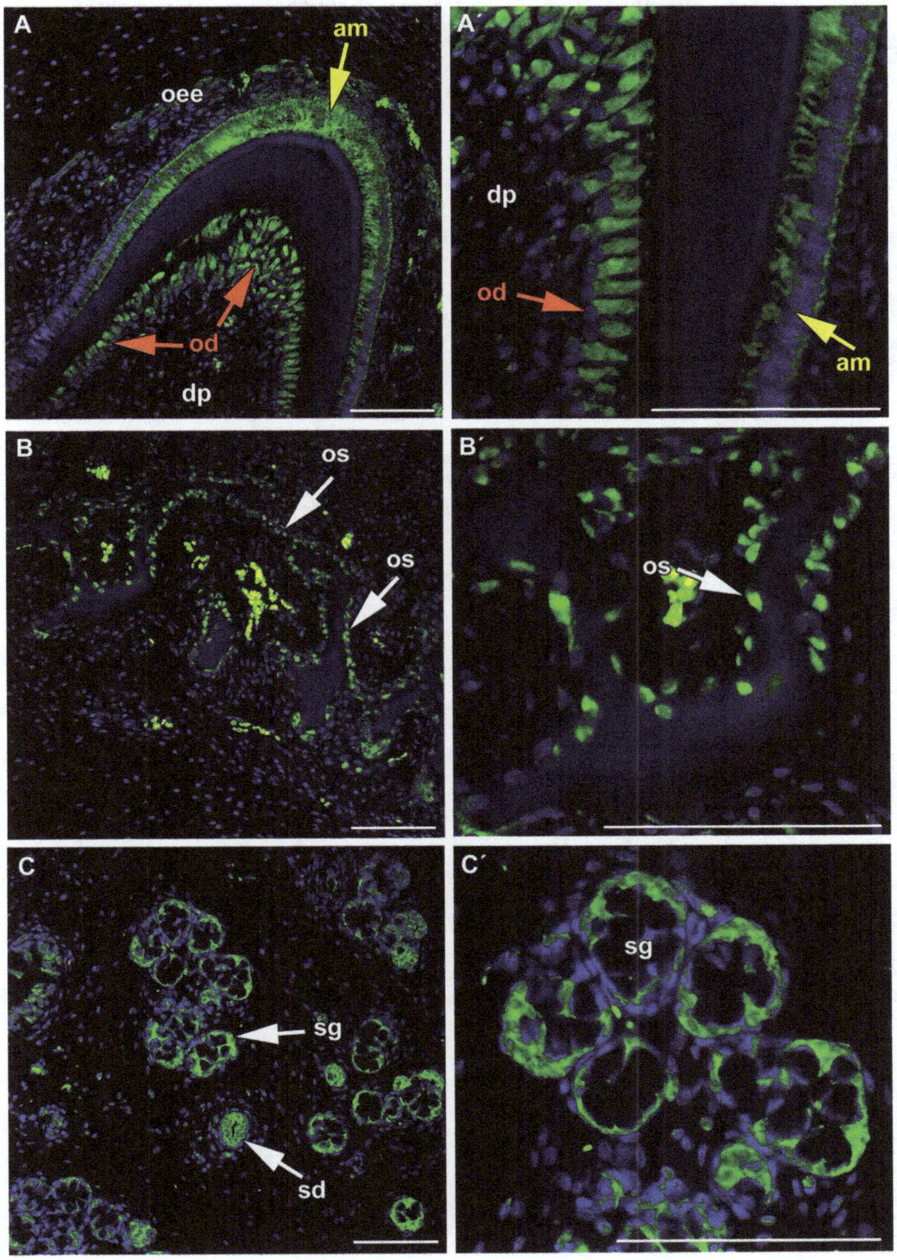

FIGURE 5 | FZD6 in differentiated ameloblasts and odontoblasts. (A,A′) Differentiated and secretory ameloblasts were FZD6-positive while non-differentiated cells of the inner enamel epithelium were negative. Similar pattern was observed in the dental papilla where differentiated odontoblasts exhibiting dentin production were FZD6-positive. FZD6 signal was localized at different stages of ameloblasts differentiation after their elongation. **(B,B′)** FZD6 signal was located also in the structures surrounding teeth such as alveolar bone where osteoblasts were positive and secretory cells of salivary gland or their ducts **(C,C′)**. am, ameloblast; dp, dental papilla; od, odontoblast; oee, outer enamel epithelium; sg, salivary gland. Scale bar = 100 μm.

While the tooth phenotype of FZD6 mutant mice has not yet been described, *Wnt5a*-deficient mice exhibit delayed odontoblast differentiation (Lin et al., 2011). Abnormal morphology of ameloblasts and defective odontoblast differentiation with absence of predentin formation were also found in *Ror2* mutant mice (Lin et al., 2011) in which ROR2 can serve as an alternative WNT receptor (Oishi et al., 2003). Odontoblasts in *Wnt5a*-deficient mice were shorter and thicker than in control animals. Similarly in *Ror2*-deficient mice, odontoblasts were polarized but appeared to be shorter in comparison to littermate control animals (Lin et al., 2011). While *Wnt5a* is expressed in the dental mesenchyme, its receptor is also expressed in the epithelium. It was proposed that another receptor must be involved in WNT5a-mediated signaling as

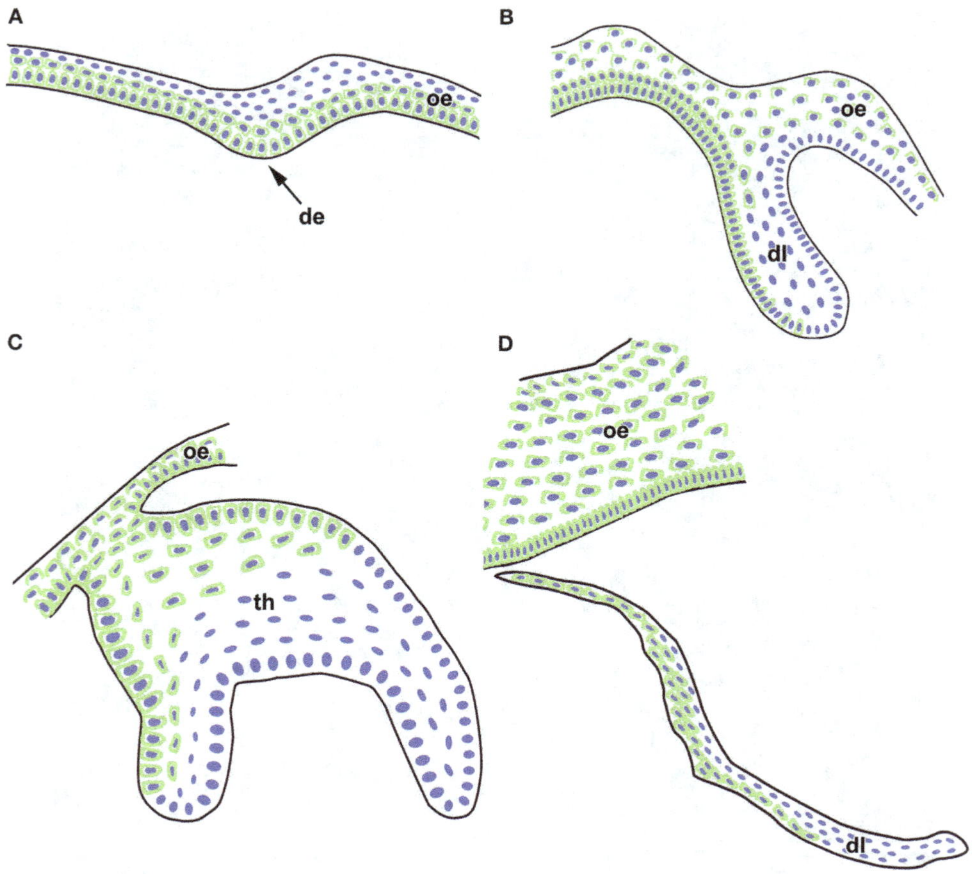

FIGURE 6 | Schema of FZD6 protein expression through odontogenesis. (A) At the epithelial thickening stage, a strong FZD6 signal was apparent especially in basal layers of the oral and future dental epithelium. **(B)** Later, FZD6-positivity was detected in the dental lamina with stronger expression on the labial side. **(C)** At the bell stage, distinct expression was found throughout the oral epithelium and in the labial cervical loop area. Almost no signal was visible in the stellate reticulum. **(D)** The tip of successional dental lamina was FZD6-negative while cells in the superficial part of the lamina were FZD6-positive. Nuclei are labeled by blue and FZD6 expression in green through the epithelial tissues. de, dental epithelium; dl, dental lamina; oe, oral epithelium; th, tooth.

defects in tooth development in *Ror2* mutants occur much later than observed in WNT5a-deficient mice (Lin et al., 2011). Based on our observations, FZD6 could be one of these receptors.

Odontoblasts and ameloblasts are highly polarized cells with a characteristic morphology and arrangement of cellular compartments. In odontoblasts, FZD6 was expressed asymmetrically only on the side facing the dentin (**Figures 5A,A′**). In ameloblasts, FZD6 was observed on both sides of differentiated cells, and later, the signal showed a more uniform distribution through the cells. Differentiation of ameloblasts and odontoblasts is characterized by elongation of the cells and establishment of their polarity. Actin filament bundles exhibit a polarized distribution in rat ameloblasts and are abundant at the ameloblast junction area (Nishikawa and Kitamura, 1985, 1986). As actin cytoskeleton organization is downstream of the PCP signaling pathway, it is possible that FZD6 can be involved in the rearrangement of cellular polarity in the odontoblasts and ameloblasts during their differentiation.

CONCLUSIONS

In summary, FZD6 was expressed asymmetrically in the dental lamina at early as well as late stages of diphyodont dentition (**Figure 6**). We observed significant differences in the level of FZD6 expression in distinct areas of the dental lamina with stronger expression in the labial and superficial parts (**Figure 6**). The apical tip of the successional lamina was FZD6-negative. During dental lamina regression, labial cells separating from the lamina were strongly FZD6-positive similar to the stalk of very flat cells connecting the dental lamina to the tooth germ. On the other hand, FZD6 was not expressed in the areas of dental lamina with high cell proliferation or proposed localization of progenitor cells.

FZD6 expression was also switched on during the differentiation of odontoblasts, ameloblasts, and osteoblasts in minipigs at time when the production of hard tissues started. In odontoblasts, FZD6 was expressed asymmetrically only on the side facing the dentin therefore it is possible that FZD6 can be involved in the establishment of cellular polarity in the odontoblasts during their differentiation. However, the exact role of FZD6 in the growth directionality of the lamina and differentiation of hard tissue producing cells has to be proven experimentally in future.

AUTHOR CONTRIBUTIONS

MB and VB designed the project. IP, HD, ML, and JS performed and interpreted experiments. IP, MB, and JS wrote manuscript with contribution of VB. All authors approved the manuscript.

ACKNOWLEDGMENTS

This study was supported by the Czech Science Foundation (14-29273P to IP and JS) and Grant Agency of the University of Veterinary and Pharmaceutical Sciences Brno (108/2015/FVL to HD), Masaryk University (MUNI/A/0988/2016) and institutional support (RVO:67985904). This contribution is free of conflict of interest.

REFERENCES

Borello, U., Buffa, V., Sonnino, C., Melchionna, R., Vivarelli, E., and Cossu, G. (1999). Differential expression of the Wnt putative receptors Frizzled during mouse somitogenesis. *Mech. Dev.* 89, 173–177. doi: 10.1016/S0925-4773(99)00205-1

Buchtová, M., Stembirek, J., Glocová, K., Matalová, E., and Tucker, A. S. (2012). Early regression of the dental lamina underlies the development of diphyodont dentitions. *J. Dent. Res.* 91, 491–498. doi: 10.1177/0022034512442896

Cai, J., Mutoh, N., Shin, J. O., Tani-Ishii, N., Ohshima, H., Cho, S. W., et al. (2011). Wnt5a plays a crucial role in determining tooth size during murine tooth development. *Cell Tissue Res.* 345, 367–377. doi: 10.1007/s00441-011-1224-4

Chang, H., Smallwood, P. M., Williams, J., and Nathans, J. (2016). The spatio-temporal domains of Frizzled6 action in planar polarity control of hair follicle orientation. *Dev. Biol.* 409, 181–193. doi: 10.1016/j.ydbio.2015.10.027

Chien, A. J., Conrad, W. H., and Moon, R. T. (2009). A Wnt survival guide: from flies to human disease. *J. Invest. Dermatol.* 129, 1614–1627. doi: 10.1038/jid.2008.445

Cui, C. Y., Klar, J., Georgii-Heming, P., Fröjmark, A. S., Baig, S. M., Schlessinger, D., et al. (2013). Frizzled6 deficiency disrupts the differentiation process of nail development. *J. Invest. Dermatol.* 133, 1990–1997. doi: 10.1038/jid.2013.84

Dijksterhuis, J. P., Petersen, J., and Schulte, G. (2016). WNT/Frizzled signalling: receptor-ligand selectivity with focus on FZD-G protein signalling and its physiological relevance: IUPHAR Review 3. *Br. J. Pharmacol.* 171, 1195–1209. doi: 10.1111/bph.12364

Du, Y., Ling, J., Wei, X., Ning, Y., Xie, N., Gu, H., et al. (2012). Wnt/β-catenin signaling participates in cementoblast/osteoblast differentiation of dental follicle cells. *Connect. Tissue Res.* 53, 390–397. doi: 10.3109/03008207.2012.668980

Fischer, T., Guimera, J., Wurst, W., and Prakash, N. (2007). Distinct but redundant expression of the Frizzled Wnt receptor genes at signaling centers of the developing mouse brain. *Neuroscience* 147, 693–711. doi: 10.1016/j.neuroscience.2007.04.060

Fröjmark, A. S., Schuster, J., Sobol, M., Entesarian, M., Kilander, M. B., Gabrikova, D., et al. (2011). Mutations in Frizzled 6 cause isolated autosomal-recessive nail dysplasia. *Am. J. Hum. Genet.* 88, 852–860. doi: 10.1016/j.ajhg.2011.05.013

Gaete, M., and Tucker, A. S. (2013). Organized emergence of multiple-generations of teeth in snakes is dysregulated by activation of Wnt/β-catenin signalling. *PLoS ONE* 8:e74484. doi: 10.1371/journal.pone.0074484

Grigoryan, T., Wend, P., Klaus, A., and Birchmeier, W. (2008). Deciphering the function of canonical Wnt signals in development and disease: conditional loss- and gain-of-function mutations of β-catenin in mice. *Genes Dev.* 22, 2308–2341. doi: 10.1101/gad.1686208

Grumolato, L., Liu, G., Mong, P., Mudbhary, R., Biswas, R., Arroyave, R., et al. (2010). Canonical and noncanonical Wnts use a common mechanism to activate completely unrelated coreceptors. *Genes Dev.* 24, 2517–2530. doi: 10.1101/gad.1957710

Gubb, D., and García-Bellido, A. (1982). A genetic analysis of the determination of cuticular polarity during development in Drosophila melanogaster. *J. Embryol. Exp. Morphol.* 68, 37–57.

Guo, N., Hawkins, C., and Nathans, J. (2004). Frizzled6 controls hair patterning in mice. *Proc. Natl. Acad. Sci. U.S.A.* 101, 9277–9281. doi: 10.1073/pnas.0402802101

Handrigan, G. R., and Richman, J. M. (2010). A network of Wnt, hedgehog and BMP signaling pathways regulates tooth replacement in snakes. *Dev. Biol.* 348, 130–141. doi: 10.1016/j.ydbio.2010.09.003

Keller, R. (2002). Shaping the vertebrate body plan by polarized embryonic cell movements. *Science* 298, 1950–1954. doi: 10.1126/science.1079478

Keller, R., Davidson, L., Edlund, A., Elul, T., Ezin, M., Shook, D., et al. (2000). Mechanisms of convergence and extension by cell intercalation. *Philos. Trans. R. Soc. Lond. B Biol. Sci.* 355, 897–922. doi: 10.1098/rstb.2000.0626

Kilian, B., Mansukoski, H., Barbosa, F. C., Ulrich, F., Tada, M., and Heisenberg, C. P. (2003). The role of Ppt/Wnt5 in regulating cell shape and movement during zebrafish gastrulation. *Mech. Dev.* 120, 467–476. doi: 10.1016/S0925-4773(03)00004-2

Lin, M., Li, L., Liu, C., Liu, H., He, F., Yan, F., et al. (2011). Wnt5a regulates growth, patterning, and odontoblast differentiation of developing mouse tooth. *Dev. Dyn.* 240, 432–440. doi: 10.1002/dvdy.22550

Liu, G., Vijayakumar, S., Grumolato, L., Arroyave, R., Qiao, H., Akiri, G., et al. (2009). Canonical Wnts function as potent regulators of osteogenesis by human mesenchymal stem cells. *J. Cell Biol.* 185, 67–75. doi: 10.1083/jcb.200810137

Logan, C. Y., and Nusse, R. (2004). The Wnt signaling pathway in development and disease. *Annu. Rev. Cell Dev. Biol.* 20, 781–810. doi: 10.1146/annurev.cellbio.20.010403.113126

Mikels, A. J., and Nusse, R. (2006). Purified Wnt5a protein activates or inhibits β-catenin-TCF signaling depending on receptor context. *PLoS Biol.* 4:e115. doi: 10.1371/journal.pbio.0040115

Millar, S. E., Koyama, E., Reddy, S. T., Andl, T., Gaddapara, T., Piddington, R., et al. (2003). Over- and ectopic expression of Wnt3 causes progressive loss of ameloblasts in postnatal mouse incisor teeth. *Connect. Tissue Res.* 44(Suppl. 1), 124–129. doi: 10.1080/03008200390152205

Mitsiadis, T. A., and Luder, H. U. (2011). Genetic basis for tooth malformations: from mice to men and back again. *Clin. Genet.* 80, 319–329. doi: 10.1111/j.1399-0004.2011.01762.x

Moon, R. T., Campbell, R. M., Christian, J. L., McGrew, L. L., Shih, J., and Fraser, S. (1993). Xwnt-5A: a maternal Wnt that affects morphogenetic movements after overexpression in embryos of *Xenopus laevis*. *Development* 119, 97–111.

Naz, G., Pasternack, S. M., Perrin, C., Mattheisen, M., Refke, M., Khan, S., et al. (2012). FZD6 encoding the Wnt receptor frizzled 6 is mutated in autosomal-recessive nail dysplasia. *Br. J. Dermatol.* 166, 1088–1094. doi: 10.1111/j.1365-2133.2011.10800.x

Nemoto, E., Sakisaka, Y., Tsuchiya, M., Tamura, M., Nakamura, T., Kanaya, S., et al. (2016). Wnt3a signaling induces murine dental follicle cells to differentiate into cementoblastic/osteoblastic cells via an osterix-dependent pathway. *J. Periodont. Res.* 51, 164–174. doi: 10.1111/jre.12294

Nishikawa, S., and Kitamura, H. (1985). Three-dimensional network of microtubules in secretory ameloblasts of rat incisors. *Arch. Oral Biol.* 30, 1–11.

Nishikawa, S., and Kitamura, H. (1986). Localization of actin during differentiation of the ameloblast, its related epithelial cells and odontoblasts in the rat incisor using NBD-phallacidin. *Differentiation* 30, 237–243.

Oishi, I., Suzuki, H., Onishi, N., Takada, R., Kani, S., Ohkawara, B., et al. (2003). The receptor tyrosine kinase Ror2 is involved in non-canonical Wnt5a/JNK signalling pathway. *Genes Cells* 8, 645–654. doi: 10.1046/j.1365-2443.2003.00662.x

Peng, L., Ren, L. B., Dong, G., Wang, C. L., Xu, P., Ye, L., et al. (2010). Wnt5a promotes differentiation of human dental papilla cells. *Int. Endod. J.* 43, 404–412. doi: 10.1111/j.1365-2591.2010.01693.x

Sakisaka, Y., Tsuchiya, M., Nakamura, T., Tamura, M., Shimauchi, H., and Nemoto, E. (2015). Wnt5a attenuates Wnt3a-induced alkaline phosphatase expression in dental follicle cells. *Exp. Cell Res.* 336, 85–93. doi: 10.1016/j.yexcr.2015.06.013

Sarkar, L., Cobourne, M., Naylor, S., Smalley, M., Dale, T., and Sharpe, P. T. (2000). Wnt/Shh interactions regulate ectodermal boundary formation during mammalian tooth development. *Proc. Natl. Acad. Sci. U.S.A.* 97, 4520–4524. doi: 10.1073/pnas.97.9.4520

Sarkar, L., and Sharpe, P. T. (1999). Expression of Wnt signalling pathway genes during tooth development. *Mech. Dev.* 85, 197–200. doi: 10.1016/S0925-4773(99)00095-7

Schulte, G., and Bryja, V. (2007). The Frizzled family of unconventional G-protein-coupled receptors. *Trends Pharmacol Sci.* 28, 518–525. doi: 10.1016/j.tips.2007.09.001

Seifert, J. R., and Mlodzik, M. (2007). Frizzled/PCP signalling: a conserved mechanism regulating cell polarity and directed motility. *Nat. Rev. Genet.* 8, 126–138. doi: 10.1038/nrg2042

Simons, M., and Mlodzik, M. (2008). Planar cell polarity signaling: from fly development to human disease. *Annu. Rev. Genet.* 42, 517–540. doi: 10.1146/annurev.genet.42.110807.091432

Thesleff, I. (2003). Epithelial-mesenchymal signalling regulating tooth morphogenesis. *J. Cell Sci.* 116, 1647–1648. doi: 10.1242/jcs.00410

Thesleff, I., Vaahtokari, A., Kettunen, P., and Aberg, T. (1995). Epithelial-mesenchymal signaling during tooth development. *Connect. Tissue Res.* 32, 9–15. doi: 10.3109/03008209509013700

Topol, L., Jiang, X., Choi, H., Garrett-Beal, L., Carolan, P. J., and Yang, Y. (2003). Wnt-5a inhibits the canonical Wnt pathway by promoting GSK-3-independent β-catenin degradation. *J. Cell Biol.* 162, 899–908. doi: 10.1083/jcb.200303158

Vinson, C. R., Conover, S., and Adler, P. N. (1989). A Drosophila tissue polarity locus encodes a protein containing seven potential transmembrane domains. *Nature* 338, 263–264. doi: 10.1038/338263a0

Wang, B., Li, H., Liu, Y., Lin, X., Lin, Y., Wang, Y., et al. (2014). Expression patterns of WNT/β-CATENIN signaling molecules during human tooth development. *J. Mol. Histol.* 45, 487–496. doi: 10.1007/s10735-014-9572-5

Wang, Y., Badea, T., and Nathans, J. (2006). Order from disorder: self-organization in mammalian hair patterning. *Proc. Natl. Acad. Sci. U.S.A.* 103, 19800–19805. doi: 10.1073/pnas.0609712104

Wang, Y., Chang, H., and Nathans, J. (2010). When whorls collide: the development of hair patterns in frizzled 6 mutant mice. *Development* 137, 4091–4099. doi: 10.1242/dev.057455

Wang, Y., Chang, H., Rattner, A., and Nathans, J. (2016). Frizzled receptors in development and disease. *Curr. Top. Dev. Biol.* 117, 113–139. doi: 10.1016/bs.ctdb.2015.11.028

Wang, Y., Guo, N., and Nathans, J. (2006). The role of Frizzled3 and Frizzled6 in neural tube closure and in the planar polarity of inner-ear sensory hair cells. *J. Neurosci.* 26, 2147–2156. doi: 10.1523/JNEUROSCI.4698-05.2005

Wu, P., Wu, X., Jiang, T. X., Elsey, R. M., Temple, B. L., Divers, S. J., et al. (2013). Specialized stem cell niche enables repetitive renewal of alligator teeth. *Proc. Natl. Acad. Sci. U.S.A.* 110, E2009–E2018. doi: 10.1073/pnas.1213202110

16

A Critical Role of TRPM7 as an Ion Channel Protein in Mediating the Mineralization of the Craniofacial Hard Tissues

*Yukiko Nakano[1,2], Michael H. Le[1], Dawud Abduweli[1], Sunita P. Ho[3], Lillia V. Ryazanova[4], Zhixian Hu[4], Alexey G. Ryazanov[4], Pamela K. Den Besten[1,2] and Yan Zhang[1,2]**

[1] Department of Orofacial Sciences, University of California, San Francisco, San Francisco, CA, USA, [2] Center for Children's Oral Health Research, University of California, San Francisco, San Francisco, CA, USA, [3] Preventive and Restorative Dental Sciences, University of California, San Francisco, San Francisco, CA, USA, [4] Department of Pharmacology, Robert Wood Johnson Medical School, Piscataway, NJ, USA

***Correspondence:**
Yan Zhang
yan.zhang2@ucsf.edu

Magnesium ion (Mg^{2+}) is the fourth most common cation in the human body, and has a crucial role in many physiological functions. Mg^{2+} homeostasis is an important contributor to bone development, however, its roles in the development of dental mineralized tissues have not yet been well known. We identified that transient receptor potential cation channel, subfamily M, member 7 (TRPM7), was significantly upregulated in the mature ameloblasts as compared to other ameloblasts through our whole transcript microarray analyses of the ameloblasts. TRPM7, an ion channel for divalent metal cations with an intrinsic serine/threonine protein kinase activity, has been characterized as a key regulator of whole body Mg^{2+} homeostasis. Semi-quantitative PCR and immunostaining for TRMP7 confirmed its upregulation during the maturation stage of enamel formation, at which ameloblasts direct rapid mineralization of the enamel matrix. The significantly hypomineralized craniofacial structures, including incisors, molars, and cranial bones were demonstrated by microCT analysis, von Kossa and trichrome staining in *Trpm7*$^{\Delta kinase/+}$ mice. A previously generated heterozygous mouse model with the deletion of the TRPM7 kinase domain. Interestingly, the skeletal phenotype of *Trpm7*$^{\Delta kinase/+}$ mice resembled those found in the tissue-nonspecific alkaline phosphatase (*Alpl*) KO mice, thus we further examined whether ALPL protein content and alkaline phosphatase (ALPase) activity in ameloblasts, odontoblasts and osteoblasts were affected in those mice. While ALPL protein in *Trpm7*$^{\Delta kinase/+}$ mice remained at the similar level as that in *wt* mice, ALPase activities in the *Trpm7*$^{\Delta kinase/+}$ mice were almost nonexistent. Supplemented magnesium successfully rescued the activities of ALPase in ameloblasts, odontoblasts and osteoblasts of *Trpm7*$^{\Delta kinase/+}$ mice. These results suggested that TRPM7 is essential for mineralization of enamel as well as dentin and bone by providing sufficient Mg^{2+} for the ALPL activity, underlining the key importance of ALPL for biomineralization.

Keywords: TRPM7, enamel, dentin, bone, ion transport, biomineralization, alkaline phosphatase, magnesium homeostasis

INTRODUCTION

Magnesium is the fourth most common cation in the human body, and is the second most abundant cellular cation (Romani, 2011). Intracellularly, by binding to the enzymes, magnesium functions as an essential activator of enzymes (Cowan, 2002; Maguire and Cowan, 2002; Sreedhara and Cowan, 2002), and by binding to nucleic acids, it contributes to the second messenger systems and modification of nucleic acid structure (Neitzel et al., 1991; Barciszewska et al., 2001). Moreover, it binds to cellular membrane components, including ion channels, and affects fluidity and permeability of molecules (Wolf and Cittadini, 2003; Wolf et al., 2003). Magnesium deficiency in humans is known to be associated with skeletal diseases, including hypocalcemia and osteoporosis, due to impaired parathyroid hormone (PTH) secretion, renal and skeletal resistance to PTH and vitamin D, and increasing inflammatory cytokines, like interleukin (IL) -1 and tumor necrosis factor (TNF) -α (Weglicki et al., 1996; Rude and Gruber, 2004; Rude et al., 2004; Rude and Shils, 2006). In animal models treated with low Mg^{2+} diet, dentin and enamel mineralization defects are reported (Irving, 1940; Bernick and Hungerford, 1965; Trowbridge et al., 1971).

Transient receptor potential melastatin-subfamily member 7 (TRPM7) is a permeable ion channel for divalent metal cations, preferentially permitting the flow of Mg^{2+} and Ca^{2+} (Nadler et al., 2001; Monteilh-Zoller et al., 2003; Penner and Fleig, 2007). TRPM7 has an essential role in the regulation of both cellular and whole body Mg^{2+} homeostasis, modulating fundamental cellular processes including cell division, growth, survival, differentiation, and migration (Ryazanova et al., 2010; Yee et al., 2014). The c-terminus of TRPM7 is a serine/threonine-protein kinase domain which functions as an intracellular sensor of magnesium status, and thus, provides coordination of cellular and systemic responses to magnesium deprivation (Ryazanova et al., 2014). In the whole body, TRPM7 is ubiquitously expressed and homozygous deletion of TRPM7 kinase domain is embryonic lethal, indicating that this molecule has a fundamental and non-redundant role in cellular physiology (Nadler et al., 2001; Ryazanova et al., 2010). Heterozygous KO mice for TRPM7 kinase domain ($Trpm7^{\Delta kinase/+}$ mice) are viable, but there is a change in magnesium homeostasis or hypomagnesemia-like phenotype. Sensitivity to intracellular Mg^{2+} levels is a critical mechanism to regulate the Mg^{2+} influx through TRPM7 channel into the cells, and the $Trpm7^{\Delta kinase/+}$ mice shows increased sensitivity to the inhibition by Mg^{2+} (Ryazanova et al., 2010, 2014).

Although, the magnesium deficiency is known to cause skeletal and tooth defects, the role of TRPM7 in hard tissue formation including the tooth mineralization has not been determined. Through, two whole transcript microarray analyses of varying stages of differentiating ameloblasts, we found that *Trpm7* was upregulated in secretory ameloblasts as compared to presecretory ameloblasts (GEO accession number GSE59214; Liu et al., 2015), and in maturation as compared to secretory ameloblasts (GEO accession number GSE57224; Zhang et al., 2014). Taking into consideration the significance of the maturation stage in enamel formation, where the majority of enamel mineralization occurs (Robinson et al., 1995; Smith, 1998), together with the importance of intracellular Mg^{2+} homeostasis in the skeletogenesis, we hypothesize that TRPM7 potentially contributes to the enamel matrix mineralization. In this study, we therefore confirmed the expression and synthesis of TRPM7 in differentiating ameloblasts, and further investigated the function of TRPM7 associated with the mineralization of craniofacial hard tissues using $Trpm7^{\Delta kinase/+}$ mice model. We determined a relationship of TRPM7 and tissue-nonspecific alkaline phosphatase activity to critically regulate the mineralization of craniofacial hard tissue.

METHODS

Animals

All animal procedures were performed upon the approval by the Institutional Animal Care and Use Committee (IACUC) of the University of California, San Francisco and Rutgers Robert Wood Johnson Medical School, and adhered to the principles outlined in the National Institutes of Health Guide for the Care and Use of Laboratory Animals. $Trpm7^{\Delta kinase/+}$ and *wt* mice were provided by Dr. Alexey G. Ryazanov (Rutgers Robert Wood Johnson Medical School). As previously described, $Trpm7^{\Delta kinase/+}$ mice were genetically modified by replacing exons 32–36 of *Trpm7* gene, the kinase domain, with the Neo gene cassette (Ryazanova et al., 2010). At postnatal day 14 days, mice were euthanized, and whole heads were dissected out and fixed with 4% paraformaldehyde (PFA) overnight.

C57BL/6J female mice were maintained at the UCSF animal facility. At postnatal day 0 (P0), 5 (P5), and 10 (P10), mice were euthanized, developing first molars were harvested and processed for total RNA extraction. For immunohistochemical staining, 7-week old female C57BL/6J mice were anesthetized with 240 mg/kg tribromoethanol (Sigma-Aldrich, St. Louis, MO), fixed with 4% PFA for overnight.

Total RNA Extraction and Semi-Quantitative PCR (qPCR)

Total RNA was purified from developing molar tooth organ using the RNeasy Mini kit (Qiagen, Germantown, MD). The tooth organs were not homogenized therefore RNA would be primarily extracted from the exposed enamel epithelium overlying the tooth bud. cDNA was obtained by reverse transcription of the mRNA using Superscript III First-Strand Synthesis Supermix for qRT-PCR (Life Technologies, Grand Island, NY).

Expression of *Trpm7* was examined by semi-quantitative PCR with FastStart Universal SYBR Green Master Kit (Roche Diagnostics, Indianapolis, IN) using the ABI 7500 system (Applied Biosystems, Foster City, CA). The primer sequences for *Trpm7* are: sense 5′-ATGGCACTGTTGGAAAGTATGG-3′, antisense 5′-CGCCTTCAAATATCAAAGCCAC-3′; *Eef1a1* was used as a reference gene, the primer sequences are: sense 5′-CAA CAT CGT CGT AAT CGG ACA-3′, antisense 5′-GTC TAA GAC CCA GGC GTA CTT-3′. The expression levels of target gene was analyzed using the ΔΔCt method (Livak and Schmittgen, 2001). The relative expression levels of *Trpm7* of P5 and P10 enamel organs were calculated based on the expression levels of P0 enamel organs. Significance of differences was determined using ΔCT values by the multiple *t*-test with Bonferroni correction following ANOVA (Baker et al., 2006; Yuan et al., 2006).

Micro-Computed Tomography (MICROCT)

Whole heads from *wt* and $Trpm7^{\Delta kinase/+}$ mice were fixed in 4% PFA overnight, and then imaged using a Micro XCT-200 system (Xradia, Pleasanton, CA). All scans were done at an operating voltage of 90 KVp and 66 μA of current, at an optical magnification 2x. A binning of 2 was used for 3D image reconstruction. All scans were done using the same experimental settings, including the distances between specimen, detector, and source. Virtual sections were converted to bmp images using the Xradia TXM3DViewer 1.1.6. software. Appropriate imaging planes were selected from three orthogonal sections centered at a level containing an entire sagittal slice of the incisor or entire frontal slice of the first molar containing the mesial and buccal cusps and mesial root inside the reconstructed space using Xradia TXM3DViewer 1.1.6. software.

Immunohistochemistry

The mandibles and maxillae were decalcified in 8% EDTA (pH 7.3) at 4°C for 2 wks (7-week-old C57BL/6J mice) or 1 wk (*wt* and $Trpm7^{\Delta kinase/+}$ mice). The jaws were further dehydrated through a graded series of ethanol, followed by a routine paraffin embedding. The paraffin blocks were sectioned at the thickness of 5 μm. After dewaxing, the sections used for TRPM7 immunostaining were subjected to the antigen retrieval in 1% SDS in 0.1 M Tris-HCL buffer (pH 9.0) for 5 mins at room temperature (Brown et al., 1996; Emoto et al., 2005), and then treated with 1% H_2O_2 for 5 min at room temperature. Afterward, all sections were incubated with the blocking reagent containing 10% swine and 5% goat sera for 2 h at room temperature followed by an incubation with either rabbit anti-TRPM7 antibody (Abcam, Cambridge, United Kingdom) overnight at 4°C or rabbit anti-human ALPL (Abcam) antibody overnight at 4°C. Sections were further incubated with biotin conjugated swine anti-rabbit F(ab')$_2$ secondary antibody (Dako Denmark A/S, Glostrup, Denmark) for 1 h at room temperature. Next, the sections incubated with anti-TRPM7 antibody were incubated with intestinal alkaline phosphatase (ALPase) conjugated streptavidin (Vector Laboratories Inc., Burlingame, CA) for 30 mins, and immunoreactivity was visualized using a Vector® Red kit (Vector Laboratories Inc.) resulting in pink/red color for positive staining. To block the endogenous tissue-nonspecific ALPase activity, 1 mM levamisole was added to the visualization reagent. The sections incubated with anti-ALPL antibody were incubated with horseradish peroxidase (HRP) conjugated streptavidin (Vector Laboratories Inc.) for 30 mins, and immunoreactivity was visualized using an ImmPACT tM DAB peroxidase substrate kit

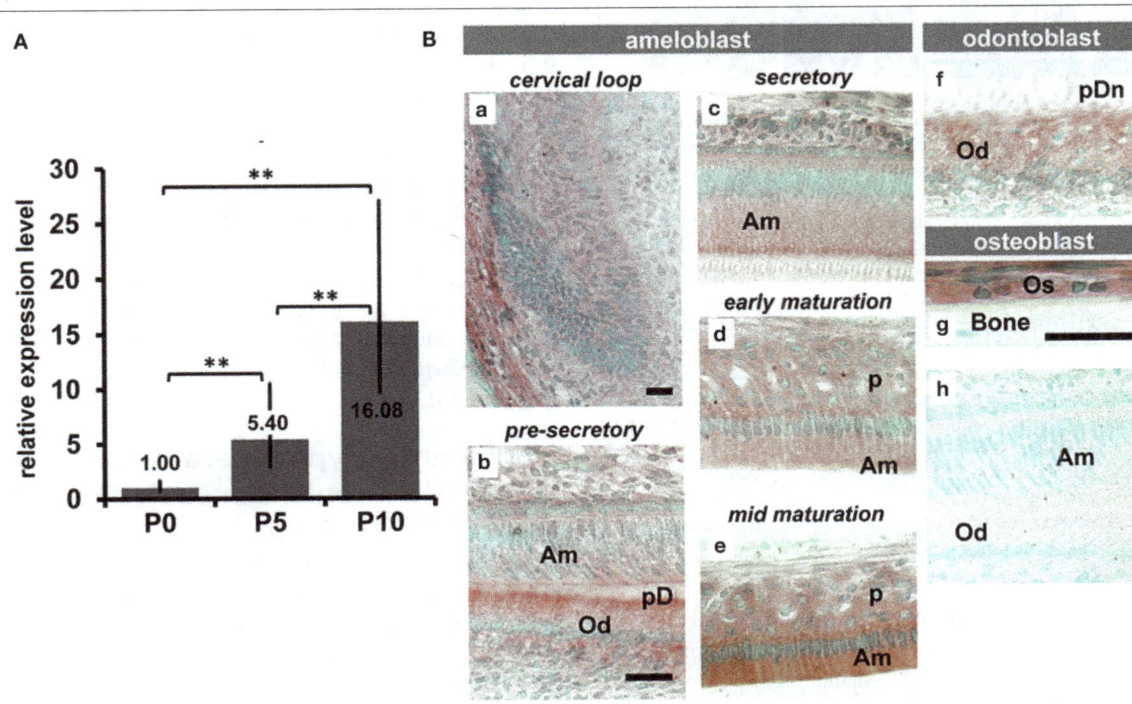

FIGURE 1 | The expression pattern of TRPM7 in craniofacial hard tissue forming cells. (A) Semi quantitive PCR analysis showed that the expression levels of TRPM7 mRNA in mouse molar enamel organ progressively increased from pre-secretoy stage (P0) to secretory stage (P5) and to early maturation stage (P10) (**$P < 0.01$). **(B)** Immunohistochemical staining for TRPM7 on incisors and surrounding alveolar bone showed an increased intensity of TRPM7 as ameloblasts progressed from precursor cells at cervical loop to maturation stage **(Ba–e)**. TRPM7 was also immunolocalized in odontoblasts **(Bb,f)**, and osteoblasts **(Bg)**. No immunoreactions were seen in those cells immunostained with non-specific rabbit IgG **(Bh)**. Scale bars: 25 μm

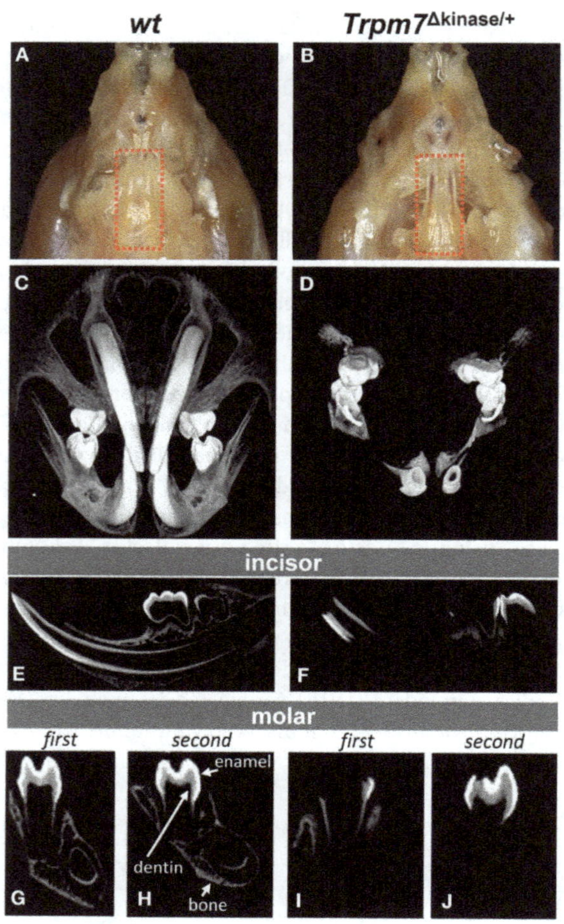

FIGURE 2 | A hypomineralized phenotype is present in enamel, dentin and cranial bones of *Trpm7*$^{\Delta kinase/+}$ mice. (A) Transluscent enamel is found in P14 *wt* mice. **(B)** The transparent mandibular incisor enamel of P14 *Trpm7*$^{\Delta kinase/+}$ mice allows the red colored pulp tissue could be seen through. **(C)** 3-D microCT images of craniofacial structure show well mineralized incisors, entire molars, and craniofacial bones in *wt* mice. **(D)** At the same intensity threshold, the mineralized tissues are only detected in the crowns of molars, a small segment of incisors near the incisal end in *Trpm7*$^{\Delta kinase/+}$. **(E)** A representive 2-D microCT image of sagittal section from P14 *wt* mouse hemimandible show the well contrasted enamel, dentin and alveolar bone. **(F)** The 2-D microCT image of sagittal section from P14 *Trpm7*$^{\Delta kinase/+}$ hemimandibles show contrasting image intensity consistent with mineralization only seen in the molar crown and incisal end of the incisor. Mineralized enamel, dentin and alveolar bone are detected in P14 *wt* first molar **(G)**, and second molar **(H)**. Clear contrasts in these tissues is only seen in part of first molar enamel, dentin and alveolar bone **(I)** and coronal enamel and dentin in the second molar **(J)** of P14 *Trpm7*$^{\Delta kinase/+}$ hemimandible.

(Vector Laboratories Inc.), resulting in dark brown color for positive staining. Nuclear counterstaining was performed with methyl green (Dako Denmark A/S). Normal rabbit IgG was used as the negative control.

Histological Analysis

The fixed mandibles and maxillae were dehydrated in acetone, and embedded in Technovit 8100 resin (Heraeus Kulzer GmbH, Hanau, Germany). Undecalcified sections were obtained at the thickness of 3 μm. Mineralization of the tissue was visualized by 2.5% silver nitrate staining (von Kossa stain). Bone and dentin mineralization was further assessed by following Goldner's Trichrome stain protocol (Goldner, 1938). For general morphological analysis, sections were stained with 1% toluidine blue.

Enzyme Histochemistry for ALPase Activity

To detect ALPase activity, the undecalcified Technovit sections were incubated with the modified Burstone's reagent comprising 1.5 mM Naphthol AS-MX phosphate, 0.5 mM Fast Red Violet LB salt and 3 mM $MgSO_4$ in 0.1 M Tris–HCl buffer (pH 9.2) at 37°C for 60 mins (Nakano et al., 2004). Some of the sections were pre-incubated with 0.1 M Tris–HCl buffer (pH 7.3) supplemented with 50 mM $MgSO_4$ for 1 day at 4°C (Yoshiki et al., 1972; Nakano et al., 2004).

RESULTS

Expression and Synthesis of Trpm7 Progressively Increased with Ameloblast Differentiation

Analysis of our previous microarray data (GSE59214 and GSE57224) revealed that expression of *Trpm7* was progressively upregulated from pre-secretory ameloblasts, to secretory ameloblasts, then to maturation ameloblasts. To confirm this, we used qPCR to compare relative *Trpm7* expression in the ameloblasts obtained from developing mouse enamel organs at three differentiation stages; pre-secretory/P0, secretory/P5 and early maturation/P10 stages. The qPCR analysis showed that the relative expression level of *Trpm7* compared with pre-secretory ameloblasts was 5.4-fold in secretory ameloblasts and 16.08-fold in maturation stage ameloblasts (**Figure 1A**). TRPM7 protein was detected in ameloblasts of all stages, and the intensity of the immunostaining increased as differentiation of ameloblasts advanced, with the highest immunostaining signal in maturation ameloblasts (**Figures 1Ba–e**). Moreover, we found that the odontoblasts (Od) and osteoblasts (Os) were also immunostained for TRPM7 (**Figures 1Bb,f,g**). No immunoreaction was detected on the negative control sections (**Figure 1Bh**).

Significantly Hypomineralized Enamel, Dentin and Cranial Bones Are Found in *Trpm7*$^{\Delta kinase/+}$ Mice

To further understand the TRPM7 functions in enamel and dentin formation, and craniofacial skeletogenesis, we compared the craniofacial structure of *Trpm7*$^{\Delta kinase/+}$ *mice* to *wt* controls. Incisors of P14 *wt* mice were hard and translucent (**Figure 2A**), whereas *Trpm7*$^{\Delta kinase/+}$ mice were soft, and the red vasculature enriched dental pulp was easily seen through the enamel and dentin layers (red box in **Figure 2B**). Moreover, craniofacial bones were also soft and easily bent like a piece of paper.

Consistent with the gross morphology, the 3D microCT of craniofacial structure showed that in *wt* mice, the well mineralized incisors, molars, and craniofacial bones were

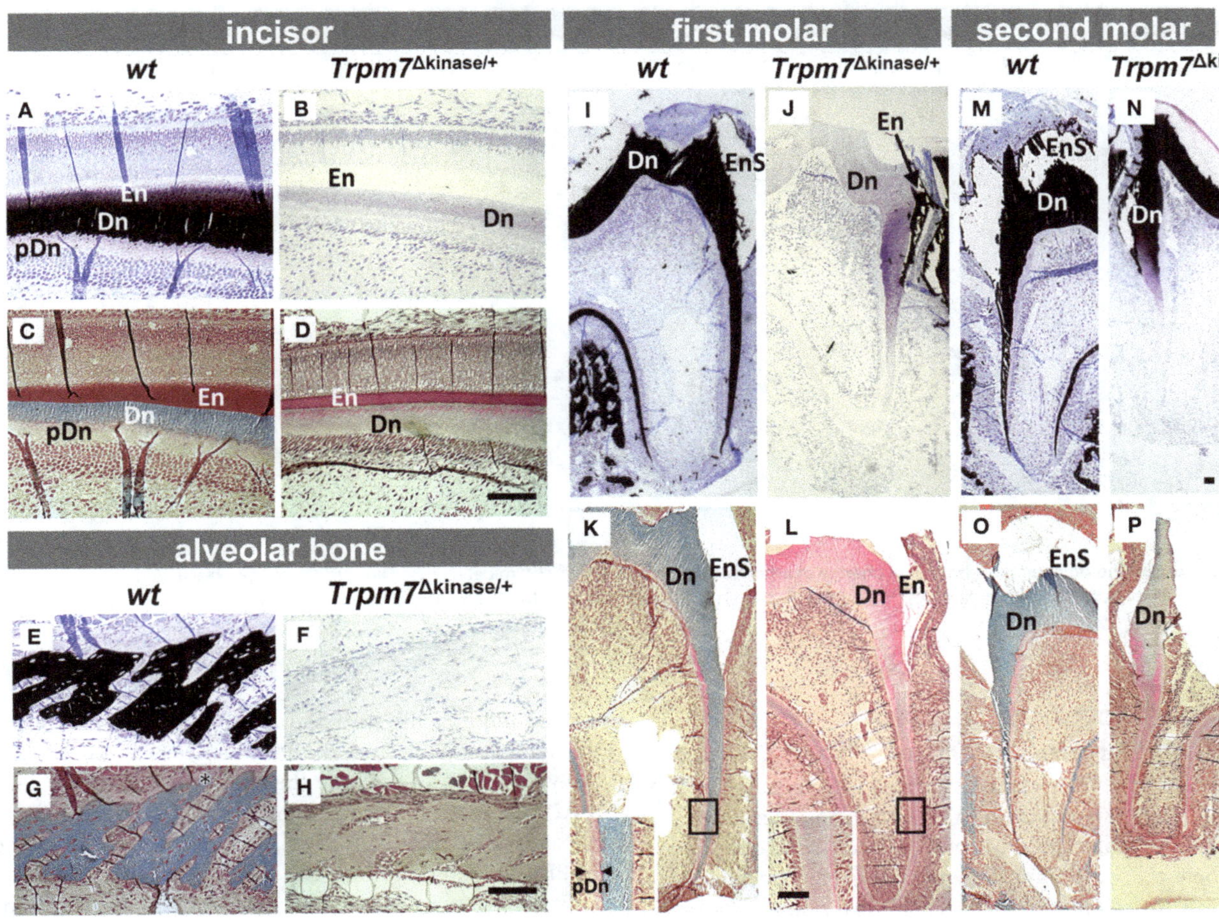

FIGURE 3 | Hypomineralization defects of enamel, dentin and alveolar bone in $Trpm7^{\Delta kinase/+}$ **mice are characterized by histological analyses.** Matrix mineralization was assessed by Von Kossa staining **(A,B,E,F,I,J,M,N)** and Goldner's Trichrome staining **(C,D,G,H,K,L,O,P).** In the *wt* incisor **(A,C)**, secretory stage enamel matrix (En) is lighty positive (black) for Von Kossa staining **(A)**, and is stained in red by Trichrome staining **(C)**. Dentin matrix (Dn) is stained in black with Von Kossa **(A)**, and is stained in blue with Trichrome staining **(C)**. Non-mineralized/Von Kossa negative pre-dentin (pDn) is stained in light pink by Trichrome staining **(C)**. In $Trpm7^{\Delta kinase/+}$ mice, both incisal enamel and dentin are negative for Von Kossa staining **(B)**, and Trichrome stains the dentin matrix in light pink, similar to the color of non-mineralized pre-dentin **(D)**. The alveolar bone matrix of *wt* mice is stained in black by Von Kossa **(E)**, and light blue by Trichrome staining **(G)**. The alveolar bone matrix of $Trpm7^{\Delta kinase/+}$ mice is negative for Von Kossa staining **(F)**, and Trichrome staining on alveolar bone showed bone in $Trpm7^{\Delta kinase/+}$ mice is light pink **(H)**, similar to osteoid. Unlike Von Kossa positive stained *wt* molar dentin **(I,M)**, the entire dentin of the $Trpm7^{\Delta kinase/+}$ first molar is negative for Von Kossa staining **(J)** and shows pink/pre-dentin status by Trichrome staining **(L)**. Interestingly, in the second molar of $Trpm7^{\Delta kinase/+}$ mice, both Von Kossa **(N)** and Trichrome **(P)** staining shows the coronal dentin as partially mineralized, but the root dentin is not mineralized. Enamel matrix of molars likely chipped off during the sectioning (seen as an enamel space/EnS), and the remaining matrix is positive for Von Kossa staining **(N)**. Scale bars: 100 μm

distinguishable at the same intensity (**Figure 2C**), while in $Trpm7^{\Delta kinase/+}$ mice, mineralization was only detected in the crowns of molars, and in smaller area of the incisors specifically at incisal end (**Figure 2D**). Virtual sagittal sections from the $Trpm7^{\Delta kinase/+}$ hemimandibles further demonstrated limited mineralization in the crown of the molar and the incisor (**Figures 2F,I,J**) as compared to *wt* controls (**Figures 2E,G,H**).

Histological assessment on the undecalcified mandibular sections showed von Kossa positive stained (in dark) enamel (En), dentin (Dn), and alveolar bone (**Figures 3A,E,I,M**), and a lack of von Kossa positive staining on the $Trpm7^{\Delta kinase/+}$ incisor enamel and dentin, molar root and alveolar bone (**Figures 3B,F,J,N**). Trichrome staining showed that dentin and bone in the *wt* mice were stained in blue (**Figures 3C,G,K,O**), while incisor dentin, molar root dentin and bones in $Trpm7^{\Delta kinase/+}$ mice were stained in pink, although the width of dentin and bone layer was comparable (**Figures 3D,H,L,P**), indicating that the dentin and bone matrix in the $Trpm7^{\Delta kinase/+}$ mice was deposited at the same levels as *wt* mice but the mineralization did not proceed normally. The coronal dentin of the first molars of $Trpm7^{\Delta kinase/+}$ mice was negative for von Kossa staining (**Figure 3J**), while the coronal dentin of the second molar was positive for the same staining (**Figure 3N**). Consistently, by staining with Trichrome, the mineralization status of the coronal dentin was also confirmed as pink/unmineralized, in the first molars (**Figure 3L**), and blue gray/mineralized, in the second molar (**Figure 3P**).

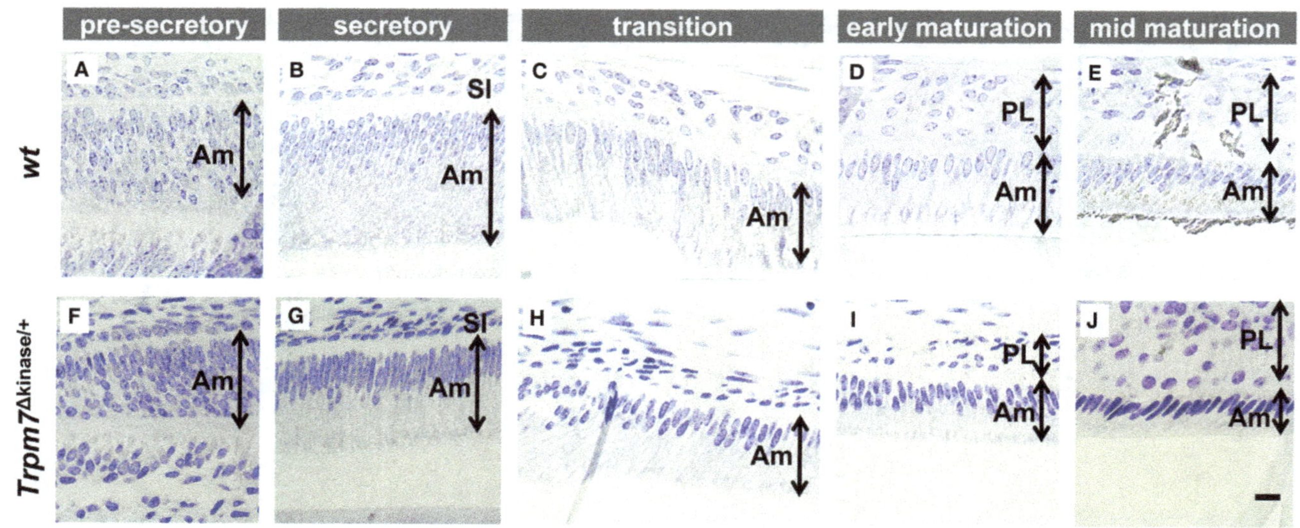

FIGURE 4 | There are no obvious morphological change in ameloblasts of *Trpm7*$^{\Delta kinase/+}$ mice. Morphodifferentiation of ameloblasts (Am) from pre-secretory stage to secretory stage in *Trpm7*$^{\Delta kinase/+}$ mice **(F–J)** is similar to that of *wt* mice **(A–E)**. Am, ameloblast; SI, stratum intermedium; PL, papillary layer; scale bars: 25 μm

Ameloblast Morphology Is Not Significantly Altered in *Trpm7*$^{\Delta kinase/+}$ Mice

The morphology of ameloblasts is associated with the functional property of each differentiation stage. As mentioned above, TRPM7 was immunolocalized in ameloblasts in a stage-specific manner. Therefore, we examined the morphology of ameloblasts by Toluidine blue staining in order to determine whether TRPM7 is critical for the morphological differentiation of ameloblasts. The morphological property of the ameloblasts in the *Trpm7*$^{\Delta kinase/+}$ mice at all stages remained similar to that of the *wt* mice throughout the differentiation. Only the height of ameloblast layer appeared to be slightly shorter (**Figure 4**).

Acellular Cementum Is Absent in *Trpm7*$^{\Delta kinase/+}$ Mice

Through further morphological studies, we found that acellular cementum in molars, normally stained as a deep blue line by toluidine blue in undecalcified sections (McKee et al., 2011; **Figures 5A,B**), was absent in the *Trpm7*$^{\Delta kinase/+}$ mice (**Figures 5C,D**). While the most of the root analog surface was covered by the acellular cementum in *wt* incisors (**Figures 5E–H**), acellular cementum was only detected near the incisal end on the incisor of *Trpm7*$^{\Delta kinase/+}$ mice (**Figures 5I–L**).

Ex vivo AlPase Activity Is Abolished in the *Trpm7*$^{\Delta kinase/+}$ Mice, But Can Be Rescued in Sections Pre-incubated with Mg^{2+} Solution

We found that the mineralization phenotypes in *the Trpm7*$^{\Delta kinase/+}$ *mice*, including hypomineralization in bone, incisor and molar root and absence of acellular cementum, resembled those of the tissue-nonspecific alkaline phosphatase (*Alpl*) KO mice (Beertsen et al., 1999; McKee et al., 2011). These phenotypes led us to examine the abundance of ALPL and *ex vivo* ALPase enzyme activity in osteoblasts (Os), odontoblasts (Od), and ameloblasts (Am). The intensity and localization of ALPL immunostaining in Os, Od, and enamel organ cells, including Am, stratum intermedium (SI) and papillary layer cells (PL), was similar in *wt* and *Trpm7*$^{\Delta kinase/+}$ *mice* (**Figure 6**). However, ALPase activity present in *wt* mice (**Figures 7A,D,G,J**) was absent in the *Trpm7*$^{\Delta kinase/+}$ mouse, except the stratum intermedium cells (**Figures 7B,E,H,K**). Nevertheless, the *ex vivo* ALPase activity was largely rescued in sections of *Trpm7*$^{\Delta kinase/+}$ mineralizing tissue by the pre-incubation of the sections with $MgSO_4$ solution prior to staining for ALPase activity (**Figures 7C,F,I,L**).

DISCUSSION

Tooth enamel is the hardest mineralized tissue in the vertebrate body comprised of 92 volume% inorganic mineral, which is higher than those in dentin and bones (61 and 64.5 volume% respectively; Kumar, 2014). Such a high mineralization rate of enamel is primarily achieved by maturation ameloblasts, which are able to efficiently remove the hydrolyzed enamel matrix proteins and deposit minerals into enamel matrix during the final phase of mineralization. We found that transient receptor potential cation channel, subfamily M, member 7 (TRPM7) was significantly upregulated in maturation ameloblasts. Characterization of craniofacial structures of mice *Trpm7*$^{\Delta kinase/+}$ mice, showed a severe hypomineralized phenotype in all mineralized tissues, indicating a universal role of TRPM7 in tissue mineralization.

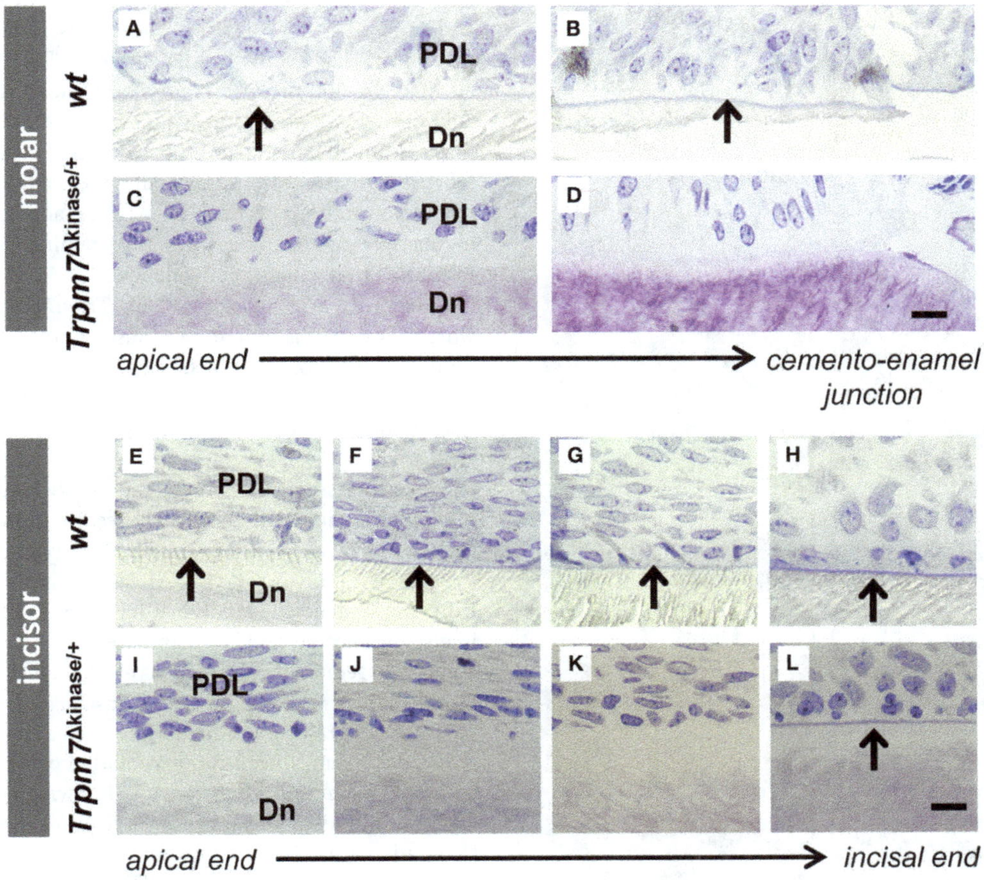

FIGURE 5 | Acellular cementum is found on the root analog of *wt* mouse incisor as well as on the molar root. Acellular cementum, ususally seen as a blue line following toluidine blue staining, is visualized between periodontal ligment (PDL) and dentin (Dn) on *wt* molar **(A,B)**. A similar staining pattern corresponding to acellular cementum can not be detected in *Trpm7*$^{\Delta kinase/+}$ mice **(C,D)**. Acellular cementum, seen as a blue line by Toluidine Blue staining, is visualized along the incisors from the apical to incisal end in P14 *wt* mice (**E–H**, indicated by black arrows). However, this line (indicated by black arrow) only appears on the surface of the incisor root analog dentin near the incisal end in *Trpm7*$^{\Delta kinase/+}$ mice **(I–L)**. Scale bars: 25 μm

Although, some unique molecular mechanisms are employed during enamel mineralization, there are many common factors that regulate the mineralization of enamel, dentin and bone. For instance, tissue-nonspecific alkaline phosphatase (ALPL) is known to be a key regulator of bone and tooth mineralization. Mice lacking *Alpl* show defects in bone, dentin and enamel mineralization and absence of acellular cementum (Waymire et al., 1995; Narisawa et al., 2001; McKee et al., 2011). In humans, mutations in *ALPL* genes cause hypophosphatasia, a rare inherited disorder characterized by deficiency of serum and bone alkaline phosphatase activity, resulting in the defective bone and tooth mineralization (Mornet, 2007). Physiological functions of ALPL are not fully understood yet, nevertheless, in bone and probably dentin, where the mineralization occurs in the type 1 collagen dominant matrix, ALPL is shown to initiate and direct mineralization by removing pyrophosphate (PPi), a mineralization inhibitor, (Addison et al., 2007) and antagonizing generation of PPi (Johnson et al., 2000; Hessle et al., 2002). Though ALPL has been shown to be present in secretory and maturation stage of ameloblasts (Bevelander and Johnson, 1949; Gomez and Boyde, 1994), the significance of ALPL in enamel formation has not been understood yet.

Divalent metal ions, including Mg^{2+}, Zn^{2+}, and Ca^{2+}, are essential for ALPase activity (Stec et al., 2000; Hoylaerts et al., 2015). Magnesium deficient rats showed significantly reduced plasma ALPase activity, which was partially restored by an *in vitro* magnesium supplementation (Heaton, 1965). TRPM family, which consists of eight members, plays an essential role for magnesium entering the cells (Ryazanova et al., 2014). In analysis of our previously published microarray data (Zhang et al., 2014; Liu et al., 2015), we identified that TRPM7 was the only gene, among the well-known magnesium transporters (such as TRPM6, MAGT1, MRS2, PPM1G, MMGT1, and NIPAL1), which was significantly upregulated in ameloblasts as compared to other epithelial cells.

Trpm7$^{\Delta kinase/+}$ mice are known to have significantly lower plasma, bone and urine magnesium levels as compared with *wt* mice, and also show behavioral defects (clasping, tremors, and seizures) and other hypomagnesemia-like phenotype (Ryazanova

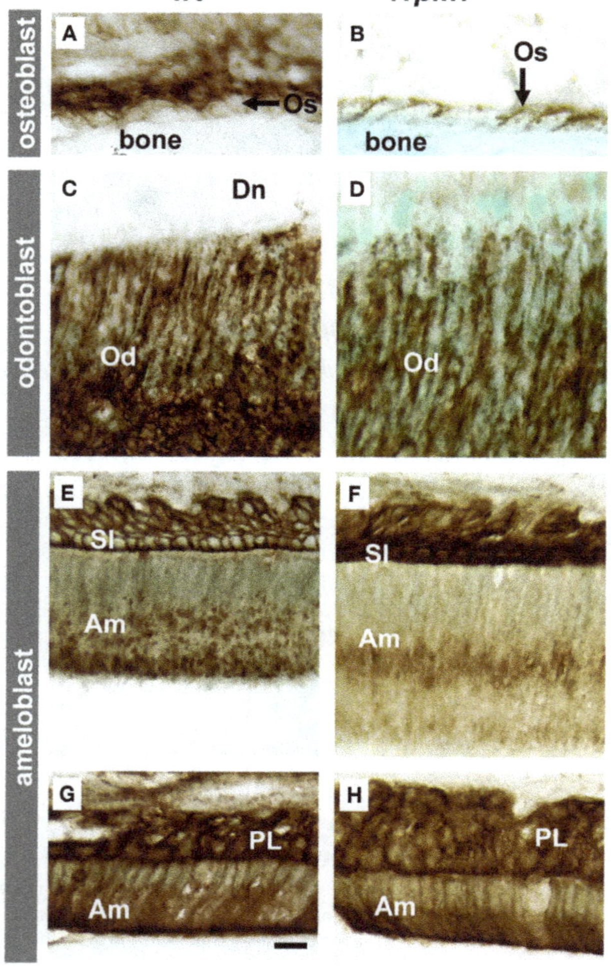

FIGURE 6 | *Trpm7* gene deficiency does not affect the abundance of ALPL protein. In both *wt* and *Trpm7*$^{\Delta kinase/+}$ mice, ALPL was immunolocalized on the basal and lateral plasma membrane of osteoblasts (Os) **(A,B)** and odontoblasts (Od) **(C,D)** at the similar levels. In enamel organs of both *wt* and *Trpm7*$^{\Delta kinase/+}$ mice, ALPL was immunolocalized on plasma membrane of stratum intermedium cells (SI) and the cytoplasm of ameloblasts (Am) at secretory stage **(E,F)**, and on the plasma membrane and cytoplasm of papillary layer cells (PL) and maturation ameloblasts **(G,H)**. There was no notable difference in immunoreactive activities between *wt* and *Trpm7*$^{\Delta kinase/+}$ mice. Scale bars: 25 μm

et al., 2010). Interestingly, a seizure is also one of the behavioral phenotypes displayed by *Alpl* KO mice, and has been linked to a lack of vitamin B6 metabolized by ALPL (Waymire et al., 1995; Whyte et al., 1995; Narisawa et al., 1997; Mackey et al., 2006). Magnesium deficiency is shown to impair vitamin B6 status by inhibiting plasma ALPase activity in rat (Planells et al., 1997), suggesting that the activity of tissue non-specific ALPase (ALPL) is repressed under hypomagnesaemia condition.

Our microCT and morphological analyses on the hemimandibles of *Trpm7*$^{\Delta kinase/+}$ mice revealed similarity in skeletal and dental phenotypes, including partially mineralized molar crowns and absence of acellular cementum, between *Alpl* KO mice (Beertsen et al., 1999; McKee et al., 2011) and *Trpm7*$^{\Delta kinase/+}$ mice. These observations suggested a possibility that ALPL in the *Trpm7*$^{\Delta kinase/+}$ mice might be affected. In support of this possibility, we found that although *Alpl* protein content was similar in *wt* and *Trpm7*$^{\Delta kinase/+}$ mouse ameloblasts, odontoblasts and osteoblasts, *ex vivo ALPase* activity was dramatically reduced in *Trpm7*$^{\Delta kinase/+}$ *mice.* Restoration of *ex vivo* ALPase activity by Mg^{2+} pre-incubation of sections prior to staining for ALP activity, indicates that magnesium deficiency is a major cause for the deficient ALPase activity of *Trpm7*$^{\Delta kinase/+}$ mice. It is worth noting that there are also numerous enzymes that require Mg^{2+} for their activities. Therefore, hypomineralized tooth and bone in the *Trpm7*$^{\Delta kinase/+}$ mice could be also due to the cumulative deficiency of some other enzymes as well.

Nevertheless, in this study, the *ex vivo* supplementation of magnesium could not completely restore the ALPase activity to the levels displayed in the *wt* cells. This phenomenon is similar to what is found in *ex vivo* ALPase activity in tissue sections from Mg^{2+} deficient rats (Heaton, 1965). The TRPM7 channel is also permeable to Ca^{2+}, and therefore the lack of TRPM7 could also reduce the amount of available intracellular calcium. Optimized Ca^{2+} is critical for ALPase activity (Hoylaerts et al., 2015), and therefore, although Mg^{2+} concentrations are restored, reduced calcium concentrations could impact ALPase activity. In addition, magnesium deficiency is known to have a secondary effect on the metabolism of Ca^{2+}, K^{+} and inorganic phosphate (Konrad et al., 2004; Rude and Shils, 2006), therefore, the hypomineralization of *Trpm7*$^{\Delta kinase/+}$ mice was also attributed to an altered intra and/or extra cellular Ca^{2+} and inorganic phosphate.

In this study, we found that TRPM7 was highly expressed by ameloblasts, odontoblasts and osteoblasts, which are cells responsible for the formation of enamel, dentin and bone respectively. All the mineralized tissues in the TRPM7 kinase domain deficient mice are hypomineralized, with reduced ALPase activity. Unlike bone and dentin, where ALPL functions in the initial phase of mineralization, in enamel formation, it is thought that ALPL functions at the maturation stage, where the final but majority of mineralization takes place (Takano and Ozawa, 1980). Our finding that ubiquitous inhibition of mineralization in all stage of enamel formation suggested that the initiation of enamel matrix mineralization at the secretory stage is also regulated by ALPL. In support of this, our immunohistochemistry showed that ALPL was apparently present in the cytoplasm of secretory ameloblasts. Therefore, similar to bone and dentin, ALPL also possibly contributes to the initiation of enamel matrix mineralization at the secretory stage by fine-tuning the local concentration of PPi.

Of course, there are also numerous enzymes that require Mg^{2+} for their activities. Therefore, hypomineralized tooth and bone in the *Trpm7*$^{\Delta kinase/+}$ mice could be also due to the cumulative deficiency of some other enzymes as well.

In conclusion, our findings suggest that TRPM7 plays a critical role in the mineralization of enamel as well as dentin and

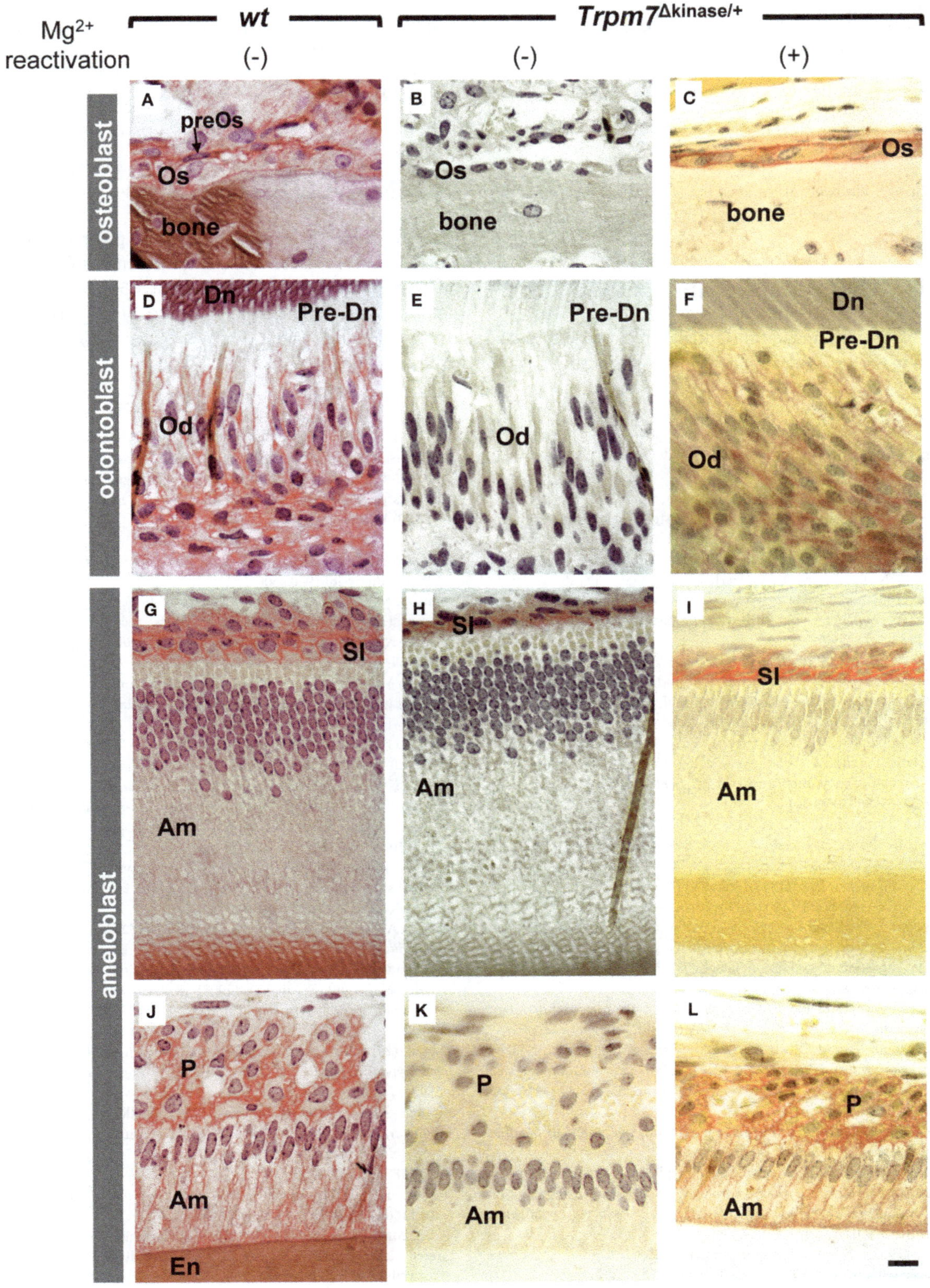

FIGURE 7 | Impaired alkaline phosphatase (ALPase) activity of osteoblasts, odotoblasts and ameloblasts in *Trpm7*$^{\Delta kinase/+}$ mice is partially retrieved by Mg^{2+} pre-treatment. (A) At the bone forming site, ALPase activity was detected (in red) on the plasma membrane of osteoblasts (Os) and its precursor cells (preOs) in *wt* mice. **(B)**There was no ALPase activity presented by osteoblasts in *Trpm7*$^{\Delta kinase/+}$ mice. **(C)** However, Mg^{2+} pre-treatment retrieved the ALPase

(Continued)

FIGURE 7 | Continued
activity on osteoblasts. **(D)** ALPase activity was detected at the basolateral surface of odontoblasts (Od) in *wt* mice. **(E)** While in $Trpm7^{\Delta kinase/+}$ mice, no ALPase activity was seen in the odontoblasts. **(F)** Mg^{2+} pre-treatment retrieved ALPase activity on odontoblasts. **(J)** ALPase activity was detected in stratum intermedium (SI), secretory ameloblasts (Am), and **(G)** papillary layer cells (P) at maturation stage in *wt* mice. In $Trpm7^{\Delta kinase/+}$ mice, ALPase activities were restricted only on the stratum intermedium at secretory stage, not in ameloblasts **(H,K)**. Mg^{2+} pre-treatment retrieved the ALPase activity on ameloblasts and papillary layer cells **(I,L)**. Dn, dentin; pre-Dn, pre-dentin; En, enamel; Scale bars: 25 μm.

craniofacial bone via regulating activity of ALPL by transporting Mg^{2+}, which is necessary for ALPL activity, into the cells.

AUTHOR CONTRIBUTIONS

All authors listed, have made substantial, direct and intellectual contribution to the work, and approved it for publication.

ACKNOWLEDGMENTS

This research was funded by NIDCR grant R03 DE019507-02 to YZ and funds from the Department of Orofacial Sciences at UCSF to YZ, YN, NIDCR grant R56 DE13508 to PD. The authors thank the Biomaterials and Bioengineering Micro-CT Imaging Facility (http://bbct.ucsf.edu) at UCSF for the use of MicroXCT-200.

REFERENCES

Addison, W. N., Azari, F., Sorensen, E. S., Kaartinen, M. T., and McKee, M. D. (2007). Pyrophosphate inhibits mineralization of osteoblast cultures by binding to mineral, up-regulating osteopontin, and inhibiting alkaline phosphatase activity. *J. Biol. Chem.* 282, 15872–15883. doi: 10.1074/jbc.M701116200

Baker, A. R., Silva, N. F., Quinn, D. W., Harte, A. L., Pagano, D., Bonser, R. S., et al. (2006). Human epicardial adipose tissue expresses a pathogenic profile of adipocytokines in patients with cardiovascular disease. *Cardiovasc. Diabetol.* 5:1. doi: 10.1186/1475-2840-5-1

Barciszewska, M. Z., Rapp, G., Betzel, C., Erdmann, V. A., and Barciszewski, J. (2001). Structural changes of tRNA and 5S rRNA induced with magnesium and visualized with synchrotron mediated hydroxyl radical cleavage. *Mol. Biol. Rep.* 28, 103–110. doi: 10.1023/A:1017951120531

Beertsen, W., VandenBos, T., and Everts, V. (1999). Root development in mice lacking functional tissue non-specific alkaline phosphatase gene: inhibition of acellular cementum formation. *J. Dent. Res.* 78, 1221–1229. doi: 10.1177/00220345990780060501

Bernick, S., and Hungerford, G. F. (1965). Effect of dietary magnesium deficiency on the bones and teeth of rats. *J. Dent. Res.* 44, 1317–1324. doi: 10.1177/00220345650440063401

Bevelander, G., and Johnson, P. L. (1949). Alkaline phosphatase in amelogenesis. *Anat. Rec.* 104, 125–135. doi: 10.1002/ar.1091040202

Brown, D., Lydon, J., McLaughlin, M., Stuart-Tilley, A., Tyszkowski, R., and Alper, S. (1996). Antigen retrieval in cryostat tissue sections and cultured cells by treatment with sodium dodecyl sulfate (SDS). *Histochem. Cell Biol.* 105, 261–267. doi: 10.1007/BF01463929

Cowan, J. A. (2002). Structural and catalytic chemistry of magnesium-dependent enzymes. *Biometals* 15, 225–235. doi: 10.1023/A:1016022730880

Emoto, K., Yamashita, S., and Okada, Y. (2005). Mechanisms of heat-induced antigen retrieval: does pH or ionic strength of the solution play a role for refolding antigens? *J. Histochem. Cytochem.* 53, 1311–1321. doi: 10.1369/jhc.5C6627.2005

Goldner, J. (1938). A modification of the masson trichrome technique for routine laboratory purposes. *Am. J. Pathol.* 14, 237–243.

Gomez, S., and Boyde, A. (1994). Correlated alkaline phosphatase histochemistry and quantitative backscattered electron imaging in the study of rat incisor ameloblasts and enamel mineralization. *Microsc. Res. Tech.* 29, 29–36. doi: 10.1002/jemt.1070290105

Heaton, F. W. (1965). Effect of magnesium deficiency on plasma alkaline phosphatase activity. *Nature* 207, 1292–1293. doi: 10.1038/2071292b0

Hessle, L., Johnson, K. A., Anderson, H. C., Narisawa, S., Sali, A., Goding, J. W., et al. (2002). Tissue-nonspecific alkaline phosphatase and plasma cell membrane glycoprotein-1 are central antagonistic regulators of bone mineralization. *Proc. Natl. Acad. Sci. U.S.A.* 99, 9445–9449. doi: 10.1073/pnas.142063399

Hoylaerts, M. F., Van Kerckhoven, S., Kiffer-Moreira, T., Sheen, C., Narisawa, S., and Millan, J. L. (2015). Functional significance of calcium binding to tissue-nonspecific alkaline phosphatase. *PLoS ONE* 10:e0119874. doi: 10.1371/journal.pone.0119874

Irving, J. T. (1940). The influence of diets low in magnesium upon the histological appearance of the incisor tooth of the rat. *J. Physiol.* 99, 8–17. doi: 10.1113/jphysiol.1940.sp003874

Johnson, K. A., Hessle, L., Vaingankar, S., Wennberg, C., Mauro, S., Narisawa, S., et al. (2000). Osteoblast tissue-nonspecific alkaline phosphatase antagonizes and regulates PC-1. *Am. J. Physiol. Regul. Integr. Comp. Phys.* 279, R1365–R1377.

Konrad, M., Schlingmann, K. P., and Gudermann, T. (2004). Insights into the molecular nature of magnesium homeostasis. *Am. J. Physiol. Renal Physiol.* 286, F599–F605. doi: 10.1152/ajprenal.00312.2003

Kumar, G. S. (2014). *Orban's Oral Histology & Embryology*. Chennai: Elsevier Health Sciences APAC.

Liu, C., Niu, Y., Zhou, X., Xu, X., Yang, Y., Zhang, Y., et al. (2015). Cell cycle control, DNA damage repair, and apoptosis-related pathways control pre-ameloblasts differentiation during tooth development. *BMC Genomics* 16:592. doi: 10.1186/s12864-015-1783-y

Livak, K. J., and Schmittgen, T. D. (2001). Analysis of relative gene expression data using real-time quantitative PCR and the $2-\Delta\Delta CT$ method. *Methods* 25, 402–408. doi: 10.1006/meth.2001.1262

Mackey, A. D., Davis, S. R., and Gregory, J. F. III (2006). "Vitamin B6," in *Modern Nutrition in Health and Disease, 10th Edn.*, eds M. E. Shils and M. Shike (Philadelphia, PA: Lippincott Williams & Wilkins), 452–461.

Maguire, M. E., and Cowan, J. A. (2002). Magnesium chemistry and biochemistry. *Biometals* 15, 203–210. doi: 10.1023/A:1016058229972

McKee, M. D., Nakano, Y., Masica, D. L., Gray, J. J., Lemire, I., Heft, R., et al. (2011). Enzyme replacement therapy prevents dental defects in a model of hypophosphatasia. *J. Dent. Res.* 90, 470–476. doi: 10.1177/0022034510393517

Monteilh-Zoller, M. K., Hermosura, M. C., Nadler, M. J., Scharenberg, A. M., Penner, R., and Fleig, A. (2003). TRPM7 provides an ion channel mechanism for cellular entry of trace metal ions. *J. Gen. Physiol.* 121, 49–60. doi: 10.1085/jgp.20028740

Mornet, E. (2007). Hypophosphatasia. *Orphanet J. Rare Dis.* 2:40. doi: 10.1186/1750-1172-2-40

Nadler, M. J., Hermosura, M. C., Inabe, K., Perraud, A. L., Zhu, Q., Stokes, A. J., et al. (2001). LTRPC7 is a Mg.ATP-regulated divalent cation channel required for cell viability. *Nature* 411, 590–595. doi: 10.1038/35079092

Nakano, Y., Beertsen, W., van den Bos, T., Kawamoto, T., Oda, K., and Takano, Y. (2004). Site-specific localization of two distinct phosphatases along the osteoblast plasma membrane: tissue non-specific alkaline phosphatase and plasma membrane calcium ATPase. *Bone* 35, 1077–1085. doi: 10.1016/j.bone.2004.07.009

Narisawa, S., Fröhlander, N., and Millán, J. L. (1997). Inactivation of two mouse alkaline phosphatase genes and establishment of a model of infantile hypophosphatasia. *Dev. Dyn.* 208, 432–446.

Narisawa, S., Wennberg, C., and Millan, J. L. (2001). Abnormal vitamin B6 metabolism in alkaline phosphatase knock-out mice causes multiple abnormalities, but not the impaired bone mineralization. *J. Pathol.* 193, 125–133. doi: 10.1002/1096-9896(2000)9999:9999<::AID-PATH722>3.0.CO;2-Y

Neitzel, J. J., Dostmann, W. R. G., and Taylor, S. S. (1991). Role of magnesium-ATP in the activation and reassociation of cAMP-dependent protein kinase I: consequences of replacing the essential arginine in cAMP-binding site A. *Biochemistry* 30, 733–739. doi: 10.1021/bi00217a023

Planells, E., Lerma, A., Sánchez-Morito, N., Aranda, P., and LLopis, J. (1997). Effect of magnesium deficiency on vitamin B2 and B6 status in the rat. *J. Am. Coll. Nutr.* 16, 352–356. doi: 10.1080/07315724.1997.10718697

Penner, R., and Fleig, A. (2007). The Mg2+ and Mg(2+)-nucleotide-regulated channel-kinase TRPM7. *Handb. Exp. Pharmacol.* 179, 313–328. doi: 10.1007/978-3-540-34891-7_19

Robinson, C., Kirkham, J., Brookes, S. J., Bonass, W. A., and Shore, R. C. (1995). The chemistry of enamel development. *Int. J. Dev. Biol.* 39, 145–152.

Romani, A. M. (2011). Cellular magnesium homeostasis. *Arch. Biochem. Biophys.* 512, 1–23. doi: 10.1016/j.abb.2011.05.010

Rude, R. K., and Gruber, H. E. (2004). Magnesium deficiency and osteoporosis: animal and human observations. *J. Nutr. Biochem.* 15, 710–716. doi: 10.1016/j.jnutbio.2004.08.001

Rude, R. K., Gruber, H. E., Norton, H. J., Wei, L. Y., Frausto, A., and Mills, B. G. (2004). Bone loss induced by dietary magnesium reduction to 10% of the nutrient requirement in rats is associated with increased release of substance P and tumor necrosis factor-alpha. *J. Nutr.* 134, 79–85.

Rude, R. K., and Shils, M. E. (2006). "Magnesium," in *Modern Nutrition in Health and Disease, 10th Edn.*, eds M. E. Shils and M. Shike (Philadelphia, PA: Lippincott Williams & Wilkins), 223–247.

Ryazanova, L. V., Hu, Z., Suzuki, S., Chubanov, V., Fleig, A., and Ryazanov, A. G. (2014). Elucidating the role of the TRPM7 alpha-kinase: TRPM7 kinase inactivation leads to magnesium deprivation resistance phenotype in mice. *Sci. Rep.* 4:7599. doi: 10.1038/srep07599

Ryazanova, L. V., Rondon, L. J., Zierler, S., Hu, Z., Galli, J., Yamaguchi, T. P., et al. (2010). TRPM7 is essential for Mg(2+) homeostasis in mammals. *Nat. Commun.* 1, 109. doi: 10.1038/ncomms1108

Smith, C. E. (1998). Cellular and chemical events during enamel maturation. *Crit. Rev. Oral Biol. Med.* 9, 128–161. doi: 10.1177/10454411980090020101

Sreedhara, A., and Cowan, J. A. (2002). Structural and catalytic roles for divalent magnesium in nucleic acid biochemistry. *Biometals* 15, 211–223. doi: 10.1023/A:1016070614042

Stec, B., Holtz, K. M., and Kantrowitz, E. R. (2000). A revised mechanism for the alkaline phosphatase reaction involving three metal ions1. *J. Mol. Biol.* 299, 1303–1311. doi: 10.1006/jmbi.2000.3799

Takano, Y., and Ozawa, H. (1980). Ultrastructural and cytochemical observations on the alternating morphologic changes of the ameloblasts at the stage of enamel maturation. *Arch. Histol. Jpn.* 43, 385–399. doi: 10.1679/aohc1950.43.385

Trowbridge, H., Louchard, W., and Jenks, P. (1971). Histochemical studies on the dentin of magnesium-deficient rats. *J. Periodont. Res.* 6, 130–139. doi: 10.1111/j.1600-0765.1971.tb00600.x

Waymire, K. G., Mahuren, J. D., Jaje, J. M., Guilarte, T. R., Coburn, S. P., and MacGregor, G. R. (1995). Mice lacking tissue non-specific alkaline phosphatase die from seizures due to defective metabolism of vitamin B-6. *Nat. Genet.* 11, 45–51. doi: 10.1038/ng0995-45

Weglicki, W. B., Dickens, B. F., Wagner, T. L., Chmielinska, J. J., and Phillips, T. M. (1996). Immunoregulation by neuropeptides in magnesium deficiency: *ex vivo* effect of enhanced substance P production on circulating T lymphocytes from magnesium-deficient mice. *Magne. Res.* 9, 3–11.

Whyte, M. P., Landt, M., Ryan, L. M., Mulivor, R. A., Henthorn, P. S., Fedde, K. N., et al. (1995). Alkaline phosphatase: placental and tissue-nonspecific isoenzymes hydrolyze phosphoethanolamine, inorganic pyrophosphate, and pyridoxal 5'-phosphate. Substrate accumulation in carriers of hypophosphatasia corrects during pregnancy. *J. Clin. Invest.* 95, 1440–1445. doi: 10.1172/JCI117814

Wolf, F. I., and Cittadini, A. (2003). Chemistry and biochemistry of magnesium. *Mol. Aspects Med.* 24, 3–9. doi: 10.1016/S0098-2997(02)00087-0

Wolf, F. I., Torsello, A., Fasanella, S., and Cittadini, A. (2003). Cell physiology of magnesium. *Mol. Aspects Med.* 24, 11–26. doi: 10.1016/S0098-2997(02)00088-2

Yee, N. S., Kazi, A. A., and Yee, R. K. (2014). Cellular and developmental biology of TRPM7 channel-kinase: implicated roles in cancer. *Cells* 3, 751–777. doi: 10.3390/cells3030751

Yoshiki, S., Umeda, T., and Kurahashi, Y. (1972). An effective reactivation of alkaline phosphatase in hard tissues completely decalcified for light and electron microscopy. *Histochemie* 29, 296–304.

Yuan, J., Reed, A., Chen, F., and Stewart, C. N. (2006). Statistical analysis of real-time PCR data. *BMC Bioinformatics* 7:85. doi: 10.1186/1471-2105-7-85

Zhang, Y., Kim, J. Y., Horst, O., Nakano, Y., Zhu, L., Radlanski, R. J., et al. (2014). Fluorosed mouse ameloblasts have increased satb1 retention and galphaq activity. *PLoS ONE* 9:e103994. doi: 10.1371/journal.pone.0103994

17

Mesenchymal Remodeling during Palatal Shelf Elevation Revealed by Extracellular Matrix and F-Actin Expression Patterns

Matthias Chiquet[1], Susan Blumer[1], Manuela Angelini[1], Thimios A. Mitsiadis[2] and Christos Katsaros[1]*

[1] Department of Orthodontics and Dentofacial Orthopedics, Medical Faculty, School of Dental Medicine, University of Bern, Bern, Switzerland, [2] Orofacial Development and Regeneration, Center for Dental Medicine, Institute for Oral Biology, University of Zurich, Zurich, Switzerland

Correspondence:
Matthias Chiquet
matthias.chiquet@zmk.unibe.ch

During formation of the secondary palate in mammalian embryos, two vertically oriented palatal shelves rapidly elevate into a horizontal position above the tongue, meet at the midline, and fuse to form a single entity. Previous observations suggested that elevation occurs by a simple 90° rotation of the palatal shelves. More recent findings showed that the presumptive midline epithelial cells are not located at the tips of palatal shelves before elevation, but mostly toward their medial/lingual part. This implied extensive tissue remodeling during shelf elevation. Nevertheless, it is still not known how the shelf mesenchyme reorganizes during this process, and what mechanism drives it. To address this question, we mapped the distinct and restricted expression domains of certain extracellular matrix components within the developing palatal shelves. This procedure allowed to monitor movements of entire mesenchymal regions relative to each other during shelf elevation. Consistent with previous notions, our results confirm a flipping movement of the palatal shelves anteriorly, whereas extensive mesenchymal reorganization is observed more posteriorly. There, the entire lingual portion of the vertical shelves moves close to the midline after elevation, whereas the mesenchyme at the original tip of the shelves ends up ventrolaterally. Moreover, we observed that the mesenchymal cells of elevating palatal shelves substantially align their actin cytoskeleton, their extracellular matrix, and their nuclei in a ventral to medial direction. This indicates that, like in other morphogenetic processes, actin-dependent cell contractility is a major driving force for mesenchymal tissue remodeling during palatogenesis.

Keywords: palate morphogenesis, palatal shelf elevation, extracellular matrix, actin, tissue remodeling, mouse embryo

INTRODUCTION

The secondary palate, which separates the oral cavity from the nasal cavity, is a specific feature of mammals (Ferguson, 1988). Cleft lip/palate is the most frequent craniofacial malformation in humans (Jugessur et al., 2009a; Mossey et al., 2009; Dixon et al., 2011). Formation of the secondary palate during embryogenesis is a complex process involving extensive tissue growth and remodeling (Gritli-Linde, 2008; Jugessur et al., 2009b; Bush and Jiang, 2012). Palate development starts from the palatal shelves, extensions of the maxillary processes that are located left and right from the tongue. The palatal shelves initially have a vertical orientation, but around the 6th week of gestation in humans, or at embryonic day 14.5 (E14.5) in mice, they elevate rapidly into a horizontal position above the tongue. The shelves meet medially, and fuse by disappearance of the midline epithelium and merging of the mesenchyme (Gritli-Linde, 2007; Bush and Jiang, 2012). While much information exists concerning the mechanism of palatal shelf fusion (Kaartinen et al., 1995; Proetzel et al., 1995) (Jin et al., 2014), the process of shelf elevation still remains elusive, and knowledge about its cellular and molecular basis is scarce (Bush and Jiang, 2012).

Palatal shelves are known to be divided into distinct regions along their anterior-posterior axis. Their frontal and medial parts will give rise to the hard palate, their posterior part to the soft palate (Yu and Ornitz, 2011; Smith et al., 2012). It was debated whether palatal shelves elevate and fuse first from the front or from the back (reviewed in Brinkley and Vickerman, 1979). *In vitro,* their medial parts elevate first (Brinkley and Vickerman, 1979), whereas in the embryo, tongue movements strongly affect shelf elevation (Iseki et al., 2007; Kouskoura et al., 2016). This causes a remarkable variability in the time course of elevation *in vivo* between siblings, and even between the two shelves of one embryo (Luke, 1984; Iseki et al., 2007; Yu and Ornitz, 2011). A recent histomorphometric analysis concludes that in the embryo, elevation usually starts at the medial to posterior part of the palatal shelves, which then zipper in both directions (Yu and Ornitz, 2011).

The above findings imply that all parts of the palatal shelves have an intrinsic capability to elevate. However, it has been debated how this reshaping occurs, and several reports indicated regional differences in tissue reorganization during shelf elevation. Histological observations suggested that anteriorly, the palatal shelves perform a simple flipping movement (Coleman, 1965). However, other reports indicated that the medial and posterior parts of the shelves remodel extensively during elevation, such that their lingual side protrudes whereas the ventral tip regresses (Brinkley and Vickerman, 1979; Chou et al., 2004). A recent study used the expression of the *Mmp13* gene to determine the origin of midline epithelial cells during palatal shelf elevation. Its results supported a flipping movement of the shelves in the front and extensive remodeling posteriorly (Jin et al., 2010), which was confirmed by careful histomorphometric analysis (Yu and Ornitz, 2011).

Although there is general agreement that extensive remodeling of the palatal shelves occurs during elevation, it is not known how different regions of the palatal mesenchyme move relative to each other. Moreover, the forces that drive tissue remodeling in the elevating shelves are still unknown. Distinct patterns of cell proliferation (Sasaki et al., 2004) and density (Brinkley and Bookstein, 1986) are unlikely to contribute substantially to the remodeling process, since it occurs in less than 1 day in mouse embryos (Yu and Ornitz, 2011). The finding of hyaluronidase-sensitive material in the "hinge" region of palatal shelves led to the hypothesis that rapid accumulation of hyaluronic acid or other glycosaminoglycans might provide the driving force for shelf elevation, by generating osmotic swelling pressure (Brinkley and Morris-Wiman, 1987). Alternatively, this process might be powered by coordinated cytoskeletal contractions of both epithelium and mesenchyme, similar to what is observed in many other morphogenetic tissue rearrangements (Wozniak and Chen, 2009). Although an early report suggested a role for actin-based contractility in palatal shelf elevation (Lessard et al., 1974), to our knowledge this idea has never been followed up.

Therefore, in the present study we address two important questions concerning the process of palatal shelf elevation. Firstly, is it possible to detect rearrangements of different parts of the palatal mesenchyme relative to each other during the elevation process? Secondly, can we find any evidence for actin-based contractility in the remodeling of palatal mesenchyme during elevation? To address these points, we took advantage of the fact that certain extracellular matrix (ECM) components have a restricted expression in defined regions of the palatal mesenchyme, which can be followed during shelf elevation. Furthermore, we stained sections through elevating palatal shelves for F-actin, and detected elongated cell nuclei that aligned with the actin network. Our results confirm and refine previous findings of extensive remodeling of the palatal mesenchyme at medial and posterior levels, and provide the first evidence for tensile stress acting within this tissue during the process of shelf elevation.

MATERIALS AND METHODS

Animals, Embryonic Tissues, and Cryosectioning

C57BL/6 wild-type mouse embryos were obtained from J.-F. Spetz at the Friedrich-Miescher Institute for Biomedical Research in Basel, Switzerland, or from in house breeding at the central animal facilities, Department of Clinical Research, University of Bern. After mating, appearance of a vaginal plug was considered embryonic day 0.5 (E0.5). Pregnant females were sacrificed at the desired stage (E13.5–E14.5), embryos were removed from the uterus and decapitated. Animal experiments were approved by the Cantonal Veterinary Offices of Basel, Zurich and Bern, Switzerland. The embryo heads were washed in ice-cold PBS, fixed in 4% paraformaldehyde in phosphate buffered saline (PBS; 150 mM NaCl, 20 mM Na-phosphate, pH 7.4) overnight, soaked for 24 h in 30% sucrose in PBS, embedded in Tissue Tek (O.C.T. compound; Sakura Finetek Europe B.V., Zoeterwoude, Netherlands), and frozen on an aluminum block cooled to −80°C. Frozen heads were stored at −80°C before sectioning. Serial frontal sections (12 μm thick) were prepared on a Cryocut E cryomicrotome (Reichert-Jung, Leica Microsystems, Heerbrugg, Switzerland). Sections were dried at 37°C for 1–5 min, and stored at −80°C for further use.

Gene-Specific RNA Probes and *In situ* Hybridization

Total RNA was isolated from E14.5 C57BL/6 wildtype mouse embryos using an RNAeasy Mini Kit (Qiagen, Hombrechtikon,

Switzerland), and reverse transcribed to cDNA using Moloney murine leukemia virus reverse transcriptase (Promega, Dübendorf, Switzerland). Gene-specific primers (Microsynth, Balgrach, Switzerland) were designed using free NCBI software (http://www.ncbi.nlm.nih.gov/tools/primer-blast/index.cgi?LINK_LOC=BlastHome). Primers were fitted with BamH1 (forward primers) or HindIII (reverse primers) restriction sites at their 5′ ends, respectively. With these primers (**Table 1**), specific products were amplified from E14.5 mouse cDNA by PCR using Go Taq polymerase (Promega), cut with respective restriction enzymes, and cloned into pBluescript SK+ plasmid (Stratagene/Agilent, Santa Clara, USA). In the case of mouse *tenascin-C* (*Tnc*) and *tenascin-W* (gene name *Tnn*), full-length cDNA clones were obtained from R. Chiquet-Ehrismann (Friedrich Miescher Institute for Biomedical Research, Basel, Switzerland), and restriction fragments of suitable size (**Table 1**) were cloned into pBluescript SK+. Plasmids were linearized by cutting upstream or downstream of the insert, respectively, and digoxygenin-labeled anti-sense or sense RNA probes were synthesized (Koch et al., 1995) with a labeling kit from Roche Diagnostics using T3 or T7 RNA polymerase (Promega). *In situ* hybridization was done with the labeled probes as published in detail before (Flück et al., 2000). After incubation with alkaline phosphatase conjugated anti-digoxygenin antibody (Roche Diagnostics), a color substrate solution was used to which 10% polyvinyl alcohol (MW 31′000-50′000; Sigma-Aldrich, Buchs, Switzerland) was added (Shen, 2001). After development, the sections were counterstained with Nuclear Fast Red (Sigma).

Fluorescence Labeling of Tissue Sections

Monoclonal antibody mTn12 against mouse tenascin-C (Aufderheide and Ekblom, 1988) was obtained from R. Chiquet-Ehrismann (Friedrich Miescher Institute for Biomedical Research, Basel, Switzerland). Cryosections from paraformaldehyde-fixed mouse embryo heads were blocked with 3% bovine serum albumin in phosphate-buffered saline (BSA/PBS) and incubated with anti-tenascin antibody (1:100 in BSA/PBS) for 1 h at room temperature. After washing with PBS containing 0.2% Tween-20, sections were incubated with Alexa488-labeled secondary antibody (Invitrogen; 1:1000 in BSA/PBS). For labeling the F-actin network on the same section, 1 μg/ml rhodamine-phalloidin (Sigma) was added to the secondary antibody solution. After washing again with PBS/Tween, sections were embedded in phosphate-buffered glycerol (pH 7.4) containing 1 μg/ml DAPI stain (Sigma) to label nuclei.

TABLE 1 | Gene-specific RNA probes for *in situ* hybridization.

MOUSE PERIOSTIN (Postn: NM_015784.3)
Forward primer: 5′CCGGATCCGCAGCCGCCATCACCTCTGAC 3′ (nucleotide: 196-216)
Reverse primer: 5′ CCAAGCTTGCTTGTCTTGCCGCAGCTTGT 3′ (nucleotide: 964-944)
PCR product/probe length (without restriction sites): 769 bp
MOUSE TENASCIN-C (Tnc: D_90343.1)
Restriction fragment: Sac1 (nucleotide 5862)–EcoR1 (nucleotide 6813)
Probe length: 950 bp
MOUSE TENASCIN-W (Tnn: AJ_580920.1)
Restriction fragment: HindIII (nucleotide 1190)–BamH1 (nucleotide 1440)
Probe length: 250 bp
MOUSE SMOC-2 (Smoc2: NM_022315.2)
Forward: 5′ CCGGATCCCAGGTGCCCCGGTTCAA 3′ (nucleotide: 661-679)
Reverse: 5′ CCAAGCTTCCAGGGTGTGGCTGGGGT 3′ (nucleotide: 1253-1235)
PCR product/probe length (without restriction sites): 593 bp
MOUSE TRANSFORMING GROWTH FACTOR-β3 (Tgfb3: NM 009368.3)
Forward primer: 5′ CCGGATCCCAACCCCAGCTCCAAGCG 3′ (nucleotide: 1578-1597)
Reverse primer: 5′ CCAAGCTTCCAGGTTGCGGAAGCAGT 3′ (nucleotide: 2046-2026)
PCR product/probe length (without restriction sites): 469 bp

Microscopy

Slides processed for *in situ* hybridization were viewed under bright field optics with 4x or 10x objectives on an Olympus BX-51 microscope. Slides triple-labeled with fluorescent dyes were observed on the same microscope by epifluorescence optics, using 10x and 20x fluorescence objectives and the following Olympus filter/mirror series: U-MWIBA3 for Alexa488; U-MWIGA3 for rhodamine; U-MNUA2 for DAPI. Digital images were recorded using a ProgRes CT3 CMOS camera and ProgRes Capture Pro software (Jenoptik, Jena, Germany). Slides from one experiment were photographed at identical camera settings, and resulting images were processed identically.

Image Analysis

DAPI-labeled nuclei on tissue sections were color-coded depending on their aspect ratio (ratio of x to y axis) in the following way. Images were imported into ImageJ, binarized, and the Watershed tool was used to separate touching/overlapping nuclei. Particles (i.e., DAPI-stained nuclei) were fitted with ellipses, and their aspect ratio was analyzed. A ROI (region of interest) color coder plugin with the "Phase" LUT (look up table) was then used to color-code all nuclei with an aspect ratio of >2.5 and above in red, 2.0–2.5 in pink, and <2.0 in blue.

RESULTS

Periostin as a Mesenchymal Marker for Palatal Shelves during Elevation

To generate a fate map of palatal mesenchyme and epithelium during the process of shelf elevation, we screened the expression patterns of more than 20 ECM components by *in situ* hybridization on frontal sections of wild-type C56/BalbC mouse embryo heads during the relevant stages, i.e., E13.5–E14.5. Of these genes, the expression of eight was highly enriched in either all or just a specific region of the palatal shelves compared to the surrounding maxillary tissue: Periostin, tenascin-C, tenascin-W, collagen types II, IX, XI, and XIV, and SMOC-2.

Periostin (gene name *Postn*) is an ECM component belonging to the "matricellular" proteins (Murphy-Ullrich and Sage, 2014) and known to be involved in morphogenesis and wound healing (Walker et al., 2016). Periostin protein was demonstrated in mouse palatal shelves by immunofluorescence (Oka et al.,

2012). Here, we used *in situ* hybridization to reveal the expression pattern of *Postn* mRNA in palatal shelves of wild-type mouse embryos immediately before (E13.5) and after (E14.5) elevation. Serial frontal cryosections through palatal shelves were hybridized with *Postn*-specific RNA probe at three levels: anterior (future anterior hard palate), medial (future posterior hard palate), and posterior (future soft palate). Anteriorly, *Postn* mRNA was expressed in a broad layer of mesenchyme on both the buccal (ventrolateral) and lingual (medial) aspect of E13.5 palatal shelves (**Figure 1A**). After shelf elevation (E14.5), the layer of *Postn* expression was located ventrolaterally in the shelves, and filled their medial tips (**Figure 1B**). At the medial level, a strong *Postn* signal covered the entire mesenchymal area of vertical palatal shelves at E13.5 (**Figure 1C**). After elevation at this level, *Postn* expression was observed in a broad area around the midline, from where it extended into a ventral stripe facing the oral cavity (**Figure 1D**). In contrast and remarkably, the dorsolateral regions of the elevated shelves were free of *Postn* signal (**Figure 1D**). A similar distribution was seen at the posterior level both before and after elevation, except that the signal was weaker in the central mesenchyme region of the shelves (**Figures 1E,F**).

Tenascin-C Expression in the Medial Palatal Mesenchyme Both before an after Shelf Elevation

Tenascin-C (gene name *Tnc*) is another "matricellular" ECM protein with highly regulated patterns of expression in vertebrate morphogenesis and pathologies (Chiquet-Ehrismann and Chiquet, 2003). Like periostin, tenascin-C protein has been detected in the developing secondary palate before by immunofluorescence (Ferguson, 1988). At the anterior level at E13.5, the *Tnc* mRNA expression pattern resembled that of periostin: In vertical shelves, the signal was found in the sub-epithelial mesenchyme both on the lingual (medial) and the buccal (ventrolateral) aspect (**Figure 2A**). After elevation, *Tnc* mRNA was concentrated at the tips of the shelves and extended laterally into the subepithelial mesenchyme both dorsally and ventrally (**Figure 2B**). A different distribution was observed at the medial level, i.e., in the future posterior hard palate. There, *Tnc* expression covered the entire lingual half of the vertical shelves at E13.5, whereas the buccal half was devoid of signal except for a thin stripe underneath the epithelium (**Figure 2C**). In elevated shelves (E14.5) at this level, *Tnc* mRNA was observed in a broad mesenchymal region that extended from dorsal to ventral around the midline, and in a thin stripe underneath the ventral epithelium (**Figure 2D**). A similar distribution was seen for *Tnc* at the posterior level (future soft palate), although the signal was weaker (**Figures 2E,F**).

Dorsomedial Tenascin-W Expression in Palatal Shelves Both before and after Shelf Elevation

Tenascin-W (gene name *Tnn*) is the latest member of this family of ECM proteins (Scherberich et al., 2004). During embryogenesis, its expression partially overlaps with that of tenascin-C but is even more restricted. Notably, tenascin-W was shown to be involved in osteogenesis (Martina et al., 2010) and is a marker for osteogenic areas in embryos (Scherberich et al., 2004). In anterior palatal shelves at E13.5, we found *Tnn* to be expressed exclusively in the dorsomedial quadrant of the mesenchyme, whereas the tips of the vertical shelves were devoid of signal (**Figure 3A**). At E14.5, the *Tnn* signal was restricted to the dorsal mesenchyme around the midline of the elevated shelves (**Figure 3B**). A similar distribution was found at the medial level both at E13.5 and E14.5, except that in the elevated shelves the area of *Tnn* expression was spread out laterally and filled the entire dorsal half of the shelf mesenchyme (**Figures 3C,D**). More posteriorly, the Tnn signal was present in addition around the developing os palatinum (**Figures 3E,F**).

SMOC-2 Expression at Palatal Shelf Tips before, but Not at the Midline after Elevation

SMOC-2 (SPARC related modular calcium binding 2; gene name *Smoc2*) belongs to the SPARC/Osteonectin family of matricellular proteins (Vannahme et al., 2003) and is involved in keratinocyte migration (Maier et al., 2008) and angiogenesis (Rocnik et al., 2006). In mouse embryos, *Smoc2* is prominently expressed in perichondrial mesenchyme (**Figure 4A**). Surprisingly, *Smoc2* mRNA is also detected in defined areas of the oral epithelium. At a medial to posterior level before elevation (E13.5), the *Smoc2* signal outlines the buccal surface of the palatal shelves and extends into the epithelium at their tips, but finishes abruptly at the lower end of their lingual aspect (**Figure 4A**). At E14.5, *Smoc2* mRNA is present in the entire ventral epithelium of the elevated shelves, but stops shortly before the midline (**Figure 4B**). A similar expression pattern in palatal epithelium before and after elevation was found for type XIV collagen, also named undulin, a minor fibril-associated collagen (Ricard-Blum, 2011) (not shown). For comparison, sections from a similar level were hybridized with a *Tgfβ3* probe. This growth factor is secreted by midline epithelial cells and required for palatal shelf fusion (Kaartinen et al., 1995). At E13.5, *Tgfβ3* mRNA extended from the shelf tip about halfway up the lingual epithelium (**Figure 4C**), and at E14.5 was found at the midline (**Figure 4D**). Thus, *Smoc2* and *Tgfb3* exhibit a reciprocal expression pattern in the palatal epithelium, except for a short overlap at the shelf tip before, or close to the ventral midline after elevation, respectively.

Mesenchymal and Epithelial Rearrangements during Palatal Shelf Elevation at the Medial Level

Since the mRNAs of the chosen ECM genes were enriched in distinct areas of the palatal shelves before and after elevation, this allowed the mapping of their combined expression patterns (**Figure 5**; compare with **Figures 1–4**). At the medial level, the combined results implied that elevation is not due to a simple rotation of the palatal shelves from the vertical into the horizontal plane. If this were the case, the *Tnc*-expressing lingual half of the vertical shelves should end up dorsally in the elevated secondary palate. Instead, the *Tnc*-expressing

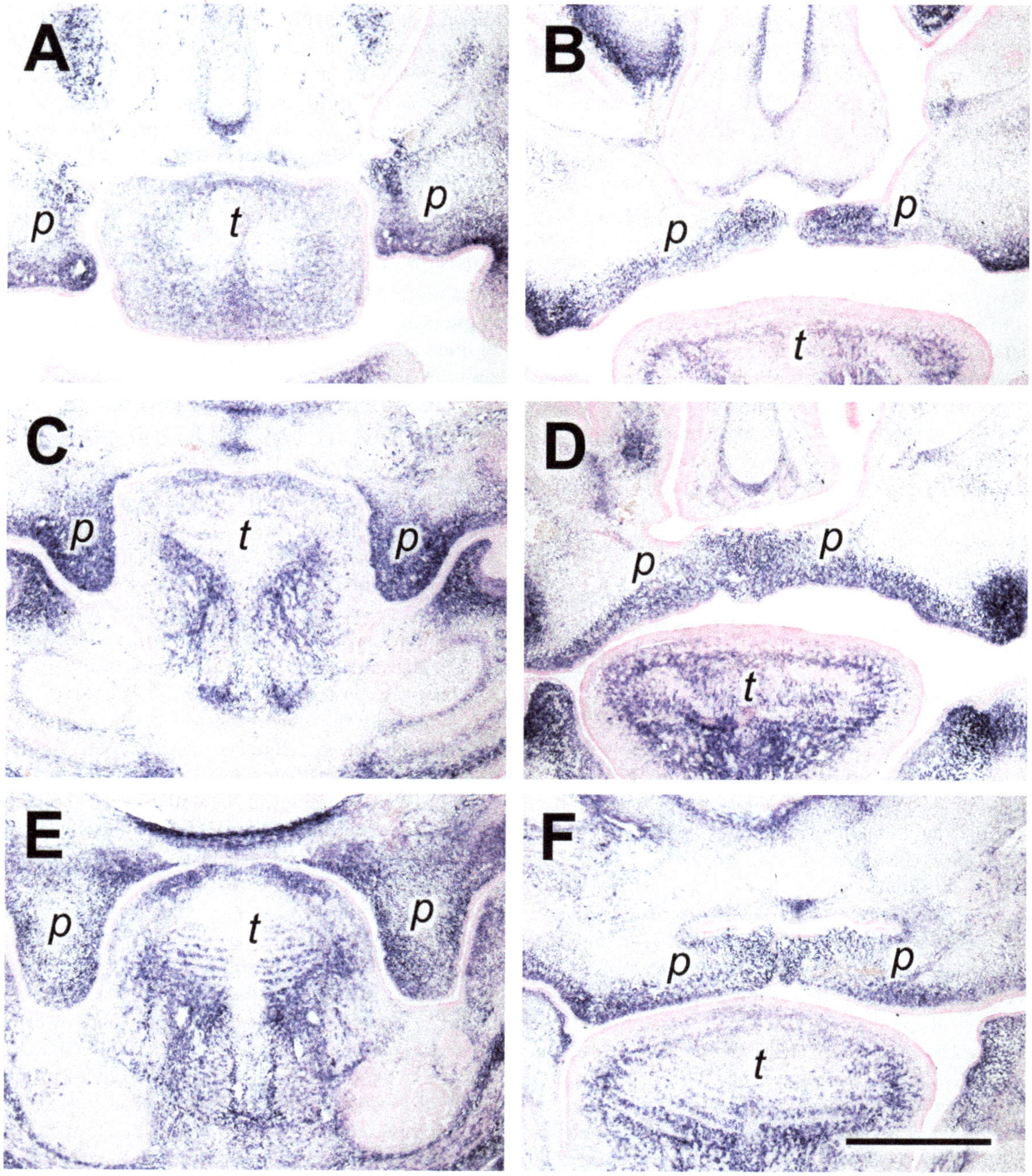

FIGURE 1 | *Periostin* expression as a marker for palatal shelves during elevation. *In situ* hybridization for *Postn* mRNA on frontal sections of palatal shelves from wild-type mouse embryos at the anterior **(A,B)**, medial **(C,D)**, and posterior **(E,F)** level. Serial sections were obtained from an E13.5 **(A,C,E)** and an E14.5 **(B,D,F)** embryo, respectively. For description, see text. Abbreviations: palatal shelf (p), tongue (t). Bar, 400 μm.

area had moved to a broad zone at the midline, whereas the lateral parts of the elevated shelves were devoid of *Tnc* signal. The *Postn* signal, which filled the entire shelves at E13.5, was drawn out after elevation into a broad tringle that filled the entire mesenchyme around the midline, and tapered on the ventrolateral aspect of the shelves (cf. **Figure 1D**). Mesenchyme around the nasopharyngeal fold that forms at E.14.5 lacked expression of *Postn* (**Figure 5**), suggesting that maxillary tissue originally outside the palatal shelf proper is drawn into the elevated shelves at E14.5. Thus, at this level the palatal shelf bulges out medially whereas the original tip retracts during elevation. This involves massive reorganization of the palatal mesenchyme: The lingual mesenchyme of the E13.5 shelf, rather than that at the distal tip, forms the tissue around the midline at E14.5. The mesenchyme at the original tip ends up more laterally after elevation, whereas the originally buccal mesenchyme distorts and

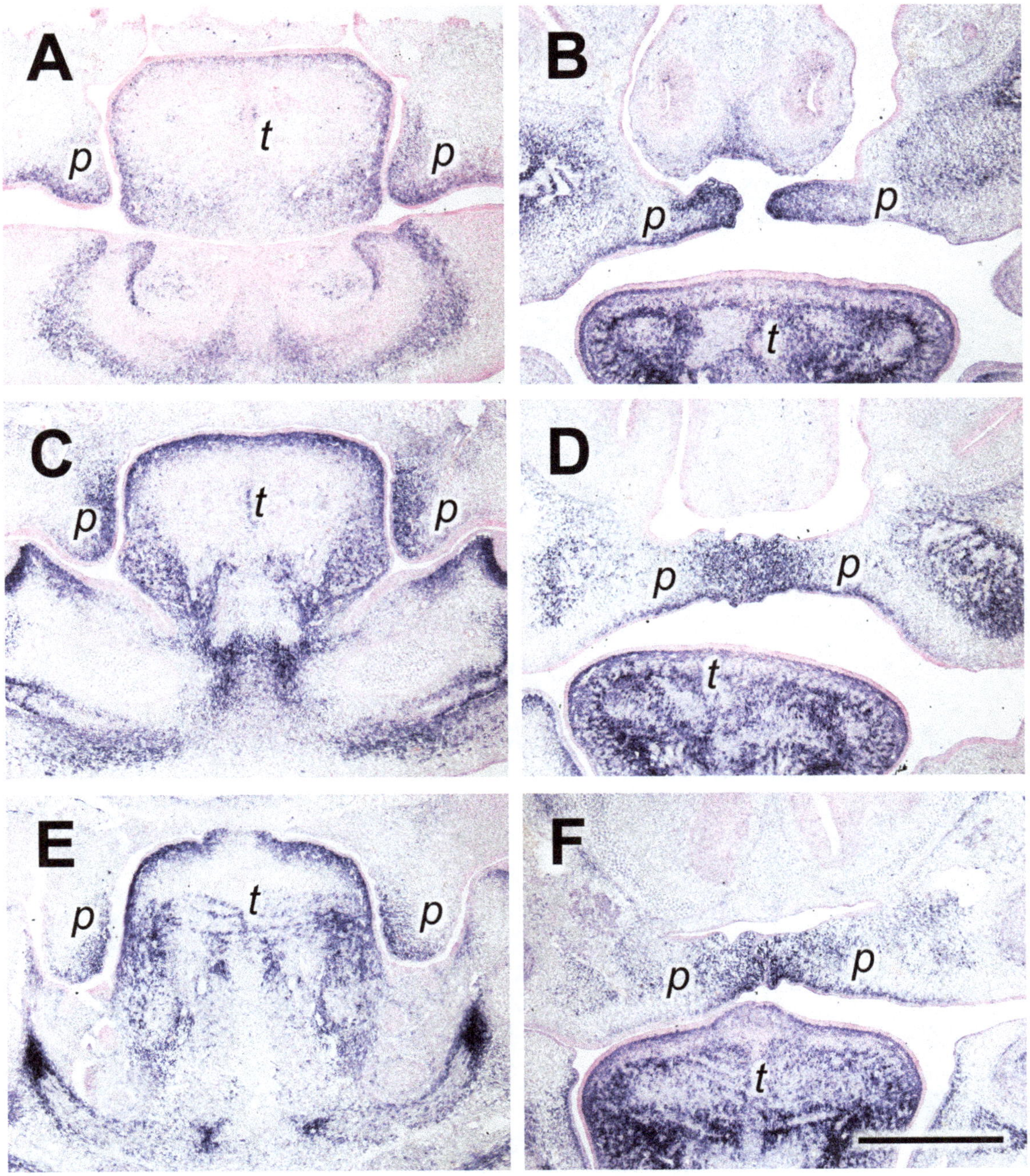

FIGURE 2 | *Tenascin-C* expression primarily in the lingual/medial half of palatal shelves both before and after shelf elevation. *In situ* hybridization for *Tnc* mRNA on frontal sections of palatal shelves from wild-type mouse embryos at the anterior **(A,B)**, medial **(C,D)**, and posterior **(E,F)** level. Serial sections were obtained from an E13.5 **(A,C,E)** and an E14.5 **(B,D,F)** embryo, respectively. For description, see text. Abbreviations: palatal shelf (p), tongue (t). Bar, 400 μm.

spreads out along the ventrolateral aspect of the elevated shelves. Remodeling of the mesenchyme is paralleled by reorganization of the palatal epithelium. *Smoc2* mRNA was detected in shelf tip epithelium before, but not in midline epithelium after elevation. Conversely, *Tgfβ3* was expressed primarily in lingual epithelium of shelves before, and in midline epithelium after elevation (**Figures 4, 5**).

Anterior to Posterior Differences in ECM Rearrangement during Shelf Elevation

In wild-type Balb/C litters collected at E14.5, it is quite frequent to find embryos in which either one or both of the palatal shelves have not elevated yet (Luke, 1984; Yu and Ornitz, 2011). These mice can be compared to their siblings with already elevated shelves, and one representative example is shown in

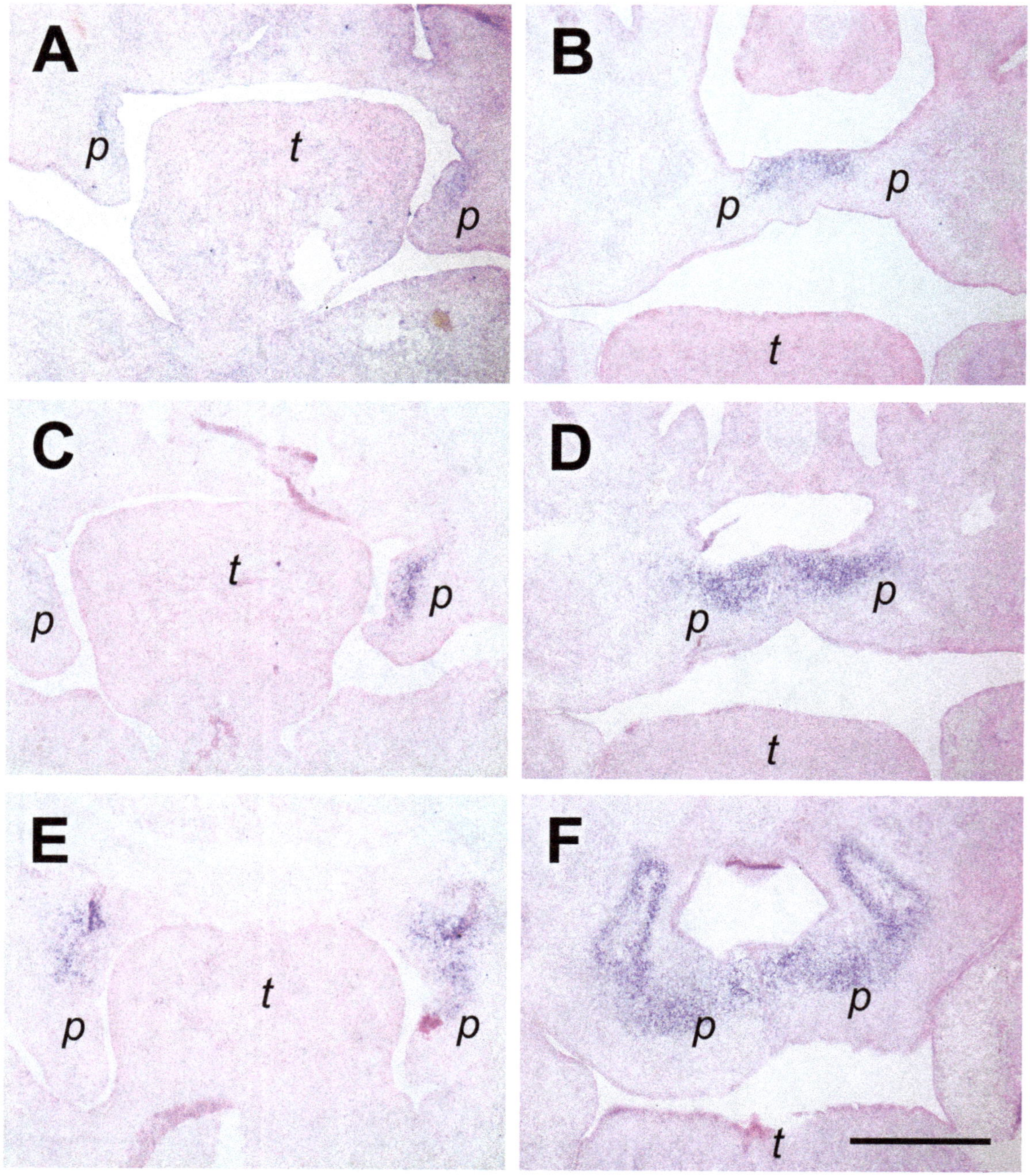

FIGURE 3 | *Tenascin-W* expression in the dorsomedial quadrant of palatal shelves both before and after elevation. *In situ* hybridization for *tenascin-W/Tnn* mRNA on frontal sections of palatal shelves from wild-type mouse embryos at the anterior **(A,B)**, medial **(C,D)**, and posterior **(E,F)** level. Serial sections were obtained from an E13.5 **(A,C,E)** and an E14.5 **(B,D,F)** embryo, respectively. For description, see text. Abbreviations: palatal shelf (p), tongue (t). Bar, 400 μm.

Figure 6. The images show frontal sections at three levels through the palatal shelves of two different E14.5 embryos from the same litter, stained by fluorescence for actin (red) and tenascin-C (green). **Figure 6A** shows a still vertical palatal shelf of one E14.5 embryo at the anterior level, and it is noteworthy that a prominent epithelial invagination has formed on its buccal side. Staining for tenascin-C protein largely fills the shelf mesenchyme, except for its central area. At the same level in the sibling (**Figure 6B**), its elevated shelf occupies the space between nasal process and tongue, and the epithelial invagination has disappeared. Tenascin-C is present in the medial and ventrolateral parts of the shelf. Since tenascin-C positive regions largely correspond to each other before and after elevation, these observations agree with a flipping movement of the anterior palatal shelves. On the other hand, comparison of shelves from the same two embryos also confirms that

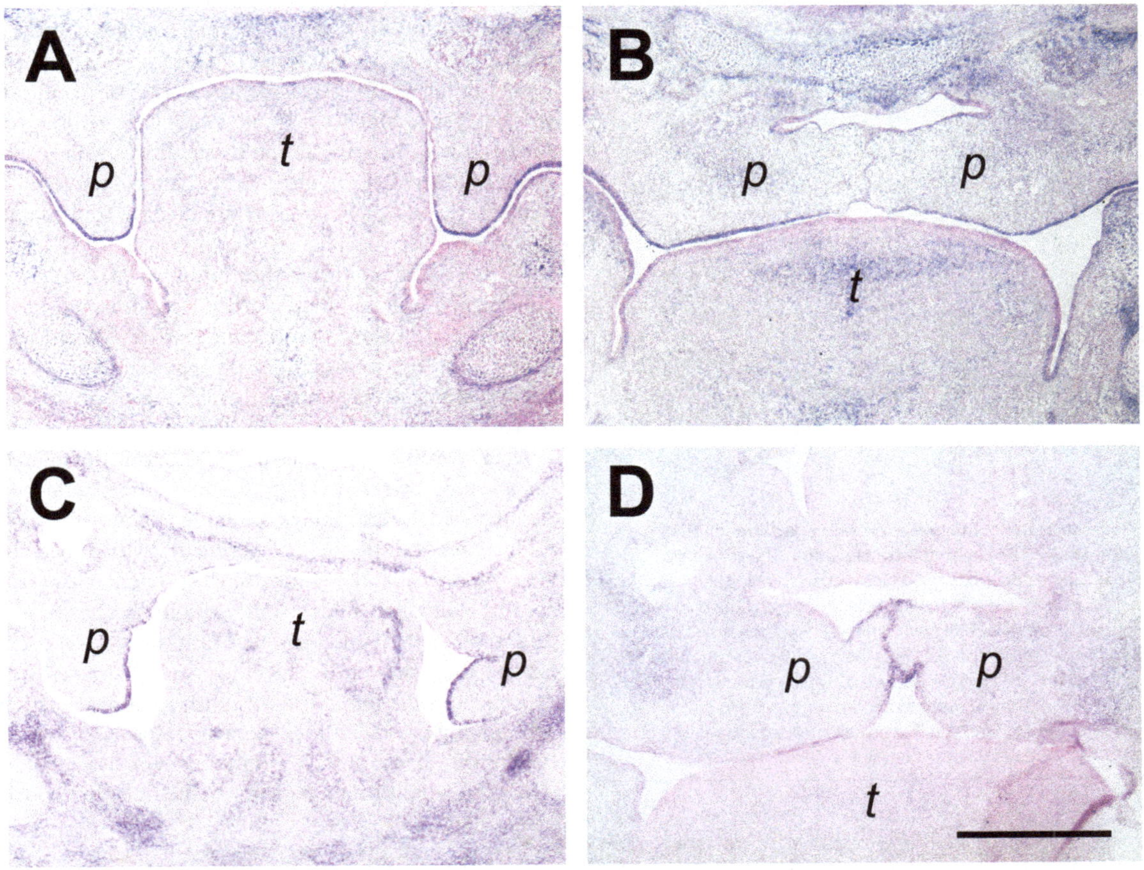

FIGURE 4 | *Smoc2* expression in palatal tip epithelium before, but not midline epithelium after elevation. *In situ* hybridization for *Smoc2* **(A,B)** or *Tgfβ3* **(C,D)** mRNA, respectively, on frontal sections at the medial level of palatal shelves from wild-type mouse embryos. Serial sections were obtained from an E13.5 **(A,C,E)** and an E14.5 **(B,D,F)** embryo, respectively. For description, see text. Abbreviations: palatal shelf (p), tongue (t). Bar, 400 μm.

extensive mesenchymal reorganization takes place at the medial and posterior level during elevation. At the medial level, a small protrusion has formed on the dorsolingual aspect of the still vertical shelf (**Figure 6C**). Tenascin-C is found primarily in the lingual half of the shelf mesenchyme, with only a narrow ribbon underneath the buccal epithelium. In case of the elevated shelf at the same level (**Figure 6D**), the entire tenascin-C containing mesenchymal shelf ECM between the original tip and the dorsolingual protrusion appears compressed between nasal process and tongue. Remarkably, the palatal artery appears circular in cross-section by actin staining before elevation, but is flattened in the vertical direction after elevation (c.f. **Figures 6C,D**). At the posterior level, the dorsolingual protrusion is very prominent on the not yet elevated shelf, forming a second tip (**Figure 6E**). Tenascin-C protein is enriched in the mesenchyme between the two shelf tips, rather than at the tips themselves. At this level, it is most obvious that the entire tenascin-C containing mesenchyme has moved to the midline after elevation (**Figure 6F**). Rather than a flipping movement as seen at the front, this again implies a slug-like reshaping of the medial/posterior palatal shelf, with a deformation and medial movement of the lingual mesenchyme (including the palatine artery) and a retraction of the original shelf tip.

Orientation of Actin Fibers and Nuclei in Palatal Mesenchyme during Elevation

Fluorescently labeled phalloidin is a specific marker for actin stress fibers of cells in culture (Small et al., 1999), and can also be used to label the cytoskeletal F-actin network of embryonic tissues (**Figures 7A,B**). As a major component of the contractile apparatus, actin stress fibers are known to align with the major direction of strain within a cell (Burridge and Wittchen, 2013). In **Figure 7A**, a higher magnification of a E14.5 palatal shelf at the medial level just before elevation (c.f. **Figure 6C**) is shown after phalloidin labeling. Note that the F-actin network of mesenchymal cells is aligned within this shelf, pointing toward the original ventral tip and the newly forming lingual protrusion, and forming an arc between them. In already elevated shelves of the same stage, the cellular actin network appears less organized, and no preferred direction is apparent in the shelf proper (**Figure 7B**). We also determined, on the same sections, the deformation of DAPI-labeled cell nuclei in the palatal mesenchyme. Using ImageJ, the ellipticity

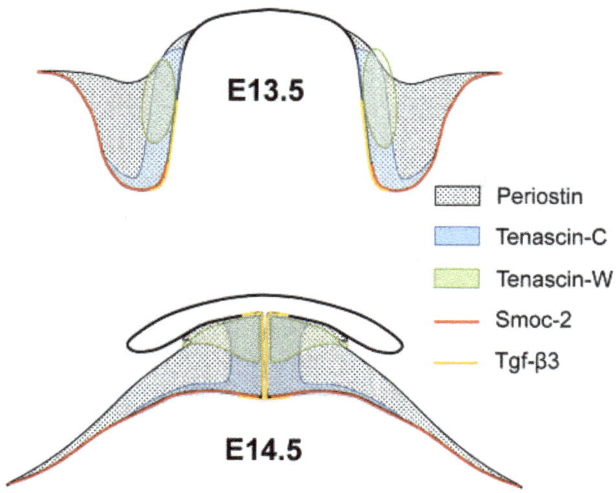

FIGURE 5 | Scheme of the combined expression patterns of ECM genes in palatal shelves before and after elevation. The schematic drawings represent palatal shelves of wild-type mouse embryos at the medial level before (E13.5; above) and after (E14.5; below) elevation. The approximate areas of mesenchymal expression of *periostin*, *tenascin-C*, *tenascin-W*, and epithelial expression of *Smoc2* and *Tgfβ3* are indicated. Note that *tenascin-C*, *tenascin-W*, and *Tgfβ3* expressing areas all end up at the midline after elevation, although their center of expression does not localize to the shelf tip before elevation. Conversely, *Smoc2* mRNA is epithelially expressed at the shelf tip before, but excluded from midline epithelium after elevation.

of stained nuclei was measured, and nuclei with an aspect ratio of >2.5 were labeled in red. As can be seen in **Figure 7C**, elongated (red) nuclei are enriched in, and align with, the arc-like F-actin network that is visible between the ventral and the lingual tips of this shelf before elevation. In contrast, elongated nuclei appear sparse and have no preferred direction in the elevated shelf (**Figure 7D**); they are more frequent in lateral maxillary mesenchyme. Note further that antibody to tenascin-C labels an ECM meshwork that lies parallel to the actin arc and the elongated nuclei in elevating shelves (**Figure 7E**). After elevation, the tenascin-C positive ECM has moved toward the midline as seen before, and the ECM fibrils appear randomly arranged (**Figure 7F**). These observations suggest that tensile stress builds up in the palatal shelves before elevation, which is released after the shelves have reached the horizontal position.

DISCUSSION

Remodeling of Palatal Shelf Mesenchyme during Elevation Revealed by ECM Expression Patterns

In the present study, we took advantage of the differential expression patterns of certain ECM genes to monitor tissue rearrangements during palatal shelf elevation. After screening over 20 ECM genes by *in situ* hybridization before and after elevation, we identified a few that exhibited expression patterns restricted to specific areas of the shelf mesenchyme or epithelium. Genes for ECM components are strongly expressed, and the turnover of their mRNAs is relatively slow (Eckes et al., 1996). We therefore argue that the observed changes in ECM expression patterns reflect morphogenetic rearrangements of palatal shelf tissue, rather than alterations in the rate of gene transcription. In the case of tenascin-C, *in situ* hybridization results were further confirmed by antibody stainings. This makes it even more unlikely that the observed dynamic changes in tenascin-C patterns during shelf elevation are due to rapid alterations in its synthesis.

Our results confirm the findings of Jin et al. (2010) concerning palatal shelf remodeling during elevation (see below). In addition, they extend earlier studies by providing more detailed information on the reshaping and medial translocation of the lingual shelf mesenchyme during this morphogenetic process. A further observation is noteworthy: During elevation, epithelial folds form dorsolaterally from the palatal shelves; these folds mark the lateral edges of the nasal cavity. Interestingly, the mesenchyme surrounding these folds express little or no periostin, which before elevation is a marker for the entire shelf proper. This suggests that at the epithelial folds, some originally nasal mesenchyme might be pulled into the elevating shelves. We have shown before that the epithelial folds are characterized by high expression of *Mmp2* mRNA and gelatinase activity, which presumably is needed there to avoid closure of the nasal cavity (Gkantidis et al., 2012). From our results, these specialized structures might originate from tissue outside the original shelf proper.

The mechanism of shelf elevation during secondary palate formation in mammals has been disputed (Brinkley and Vickerman, 1979; Jin et al., 2010; Bush and Jiang, 2012). Early reports favored a simple flipping movement of the vertical palatal shelves into a horizontal position (Coleman, 1965), but it was soon postulated that posteriorly the palatal shelves reorganize differently. From histological observations, it appeared that their lingual/medial aspect bulged out whereas their original ventral tip retracted (Brinkley and Vickerman, 1979). This process requires extensive remodeling of the entire shelf, but the underlying mechanism remained obscure. Recently, Jin et al. (2010) found that matrix metalloproteinase *Mmp13*, a specific marker for midline epithelial cells, was expressed in still vertical E14.5 shelves posteriorly not at their tip but on their lingual/medial aspect, whereas anteriorly the *Mmp13* signal extended into the shelf tip. The authors concluded that only anteriorly, the original tip epithelium will form the midline of elevated palatal shelves, whereas in middle and posterior regions, the midline epithelial cells are derived from the lingual epithelium of vertical shelves (Jin et al., 2010). These findings were in agreement with the earlier hypothesis that upon elevation, shelves undergo a flipping motion anteriorly, and a reshaping in middle and posterior regions.

(Jin et al., 2010) also showed that the mesenchymal transcription factor *Goosecoid* was expressed around the midline in E14.5 embryos, but in the lingual rather than the tip mesenchyme of non-elevated shelves of the same stage. This provided the first indication for large scale reorganization of

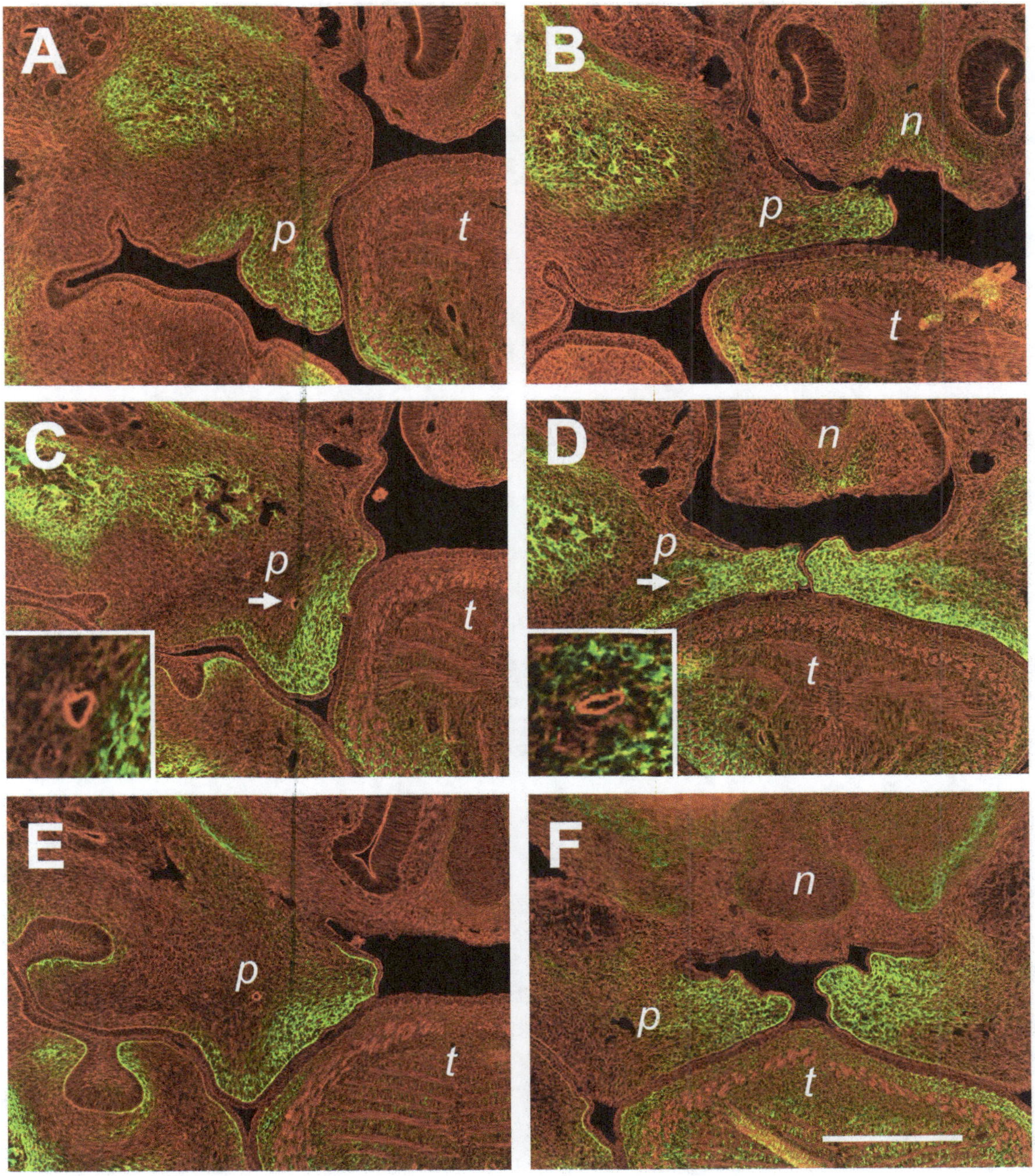

FIGURE 6 | Differences in tissue rearrangements between anterior, medial, and posterior palatal shelves during elevation. Serial sections through E14.5 palatal shelves at the anterior **(A,B)**, medial **(C,D)**, and posterior **(E,F)** level were double-stained with rhodamine-phalloidin for actin (red) and antibody to tenascin-C (green), and viewed in a fluorescence microscope. Sections were obtained from two embryos of the same E14.5 litter; one in which the shelves had just started to elevate **(A,C,E)**, and one in which they had already risen above the tongue **(B,D,F)**. Abbreviations: palatal shelf (p), tongue (t), nasal septum (n). The palatine artery is marked with an arrow in **(C,D)**, and shown enlarged in the inserts. Bar, 400 μm.

pre-existing mesenchyme during shelf elevation, rather than for differential cell growth as it has been suggested (Brinkley and Bookstein, 1986; Sasaki et al., 2004). In any case, the rapid and often asynchronous time course of shelf elevation (Yu and Ornitz, 2011), as well as our present results, strongly argue against differential cell growth as a mechanism for palatal shelf remodeling.

Actin-Based Cellular Contractility Combined with Differential ECM Stiffness as a Possible Mechanism for Shelf Remodeling during Elevation

Cells attach to the ECM via integrins, which in turn are linked to the intracellular actin cytoskeleton. Embryonic cells and their

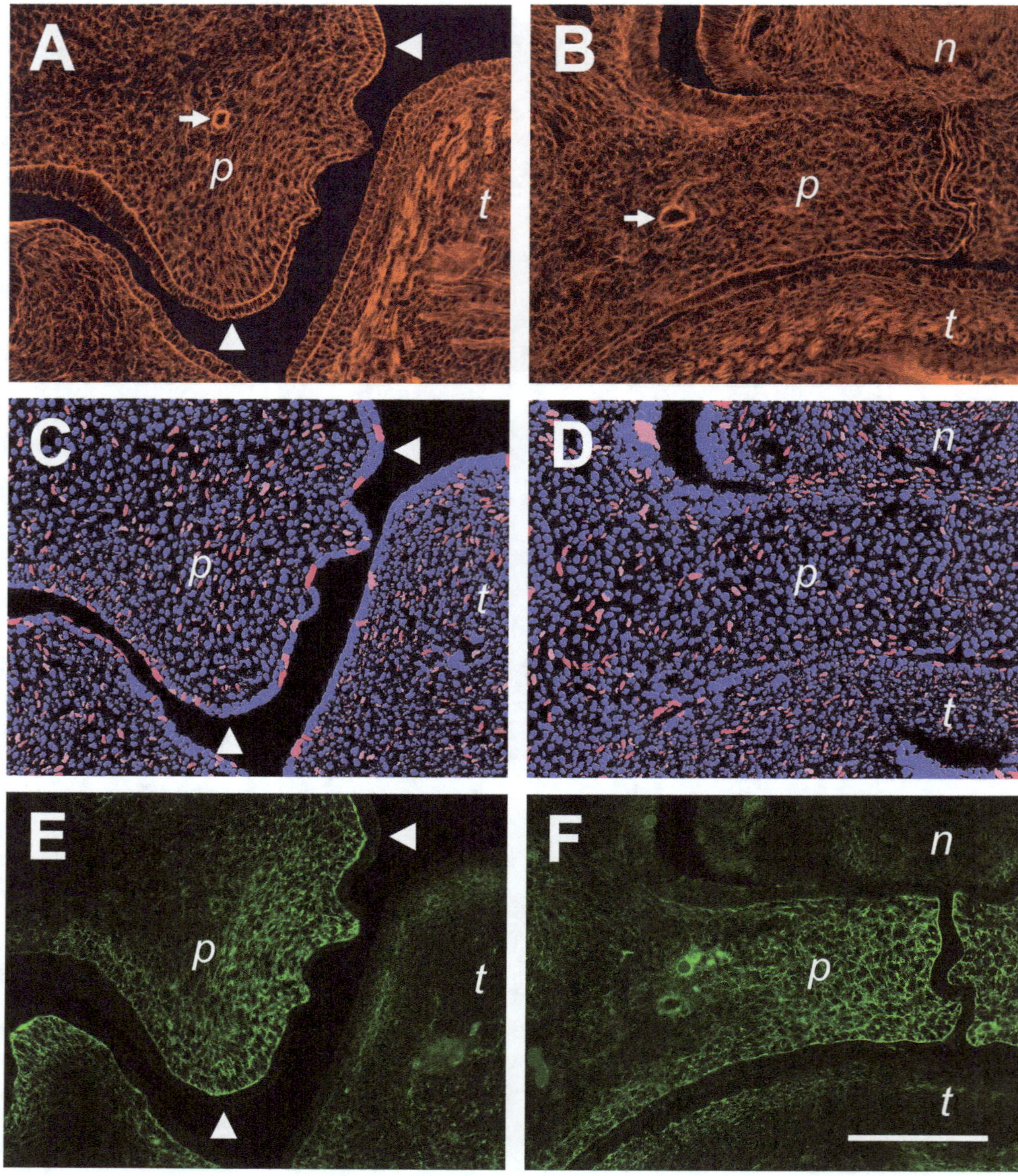

FIGURE 7 | Actin fiber and nuclear orientation in the mesenchyme of the posterior palate during elevation. Representative sections through E14.5 palatal shelves were triple-stained with phalloidin for actin **(A,B)**, DAPI for nuclei **(C,D)**, and antibody to tenascin-C **(E,F)**, respectively, and viewed in a fluorescence microscope. On the left **(A,C,E)**, a shelf just before elevation is shown, and on the right **(B,D,F)** an already elevated shelf from an embryo of the same litter. The images **(C,D)** were processed by ImageJ, such that all elongated nuclei with an aspect ratio above 2.5 are false-colored in red, those with 2.0–2.5 in pink. Roundish nuclei (aspect ratio <2.0) are blue. Note that before elevation **(C)**, many elongated (red/pink) nuclei are present between the original tip and the medial protrusion of the elevating shelf (arrowheads in **A,C,E**), and that their direction parallels that of the actin **(A)** and ECM **(E)** meshwork. The palatine artery is marked with an arrow in **(A,B)**. Abbreviations: palatal shelf (p), tongue (t), nasal septum (n). Bar, 200 μm.

ECM thereby form a mechanical continuum, in which actin-generated tensile stresses are transmitted from one cell to the next (Wozniak and Chen, 2009). Stresses align the intracellular F-actin, and also reorient and organize extracellular ECM fibers (Burridge and Wittchen, 2013). Moreover, cell nuclei are mechanically connected to the actin cytoskeleton and deformed by tensile stresses that pull on the cell (Brosig et al., 2010). Thus, preferred orientations of the interconnected actin-integrin-ECM meshwork, together with elongated cell nuclei, reflect vectors of tensile stress that act within embryonic mesenchyme. The fungal toxin phalloidin specifically binds to cellular F-actin (Small et al., 1999). Tenascin-C is known to decorate ECM fibrils in embryonic tissues (Chiquet-Ehrismann and Chiquet, 2003). We used these two tools, together with measurements of the ellipticity of cell nuclei, to determine whether tensile stresses might occur in palatal shelves during their elevation. Our results clearly indicate that in the medial and posterior parts of the elevating shelf, the mesenchyme is tensed between the original tip and the newly forming lingual/medial protrusion. It is more than likely that such tensile stress is generated by F-actin dependent contraction of the shelf mesenchymal cells themselves, and that it is transmitted onto the ECM in which they are embedded.

Despite of several hypotheses that have been put forward over the years, the forces driving palatal shelf elevation were essentially unknown. Walker and Fraser (1956) first postulated an "internal shelf force." A popular hypothesis, still cited in recent reviews (Gritli-Linde, 2007), postulated that a cushion of hyaluronic acid in the "hinge" region of the palatal shelves provides a swelling force by generating osmotic pressure, which pushes up the shelf (Brinkley and Morris-Wiman, 1987). This idea was based on the presence of hyaluronidase-sensitive material in the respective region of the palatal shelf (Brinkley and Morris-Wiman, 1987), and on the fact that a glycosaminoglycan synthesis inhibitor caused cleft palate in mice (Brinkley and Vickerman, 1982). However, the main effect of the inhibitor was to cause a substantial shrinkage in shelf size compared to controls (Brinkley and Vickerman, 1982). Therefore, the inhibitor was likely to cause its damage long before shelf elevation occurred. In essence, there is no direct evidence that hyaluronic acid or other glycosaminoglycans are involved in generating the forces for shelf elevation.

Actin-based cellular contractility is well recognized for driving diverse morphogenetic movements during embryogenesis of both vertebrate and non-vertebrate species (Wozniak and Chen, 2009). Compared to alternatives such as differential cell growth or accumulation of ECM, this mechanism has a large advantage for the involved cells. Namely, they can control it rapidly and precisely in time and space, by activating the intracellular RhoA/ROCK signaling pathway that triggers actomyosin contraction (Burridge and Wittchen, 2013). Surprisingly, although actin contractility has been suggested as a mechanism for palatal shelf elevation early on (Lessard et al., 1974), this idea has apparently not been followed up in more recent years, but is now strongly supported by our current findings.

An actin-based mechanism for palatal shelf reorganization by no means implies that ECM itself has no function in the process. ECM sustains and counteracts forces generated by cellular contractility, and its local stiffness determines to which extent embedded cells are able to deform the tissue (Shawky and Davidson, 2015). Thus, if palatal shelf elevation is driven by cellular actin contraction, differences in ECM composition and stiffness within the shelf might have substantial effects on reshaping of the tissue. Moreover, specific ECM components can modulate cell adhesion, and thereby affect cell contractility. For example, tenascin-C inhibits RhoA/ROCK signaling (and thus actomyosin contraction) by interfering with cell adhesion to fibronectin (Midwood and Schwarzbauer, 2002). It can therefore be speculated that cell contraction is diminished in tenascin-C rich regions within the palatal mesenchyme. Future studies involving a careful mapping of F-actin dynamics, as well as of ECM composition and stiffness, within elevating palatal shelves will be required to fully understand this complex morphogenetic process.

AUTHOR CONTRIBUTIONS

MC, SB, TM, and CK contributed to the conception and design of the work; MC, SB, and MA were responsible for data acquisition, analysis, and interpretation; MC drafted the manuscript; SB, MA, TM, and CK critically revised the manuscript; MC, SB, MA, TM, and CK approved the manuscript; MC, SB, MA, TM, and CK agreed to be accountable for all aspects of the work.

ACKNOWLEDGMENTS

We are grateful to François Spetz and Dr. Ruth Chiquet-Ehrismann (Friedrich Miescher Institute for Biomedical Research, Basel, Switzerland), Dr. Daniel Graf (University of Alberta, Edmonton, Canada), and Younes El Fersioui (Department of Orthodontics and Dentofacial Orthopedics, University of Bern, Switzerland) for providing us with tissue and reagents for this study. We thank Sabrina Ruggiero for technical help. MC would like to express his profound gratitude to Ruth Chiquet-Ehrismann, close collaborator, friend and partner for more than 30 years, for her unfailing support throughout his career. Ruth sadly and unexpectedly died on September 4, 2015.

REFERENCES

Aufderheide, E., and Ekblom, P. (1988). Tenascin during gut development: appearance in the mesenchyme, shift in molecular forms, and dependence on epithelial-mesenchymal interactions. *J. Cell Biol.* 107, 2341–2349. doi: 10.1083/jcb.107.6.2341

Brinkley, L. L., and Bookstein, F. L. (1986). Cell distribution during mouse secondary palate closure. II. Mesenchymal cells. *J. Embryol. Exp. Morphol.* 96, 111–130.

Brinkley, L. L., and Morris-Wiman, J. (1987). Computer-assisted analysis of hyaluronate distribution during morphogenesis of the mouse secondary palate. *Development* 100, 629–635.

Brinkley, L. L., and Vickerman, M. M. (1979). Elevation of lesioned palatal shelves *in vitro*. *J. Embryol. Exp. Morphol.* 54, 229–240.

Brinkley, L. L., and Vickerman, M. M. (1982). The effects of chlorcyclizine-induced alterations of glycosaminoglycans on mouse palatal shelf elevation *in vivo* and *in vitro*. *J. Embryol. Exp. Morphol.* 69, 193–213.

Brosig, M., Ferralli, J., Gelman, L., Chiquet, M., and Chiquet-Ehrismann, R. (2010). Interfering with the connection between the nucleus and the cytoskeleton affects nuclear rotation, mechanotransduction and myogenesis. *Int. J. Biochem. Cell Biol.* 42, 1717–1728. doi: 10.1016/j.biocel.2010.07.001

Burridge, K., and Wittchen, E. S. (2013). The tension mounts: stress fibers as force-generating mechanotransducers. *J. Cell Biol.* 200, 9–19. doi: 10.1083/jcb.201210090

Bush, J. O., and Jiang, R. (2012). Palatogenesis: morphogenetic and molecular mechanisms of secondary palate development. *Development* 139, 231–243. doi: 10.1242/dev.067082

Chiquet-Ehrismann, R., and Chiquet, M. (2003). Tenascins: regulation and putative functions during pathological stress. *J. Pathol.* 200, 488–499. doi: 10.1002/path.1415

Chou, M. J., Kosazuma, T., Takigawa, T., Yamada, S., Takahara, S., and Shiota, K. (2004). Palatal shelf movement during palatogenesis: a fate map of the fetal mouse palate cultured *in vitro*. *Anat. Embryol.* 208, 19–25. doi: 10.1007/s00429-004-0379-0

Coleman, R. D. (1965). Development of the rat palate. *Anat. Rec.* 151, 107–117. doi: 10.1002/ar.1091510202

Dixon, M. J., Marazita, M. L., Beaty, T. H., and Murray, J. C. (2011). Cleft lip and palate: understanding genetic and environmental influences. *Nat. Rev. Genet.* 12, 167–178. doi: 10.1038/nrg2933

Eckes, B., Mauch, C., Hüppe, G., and Krieg, T. (1996). Differential regulation of transcription and transcript stability of pro-alpha 1(I) collagen and fibronectin in activated fibroblasts derived from patients with systemic scleroderma. *Biochem. J.* 315(Pt 2), 549–554.

Ferguson, M. W. (1988). Palate development. *Development* 103(Suppl.), 41–60.

Flück, M., Tunc-Civelek, V., and Chiquet, M. (2000). Rapid and reciprocal regulation of tenascin-C and tenascin-Y expression by loading of skeletal muscle. *J. Cell Sci.* 113(Pt 20), 3583–3591.

Gkantidis, N., Blumer, S., Katsaros, C., Graf, D., and Chiquet, M. (2012). Site-specific expression of gelatinolytic activity during morphogenesis of the secondary palate in the mouse embryo. *PLoS ONE* 7:e47762. doi: 10.1371/journal.pone.0047762

Gritli-Linde, A. (2007). Molecular control of secondary palate development. *Dev. Biol.* 301, 309–326. doi: 10.1016/j.ydbio.2006.07.042

Gritli-Linde, A. (2008). The etiopathogenesis of cleft lip and cleft palate: usefulness and caveats of mouse models. *Curr. Top. Dev. Biol.* 84, 37–138. doi: 10.1016/S0070-2153(08)00602-9

Iseki, S., Ishii-Suzuki, M., Tsunekawa, N., Yamada, Y., Eto, K., and Obata, K. (2007). Experimental induction of palate shelf elevation in glutamate decarboxylase 67-deficient mice with cleft palate due to vertically oriented palatal shelf. *Birth Defects Res. Part A Clin. Mol. Teratol.* 79, 688–695. doi: 10.1002/bdra.20400

Jin, J. Z., Tan, M., Warner, D. R., Darling, D. S., Higashi, Y., Gridley, T., et al. (2010). Mesenchymal cell remodeling during mouse secondary palate reorientation. *Dev. Dyn.* 239, 2110–2117. doi: 10.1002/dvdy.22339

Jin, J. Z., Warner, D. R., Lu, Q., Pisano, M. M., Greene, R. M., and Ding, J. (2014). Deciphering TGF-beta3 function in medial edge epithelium specification and fusion during mouse secondary palate development. *Dev. Dyn.* 243, 1536–1543. doi: 10.1002/dvdy.24177

Jugessur, A., Farlie, P. G., and Kilpatrick, N. (2009a). The genetics of isolated orofacial clefts: from genotypes to subphenotypes. *Oral Dis.* 15, 437–453. doi: 10.1111/j.1601-0825.2009.01577.x

Jugessur, A., Shi, M., Gjessing, H. K., Lie, R. T., Wilcox, A. J., Weinberg, C. R., et al. (2009b). Genetic determinants of facial clefting: analysis of 357 candidate genes using two national cleft studies from Scandinavia. *PLoS ONE* 4:e5385. doi: 10.1371/journal.pone.0005385

Kaartinen, V., Voncken, J. W., Shuler, C., Warburton, D., Bu, D., Heisterkamp, N., et al. (1995). Abnormal lung development and cleft palate in mice lacking TGF-beta 3 indicates defects of epithelial-mesenchymal interaction. *Nat. Genet.* 11, 415–421. doi: 10.1038/ng1295-415

Koch, M., Bohrmann, B., Matthison, M., Hagios, C., Trueb, B., and Chiquet, M. (1995). Large and small splice variants of collagen XII: differential expression and ligand binding. *J. Cell Biol.* 130, 1005–1014. doi: 10.1083/jcb.130.4.1005

Kouskoura, T., El Fersioui, Y., Angelini, M., Graf, D., Katsaros, C., and Chiquet, M. (2016). Dislocated tongue muscle attachment and cleft palate formation. *J. Dent. Res.* 95, 453–459. doi: 10.1177/0022034515621869

Lessard, J. L., Wee, E. L., and Zimmerman, E. F. (1974). Presence of contractile proteins in mouse fetal palate prior to shelf elevation. *Teratology* 9, 113–125. doi: 10.1002/tera.1420090114

Luke, D. A. (1984). Epithelial proliferation and development of rugae in relation to palatal shelf elevation in the mouse. *J. Anat.* 138(Pt 2), 251–258.

Maier, S., Paulsson, M., and Hartmann, U. (2008). The widely expressed extracellular matrix protein SMOC-2 promotes keratinocyte attachment and migration. *Exp. Cell Res.* 314, 2477–2487. doi: 10.1016/j.yexcr.2008.05.020

Martina, E., Chiquet-Ehrismann, R., and Brellier, F. (2010). Tenascin-W: an extracellular matrix protein associated with osteogenesis and cancer. *Int. J. Biochem. Cell Biol.* 42, 1412–1415. doi: 10.1016/j.biocel.2010.06.004

Midwood, K. S., and Schwarzbauer, J. E. (2002). Tenascin-C modulates matrix contraction via focal adhesion kinase- and Rho-mediated signaling pathways. *Mol. Biol. Cell* 13, 3601–3613. doi: 10.1091/mbc.E02-05-0292

Mossey, P. A., Little, J., Munger, R. G., Dixon, M. J., and Shaw, W. C. (2009). Cleft lip and palate. *Lancet* 374, 1773–1785. doi: 10.1016/S0140-6736(09)60695-4

Murphy-Ullrich, J. E., and Sage, E. H. (2014). Revisiting the matricellular concept. *Matrix Biol.* 37, 1–14. doi: 10.1016/j.matbio.2014.07.005

Oka, K., Honda, M. J., Tsuruga, E., Hatakeyama, Y., Isokawa, K., and Sawa, Y. (2012). Roles of collagen and periostin expression by cranial neural crest cells during soft palate development. *J. Histochem. Cytochem.* 60, 57–68. doi: 10.1369/0022155411427059

Proetzel, G., Pawlowski, S. A., Wiles, M. V., Yin, M., Boivin, G. P., Howles, P. N., et al. (1995). Transforming growth factor-beta 3 is required for secondary palate fusion. *Nat. Genet.* 11, 409–414. doi: 10.1038/ng1295-409

Ricard-Blum, S. (2011). The collagen family. *Cold Spring Harb. Perspect. Biol.* 3:a004978. doi: 10.1101/cshperspect.a004978

Rocnik, E. F., Liu, P., Sato, K., Walsh, K., and Vaziri, C. (2006). The novel SPARC family member SMOC-2 potentiates angiogenic growth factor activity. *J. Biol. Chem.* 281, 22855–22864. doi: 10.1074/jbc.M513463200

Sasaki, Y., Tanaka, S., Hamachi, T., and Taya, Y. (2004). Deficient cell proliferation in palatal shelf mesenchyme of CL/Fr mouse embryos. *J. Dent. Res.* 83, 797–801. doi: 10.1177/154405910408301012

Scherberich, A., Tucker, R. P., Samandari, E., Brown-Luedi, M., Martin, D., and Chiquet-Ehrismann, R. (2004). Murine tenascin-W: a novel mammalian tenascin expressed in kidney and at sites of bone and smooth muscle development. *J. Cell Sci.* 117, 571–581. doi: 10.1242/jcs.00867

Shawky, J. H., and Davidson, L. A. (2015). Tissue mechanics and adhesion during embryo development. *Dev. Biol.* 401, 152–164. doi: 10.1016/j.ydbio.2014.12.005

Shen, M. M. (2001). Identification of differentially expressed genes in mouse development using differential display and *in situ* hybridization. *Methods* 24, 15–27. doi: 10.1006/meth.2001.1152

Small, J., Rottner, K., Hahne, P., and Anderson, K. I. (1999). Visualising the actin cytoskeleton. *Microsc. Res. Tech.* 47, 3–17.

Smith, T. M., Lozanoff, S., Iyyanar, P. P., and Nazarali, A. J. (2012). Molecular signaling along the anterior-posterior axis of early palate development. *Front. Physiol.* 3:488. doi: 10.3389/fphys.2012.00488

Vannahme, C., Gösling, S., Paulsson, M., Maurer, P., and Hartmann, U. (2003). Characterization of SMOC-2, a modular extracellular calcium-binding protein. *Biochem. J.* 373, 805–814. doi: 10.1042/bj20030532

Walker, B. E., and Fraser, F. C. (1956). Closure of the secondary palate in three strains of mice. *J. Embryol. Exp. Morph.* 4, 176–189.

Walker, J. T., McLeod, K., Kim, S., Conway, S. J., and Hamilton, D. W. (2016). Periostin as a multifunctional modulator of the wound healing response. *Cell Tissue Res.* doi: 10.1007/s00441-016-2426-6. [Epub ahead of print].

Wozniak, M. A., and Chen, C. S. (2009). Mechanotransduction in development: a growing role for contractility. *Nat. Rev. Mol. Cell Biol.* 10, 34–43. doi: 10.1038/nrm2592

Yu, K., and Ornitz, D. M. (2011). Histomorphological study of palatal shelf elevation during murine secondary palate formation. *Dev. Dyn.* 240, 1737–1744. doi: 10.1002/dvdy.22670

18

Calvarial Suture-Derived Stem Cells and their Contribution to Cranial Bone Repair

*Daniel H. Doro, Agamemnon E. Grigoriadis and Karen J. Liu**

Centre for Craniofacial and Regenerative Biology, King's College London, Guy's Hospital, London, United Kingdom

Correspondence:
Karen J. Liu
karen.liu@kcl.ac.uk

In addition to the natural turnover during life, the bones in the skeleton possess the ability to self-repair in response to injury or disease-related bone loss. Based on studies of bone defect models, both processes are largely supported by resident stem cells. In the long bones, the source of skeletal stem cells has been widely investigated over the years, where the major stem cell population is thought to reside in the perivascular niche of the bone marrow. In contrast, we have very limited knowledge about the stem cells contributing to the repair of calvarial bones. In fact, until recently, the presence of specific stem cells in adult craniofacial bones was uncertain. These flat bones are mainly formed via intramembranous rather than endochondral ossification and thus contain minimal bone marrow space. It has been previously proposed that the overlying periosteum and underlying dura mater provide osteoprogenitors for calvarial bone repair. Nonetheless, recent studies have identified a major stem cell population within the suture mesenchyme with multiple differentiation abilities and intrinsic reparative potential. Here we provide an updated review of calvarial stem cells and potential mechanisms of regulation in the context of skull injury repair.

Keywords: skull, calvaria, bone, stem cells, repair, cranial

INTRODUCTION: SKELETAL STEM CELLS (SSCs)

Skeletal stem cells (SSCs) provide the bones with a supply of osteochondroprogenitors during development, modeling and life-long homeostasis (Park et al., 2012). More importantly, these cells are crucial for appropriate self-healing in response to injury or general bone loss. Bone marrow (BM) residing stem cells have been suggested to assist the repair by establishing a pro-regenerative hematopoietic microenvironment, but also by supplying progenitors for all the newly formed skeletal components (Grcevic et al., 2012; Park et al., 2012).

Defining specific stem cell subsets and their ontogeny within the stromal system remains a challenge, as the discovery of numerous markers and isolation methods reveals a large phenotypic heterogeneity of the SSC population (Bianco and Robey, 2015). Fundamental studies leading to the initial characterization of SSCs were based on heterotopic transplantation of bone marrow cell suspensions or bone-devoid BM explants into extramedullary sites. Both populations were able to generate an ectopic ossicle, similar in tissue composition and architecture to trabecular bone and its stroma, fulfilling the first of two essential criteria that define a stem cell population—the *in vivo* multipotency (Friedenstein et al., 1968; Tavassoli and Crosby, 1968). The second criterion, self-renewal capacity, was met later as isolated clonogenic cells were found able to reconstitute progenitors with identical phenotype, potency and equivalent anatomical location within the ectopic bony structure formed (Friedenstein et al., 1974; Kuznetsov et al., 1997). Further knowledge about phenotypic identity and anatomical location of SSCs has been accumulated upon discovery of cell-surface markers like human-CD146 (Sacchetti et al., 2007) and mouse-CD45/CD200 (Chan et al., 2015), or even proteins expressed by specific SSC subpopulations like NESTIN (Méndez-Ferrer et al., 2010) and GREM1 (Worthley et al., 2015). Taken together, these studies agree on the widely reported perivascular niche of SSCs in the long bone marrow (**Figure 1**). Cells labeled with the CD146 marker are found in the adventitial layer of sinusoidal walls with typical reticular morphology, reminiscent of previously described ARCs (adventitial reticular cells) (Sacchetti et al., 2007).

Across studies, however, the distinctively identified populations vary in their multipotency, as some of them can generate *in vivo* osteoblasts, chondrocytes and stromal cells, but not adipocytes (Worthley et al., 2015). Rather than conflicting findings, these results point toward phenotypic heterogeneity of the SSCs, revealing that what were once generically called bone marrow mesenchymal stem cells actually comprise a number of subsets with subtly different properties. Many aspects regarding ontogeny and regulatory networks in long bone stromal SSCs have yet to be elucidated. Nevertheless, the knowledge accumulated over the years far exceeds that of stem cell populations serving the calvarial bones, which only recently started to be characterized in detail. Our aim here is to provide a comprehensive summary of recently reported stem cell populations within the cranial suture mesenchyme, their roles during postnatal turnover and wound repair and proposed mechanisms of regulation.

LONG BONE SSCs: WHERE DO THEY COME FROM?

Embryonic development of the long bones occurs via endochondral ossification and begins with the condensation of mesenchymal cells derived from lateral plate or paraxial mesoderm (reviewed in Olsen et al., 2000). These cells differentiate into chondrocytes and lay down a cartilaginous anlagen, which is later replaced by the osteoblasts and bone formation (see **Figure 1**). Chondrocytes in the center enlarge to a hypertrophic state allowing bone growth and inducing ossification in the peripheral layer of undifferentiated cells around the cartilage, the perichondrium (Kronenberg, 2003). Secretion of vascular endothelial growth factor (VEGF) attracts blood vessels and chondroclasts, cells specialized in digesting the cartilage matrix, which will then invade the ossified bone collar (Arai et al., 2002). Upon apoptosis of the hypertrophic chondrocytes, the hollow cavities left in the matrix are invaded by blood vessels and osteoblasts, which will lay down bone matrix on top of a calcified cartilage scaffold to form primary spongy or trabecular bone. Once the marrow space is established, the bone is finally invaded by stromal osteoprogenitors, some of which are recruited to the perivascular niche of large caliber sinusoids where they will reside as bone marrow skeletal stem cells. Prior to invasion and formation of bone marrow stroma, these cells are reportedly derived from proliferating perichondrial precursors. Phenotypic similarity of cells in the perichondrium with primitive stromal cells was observed in early studies (Bianco et al., 1993). Their origin was later confirmed by immunostaining of the perichondrial marker ALCAM (activated leukocyte cell adhesion molecule) (ALCAM). FAC-sorted ALCAM positive cells showed characteristics of mesenchymal stem cells and ability to differentiate into all skeletal lineages (Arai et al., 2002). Moreover, osterix expressing perichondrial/periosteal cells, labeled prior to vascular invasion, give rise to trabecular osteoblasts, osteocytes and stromal cells inside the developing bone, confirming the unequivocal origin of skeletal stem cells in the undifferentiated perichondrium (Maes et al., 2010; Staines et al., 2013).

ANATOMICAL AND DEVELOPMENTAL DIFFERENCES POINT TO DISTINCT STEM CELL NICHE IN CALVARIAL BONES

In contrast with the extensively studied stem cell niche in the endochondral bones, the source of SSCs in cranial bones was, until recent years, neglected or generally assumed to be identical to the long bones. Given the limited bone marrow space in these bones and very distinct developmental history, it is unsurprising that the local stem cell population would reside in a different compartment (**Figure 1**). The majority of craniofacial bones derive from the neural crest, with a few exceptions like mesodermally-derived parietal bones (Jiang et al., 2002). The latter will compose, together with crest-derived frontal bones, the top part of the skull called the cranial vault, or calvaria, which is fully made via intramembranous ossification. Although early mesenchymal condensations are also required in membranous bone formation (Hall and Miyake, 2000), these cells do not assume a chondrogenic fate or lay down cartilaginous scaffolds as in endochondral bones. Rather, upon expansion of the condensed mesenchyme, the cells in the center differentiate directly into osteoblasts, which will then secrete unossified matrix (osteoid) that will be later mineralized into compact bone. Growth of the immature bone then occurs at the leading edges of separate bones, dependent on proliferation and subsequent differentiation of osteoprogenitors at the commonly called osteogenic front (Rice et al., 2003). As the osteogenic fronts of two bones approach each other, they are interposed by undifferentiated mesenchyme, forming fibrous joints called sutures. Throughout embryonic and postnatal development, the sutures remain as an active site of bone formation in the expanding skull. The studies of Lana-Elola et al. (2007) helped to elucidate the mechanisms of bone growth and the contribution of different lineages within the suture environment. Using vital dye labeling, it was found that the primary mechanism for parietal bone growth is via proliferation and differentiation of leading edge osteoprogenitors with a surprisingly minor contribution of sutural mesenchymal cells, provided they are adjacent to the osteogenic fronts (Lana-Elola et al., 2007). Growth at the suture is also finely controlled by signaling from the underlying dura mater (Kim et al., 1998). Absence of dura mater leads to osseous obliteration of the coronal

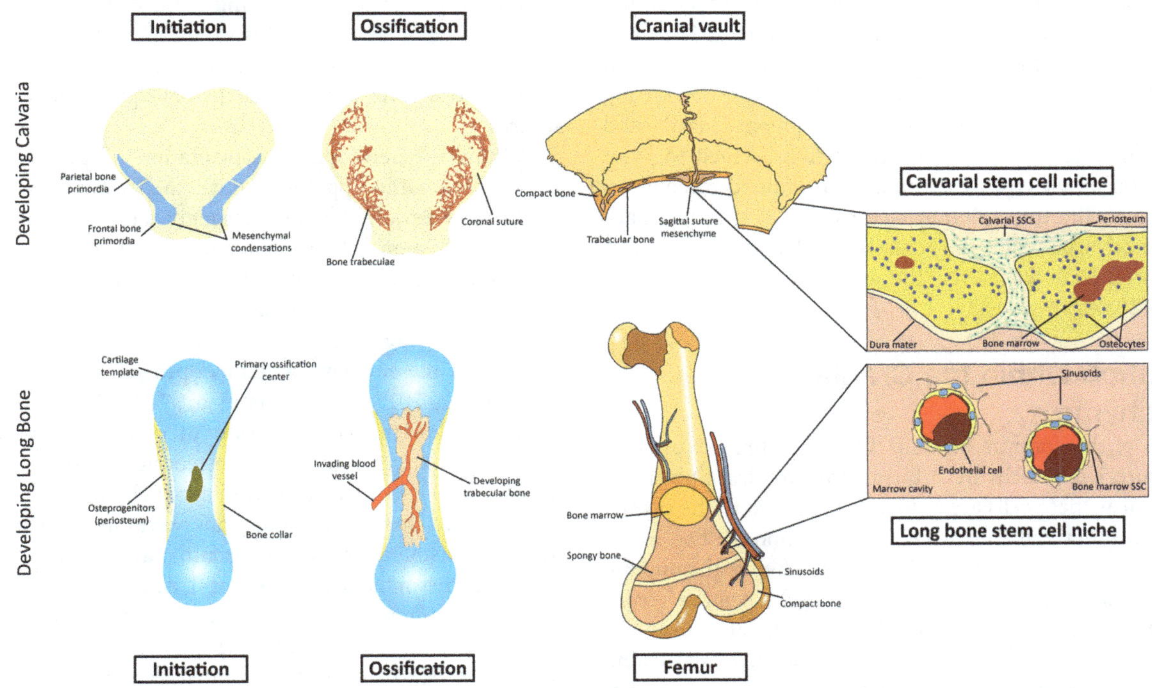

FIGURE 1 | Schematic representation of intramembranous and endochondral ossification. Top row: Initiation and development of the intramembranous calvarial bone. The calvarial stem cell resides primarily in the sutural mesenchyme. Bottom row: Initiation and development of endochondral bone. The stem cell niche in endochondral bone is more complex, residing in the marrow cavity.

suture, arresting the active growth at that site (Opperman et al., 1995). Moreover, the orientation of the dura mater under the cranial vault is critical for temporal control over suture patency or fusion (Levine et al., 1998). Growth and remodeling of the skull is also influenced by the overlying periosteum, a stratified membrane of mesenchymal cells including fibroblasts and osteoprogenitors (Brey et al., 2007). Mechanisms of periosteal activity during appositional growth and bone resorption of the cranial vault remain unclear. However, the membrane has been suggested to regulate osteogenesis via paracrine signaling (Cadet et al., 2003) and to provide osteoprogenitors that support craniofacial repair (Ochareon and Herring, 2011). Unlike the thoroughly described bone marrow-residing SSCs as the main source of osteoprogenitors during long bone repair (Zhou et al., 2014), the contribution of calvarial specific stem cells for cranial regeneration was unknown until very recently. Although a clonal population with multipotent MSC differentiation properties has long been isolated from rat calvaria (Grigoriadis et al., 1988), the visual evidence of the niche where the calvarial SSCs reside was only provided in the last few years.

SSCs RESIDING IN THE CRANIAL SUTURE ARE THE MAJOR CONTRIBUTORS TO INJURY REPAIR

In the same way as BM-SSCs, calvarial stem cell research was largely propelled by the identification of specific markers expressed by resident populations. Only in the last 2 years, three populations were identified within the sutural mesenchyme and proposed as major calvarial skeletal stem cells, or subsets of it. Namely, *Gli1* positive (*Gli1*+), *Axin2*-expressing (*Axin2*+) and postnatal *Prx1*-expressing (*Prx1*+) cells, as per definition in the original references (Zhao et al., 2015; Maruyama et al., 2016; Wilk et al., 2017). The authors used similar approaches to characterize the suspected SSC population with regards to location, stem cell-like properties and other features shared by the cells described which we attempt to summarize in this section.

Finding a Good Calvarial Stem Cell Marker

Zhao et al. (2015) hypothesized that *Gli1* expressing cells were the MSCs for craniofacial bones, as they were for the incisor mesenchyme they reported earlier (Zhao et al., 2014). The zinc finger protein GLI1 is a well-known transcriptional effector of Hedgehog signaling (Hooper and Scott, 2005). Seidel et al. (2010) had previously proposed it as a dental stem cell marker upon discovery of Hh responsiveness ($Gli1^{lacZ}$) from slow cycling cells of the dental epithelium (Seidel et al., 2010). The stem cell identity of these cells was later confirmed in the studies of Zhao et al. (2014). The AXIN2 protein, a negative regulator of Wnt signaling, was previously implicated in calvarial morphogenesis with *Axin2* knockout mice showing craniosynostosis (Yu et al., 2005). Maruyama et al. (2011) described the essential role of AXIN2 in orchestrating the signaling network (Wnt, BMP, FGF) that regulates mesenchymal cell fate determination (Maruyama et al., 2011). The protein was recently proposed as a calvarial stem cell marker as *Axin2*-expressing cells in the midline of the suture mesenchyme were found slow-cycling in nature (Maruyama et al., 2016). Finally, the transcription factor *Prx1* (also referred to as *Prrx1*) was previously shown to be highly expressed during limb bud formation and craniofacial development (Martin and Olson, 2000). Interestingly, PRX1 expression seemed to avert differentiation of early progenitors into committed osteoblasts, suggesting that the transcription factor could potentially mark SSCs in the calvarial bones (Lu et al., 2011). This hypothesis was successfully tested in the latest of the above-mentioned studies by Wilk et al. (2017).

Distribution within the Cranial Mesenchyme

Gli1+ cells of the cranium are found in the entire periosteum, dura and suture mesenchyme at birth. However, from postnatal day 21 onwards these cells are gradually restricted to the cranial sutures where they remain throughout adulthood (Zhao et al., 2015). *Axin2* was previously found to be expressed in the midline of sagittal suture skeletogenic mesenchyme. In a more recent study, *Axin2* expression was reported in all calvarial sutures, co-localizing with slow cycling cells that retained EdU (Maruyama et al., 2016). Unlike the *Gli1*+ cells, no obvious mention or visual evidence of early expression in the dura or periosteum is seen. In fact, *Axin2* expression is reportedly restricted to the midline of the sutural mesenchyme from postnatal day 10, whereas *Gli1*+ tracing seems to target a larger area within the suture. Wilk et al. (2017) investigated postnatal *Prx1*+ cells and found them exclusively in the calvarial sutures from 2 weeks of age until late adulthood. Like *Axin2*-expressing cells, *Prx1*+ were also not found in the periosteum or dura mater, although no mention or visual evidence of early postnatal expression is given (as in Zhao et al., 2015). Overall, the markers described seem to identify cells in a common niche. Whether the populations overlap in identity and function, or represent distinct functional subsets of a main stem cell source is still under debate as further discussed below. No expression of the above mentioned markers was detected in the posterior frontal suture, which likely correlates with the fact that this is the only calvarial suture fused at that stage in mouse development.

Self-Renewal and Ability to Generate All Calvarial Tissues

As previously mentioned in this review, self-renewal ability and *in vivo* multipotency are the cardinal requirements of a *bone fide* stem cell. While the *in vivo* differentiation potential can be assessed in many ways, some authors argue that self-renewal should only be assessed via heterotopic transplantation of non-induced cultures (Bianco and Robey, 2015). A typical SSC after being cultured and clonally isolated should still be able to generate all the skeletal compartments (multipotency) and "a cell compartment anatomically, phenotypically and functionally equivalent to the one originally explanted" (self-renewal) (Bianco and Robey, 2015). This remains the mainstay of MSC investigation criteria, as it honors the concept of stem cell autonomy in making, without the need for any artificial cues, organized skeletal tissue, including a reservoir of stem cells. In the case of calvarial stem cells, this would mean the ability to make *in vivo*, after culture and clonal isolation, all the components of a membranous bone and a mesenchymal equivalent to the cranial sutures.

Although heterotopic transplantation of putative calvarial SSCs was not the approach taken, the evidence presented in the studies reviewed herein strongly supports the ability of the putative stem cells to generate all calvarial compartments *in vivo*. Firstly, single pulse labeling (induced by tamoxifen in *Gli1-CreERT2* and *Prx1-creER* mice, or doxycycline in *Axin2-cre-Dox*) provides that only the cells initially labeled within the sutural mesenchyme and their progeny are being tracked (Zhao et al., 2015; Maruyama et al., 2016; Wilk et al., 2017). In all studies, the co-expression of osteogenic markers like runx2, osterix, collagen type 1, osteocalcin and sclerostin was not observed in the labeled suture mesenchyme, confirming that the proposed stem cell populations were undoubtedly distinct from any postnatal preosteoblasts and mature osteoblasts. *Gli1*+ cells were permanently labeled at 1 month of age and found increasingly abundant in the suture mesenchyme, periosteum, dura mater and parts of the calvarial bones up to 8 months of age (Zhao et al., 2015). In a similar manner, derivatives of the *Axin2*+ cells permanently labeled at 1 month, accumulated continuously in the sagittal suture until after 1 year of development, with a small number of cells found embedded in the bone matrix near the osteogenic fronts. However, this study did not report any contributions of the cells in question to the mature bone and surrounding tissues (dura mater and periosteum). Conversely, a large contribution of *Prx1*+ cells to all calvarial tissues, except bone marrow osteoblasts, was observed in 6–8 week old mice (Wilk et al., 2017). *Prx1* expression is detected as early as embryonic day 15, if not earlier, in the developing skull (Ouyang et al., 2013). Unfortunately, the conclusions about postnatal *Prx1*+ contribution to adult tissues were drawn from constitutive *Prx1-cre* lineage tracing analysis. This could include, although unlikely, cells that were specified immediately before the formation, or turn-over of the calvarial components analyzed, without definitive proof that they came from the sutural niche. Moreover, although Zhao and Wilk make no specific claims about self-renewal properties of the stem cell populations reported, Maruyama goes so far as to say that the accumulation of *Axin2*+ cells within the 1 year period reflects a self-renewal capability of those cells (Maruyama et al., 2016); however, this could also be due to a high proliferation capacity (Bianco and Robey, 2015). Nonetheless, Maruyama provides rigorous and more compelling evidence of *in vivo* stem cell behavior by transplanting isolated multi-colored (*R26R^{Confetti}*) *Axin2$^+$* cells to an extra-skeletal site (kidney capsule), which the other authors did not attempt. Ectopic bones labeled by single fluorescent colors were observed 3 weeks after transplantation, indicating that these cells can clonally expand *in vivo* and differentiate autonomously into the osteogenic lineage (Maruyama et al., 2016). However, contrary to bone marrow residing skeletal stem cells, *Axin2$^+$* SCs from the suture were not able to generate cartilage, unless artificially stimulated by BMP2, which drifts away from the principle of non-cued multipotency toward skeletal lineages expected from *bona fide* SSCs. While this could be a specific feature of membranous bone residing stem cells, ectopic chondrogenesis has been previously reported in the sutural mesenchyme, suggesting that they possess the intrinsic ability to differentiate into the chondrogenic lineage (Grigoriadis et al., 1988; Maruyama et al., 2011).

MSC *In vitro/Ex vivo* Behavior

Aside from rigorously established criteria, MSCs are popularly defined by their *in vitro* culture properties, including the ability to differentiate into various cell types (osteoblasts, chondrocytes, adipocytes and, arguably, neurons) (Keating, 2012). Likewise, although with considerable disagreement within the stem cell field, MSCs are loosely defined based on the expression profile of numerous surface markers (Dominici et al., 2006). Typical MSC markers CD90, CD73, CD44, *Sca1*, and CD146 were not detected in the majority of *Gli1*$^{+}$ cells *in vivo*. However, after 1 week of culture, fluorescent-activated *Gli1*$^{+}$ sorted cells express high levels of such MSC markers. *Gli1*$^{+}$ cells are also clonogenic *in vitro* and subcultured clones were successfully differentiated into osteo-, chondro-, and adipogenic lineages under appropriate conditions (Zhao et al., 2015). With the exception of the recently reported Leptin receptor (Zhou et al., 2014), none of the bone marrow SSC markers investigated by Maruyama was distinctively expressed in the *Axin2*$^{+}$ cells of the suture (*Mcam/CD146, Nestin and Gremlin1*). Moreover, the *in vitro* differentiation ability of these cells was not assessed in this particular study. *Axin2*$^{+}$ isolated cells were, nevertheless, able to form colonies *in vitro* and to differentiate, after heterotopic transplantation, into the osteogenic lineage and into chondrogenic, although only upon external stimulation (BMP2), as previously mentioned (Maruyama et al., 2016). Postnatal *Prx1*$^{+}$ cells are also clonogenic and exhibit a SSC-like profile *ex vivo*, including: upregulation of SSC markers *Pdgfrα* and *Mcam/CD146;* downregulation of cell cycle and DNA replication markers *Ccne2*, *Mcm4*, and *Pcna*—typical of quiescent cells; and high levels of transcripts associated with stem cell homing (*Itga2, Itga3,* and *Itga6*). Upon *in vitro* and *in vivo* stimulation with recombinant WNT3A, these cells are pushed toward osteogenic differentiation, judging by upregulated *Osx* and *Col1* and reduced expression of chondrogenic markers *Sox9* and *Col2* (Wilk et al., 2017). Altogether, the variable approaches, contrasting profiles and requirement of cueing factors for multi-differentiation in these studies points to the unreliability of loosely defined criteria to identify SSCs, based on which virtually every tissue can provide "stem cell" equivalents.

Contribution to Repair

The notion that skeletal stem cells work as postnatal contributors for tissue regeneration represents not only a general understanding of the organ physiology, but the very motivation for cautious and rigorous investigation of the stem cell populations, aiming at their translational potential. Although classically established requirements for SSCs do not include their regenerative properties, more than it does their multi-lineage differentiation ability in the context of organogenesis and postnatal turn-over, investigating the role of these cells during injury repair is essential, as the pursuit for stem cell-based therapies demand such knowledge. Therefore, the mechanisms of SSC recruitment and contribution to calvarial wound repair should accompany the research of any reported populations, as the three current studies highlighted here have done well to address. *Gli1*$^{+}$ cells respond immediately to injury in the suture by rapidly activating proliferation within 24 h post incision at the sagittal midline. Contribution of *Gli1*$^{+}$ cells to calvarial repair is observed in the vast infiltration of conditionally labeled cells into a 1 mm wide parietal wound situated 2 mm away from the sagittal suture. Two weeks after the injury is made, the majority of cells in the area are strongly labeled and, at 1 month, the repaired bone is mostly composed of *Gli1*$^{+}$ osteocytes as well as positively labeled periosteum and dura mater. Orthotopic transplantation of a lineage traced calvarial bone piece containing sagittal suture into a 4mm defect, revealed a significant number of labeled cells within 1 month-regenerated periosteum, dura mater and bone, whereas an explant lacking the suture failed to generate any of these components. Even with intact dura mater and periosteum, calvarial explants devoid of suture were incapable of regenerating the wounded bone in the recipient mice. The results indicate that, contrary to the previous idea that progenitors involved in cranial repair mainly resided in the periosteum, the sutural mesenchyme and not the surrounding membranes possesses the regenerative capacity (Zhao et al., 2015). Similarly to the *Gli1*+ population, *Axin2*+ lineage traced cells here drastically expanded in the sutural mesenchyme in response to a 1.4 mm parietal bone defect. Four weeks after the surgical procedure, large infiltration of the injury site by *Axin2*$^{+}$ cells is observed and co-localization with OSX (osteoprogenitors) and SOST (osteocytes) expression strongly indicates direct contribution to bone repair. *Axin2*$^{+}$ cells were also shown to improve injury repair when directly transplanted into the wound site. While *Axin2* negative cells from the suture mesenchyme provide no better healing than that seen in non-transplanted injuries, *Axin2*$^{+}$ cell transplantation significantly increased the repaired area 2 and 4 weeks after surgery. As in the previous experiment, the lineage labeling overlapped with markers of osteoprogenitors and osteocytes, confirming direct contribution of the *Axin2*+ population to repair of the wounded area (Maruyama et al., 2016).

Finally, *Prx1*$^{+}$ cells actively contributed to regeneration of subcritical size defects in both frontal and parietal bones, although in this study a smaller 100 μm wide injury was made. Nevertheless, lineage traced *Prx1*$^{+}$ cells were increasingly present in the wound area 5, 10, and 30 days post-surgery, when they co-localized to osteoblasts and osteocytes embedded in the newly formed bone. Moreover, the regeneration of, questionably, critical-sized (2 mm) defects was greatly improved by heterotopic transplantation of minced sutures into the wound, where *Prx1* labeling was seen in the majority of cells integrating the repaired bone 4 weeks after surgery. Interestingly, the repair of parietal subcritical defect did not occur in suturectomized mice after 4 weeks, whereas the 0.5 mm wound is fully repaired in mice with intact sagittal and coronal sutures (Wilk et al., 2017). Taken together, these studies confirm the unequivocal and potentially exclusive contribution of the sutural mesenchyme to calvarial injury repair.

Requirement for Development, Homeostasis and Injury Repair

Overall, the studies described provide compelling evidence for direct (by providing osteoprogenitors) as well as indirect (via paracrine signaling) contribution of the putative stem cell populations to calvarial repair. Predominant infiltration of *Gli1*$^+$/*Axin2*$^+$/*Prx1*$^+$ cells is seen in all the subcritical size defect assays, whereby the healing process should be accomplished by natural mechanisms occurring during normal bone physiology. Moreover, transplantation of these cells to the wound site showed significant repair improvement in all the attempts described in the previous section, supporting the translational potential of calvarial SSCs in a number of clinical scenarios. In two of the studies, notwithstanding, the authors found it appropriate to investigate whether the stem cell population described was indispensable for skull development, homeostasis and injury repair. While this is not a particular requirement for determining a resident stem cell, the findings provide valuable information on the ontogeny of the sutural niche and other calvarial compartments, as well as potential mechanisms of congenital disorders like craniosynostosis. Conditional ablation of *Gli1*$^+$ *cells*, for instance, led to severe craniofacial phenotypes in *Gli1-Cre*^{ERT2}; *DTA*$^{flox/flox}$ mice (diphtheria toxin A). When ablation was induced at 1 month of age, fusion of ordinarily patent coronal and frontal-premaxilla sutures was observed after 1 month, leading to general reduction of DTA-mice body size at 2 months post-induction. At this stage, all the craniofacial sutures were fused and the bones of *Gli1*$^+$ ablated mice presented severe osteoporosis. Repair of 1mm parietal defects was also compromised in DTA mice when compared to fully regenerated controls. Altogether, the results indicate that *Gli1*$^+$ cells are largely required for craniofacial bone turnover and injury healing. Moreover, pathological fusion of the cranial sutures in *Gli1*-ablated mice suggests that a deficient supply of undifferentiated mesenchymal cells hinders the patency expected in calvarial sutures of adult mice (Zhao et al., 2015).

Two different strategies confirmed *Prx1*$^+$ SSCs requirement for injury repair. Firstly, 8 week-old *Prx1-cre*^{ER}; *Rosa26*$^{DTA/+}$ mice were used to perform global ablation of *Prx1*$^+$ cells during 5 days before and 5 days after 0.5 mm parietal wound surgery. Twenty 8 days later, micro-computed tomography and histological analysis showed drastic healing impairment in *Prx1*$^+$ ablated mice against complete regeneration in the controls. Even in mice injured 2 months after ablation, parietal defects failed to regenerate as non-ablated mice. Secondly, excision of sagittal and right coronal sutures yielded non-regenerated wound in the right parietal bone, whereas removal of the opposing sutures (frontal and left coronal) did not affect the healing of parietal subcritical defect. This strongly suggests that calvarial bones depend on the SSCs of adjacent sutures to perform injury repair. Unlike *Gli1*$^+$ SSCs, however, global ablation of postnatal *Prx1*$^+$ cells did not result in craniosynostosis or any other major craniofacial phenotype. Indeed, *Gli1* expression is thought to identify a broadly distributed population of stem cells in the suture mesenchyme, of which *Prx1*+ cells constitute a subset seemingly dispensable for postnatal development and turnover. Ablation of embryonic *Prx1*+ cells leads to incomplete calvarial bone formation, suggesting that this specific subpopulation might only be required in earlier stages of development (Wilk et al., 2017). Whereas Maruyama did not perform any *Axin2*$^+$ SSC ablation studies, *Axin2*-null mice are known to exhibit premature fusion of the cranial sutures (Yu et al., 2005), although this does not necessarily correlate with any particular requirement of the population concerned. Reduction of *Axin2*-expressing cells is seen upon ossification of the frontal suture (Maruyama et al., 2016). However, this is likely an effect on the entire undifferentiated mesenchyme at the interfrontal suture as it commits to the osteogenic lineage and promotes the fusion of the osteogenic fronts.

Aspects of Regulatory Signaling

Throughout the skeleton, as a local niche is established, mesenchymal stem cells are subject to recruitment, proliferation, induction of mitotic quiescence and lineage commitment. Over the years, extensive research of bone marrow SSCs has shown that these steps are regulated by largely convoluted signaling pathways including: platelet-derived growth factor (PDGF) during perivascular recruitment (Sacchetti et al., 2007); parathyroid hormone (PTH) during expansion of the bone marrow stroma (Kuznetsov et al., 2004); TGF-β1 as the cells are maintained in a quiescent state (reviewed in Pepper, 1997; Jain, 2003) and extensive crosstalk between TGFβ/BMP, Wnt/β-catenin, FGF and Hedgehog pathways, which generally control MSCs lineage fate decision (reviewed in Cook and Genever, 2013). Given the complexity of the network necessary for developing and maintaining a stem cell niche, it is no surprise that regulatory signaling receives little attention in recent papers that attempt to describe calvarial SSCs. In fact, most of the preliminary evidence regarding regulation of calvarial SSCs arose from *in vitro* or unconvincing *in vivo* assays that were based on mechanisms previously established for stem cells in the long bones. Zhao et al. set out to investigate whether *Gli1*$^+$ cells were, like BM-SSCs, regulated by hedgehog signaling in the context of lineage commitment. No Sonic hedgehog (Shh) signal was detected in the suture region using a R26Tdtomato reporter. However, Indian hedgehog (Ihh), a regulator of skeletal development, was found in cells of the osteogenic fronts flanking the cranial sutures. Deletion of the hedgehog receptor Smoothened (*Smo*) in *Gli1*$^+$ cells did not affect suture patency, proliferation of *Gli1*$^+$ cells, or their ability to generate periosteum, dura and osteocytes; nor did it induce apoptosis in the sagittal suture. Nonetheless, all the craniofacial bones in *SmoKO*$^{Gli1-cre}$ mice exhibited severe osteoporosis and reduced bone volume after 8 months. *In vitro* analysis of sutural mesenchyme cells revealed up-regulated *Gli1* expression, increased osteogenic activity and upregulation of osteodifferentiation markers upon IHH treatment, whereas the hedgehog inhibitor GDC0449 induced the opposite effects. Neither treatment affected proliferation or apoptosis of cultured mesenchymal cells, suggesting that Hedgehog signaling might be important for regulation of *Gli1*$^+$ SSC differentiation, but not their maintenance (Zhao et al., 2015). Maruyama and Wilk's insights on regulation of *Axin2*$^+$ and *Prx1*+ cells, respectively, are merely suggestive, as these cells present *in vivo* expression of canonical Wnt inhibitors in their quiescent state and lineage fate decision changes upon exogenous activation of Wnt or BMP signaling. Transplanted *Axin2*$^+$ cells were able to generate ectopic mineralized bone, but no cartilage after 7 days, contrasting the multi-lineage potential of long bone marrow SSCs. However, exogenous stimulation with BMP2 shifted *Axin2*$^+$ cells from an osteogenic to a chondrogenic fate, shown by detection of Alcian blue (cartilage), but not von Kossa (bone) staining in the structure generated (Maruyama et al., 2016). Expression of Wnt inhibitors *Dkk1* and *Sost* by *Prx1*$^+$ sorted cells supports the well-established idea that skeletal progenitors are maintained in an undifferentiated status, or yield chondrogenic differentiation in the absence of canonical Wnt activation (Day et al., 2005; Hill et al., 2005). Indeed, *in vivo* expression of chondrogenic markers *Sox9* and *Col2* was diminished in pnPRX1$^+$ cells upon subperiosteal injection of Wnt agonist WNT3A to the cranial sutures, whereas osteogenic markers Osx and Col1 were significantly upregulated. Commitment to the osteogenic fate has also observed when these cells were treated in culture with recombinant WNT3A, endorsing the previously described role of Wnt/β-catenin pathway in differentiation of mesenchymal progenitors (Wilk et al., 2017). Altogether, recently published studies provide informative, yet inconclusive findings to characterize molecular regulation of calvarial SSCs, leaving exciting open prospects for future stem cell research.

DISCUSSION

As once wisely stated, "All definitions of stem cells are functional in nature, and all types of stem cells are defined by functional assays" (Bianco et al., 2013). That is, one must see that hasty and careless attempts to identify stem cells in the adult body will not prompt us to replace rigorously established criteria with simple surface marker profiling, or loosely defined *in vitro* properties. From the very concept of stemness, proposing a stem cell candidate requires that a single cell within the niche described can generate multiple and fully differentiated tissues *in vivo* and produce a reservoir of cells with identical phenotype and multipotency. At the risk of raising unrealistic expectations for the clinical use of stem cells, many authors over the years claimed to have isolated post-natal fibroblastic populations from virtually every tissue with differentiation abilities that extrapolate the tissue-specific potential of the identified progenitor, much like an embryonic stem cell (da Silva Meirelles et al., 2006). This apparent "pluripotency" attributed to putative post-natal stem cells is often based on chemically induced *in vitro* differentiation studies (Robey et al., 2014), which more accurately describe the artificial reprogramming of a cell than its *in vivo* potency. The very use of the term mesenchymal stem cell (MSC) to describe bone marrow stromal progenitors is misleading in that it is based on the erroneous and unproven hypothesis that stem cells in the bone marrow could generate various differentiated tissues beyond the skeletal lineages. It also assumes that MSCs throughout the body have a common developmental origin (Caplan, 1991) and can be found in a number of different organs sharing the same differentiation potential as BMSCs and, as previously hypothesized, equivalent perivascular niche (Chen et al., 2012). In reality, evidence originating from more stringent *in vivo* assays indicates that the bone marrow harbors stem cells exclusively for skeletal-tissues, namely, bone, cartilage, adipose tissue and stroma (Owen and Friedenstein, 1988; Sacchetti et al., 2007). Therefore, as previously proposed (Bianco et al., 2008), "skeletal stem cell" is a more adequate designation, for it describes the real potential of the so called bone marrow stromal cells and implies that stem cell populations identified in other tissues are not expected to behave exactly like SSCs in the long bones. In fact, the concept of tissue-specific stem cells as opposed to a homogeneous MSC population with multiple locations, accords with a more reasonable prediction that most adult tissues would maintain a stock of undifferentiated yet committed progenitors to support physiological turn-over and regeneration in response to injury.

The search for a calvarial stem cell then must indeed be grounded on very stringent criteria. However, the assessment of *in vivo* multipotency and self-renewal in this population need not be guided inflexibly by the sequential assays classically employed for BM-SSCs investigation (Bianco et al., 2013; Bianco and Robey, 2015), lest one must conclude that: either the membranous bones in the skull lack a resident stem cell population, or the well supported contribution of sutural mesenchymal progenitors to all calvarial components reflects a distinct role/mechanism of skeletal turn-over and injury repair, even though the same is performed by bone marrow SSCs in the long bones. For instance, it is fair to require that *in vivo* multipotency is assessed exclusively by heterotopic transplantation of clonally isolated calvarial cells rather than alternate *in vitro* assays. But, to expect the formation of an ectopic ossicle with all the compartments of an endochondral bone, contradicts the idea of organ-specific stem cells and resonates with the old farfetched concept of "pluripotent" MSCs. Moreover, the ability to self-renew is easily observed in ectopically transplanted BM-SSCs, as these cells generate organized bone marrow tissue and reconstitute a pool of identical undifferentiated progenitors (Sacchetti et al., 2007). However, since the stem cells committed to an intramembranous fate will not generate the compartments produced during an endochondral ossification, a different readout must be required as proof of self-renewal ability. Maruyama has shown that ectopically transplanted *Axin2*$^+$ sutural SCs can clonally expand *in vivo*, but also generate bony structures, judging by monochromatic expansion of *R26-confetti* traced cells (Maruyama et al., 2016). Whether this could be taken as convincing evidence of stemness is still debatable, although it is surely more rigorous than otherwise defined *in vitro* MSC criteria (Dominici et al., 2006). Also, lineage-tracing approaches like the ones employed for the calvarial stem cell niche investigation might not be the mainstay for assessing *bona fide* stem cell criteria. Nonetheless, the conclusions drawn with regards to multi-lineage differentiation ability and injury repair contribution *in vivo* are well supported with single-pulse conditional labeling methods.

In summary, the stringent criteria defended by "rigorous *in vivo* assay" apologists stems from a genuine concern about negligent clinical application of poorly characterized stem cell candidates. Experienced stem cell scholars report the uprising of unrealistic expectations of systemic regenerative therapy using bone marrow stromal cells, when in fact, effective translational success, to date, was always obtained from local transplantation of organ-specific progenitors [e.g., bone marrow orthotopic transplantation (Horwitz et al., 2002); skin regeneration (Green, 1989; De Luca et al., 2006); cornea regeneration (Pellegrini et al., 1997; Rama et al., 2010)]. More importantly, stem cell investigation must be guided by translational demands, in which the primary ambition is to find: cells that can be easily isolated, whether prospectively (based on surface markers), or by plastic adherence of clonal populations; cells that can be clonally expanded *in vitro*; cells that can be locally and not systemically delivered and that will directly engraft or at least support regeneration by establishing a healing microenvironment; or ideally cells that can be regulated *in vivo* by pharmacological stimulation. With that in mind, the recent discovery of the calvarial stem cell niche is well evidenced and presents putative populations that fulfill the basic stem cell criteria, as dictated by translational demands. Whereas *Gli1*$^+$ cells are distributed across a large portion of the sutural mesenchyme, expression of *Axin2* and *Prx1* seems to identify more discrete subsets that may or may not be part of a major population (Wilk et al., 2017). Partial overlapping of the proposed markers and slight differences in functional assays should not imply contradictions in calvarial stem cell properties. Rather, the suture mesenchyme most likely comprises a heterogeneous niche in which distinct stem cell subsets can be identified, isolated and characterized with clinical application purposes. Since all recent studies reported *in vitro* clonogenicity of the candidate populations described, a step forward in understanding their biology and potency would be to transplant the expanded colonies to an ectopic site, as the approach addresses the autonomy of the cells in a non-skeletogenic environment.

In humans, while the existence of a calvarial niche residing in the sutural mesenchyme has not been examined, expression of these putative stem cell markers (*Gli1*, *Axin2*, and *Prx1*) is well predicted based on fetal studies (Homayounfar et al., 2015), analyses of pathogenic skull bones (Coussens et al., 2007) and on our knowledge of signaling pathways crucial in calvarial development. Clearly, the calvarial stem cell niche needs to be further defined in humans if we are to harness these cells for improved skull repair. Isolation and thorough analysis of these cells will then allow us to design new therapies, including introduction of synthetic scaffolds designed to enrich for these cells, or carrying chemotactic cues for to attract these cells to the wound site. Moreover, from the perspective of future clinical translation, two potential autologous stem cell sources are the bone marrow and adipose-derived stem cells. Both of these are heterogenous populations which could be further examined for expression of *Gli1*, *Axin2*, and *Prx1* positive sub-populations. These markers have not been well characterized in human stem cell populations, although the relevant signaling pathways are implicated in cancer stem cells.

Finally, although the mesenchyme interposing all calvarial bones is predominantly neural crest derived, very little attention was given in the studies reviewed to the distinct embryonic origins of frontal and parietal bones and how this might determine how surrounding stem cells are regulated. Even the mesoderm derived bone is hypothesized to require neural crest (*Sox10+*) lineages residing in the periosteum (Isern et al., 2014). Thus, given the inherent multi-potency of the neural crest cells, osteoblasts derived from that lineage may provide a more plastic milieu than the mesoderm.

AUTHOR CONTRIBUTIONS

DD, AG, and KL sketched out the initial draft of the review. DD wrote the review and designed the figure. AG and KL revised and edited the review.

REFERENCES

Arai, F., Ohneda, O., Miyamoto, T., Zhang, X. Q., and Suda, T. (2002). Mesenchymal stem cells in perichondrium express activated leukocyte cell adhesion molecule and participate in bone marrow formation. *J. Exp. Med.* 195, 1549–1563. doi: 10.1084/jem.20011700

Bianco, P., Cao, X., Frenette, P. S., Mao, J. J., Robey, P. G., Simmons, P. J., et al. (2013). The meaning, the sense and the significance: translating the science of mesenchymal stem cells into medicine. *Nat. Med.* 19, 35–42. doi: 10.1038/nm.3028

Bianco, P., Riminucci, M., Bonucci, E., Termine, J. D., and Robey, P. G. (1993). Bone Sialoprotein (BSP) secretion and osteoblast differentiation: relationship to bromodeoxyuridine incorporation, alkaline phosphatase, and matrix deposition. *J. Histochem. Cytochem.* 41, 183–191. doi: 10.1177/41.2.8419458

Bianco, P., and Robey, P. G. (2015). Skeletal stem cells. *Development* 142, 1023–1027. doi: 10.1242/dev.102210

Bianco, P., Robey, P. G., and Simmons, P. J. (2008). Commentary mesenchymal stem cells : revisiting history, concepts, and assays. *Cell Stem Cell* 2, 313–319. doi: 10.1016/j.stem.2008.03.002

Brey, E. M., Cheng, M. H., Allori, A., Satterfield, W., Chang, D. W., Patrick, C. W., et al. (2007). Comparison of guided bone formation from periosteum and muscle fascia. *Plast. Reconstr. Surg.* 119, 1216–1222. doi: 10.1097/01.prs.0000254361.74614.bb

Cadet, E. R., Gafni, R. I., McCarthy, E. F., McCray, D. R., Bacher, J. D., Barnes, K. M., et al. (2003). Mechanisms responsible for longitudinal growth of the cortex: coalescence of trabecular bone into cortical bone. *J. Bone Joint Surg.* 85-A, 1739–1748.

Caplan, A. I. (1991). Mesenchymal stem cells. *J. Orthopaed. Res.* 9, 641–650. doi: 10.1002/jor.1100090504

Chan, C. K., Seo, E. Y., Chen, J. Y., Lo, D., McArdle, A., Sinha, R., et al. (2015). Identification and specification of the mouse skeletal stem cell. *Cell* 160, 285–298. doi: 10.1016/j.cell.2014.12.002

Chen, C. W., Corselli, M., Péault, B., and Huard, J. (2012). Human blood-vessel-derived stem cells for tissue repair and regeneration. *J. Biomed. Biotechnol.* 2012:597439. doi: 10.1155/2012/597439

Cook, D., and Genever, P. (2013). Regulation of mesenchymal stem cell differentiation. *Adv. Exp. Med. Biol.* 786, 213–229. doi: 10.1007/978-94-007-6621-1_12

Coussens, A. K., Wilkinson, C. R., Hughes, I. P., Morris, C. P., van Daal, A., Anderson, P. J., et al. (2007). Unravelling the molecular control of calvarial suture fusion in children with craniosynostosis. *BMC Genomics* 8:458. doi: 10.1186/1471-2164-8-458

da Silva Meirelles, L., Chagastelles, P. C., and Nardi, N. B. (2006). Mesenchymal stem cells reside in virtually all post-natal organs and tissues. *J. Cell Sci.* 119, 2204–2213. doi: 10.1242/jcs.02932

Day, T. F., Guo, X., Garrett-Beal, L., and Yang, Y. (2005). Wnt/β-catenin signaling in mesenchymal progenitors controls osteoblast and chondrocyte differentiation during vertebrate skeletogenesis. *Dev. Cell* 8, 739–750. doi: 10.1016/j.devcel.2005.03.016

De Luca, M., Pellegrini, G., and Green, H. (2006). Regeneration of Squamous epithelia from stem cells of cultured grafts. *Regen. Med.* 1, 45–57. doi: 10.2217/17460751.1.1.45

Dominici, M., Le Blanc, K., Mueller, I., Slaper-Cortenbach, I., Marini, F., Krause, D., et al. (2006). Minimal criteria for defining multipotent mesenchymal stromal cells. The international society for cellular therapy position statement. *Cytotherapy* 8, 315–317. doi: 10.1080/14653240600855905

Friedenstein, A. J., Chailakhyan, R. K., Latsinik, N. V., Panasyuk, A. F., and Keiliss-Borok, I. V. (1974). Stromal cells responsible for transferring the microenvironment of the hemopoietic tissues. cloning *in vitro* and retransplantation *in vivo*. *Transplantation.* 17, 331–340. doi: 10.1097/00007890-197404000-00001

Friedenstein, A. J., Petrakova, K. V., Kurolesova, A. I., and Frolova, G. P. (1968). Heterotopic transplants of bone marrow. *Transplantation* 6, 230–247. doi: 10.1097/00007890-196803000-00009

Grcevic, D., Pejda, S., Matthews, B. G., Repic, D., Wang, L., Li, H., et al. (2012). *In vivo* fate mapping identifies mesenchymal progenitor cells. *Stem Cells* 30, 187–196. doi: 10.1002/stem.780

Green, H. (1989). Regeneration of the skin after grafting of epidermal cultures. *Lab. Invest.* 60, 583–584.

Grigoriadis, A. E., Heersche, J. N., and Aubin, J. E. (1988). Differentiation of muscle, fat, cartilage, and bone from progenitor cells present in a bone-derived clonal cell population: effect of dexamethasone. *J. Cell Biol.* 106, 2139–2151. doi: 10.1083/jcb.106.6.2139

Hall, B. K., and Miyake, T. (2000). All for one and one for all: condensations and the initiation of skeletal development. *Bioessays* 22, 138–147. doi: 10.1002/(SICI)1521-1878(200002)22:2<138::AID-BIES5>3.0.CO;2-4

Hill, T. P., Später, D., Taketo, M. M., Birchmeier, W., and Hartmann, C. (2005). Canonical Wnt/β-catenin signaling prevents osteoblasts from differentiating into chondrocytes. *Dev. Cell* 8, 727–738. doi: 10.1016/j.devcel.2005.02.013

Homayounfar, N., Park, S. S., Afsharinejad, Z., Bammler, T. K., Macdonald, J. W., Farin, F. M., et al. (2015). Transcriptional analysis of human cranial compartments with different embryonic origins. *Arch. Oral Biol.* 60, 1450–1460. doi: 10.1016/j.archoralbio.2015.06.008

Hooper, J. E., and Scott, M. P. (2005). Communicating with hedgehogs. *Nat. Rev.* 6, 306–317. doi: 10.1038/nrm1622

Horwitz, E. M., Gordon, P. L., Koo, W. K., Marx, J. C., Neel, M. D., McNall, R. Y., et al. (2002). Isolated allogeneic bone marrow-derived mesenchymal cells engraft and stimulate growth in children with osteogenesis imperfecta: implications for cell therapy of bone. *Proc. Natl. Acad. Sci. U.S.A.* 99, 8932–8937. doi: 10.1073/pnas.132252399

Isern, J., García-García, A., Martín, A. M., Arranz, L., Martín-Pérez, D., Torroja, C., et al. (2014). The neural crest is a source of mesenchymal stem cells with specialized hematopoietic stem cell niche function. *Elife* 3:e03696. doi: 10.7554/eLife.03696

Jain, R. K. (2003). Molecular regulation of vessel maturation. *Nat. Med.* 9, 685–693. doi: 10.1038/nm0603-685

Jiang, X., Iseki, S., Maxson, R. E., Sucov, H. M., and Morriss-Kay, G. M. (2002). Tissue origins and interactions in the mammalian skull vault. *Dev. Biol.* 241, 106–116. doi: 10.1006/dbio.2001.0487

Keating, A. (2012). Perspective mesenchymal stromal cells : new directions. *Stem Cell* 10, 709–716. doi: 10.1016/j.stem.2012.05

Kim, H.-J., Rice, D. P. C., Kettunen, P. J., and Thesleff, I. (1998). FGF-, BMP- and Shh-mediated signalling pathways in the regulation of cranial suture morphogenesis and calvarial bone development. *Development* 1251, 1241–1251.

Kronenberg, H.M. (2003). Developmental regulation of the growth plate. *Nature* 423, 332–336. doi: 10.1038/nature01657

Kuznetsov, S. A., Krebsbach, P. H., Satomura, K., Kerr, J., Riminucci, M., Benayahu, D., et al. (1997). Single-colony derived strains of human marrow stromal fibroblasts form bone after transplantation *in vivo*. *J. Bone Mineral Res.* 12, 1335–1347. doi: 10.1359/jbmr.1997.12.9.1335

Kuznetsov, S. A., Riminucci, M., Ziran, N., Tsutsui, T. W., Corsi, A., Calvi, L., et al. (2004). The interplay of osteogenesis and hematopoiesis. *J. Cell Biol.* 167, 1113–1122. doi: 10.1083/jcb.200408079

Lana-Elola, E., Rice, R., Grigoriadis, A. E., and Rice, D. P. (2007). Cell fate specification during calvarial bone and suture development. *Dev. Biol.* 311, 335–346. doi: 10.1016/j.ydbio.2007.08.028

Levine, J. P., Bradley, J. P., Roth, D. A., McCarthy, J. G., and Longaker, M. T. (1998). Studies in cranial suture biology: regional dura mater determines overlying suture biology. *Plast. Reconstr. Surg.* 101, 1441–1447. doi: 10.1097/00006534-199805000-00002

Lu, X., Beck, G. R., Gilbert, L. C., Camalier, C. E., Bateman, N. W., Hood, B. L., et al. (2011). Identification of the homeobox protein Prx1 (MHox, Prrx-1) as a regulator of osterix expression and mediator of tumor necrosis factor? Action in Osteoblast Differentiation. *J. Bone Mine. Res.* 26, 209–219. doi: 10.1002/jbmr.203

Maes, C., Kobayashi, T., Selig, M. K., Torrekens, S., Roth, S. I., Mackem, S., et al. (2010). Osteoblast precursors, but not mature osteoblasts, move into developing and fractured bones along with invading blood vessels. *Dev. Cell* 19, 329–344. doi: 10.1016/j.devcel.2010.07.010

Martin, J. F., and Olson, E. N. (2000). Identification of a *prx1* Limb Enhancer. *Genesis* 26, 225–229. doi: 10.1002/(SICI)1526-968X(200004)26:4<225::AID-GENE10>3.0.CO;2-F

Maruyama, T., Jeong, J., Sheu, T. J., and Hsu, W. (2016). Stem cells of the suture mesenchyme in craniofacial bone development, repair and regeneration. *Nat. Commun.* 7:10526. doi: 10.1038/ncomms10526

Maruyama, T., Mirando, A. J., Deng, C. X., and Hsu, W. (2011). The balance of WNT and FGF signaling influences mesenchymal stem cell fate during skeletal development. *Sci. Signal.* 3:ra40. doi: 10.1126/scisignal.2000727

Méndez-Ferrer, S., Michurina, T. V., Ferraro, F., Mazloom, A. R., Macarthur, B. D., Lira, S. A., et al. (2010). Mesenchymal and haematopoietic stem cells form a unique bone marrow niche. *Nature* 466, 829–834. doi: 10.1038/nature09262

Ochareon, P., and Herring, S. W. (2011). Cell replication in craniofacial periosteum: appositional vs. resorptive sites. *J. Anat.* 218, 285–297. doi: 10.1111/j.1469-7580.2010.01336.x

Olsen, B. R., Reinato, A. M., and Wang, W. (2000). Bone development. *Annu. Rev. Cell Dev. Biol.* 16, 191–220. doi: 10.1146/annurev.cellbio.16.1.191

Opperman, L. A., Passarelli, R. W., Morgan, E. P., Reintjes, M., and Ogle, R. C. (1995). Cranial sutures require tissue interactions with dura mater to resist osseous obliteration *in vitro*. *J. Bone Mine. Res.* 10, 1978–1987. doi: 10.1002/jbmr.5650101218

Ouyang, Z., Chen, Z., Ishikawa, M., Yue, X., Kawanami, A., Leahy, P., et al. (2013). *Prx1* and 3.2kb *Col1a1* promoters target distinct bone cell populations in transgenic mice. *Bone* 58, 136–145. doi: 10.1016/j.bone.2013.10.016

Owen, M., and Friedenstein, A. J. (1988). Stromal stem cells: marrow-derived osteogenic precursors. *Ciba Found. Symp.* 136, 42–60.

Park, D., Spencer, J. A., Koh, B. I., Kobayashi, T., Fujisaki, J., Clemens, T. L., et al. (2012). Endogenous bone marrow MSCs are dynamic, fate-restricted participants in bone maintenance and regeneration. *Cell Stem Cell* 10, 259–272. doi: 10.1016/j.stem.2012.02.003

Pellegrini, G., Traverso, C. E., Franzi, A. T., Zingirian, M., Cancedda, R., and De Luca, M. (1997). Long-term restoration of damaged corneal surfaces with autologous cultivated corneal epithelium. *Lancet* 349, 990–993. doi: 10.1016/S0140-6736(96)11188-0

Pepper, M. S. (1997). Transforming growth factor-beta: vasculogenesis, angiogenesis, and vessel wall integrity. *Cytokine Growth Factor Rev.* 8, 21–43. doi: 10.1016/S1359-6101(96)00048-2

Rama, P., Matuska, S., Paganoni, G., Spinelli, A., De Luca, M., and Pellegrini, G. (2010). Limbal stem-cell therapy and long-term corneal regeneration. *N. Engl. J. Med.* 363, 147–155. doi: 10.1056/NEJMoa0905955

Rice, D. P., Rice, R., and Thesleff, I. (2003). Molecular mechanisms in calvarial bone and suture development, and their relation to craniosynostosis. *Eur. J. Orthod.* 25, 139–148. doi: 10.1093/ejo/25.2.139

Robey, P. G., Kuznetsov, S. A., Riminucci, M., and Bianco, P. (2014). Bone marrow stromal cell assays: *in vitro* and *in vivo*. *Methods Mol. Biol.* 1130, 279–293. doi: 10.1007/978-1-62703-989-5_21

Sacchetti, B., Funari, A., Michienzi, S., Di Cesare, S., Piersanti, S., Saggio, I., et al. (2007). Self-renewing osteoprogenitors in bone marrow sinusoids can organize a hematopoietic microenvironment. *Cell* 131, 324–336. doi: 10.1016/j.cell.2007.08.025

Seidel, K., Ahn, C. P., Lyons, D., Nee, A., Ting, K., Brownell, I., et al. (2010). Hedgehog signaling regulates the generation of ameloblast progenitors in the continuously growing mouse incisor. *Development* 137, 3753–3761. doi: 10.1242/dev.056358

Staines, K. A., Pollard, A. S., McGonnell, I. M., Farquharson, C., and Pitsillides, A. A. (2013). Cartilage to bone transitions in health and disease. *J. Endocrinol.* 219, R1–R12. doi: 10.1530/JOE-13-0276

Tavassoli, M., and Crosby, W. H. (1968). Transplantation of marrow to extramedullary sites. *Science* 161, 7–10. doi: 10.1126/science.161.3836.54

Wilk, K., Yeh, S. A., Mortensen, L. J., Ghaffarigarakani, S., Lombardo, C. M., Bassir, S. H., et al. (2017). Postnatal calvarial skeletal stem cells expressing PRX1 reside exclusively in the calvarial sutures and are required for bone regeneration. *Stem Cell Rep.* 8, 933–946. doi: 10.1016/j.stemcr.2017.03.002

Worthley, D. L., Churchill, M., Compton, J. T., Tailor, Y., Rao, M., Si, Y., et al. (2015). Gremlin 1 identifies a skeletal stem cell with bone, cartilage, and reticular stromal potential. *Cell* 160, 269–284. doi: 10.1016/j.cell.2014.11.042

Yu, H. M., Jerchow, B., Sheu, T. J., Liu, B., Costantini, F., Puzas, J. E., et al. (2005). The role of Axin2 in calvarial morphogenesis and craniosynostosis. *Development* 132, 1995–2005. doi: 10.1242/dev.01786

Zhao, H., Feng, J., Ho, T. V., Grimes, W., Urata, M., and Chai, Y. (2015). The suture provides a niche for mesenchymal stem cells of craniofacial bones. *Nat. Cell Biol.* 17, 386–396. doi: 10.1038/ncb3139

Zhao, H., Feng, J., Seidel, K., Shi, S., Klein, O., Sharpe, P., et al. (2014). Secretion of Shh by a neurovascular bundle niche supports mesenchymal stem cell homeostasis in the adult mouse incisor. *Cell Stem Cell* 14, 160–173. doi: 10.1016/j.stem.2013.12.013

Zhou, J., Chen, Y., Cao, C., Chen, X., Gao, W., and Zhang, L. (2014). Inactivation of glycogen synthase kinase-3β up-regulates β-catenin and promotes chondrogenesis. *Cell Tissue Bank.* 16, 135–142. doi: 10.1007/s10561-014-9449-6

19

Detection of a Novel *DSPP* Mutation by NGS in a Population Isolate in Madagascar

Agnès Bloch-Zupan[1,2,3], Mathilde Huckert[1,4], Corinne Stoetzel[4], Julia Meyer[1], Véronique Geoffroy[4], Rabisoa W. Razafindrakoto[5], Saholy N. Ralison[5], Jean-Claude Randrianaivo[5], Georgette Ralison[5], Rija O. Andriamasinoro[5], Rija H. Ramanampamaharana[5], Solofomanantsoa E. Randrianazary[5], Louise H. Ralimanana[5], Béatrice Richard[6], Philippe Gorry[7], Marie-Cécile Manière[1,2], Jeanne A. Rasoamananjara[5], Simone Rakoto Alson[5] and Hélène Dollfus[4]*

[1] Faculté de Chirurgie Dentaire, Université de Strasbourg, Strasbourg, France, [2] Centre de Référence des Manifestations Odontologiques des Maladies Rares, Hôpitaux Universitaires de Strasbourg, Pôle de Médecine et Chirurgie Bucco-dentaires Hôpital Civil, Strasbourg, France, [3] Centre National de la Recherche Scientifique-UMR7104, Institut de Génétique et de Biologie Moléculaire et Cellulaire, Institut National de la Santé et de la Recherche Médicale U 964, Université de Strasbourg, Illkirch, France, [4] Laboratoire de Génétique Médicale, Faculté de Médecine, Institut National de la Santé et de la Recherche Médicale U 1112, Université de Strasbourg, Strasbourg, France, [5] Institut d'Odonto-Stomatologie Tropicale de Madagascar, Université de Mahajanga, Mahajanga, Madagascar, [6] UFR Odontologie de Lyon, Université Claude Bernard, Lyon, France, [7] Research Unit of Theoretical & Applied Economics, GREThA (UMR Centre National de la Recherche Scientifique 5113), Université de Bordeaux, Pessac, France

Correspondence:
Agnès Bloch-Zupan
agnes.bloch-zupan@unistra.fr

A large family from a small village in Madagascar, Antanetilava, is known to present with colored teeth. Through previous collaboration and 4 successive visits in 1994, 2004, 2005, and 2012, we provided dental care to the inhabitants and diagnosed dentinogenesis imperfecta. Recently, using whole exome sequencing we confirmed the clinical diagnosis by identifying a novel single nucleotide deletion in exon 5 of *DSPP*. This paper underlines the necessity of long run research, the importance of international and interpersonal collaborations as well as the major contribution of next generation sequencing tools in the genetic diagnosis of rare oro-dental anomalies. This study is registered in ClinicalTrials (https://clinicaltrials.gov) under the number NCT02397824.

Keywords: rare disease, dentinogenesis imperfecta, dental anomalies, dentin, mutations, NGS, human

INTRODUCTION

Dentinogenesis imperfecta (DI) belongs to a group of rare genetic diseases affecting the formation/mineralization of tooth dentin and is transmitted, as recorded so far, in an autosomal dominant manner (Barron et al., 2008). A dominant negative effect of a modified dentin sialophosphoprotein (DSPP) has been suggested as the pathogenic mechanism underlying DI (Wang et al., 2011).

These disorders exist either in isolation, with clinical manifestations limited to the oral cavity and are named dentinogenesis imperfecta type II (DGI-II) or hereditary opalescent dentin (OMIM #125490) also called dentinogenesis imperfecta 1 (DGI-1) or Capdepont teeth, and dentinogenesis imperfecta type III (DGI-III; OMIM # 125500) (Shields et al., 1973; Kim and Simmer, 2007; Barron et al., 2008; de la Dure-Molla et al., 2015). They can be associated with other symptoms like progressive sensorineural hearing loss (OMIM # 605594) (Xiao et al., 2001) or encountered in syndromes like osteogenesis imperfecta and Goldblatt syndrome for example in which bone defects (a tissue similar to dentin) are key features of the clinical synopsis (Bloch-Zupan et al., 2012; Bloch-Zupan, 2014). Mutations described so far occur in one single gene *DSPP* (4q21.3), belonging to the SIBLINGs family and encoding three major non-collagenous dentin matrix proteins- dentin sialoprotein (DSP), dentin glycoprotein (DGP) and dentin phosphoprotein (DPP) (Zhang et al., 2001; MacDougall, 2003; Kim et al., 2005; Lee et al., 2008, 2009, 2011a, 2013).

In this paper, we focus on a large family from a small village in Madagascar, Antanetilava, known to present with colored teeth. The aim of the study is, through phenotyping and genotyping, to unravel the diagnosis and genetic origin of this rare familial condition. Through previous collaboration (1996) and successive visits in 2004, 2005 and 2012, we provided dental care to the inhabitants and linked the discoloration diagnosis to dentinogenesis imperfecta. Recently, using whole exome sequencing we confirmed this diagnosis by identifying a novel *DSPP* mutation segregating with the disease in this family.

MATERIALS AND METHODS

Patients

In 1996 (Razafindrakoto et al., 1996), the Strasbourg Faculty of Dentistry and the INSERM_U424 (JV Ruch) were contacted by colleagues from l'IOSTM (Institut d'Odonto-Stomatologie Tropicale de Madagascar) of Mahajanga University to help in disseminating scientific data related to a specific family originating from the small isolated village of Antanetilava (18°58′42.2″S 47°14′01.9″E), in the middle of the luxuriant tropical forest, in the Toamasina province, located 40 km North-West from the city of Toamasina. This region on the East coast of Madagascar is known for its hot and humid climate. It is a rural area devoted essentially to agriculture where rice, manioc, potatoes, banana and yam are cultivated. Colleagues visited Antanetilava in 1994, when a total of 110 inhabitants lived there. Problems related to inherited tooth anomalies in the population of Antanetilava had been previously noticed and the aim of this first visit was to determine what the tooth defects were, to follow the disorder in the families and to estimate its frequency.

At that time 50 people (28 females and 22 males) belonging to 22 of 26 households in the village were examined. Eleven individuals (22%, 6 females and 5 males) presented with this colored teeth anomaly affecting both the primary and permanent dentition. Clinical examination revealed brown to blue-gray discoloration of the crowns. Severe attrition due to early enamel chipping was visible. A clinical diagnosis of dentinogenesis imperfecta type II was proposed. Radiographic examination was possible for one 23 year-old patient in the nearest local hospital of Toamasina. Progressive pulp chamber obliterations as well as absent root canals were noticed, confirming the diagnosis. A first pedigree was drawn and demonstrated that the genetic disease affected 5 generations and 46.7% of the family members.

After a 2004 preparatory mission, JM returned to Mahajanga and visited Antanetilava in 2005 after a difficult journey consisting of 6 h of bus, 8 h of bush taxi, 1 dugout canoe river crossing and a further hour of walking.

Twenty seven participants (25 affected) and 2 non-affected family members were examined during this 2005 visit. Affected and unaffected family members gave written informed consent and, the study was approved by the village council. The orodental phenotypes were documented using the D[4]/phenodent registry: a Diagnosing Dental Defects Database (see www.phenodent.org, to access assessment form). This registry allows the standardization of data collection and assists in orodental phenotyping. It also facilitates providing clinical care to patients, a basis for genotype/orodental phenotype correlations, and sharing of data and clinical material between clinicians. D[4]/phenodent registry is approved by CNIL (French National commission for informatics and liberty) under the following number 908416.

This clinical study has been registered in Clinical trials (https://clinicaltrials.gov) under the number NCT02397824 and is registered by the French Ministère de l'enseignement supérieur et de la recherche, DGRI/Cellule de bioéthique (bioethics committee) under DC-2012-1677. It was acknowledged by the CPP (person protection committee) Est IV on the 11/12/2012.

Mutation Analysis

JM collected DNA samples using Whatman FTA cards and Oragene® DNA kits.

Genomic DNA was isolated from the saliva of 14 family members (9 affected and 5 unaffected), during the 2012 mission, using the prepIT-L2P OG-250 Oragene® DNA kit (DNA Genotek Inc., Ontario, Canada) according to standard protocols.

A few attempts of direct *DSPP* Sanger sequencing were unsuccessful.

We performed whole-exome sequencing (IntegraGen, Evry, France) for five affected patients (III.15, III.32, IV.26, IV.57, and IV.65) and one healthy individual (IV.22). Exons of DNA samples were captured using in-solution enrichment methodology (SureSelect Human All Exon Kits Version 3, Agilent, Massy, France) with the company's biotinylated oligonucleotide probe library (Human All Exon v5+UTR—75 Mb, Agilent). The genomic DNA was then sequenced on a sequencer as paired-end 2X75 base pair reads (Illumina HISEQ2000, Illumina, San Diego, USA) resulting in an average coverage of 200X. Image analysis and base calling was performed using Real Time Analysis (RTA) Pipeline version 1.9 with default parameters (Illumina). The bioinfomatic analysis of sequencing raw data was based on the pipeline provided by the company (CASAVA 1.8, Illumina and finally detects from 80965 to 82263 variants (SNPs and Indels) per proband (**Table 1**). Annotation, ranking, and filtering of genetic variants were performed with the VaRank program (Geoffroy et al., 2015). Very stringent criteria were used for excluding non-pathogenic variants, in particular: (1) variants represented with an allele frequency of more than 1% in dbSNP 138, the EXAC database or the NHLBI Exome Sequencing Project Exome Variant Server (EVS), (2) variants found at the homozygous state or more than once at the heterozygous state in 48 control exomes, (3) variants in the 5′ or 3′ UTR, (4) variants with intronic locations and no prediction of local splice effect, and (5) synonymous variants without prediction of local splice effect.

TABLE 1 | Summary of the exome sequencing results.

Individuals	III.15		III.32		IV.22		IV.26		IV.57		IV.65	
Type of sequence variant	**SNV**	**Indel**	**SNV**	**Indel**	**SNV**	**Indel**	**SNV**	**Indel**	**SNV**	**Indel**	**SNV**	**Indel**
Total number of variants	72429	9001	72273	8692	72638	8960	73233	9030	72480	8908	72212	8970
After exclusion of non-pathogenic variants (as determined from the ClinicalSignificance field in dbSNP) validated by at least 2 methods in dbSNP (as determined from the "Validation Status" field)	8767	4955	8617	4658	8745	4898	8758	4940	8576	4812	8564	4852
After exclusion of variants with an allele frequency > 1% (extracted from the EXAC database, the Exome Variant Server and the dbSNP database)	5734	3122	5653	3035	5792	3117	5703	3162	5675	3106	5648	3091
After exclusion of variants found in the homozygous state or more than once in the heterozygous state in 70 control exomes	1972	843	1998	910	2041	888	1990	901	2115	923	2234	884
After exclusion of 5′UTR, 3′UTR, downstream, upstream and intron locations without local splice effect prediction (from the "localSpliceEffect" field of Alamut-Batch)	767	123	729	132	757	119	706	120	731	122	780	119
After exclusion of synonymous variants without local splice effect prediction (from the "localSpliceEffect" field of Alamut-Batch)	571	123	563	132	571	119	520	120	569	122	592	119
Selection of variants consistent with recessive transmission	0 compound heterozygous 0 homozygous variants											
Selection of variants consistent with dominant transmission.	4 heterozygous variants (in the *DSPP*, *ABHD14A-ACY1*, *ABHD14A*, *HERC6* and *THAP9* genes)											

Sanger sequencing (GATC Biotech, Applied Biosystems ABI 3730xl^{TM}, Konstanz, Germany) was used to validate the mutations and verify segregation using the following primers.

Specific forward (F) and reverse (R) primers were designed to amplify the *DSPP* exon 5 region containing the mutation: DSPP-F (GTGACAGCAGCAATAGCAGTGATA) and DSPP-R (TCACTGGTTGAGTGGTTACTGTC) (expected product size of 376 bp (base pair). PCR amplifications were performed in a final volume of 50 µl containing 0.2 µM forward and reverse primers, 0.2 mM dNTPs, 1X GoTaq reaction buffer containing 1.5 mM MgCl2, 1.25 unit of GoTaq DNA polymerase (Promega), 50 ng of template DNA and 3% DMSO. Amplifications were performed for 40 cycles, each consisting of 30s denaturation at 94°C, 30s annealing at 64.9°C and 17s elongation at 72°C.

RESULTS

Clinical Phenotype

The family history and pedigree, as established in 1996, was updated. It then included 137 individuals spanning 5 generations (**Figure 1**) and 4 related families. 55 individuals, 31 males and 24 females, were reported as affected and presenting with DI corresponding to a 40.1% prevalence of the disease within this population (1/2 in generation I, 2/3 in generation II, 4/13 or 30.8% in generation III, 16/25 (64%) in IV, 30/64 (46.9%) in V and 2/7 (28.6%) in VI).

Medical history was collected from the 25 affected of the 27 examined persons. Patients reported only infectious episodes like malaria, measles, and fever. Some affected individuals (3) presented a triangular face shape or a facial asymmetry. Most of affected persons (23) showed blue sclera. Disturbance of hearing was recorded for 5 affected individuals. 9 patients presented articular distortions or pain and 3 had nail dysplasia.

Dental history mentioned infections, early tooth mobility and loss and tooth extractions. Both the primary and permanent dentitions were affected. Teeth presented with the amber-gray color pathognomonic of heritable dentin defects (**Figure 2**). Some tooth shape/size anomalies were observed as scoop shaped incisors, absence of convex vestibular crown surface, flat aspect of crown occlusal surfaces and supernumerary cusps. Enamel, when visible, presented an irregular appearance. Tooth wear was considerable and was visible via the colored abnormal dentin after enamel shedding. Fifteen individuals (11 adults, 4 children) suffered from tooth mobility. Nine individuals experienced dental infections. A probable diagnosis of DI was made. Three affected patients benefitted from X-ray investigations through intraoral radiographs taken in a private practice in the Antananarivo town. These pictures showed complete pulp space obliteration and globular crowns with cervical constrictions (**Figure 2**) confirming the diagnosis.

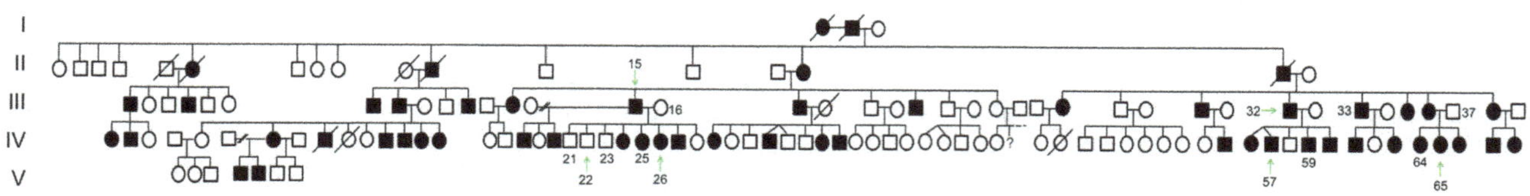

FIGURE 1 | Family pedigree. A large pedigree, spanning 5-generations with 137 individuals, of which 55 are affected, is showing a dominant inheritance pattern. Arrows point to individuals whose exomes were sequenced (affected: III.15, III.32, IV.26, IV.57, IV.65; non-affected: IV.22). Sanger sequencing was performed for the following subjects: affected (III.15, III.32, III.33, IV.25, IV.26, IV.57, IV.59, IV.64, IV.65), non-affected (III.16, III.37, IV.21, IV.22, IV.23).

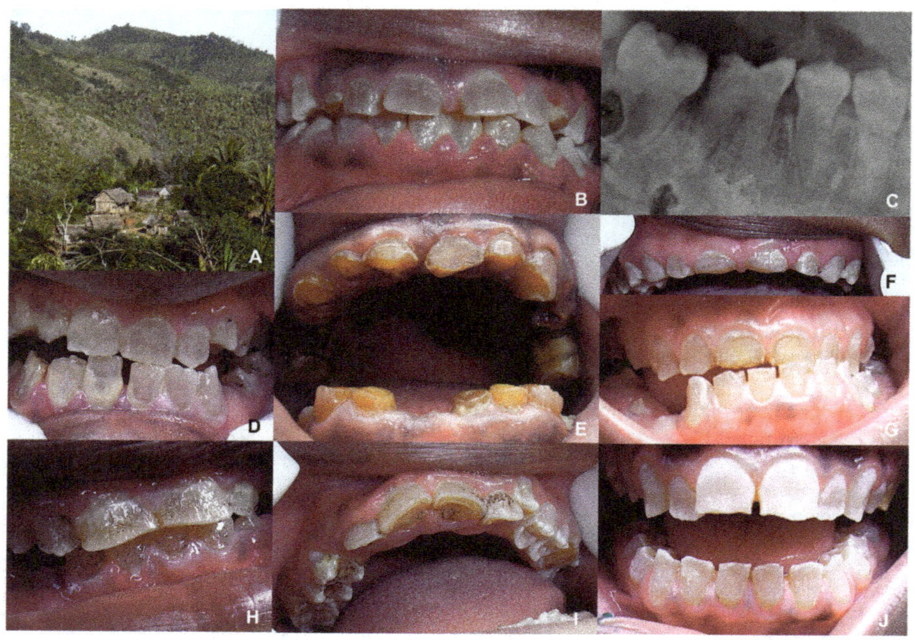

FIGURE 2 | Clinical description of the disease. (A) The remote village of Antananarivo. **(B–J)** Inhabitants'dentition showing the typical features of dentinogenesis imperfecta with the gray-brown discolouration of the dentin clearly visible after enamel cleavage and progressive tooth wear. **(C)** On the retro-alveolar radiography of the lower right premolar/molar sector of individual **(B)**, cervical constriction, short roots and the disappearance of pulp spaces due to erratic dentin formation represent the characteristic hallmarks of dentinogenesis imperfecta. **(H–J)** In addition to dentin anomalies, hypoplastic enamel defects exist, with the presence of pits, striae and flattened buccal surfaces.

Genotype

Using VaRank, to annotate rank, and filter the genetic variants, we identified, amongst 80965–82263 variants (SNPs and Indels) per proband, four candidate variants in five genes (*DSPP* [dentin sialophosphoprotein, OMIM: 125485], *ABHD14A-ACY1* [ABHD14A-ACY1 readthrough (NMD candidate)], *ABHD14A* [abhydrolase domain containing 14A], *HERC6* [HECT and RLD domain containing E3 ubiquitin protein ligase family member 6, OMIM: 609249] and *THAP9* [THAP domain containing 9, OMIM: 612537]) with heterozygous variants present only in the affected patients (**Table 1**). We then focused the subsequent study on the heterozygous variant in *DSPP*, a known causal gene for DI: a heterozygous deletion (c.3676del [p.Ser1226Alafs*88] [RefSeq NM_014208.3]). Mutation is absent from the 1000 genome, NHLBI EVS and ExAC databases.

We identified through exome sequencing and confirmed by bidirectional Sanger sequencing analysis of *DSPP*, a heterozygous deletion of 1 base pair (bp) in exon 5 (p.[Ser1226Alafs*88];[=] or c.[3676delA];[=]) in 9 affected patients (**Figure 3**). Segregation analysis validated the absence of the mutation in unaffected individuals. The deletion was absent from dbSNP and the Exome Variant Server. These mutations are predicted to cause a frameshift from codon Ser1226 producing an early stop codon 87 amino acids after the deletion and deleting the protein of an important functional domain.

DISCUSSION

This work is an extraordinary travel in time, human beliefs and mutual assistance, genetics, science, and new technologies allowing the understanding of the exceptional prevalence of DI in this remote village from Madagascar. The family believed that the tooth coloration and the disease was of nutritional origin.

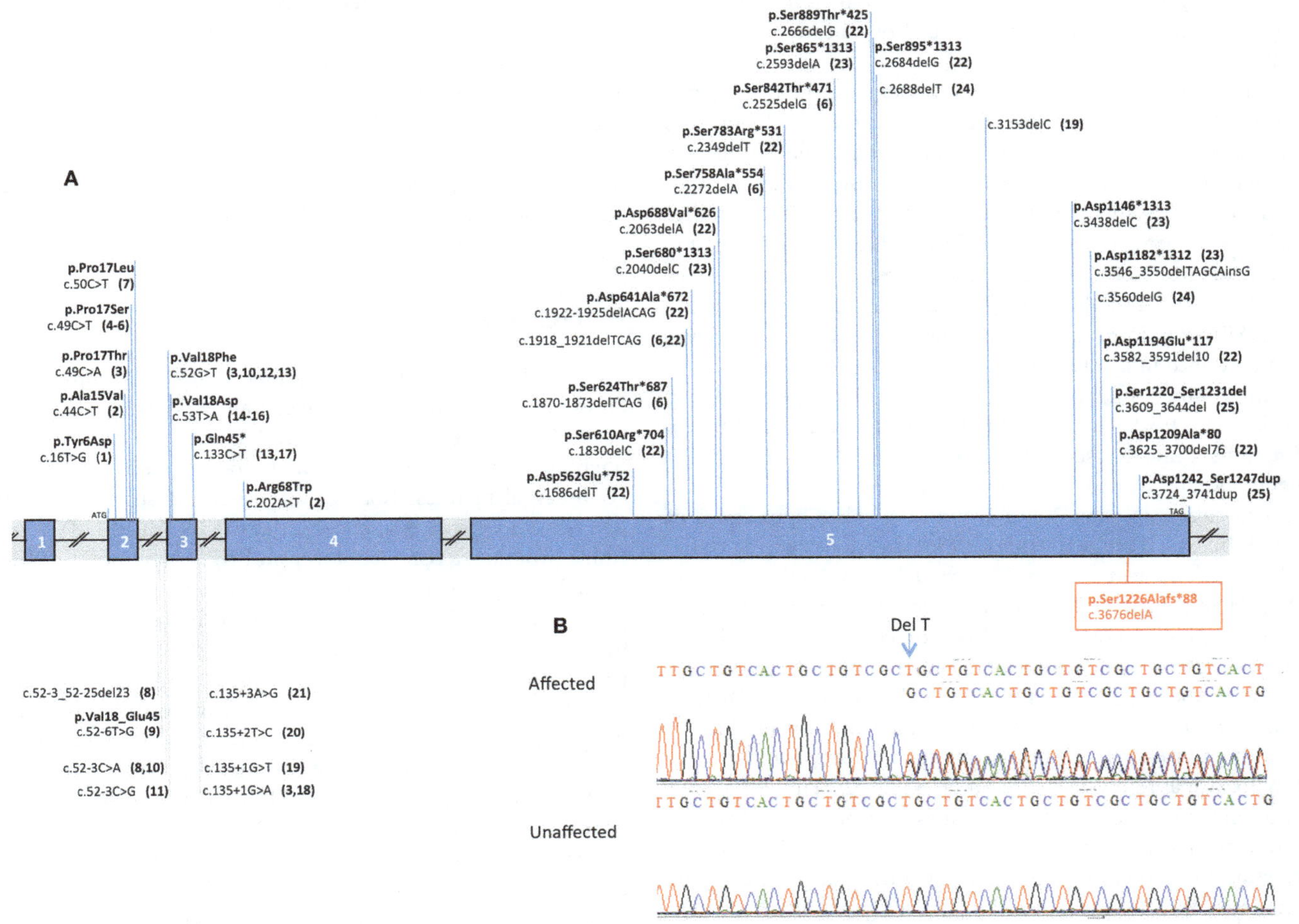

FIGURE 3 | *DSPP* mutation analysis. *DSPP* mutations are indicated against the gene structure (reference sequence: NM_014208.3). **(A)** Schematic representation of *DSPP*: this gene contains 5 exons (vertical blue hatches), the position of the start codon (ATG) and the stop codon (TAG) are indicated respectively in exon 2 and exon5. The known mutations in the *DSPP* gene are summarized against the gene structure and associated to a literature reference. The new mutation described in this paper is boxed and written in red. For example: the most 5′ *DSPP* mutation, near the initiation codon (ATG) is lying in exon 2 and described as a single nucleotide variant c.16T>G leading to the following amino acid changes in the protein p.Tyr6Asp and reported in the literature in quoted reference (Rajpar et al., 2002). **(B)** Electrophoregrams of a part of *DSPP* exon 5 showing the heterozygous mutation in an affected person and the normal sequence in an unaffected individual. The deletion of 1T is indicated with an arrow, this deletion creates a shift in the reading frame in position 3676 of the cDNA reference sequence, resulting in 2 superposed sequences. On the scheme the numbering corresponds to the following references: **1.** Rajpar et al. (2002); **2.** Malmgren et al. (2004); **3.** Xiao et al. (2001); **4.** Zhang et al. (2007) and Qu et al. (2009); **5.** Hart and Hart (2007); **6.** Mcknight et al. (2008a); **7.** Li et al. (2012) and Lee et al. (2013); **8.** Wang et al. (2009); **9.** Lee et al. (2008); **10.** Holappa et al. (2006); **11.** Kim et al. (2004); **12.** Kim et al. (2005); **13.** Song et al. (2006); **14.** Lee et al. (2011b); **15.** Kida et al. (2009); **16.** Lee et al. (2009); **17.** Zhang et al. (2001); **18.** Wang et al. (2011); **19.** Mcknight et al. (2008b); **20.** Zhang et al. (2011); **21.** Bai et al. (2010); **22.** Nieminen et al. (2011); **23.** Song et al. (2008); **24.** Lee et al. (2011a); **25.** Dong et al. (2005).

Some hypotheses were proposed like the large consumption of red rice, or drinking habits (acidic water source). Oral tradition of the family history described healthy ancestors. Tradition forbids women, after giving birth, to eat white rice and transgression of this law after a famine period was believed to be associated with the appearance of the dental defect among the population.

DI incidence is believed to reach 1 in 8000 individuals according to Barron et al. (2008). Due to the founder effect, well observed in generation I of the pedigree, and the geographic isolation of the studied population, this prevalence approximates 40% in this population.

DI is transmitted as an autosomal dominant trait and this is clearly visible with the parent to child transmission seen in the pedigree and the presence of affected members in each generation.

The medical history revealed hearing loss problems, which indeed have been reported as associated with DI and *DSPP* mutations (Xiao et al., 2001). Blue sclerae are a classical hallmark of osteogenesis imperfecta clinical synopsis and the association of DI with even a milder form of osteogenesis imperfecta was still a possible diagnosis (Wang et al., 2012).

The phenotype demonstrated both enamel and dentin defects as was previously also reported (Wang et al., 2011). *Dspp* is expressed by odontoblasts and transiently by preameloblasts (Bronckers et al., 1993; Ritchie et al., 1997; Begue-Kirn et al., 1998).

Difficulties throughout the years to sequence the *DSPP* gene, especially the *DPP* region, are due to the high GC rich contents and the number of repeats. As no mutation could be initially detected in this candidate gene and because of disease high frequency within this population we hypothesized that another unidentified gene might be involved. Thus, we used exome sequencing to look for the causative gene. But in fact, we identified a novel single base pair deletion within the end of the fifth *DSPP* exon leading to a premature stop codon. It has never been described in the literature.

Thirty nine mutations in the human *DSPP* gene causing dentin defects have been previously reported (**Figure 3**). Mutations (mostly substitutions) leading to a DI (DGI) phenotype are located mostly at the 5′ end of *DSPP* and also seem to cluster in exon 2 and around the splice boundaries of exon 3. In exon 5 at the 3′ end of *DSPP*, deletions causing frame shift mutations were responsible for DGI and dentin dysplasia (DD) (Wang et al., 2011). The mutation described herein is also localized at the end of exon 5. This exon codes for DPP (dentin phosphoprotein), which is one of the most abundant extracellular matrix components in dentin (after collagen type I COL1A1, COL1A2). DPP has a role in biomineralization by binding to collagen and calcium and promoting the nucleation and growth of hydroxyapatite crystals (Prasad et al., 2010). The discovered mutation is predicted to cause a frameshift from codon Ser1226 producing an early stop codon 87 amino acids after the deletion, depleting the protein of an important functional domain. This domain is called "Asp/Ser-rich" by UniProt (position 439-1301).

To date, only one other mutation has been identified in the 3′ end of exon 5 (Dong et al., 2005) and consisted of a 36 bp deletion and an 18 bp insertion with a phenotype of DGI type III. Authors reported affected family members with amber tooth discoloration, opalescent appearance, severe attrition of teeth, visible pulp chambers and shell teeth on radiographs differing from the DI phenotype reported in this paper.

Targeted next-generation sequencing technics for orodental disorders (Prasad et al., 2016) prove to be efficient methods to sequence *DSPP* gene allowing further mutations detection and helping providing accurate molecular and clinical diagnosis to rare disease patients. Differential clinical and molecular diagnosis between DI and mild forms of osteogenesis imperfecta presenting with opalescent teeth is important and will orientate patients toward appropriate integrated dental and medical care. These methods, as associated costs decrease, will be transposed from research results to diagnostic molecular findings.

AUTHOR CONTRIBUTIONS

JM, RWR, SNR, JCR, GR, ROA, RHR, SER, LHR, JAR collected the salivary samples and detailed the patients' phenotype. JM travelled back and forth between France and Madagascar to develop the project and gathered funding. BR, PG tried to sequence DSPP gene using conventional techniques. MH, CS, VG identified the molecular basis of the disease through NGS assays. MH, CS, VG, MCM, SRA, JAR, HD, ABZ analyzed the data and wrote the manuscript. ABZ designed the study and was involved from conception, funding seeking to drafting and critical review of the manuscript. All authors therefore contributed to conception, design, data acquisition, analysis, and interpretation, drafted and critically revised the manuscript. All authors gave final approval and agree to be accountable for all aspects of the work.

FUNDING

This work was financed by grants from: the University of Strasbourg, the Hôpitaux Universitaires de Strasbourg (API, 2009-2012, "Development of the oral cavity: from gene to clinical phenotype in Human"), the EU-funded project (ERDF) A27 "Oro-dental manifestations of rare diseases," supported by the RMT-TMO Offensive Sciences initiative, INTERREG IV Upper Rhine program, a contribution from EAPD and the INTERREG V RARENET program. This study was also supported by the grant ANR-10-LABX-0030-INRT, a French State fund managed by the Agence Nationale de la Recherche under the frame programme Investissements d'Avenir labeled ANR-10-IDEX-0002-02. ABZ is a fellow of University of Strasbourg Institute for Advanced Study (USIAS) and received USIAS Fellowship. Funding, support as well as dental materials were gathered by JM for her travels from the Conseil Départemental de l'Ordre des Chirurgiens Dentistes du Bas-Rhin, Ville de Strasbourg, Conseil Général du Bas-Rhin, Bureau de la Vie Etudiante de l'Université de Strasbourg, Association Amicale des Etudiants en Chirurgie Dentaire de Strasbourg, Henry Schein, GC Europe, Megadental, Laboratoire Unodis Haguenau, Colgate, Pierre Fabre, Alpha Omega Alsace, Laboratoire Flecher Strasbourg, Crédit Mutuel Profession de Santé. A grant was received in Madagascar from Général Randrianazary "Secrétaire d'état à la gendarmerie" in 2012, to cover travel expenses.

WEB RESOURCES

The URLs for data presented herein are as follows:

dbSNP, http://www.ncbi.nlm.nih.gov/projects/SNP/
NHLBI Exome Sequencing Project (ESP) Exome Variant Server, http://evs.gs.washington.edu/EVS/
OMIM, http://www.omim.org/
PolyPhen-2, http://genetics.bwh.harvard.edu/pph2/
RefSeq, http://www.ncbi.nlm.nih.gov/refseq/
SIFT, http://sift.bii.a-star.edu.sg/
VaRank, http://www.lbgi.fr/VaRank
UCSC Genome Browser, http://genome.ucsc.edu

ACKNOWLEDGMENTS

We are grateful to the families and village council for their participation and invaluable contribution. We are grateful to Emilson, Nirina, Liva, Judicaël, Prudence, Nelly-Olivia for their help. We would like to thank Prof. Y. Rumpler, University of Strasbourg who inspired this project and long lasting collaboration. Several persons contributed to this project, and we would like to acknowledge their contribution here: Mr. J. Zafy Jean, for guiding one of the visits, Miss Rakotonindrina Miary for transferring samples from Madagascar, Dr. C. Kaempf, president of the Conseil de l'Ordre des Chirurgiens Dentistes du Bas-Rhin, Dr. H. Randrianary and Dr. Y. Randriamahefa, presidents of the Conseil de l'Ordre des Chirurgiens-Dentistes de Madagascar and from Toamasina province in 2004, Dr. A. E. Rakotoarivony, Director of IOSTM, Dr. S. Ralison, assistant in IOSTM in 2004. Prof. C. Holmgren gave generous advises about the ART (Atraumatic Restorative treatment) technique. Prof. Y. Haikel supported this project. We would like to thank also Dr. M. K. Prasad for critical reading of the manuscript. The authors declare no potential conflict of interest with respect to the authorship and/or publication of this article.

REFERENCES

Bai, H., Agula, H., Wu, Q., Zhou, W., Sun, Y., Qi, Y., et al. (2010). A novel DSPP mutation causes dentinogenesis imperfecta type II in a large Mongolian family. *BMC Med. Genet.* 11:23. doi: 10.1186/1471-2350-11-23

Barron, M. J., McDonnell, S. T., Mackie, I., and Dixon, M. J. (2008). Hereditary dentine disorders: dentinogenesis imperfecta and dentine dysplasia. *Orphanet J. Rare Dis.* 3:31. doi: 10.1186/1750-1172-3-31

Bégue-Kirn, C., Krebsbach, P. H., Bartlett, J. D., and Butler, W. T. (1998). Dentin sialoprotein, dentin phosphoprotein, enamelysin and ameloblastin: tooth-specific molecules that are distinctively expressed during murine dental differentiation. *Eur. J. Oral Sci.* 106, 963–970. doi: 10.1046/j.0909-8836.1998.eos106510.x

Bloch-Zupan, A. (2014). "Genetic alterations: heritable dentin defects," in *The Dental Pulp: Biology, Pathology, and Regenerative Therapies, 1st Edn.*, ed M. Goldberg (Berlin; Heidelberg: Springer-Verlag), 155–168.

Bloch-Zupan, A., Sedano, H., and Scully, C. (2012). *Dento/Oro/Craniofacial Anomalies and Genetics.* London: Elsevier Inc.

Bronckers, A. L., D'souza, R. N., Butler, W. T., Lyaruu, D. M., Van Dijk, S., Gay, S., et al. (1993). Dentin sialoprotein: biosynthesis and developmental appearance in rat tooth germs in comparison with amelogenins, osteocalcin and collagen type-I. *Cell Tissue Res.* 272, 237–247. doi: 10.1007/BF00302729

de la Dure-Molla, M., Philippe Fournier, B., and Berdal, A. (2015). Isolated dentinogenesis imperfecta and dentin dysplasia: revision of the classification. *Eur. J. Hum. Genet. EJHG* 23, 445–451. doi: 10.1038/ejhg.2014.159

Dong, J., Gu, T., Jeffords, L., and MacDougall, M. (2005). Dentin phosphoprotein compound mutation in dentin sialophosphoprotein causes dentinogenesis imperfecta type III. *Am. J. Med. Genet. A* 132, 305–309. doi: 10.1002/ajmg.a.30460

Geoffroy, V., Pizot, C., Redin, C., Piton, A., Vasli, N., Stoetzel, C., et al. (2015). VaRank: a simple and powerful tool for ranking genetic variants. *PeerJ* 3:e796. doi: 10.7717/peerj.796

Hart, P. S., and Hart, T. C. (2007). Disorders of human dentin. *Cells Tissues Organs* 186, 70–77. doi: 10.1159/000102682

Holappa, H., Nieminen, P., Tolva, L., Lukinmaa, P. L., and Alaluusua, S. (2006). Splicing site mutations in dentin sialophosphoprotein causing dentinogenesis imperfecta type II. *Eur. J. Oral Sci.* 114, 381–384. doi: 10.1111/j.1600-0722.2006.00391.x

Kida, M., Tsutsumi, T., Shindoh, M., Ikeda, H., and Ariga, T. (2009). De novo mutation in the DSPP gene associated with dentinogenesis imperfecta type II in a Japanese family. *Eur. J. Oral Sci.* 117, 691–694. doi: 10.1111/j.1600-0722.2009.00683.x

Kim, J. W., Hu, J. C., Lee, J. I., Moon, S. K., Kim, Y. J., Jang, K. T., et al. (2005). Mutational hot spot in the DSPP gene causing dentinogenesis imperfecta type II. *Hum. Genet.* 116, 186–191. doi: 10.1007/s00439-004-1223-6

Kim, J. W., Nam, S. H., Jang, K. T., Lee, S. H., Kim, C. C., Hahn, S. H., et al. (2004). A novel splice acceptor mutation in the DSPP gene causing dentinogenesis imperfecta type II. *Hum. Genet.* 115, 248–254. doi: 10.1007/s00439-004-1143-5

Kim, J. W., and Simmer, J. P. (2007). Hereditary dentin defects. *J. Dent. Res.* 86, 392–399. doi: 10.1177/154405910708600502

Lee, K. E., Kang, H. Y., Lee, S. K., Yoo, S. H., Lee, J. C., Hwang, Y. H., et al. (2011a). Novel dentin phosphoprotein frameshift mutations in dentinogenesis imperfecta type II. *Clin. Genet.* 79, 378–384. doi: 10.1111/j.1399-0004.2010.01483.x

Lee, S. K., Hu, J. C., Lee, K. E., Simmer, J. P., and Kim, J. W. (2008). A dentin sialophosphoprotein mutation that partially disrupts a splice acceptor site causes type II dentin dysplasia. *J. Endod.* 34, 1470–1473. doi: 10.1016/j.joen.2008.08.027

Lee, S. K., Lee, K. E., Hwang, Y. H., Kida, M., Tsutsumi, T., Ariga, T., et al. (2011b). Identification of the DSPP mutation in a new kindred and phenotype-genotype correlation. *Oral Dis.* 17, 314–319. doi: 10.1111/j.1601-0825.2010.01760.x

Lee, S. K., Lee, K. E., Jeon, D., Lee, G., Lee, H., Shin, C. U., et al. (2009). A novel mutation in the DSPP gene associated with dentinogenesis imperfecta type II. *J. Dent. Res.* 88, 51–55. doi: 10.1177/0022034508328168

Lee, S. K., Lee, K. E., Song, S. J., Hyun, H. K., Lee, S. H., and Kim, J. W. (2013). A DSPP mutation causing dentinogenesis imperfecta and characterization of the mutational effect. *Biomed Res. Int.* 2013:948181. doi: 10.1155/2013/948181

Li, D., Du, X., Zhang, R., Shen, B., Huang, Y., Valenzuela, R. K., et al. (2012). Mutation identification of the DSPP in a Chinese family with DGI-II and an up-to-date bioinformatic analysis. *Genomics* 99, 220–226. doi: 10.1016/j.ygeno.2012.01.006

MacDougall, M. (2003). Dental structural diseases mapping to human chromosome 4q21. *Connect. Tissue Res.* 44 (Suppl. 1), 285–291. doi: 10.1080/03008200390181780

Malmgren, B., Lindskog, S., Elgadi, A., and Norgren, S. (2004). Clinical, histopathologic, and genetic investigation in two large families with dentinogenesis imperfecta type II. *Hum. Genet.* 114, 491–498. doi: 10.1007/s00439-004-1084-z

Mcknight, D. A., Simmer, J. P., Hart, P. S., Hart, T. C., and Fisher, L. W. (2008a). Overlapping DSPP mutations cause dentin dysplasia and dentinogenesis imperfecta. *J. Dent. Res.* 87, 1108–1111. doi: 10.1177/154405910808701217

Mcknight, D. A., Suzanne Hart, P., Hart, T. C., Hartsfield, J. K., Wilson, A., Wright, J. T., et al. (2008b). A comprehensive analysis of normal variation and disease-causing mutations in the human DSPP gene. *Hum. Mutat.* 29, 1392–1404. doi: 10.1002/humu.20783

Nieminen, P., Papagiannoulis-Lascarides, L., Waltimo-Siren, J., Ollila, P., Karjalainen, S., Arte, S., et al. (2011). Frameshift mutations in dentin phosphoprotein and dependence of dentin disease phenotype on mutation location. *J. Bone Miner. Res.* 26, 873–880. doi: 10.1002/jbmr.276

Prasad, M., Butler, W. T., and Qin, C. (2010). Dentin sialophosphoprotein in biomineralization. *Connect. Tissue Res.* 51, 404–417. doi: 10.3109/03008200903329789

Prasad, M. K., Geoffroy, V., Vicaire, S., Jost, B., Dumas, M., Le Gras, S., et al. (2016). A targeted next-generation sequencing assay for the molecular diagnosis of genetic disorders with orodental involvement. *J. Med. Genet.* 53, 98–110. doi: 10.1136/jmedgenet-2015-103302

Qu, E. J., Zhang, H. B., Chen, L. Y., and Gu, L. B. (2009). [Mutation analysis of a Chinese family with genetic dentinogenesis imperfecta]. *Zhonghua Yi Xue Yi Chuan Xue Za Zhi* 26, 536–538. doi: 10.3760/cma.j.issn.1003-9406.2009.05.013

Rajpar, M. H., Koch, M. J., Davies, R. M., Mellody, K. T., Kielty, C. M., and Dixon, M. J. (2002). Mutation of the signal peptide region of the bicistronic gene DSPP affects translocation to the endoplasmic reticulum and results in defective dentine biomineralization. *Hum. Mol. Genet.* 11, 2559–2565. doi: 10.1093/hmg/11.21.2559

Razafindrakoto, R. W., Rasoamananjara, J. A., Ralimanana, L. H., Randrianaivo, J. C. P., and Bloch-Zupan, A. (1996). "Dentinogenesis imperfecta: a family story," in *Abstract Book of the Congress of the European Academy of Paediatric Dentistry* (Bruges: EAPD), 89.

Ritchie, H. H., Berry, J. E., Somerman, M. J., Hanks, C. T., Bronckers, A. L., Hotton, D., et al. (1997). Dentin sialoprotein (DSP) transcripts: developmentally-sustained expression in odontoblasts and transient expression in pre-ameloblasts. *Eur. J. Oral Sci.* 105, 405–413. doi: 10.1111/j.1600-0722.1997.tb02137.x

Shields, E. D., Bixler, D., and el-Kafrawy, A. M. (1973). A proposed classification for heritable human dentine defects with a description of a new entity. *Arch. Oral Biol.* 18, 543–553. doi: 10.1016/0003-9969(73)90075-7

Song, Y., Wang, C., Peng, B., Ye, X., Zhao, G., Fan, M., et al. (2006). Phenotypes and genotypes in 2 DGI families with different DSPP mutations. *Oral Surg. Oral Med. Oral Pathol. Oral Radiol. Endod.* 102, 360–374. doi: 10.1016/j.tripleo.2005.06.020

Song, Y. L., Wang, C. N., Fan, M. W., Su, B., and Bian, Z. (2008). Dentin phosphoprotein frameshift mutations in hereditary dentin disorders and their variation patterns in normal human population. *J. Med. Genet.* 45, 457–464. doi: 10.1136/jmg.2007.056911

Wang, H., Hou, Y., Cui, Y., Huang, Y., Shi, Y., Xia, X., et al. (2009). A novel splice site mutation in the dentin sialophosphoprotein gene in a Chinese family with dentinogenesis imperfecta type II. *Mutat. Res.* 662, 22–27. doi: 10.1016/j.mrfmmm.2008.11.019

Wang, S. K., Chan, H. C., Makovey, I., Simmer, J. P., and Hu, J. C. (2012). Novel PAX9 and COL1A2 missense mutations causing tooth agenesis and OI/DGI without skeletal abnormalities. *PLoS ONE* 7:e51533. doi: 10.1371/journal.pone.0051533

Wang, S. K., Chan, H. C., Rajderkar, S., Milkovich, R. N., Uston, K. A., Kim, J. W., et al. (2011). Enamel malformations associated with a defined dentin sialophosphoprotein mutation in two families. *Eur. J. Oral Sci.* 119 (Suppl. 1), 158–167. doi: 10.1111/j.1600-0722.2011.00874.x

Xiao, S., Yu, C., Chou, X., Yuan, W., Wang, Y., Bu, L., et al. (2001). Dentinogenesis imperfecta 1 with or without progressive hearing loss is associated with distinct mutations in DSPP. *Nat. Genet.* 27, 201–204. doi: 10.1038/84848

Zhang, J., Wang, J., Ma, Y., Du, W., Zhao, S., Zhang, Z., et al. (2011). A novel splicing mutation alters DSPP transcription and leads to dentinogenesis imperfecta type II. *PLoS ONE* 6:e27982. doi: 10.1371/journal.pone.0027982

Zhang, X., Chen, L., Liu, J., Zhao, Z., Qu, E., Wang, X., et al. (2007). A novel DSPP mutation is associated with type II dentinogenesis imperfecta in a Chinese family. *BMC Med. Genet.* 8:52. doi: 10.1186/1471-2350-8-52

Zhang, X., Zhao, J., Li, C., Gao, S., Qiu, C., Liu, P., et al. (2001). DSPP mutation in dentinogenesis imperfecta Shields type II. *Nat. Genet.* 27, 151–152. doi: 10.1038/84765

20

MORN5 Expression during Craniofacial Development and its Interaction with the BMP and TGFβ Pathways

*Petra Cela[1, 2], Marek Hampl[1, 2], Katherine K. Fu[3], Michaela Kunova Bosakova[4], Pavel Krejci[4, 5], Joy M. Richman[3] and Marcela Buchtova[1, 2]**

[1] Institute of Animal Physiology and Genetics, v.v.i., Academy of Sciences of the Czech Republic, Brno, Czech Republic, [2] Department of Animal Physiology and Immunology, Institute of Experimental Biology, Masaryk University, Brno, Czech Republic, [3] Life Sciences Institute, University of British Columbia, Vancouver, BC, Canada, [4] Department of Biology, Faculty of Medicine, Masaryk University, Brno, Czech Republic, [5] International Clinical Research Center, St. Anne's University Hospital, Brno, Czech Republic

***Correspondence:**
Marcela Buchtova
buchtova@iach.cz

MORN5 (MORN repeat containing 5) is encoded by a locus positioned on chromosome 17 in the chicken genome. The MORN motif is found in multiple copies in several proteins including junctophilins or phosphatidylinositol phosphate kinase family and the MORN proteins themselves are found across the animal and plant kingdoms. MORN5 protein has a characteristic punctate pattern in the cytoplasm in immunofluorescence imaging. Previously, *MORN5* was found among differentially expressed genes in a microarray profiling experiment of the chicken embryo head. Here, we provided *in situ* hybridization to analyse, in detail, the *MORN5* expression in chick craniofacial structures. The expression of *MORN5* was first observed at stage HH17-18 (E2.5). *MORN5* expression gradually appeared on either side of the primitive oral cavity, within the maxillary region. At stage HH20 (E3), prominent expression was localized in the mandibular prominences lateral to the midline. From stage HH20 up to HH29 (E6), there was strong expression in restricted regions of the maxillary and mandibular prominences. The frontonasal mass (in the midline of the face) expressed MORN5, starting at HH27 (E5). The expression was concentrated in the corners or globular processes, which will ultimately fuse with the cranial edges of the maxillary prominences. *MORN5* expression was maintained in the fusion zone up to stage HH29. In sections *MORN5* expression was localized preferentially in the mesenchyme. Previously, we examined signals that regulate *MORN5* expression in the face based on a previous microarray study. Here, we validated the array results with *in situ* hybridization and QPCR. *MORN5* was downregulated 24 h after Noggin and/or RA treatment. We also determined that BMP pathway genes are downstream of *MORN5* following siRNA knockdown. Based on these results, we conclude that *MORN5* is both regulated by and required for BMP signaling. The restricted expression of *MORN5* in the lip fusion zone shown here supports the human genetic data in which *MORN5* variants were associated with increased risk of non-syndromic cleft lip with or without cleft palate.

Keywords: cleft lip, maxillary prominence, mandibular prominence, frontonasal mass, BMP

INTRODUCTION

The vertebrate face is formed very early in development from the paired maxillary and mandibular prominences and the single frontonasal mass surrounding the oral cavity. These facial prominences arise during early embryogenesis from interactions between neural crest derived mesenchyme and head ectoderm. The frontonasal mass grows out, contacts and fuses together with the maxillary prominences to form the upper jaw. The midline facial skeleton consisting of the nasal septum, prenasal cartilage and premaxilla are all derived from the frontonasal mass (Richman and Lee, 2003). Craniofacial development is complex process coordinated by a network of transcription factors and signaling molecules (Murray and Schutte, 2004; Chai and Maxson, 2006; Jiang et al., 2006; Brunskill et al., 2014; Kurosaka, 2015; Marcucio et al., 2015; Nimmagadda et al., 2015). Disruption of this tightly controlled cascade can result in clefts where the facial prominences fail to meet and fuse (Leslie and Marazita, 2013).

Cleft lip and/or cleft palate are the most common craniofacial birth defects in humans (Setó-Salvia and Stanier, 2014; Watkins et al., 2014). The majority of clefts appear as isolated or non-syndromic clefts, because they occur in isolation from other developmental abnormalities. The causes of clefting are thought to be multifactorial, including an interaction between genes and the environmental factors (Schutte and Murray, 1999; Dixon et al., 2011; Leslie and Marazita, 2013; Setó-Salvia and Stanier, 2014; Watkins et al., 2014). Identification of genes contributing to clefts formation is important not only for our understanding of facial development, but also for improved prevention and treatment of affected individuals. The chicken embryo is a valuable experimental model to study the signals that control lip fusion. The avian primary palate closely resembles the primary palate in mammals (Abramyan et al., 2015). Moreover, the face can be accessed directly in the living embryo through a window in the shell. The disruption of FGF (Szabo-Rogers et al., 2008), BMP (Ashique et al., 2002), SHH (Hu et al., 2015), and WNT signaling (Geetha-Loganathan et al., 2014) causes a cleft lip in chickens that resembles that of humans.

Previously, a microarray study was performed to profile gene expression in individual chicken facial prominences in stage 18 embryos (Buchtová et al., 2010). From the list of genes that were significantly more highly expressed in the maxillary prominence, we selected *MORN5* (also known as C9orf113, C9orf18 or FLJ46909) for further studies because it was described as a cleft susceptibility gene (Letra et al., 2010). Microarray analysis revealed 24 times higher expression of *MORN5* in the maxillary prominence compared to expression in the frontonasal mass at stage 18, while mandibular prominence showed 10 times higher expression than the frontonasal mass (Buchtová et al., 2010).

Members of the MORN family were named for the presence of multiple MORN motifs (Membrane Occupation and Recognition Nexus). There are five paralogous genes in the *MORN* family (MORN1-5). Limited functional information is available for a subset of MORN genes. *MORN1* has been identified in the parasite *Toxoplasma gondii* and other Apicomplexan protists where it plays role during cell division (Ferguson et al., 2008; Lorestani et al., 2010). Human *MORN2* was found to facilitate phagocytosis-mediated restriction of some bacteria in macrophages (Abnave et al., 2014). Expression of *MORN3* was detected in mouse testis, where it regulates spermatogenesis (Zhang et al., 2015). Finally, *MORN4* promotes axonal degeneration in mouse sensory axons (Bhattacharya et al., 2012).

In chicken, the *MORN5* gene is located on the forward strand of chromosome 17. On the reverse strand, *NDUFA8* and *LHX6* genes are nearby to the *MORN5* gene. The size of the *MORN5* gene is 13.5 kb and there are 6 exons (only 5 exons are coding) with four splice variants. The *MORN5* gene encodes a protein of 172 amino acids, which contains a histone H3 K4-specific methyltransferase SET7/9 N-terminal domain (SSF82185) and three MORN motifs (**Figure 1**).

As the gene expression pattern or possible function of *MORN5* during development had not been investigated in any animal model, we aim to analyzed chicken *MORN5* expression in embryos and its integration into signaling pathways.

MATERIALS AND METHODS

Embryonic Material

Fertilized chicken eggs (ISA brown) were obtained from the farm Integra (Žabčice, Czech Republic). Eggs were incubated in a humidified forced air incubator at 37.8°C. Embryos were staged and morphological characteristic were described according to Hamburger and Hamilton (1951). All procedures were conducted following a protocol approved by the Laboratory Animal Science Committee of the Institute of Animal Physiology and Genetics (Liběchov, Czech Republic).

Section *In situ* Hybridization (ISH)

Chicken *MORN5* was obtained as chicken EST clone CHEST ID 543 F09 (Biovalley, France), where the probe sequence was cloned into pBluescript II KS+ vector. The entire region containing the probe sequence flanked by T3 and T7 RNA polymerase sites was amplified using M13 primers (forward primer: 5′-GTA AAA CGA CGG CCA G-3′, reverse primer: 5′-CAG GAA ACA GCT ATG AC-3′). Then, the amplicon was isolated via gel purification (QIAquick Gell Extraction Kit, Qiagen, Germany) and this linearized DNA fragment was used in RNA polymerase reactions. DIG labeled antisense riboprobe was synthesized with T3 RNA polymerase (antisense) or with T7 polymerase (sense controls).

Embryos were fixed in 4% paraformaldehyde (PFA), processed through ethanol and xylene into paraffin, and sectioned for ISH. Hybridization was performed with RNA probe at 60°C overnight as described previously (Holland et al., 1996). Anti-digoxigenin sheep antibody conjugated with alkaline phosphatase (1:2000, Roche, USA) was applied overnight at 4°C. Visualization was achieved by incubation with substrates for alkaline phosphatase (BM Purple AP, Roche, Germany) for several days. Slides were then counterstained with eosin. ISH was carried out on at least three embryos for each stage.

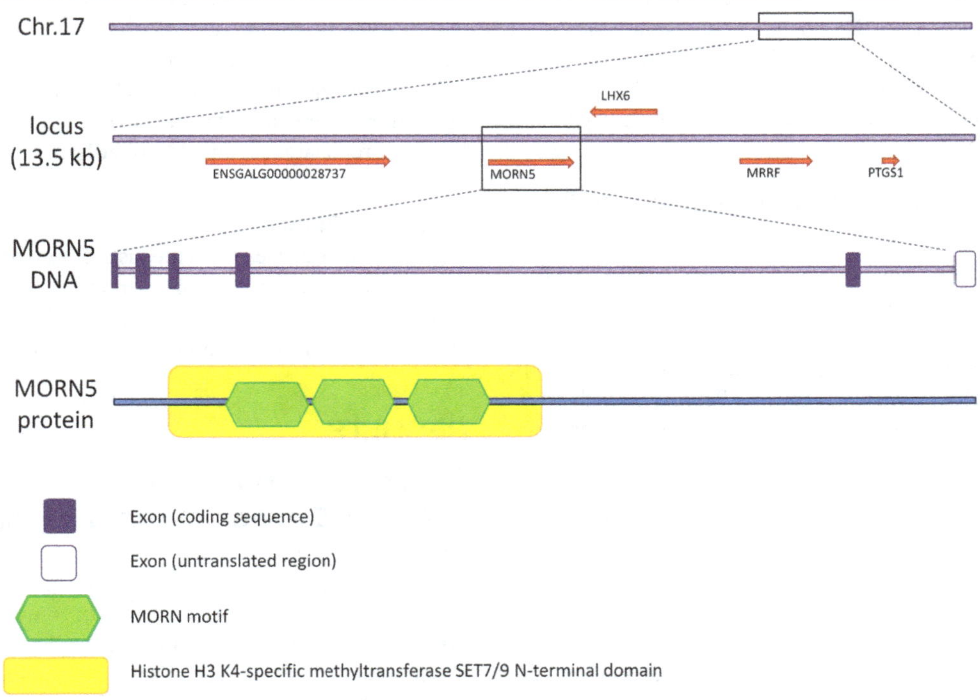

FIGURE 1 | Gene characteristics of chicken *MORN5* and domain analysis. *MORN5* gene is located on chromosome 17 of the chicken genome and its length is 13.5 kb. The gene is composed of 6 exons where the last one is non-coding. The open reading frame codes for a protein 172 amino acids in length. The gene contains SSF82185 domain and three MORN motifs.

Embryo Manipulations

Embryos were treated with beads soaked in All-trans retinoic acid (RA), Noggin protein, Tris or Dimethyl Sulfoxide (DMSO) as described (Lee et al., 2001). Since DMSO was the solvent for RA, we used DMSO bead as a control for RA treatment and Tris as a control for Noggin treatment. AG1-X2 beads (Bio-Rad Laboratories, Hercules, Canada) of 100 μm in diameter were soaked in RA (cat. No. R2625 Sigma) at a concentration of 1 mg/ml for 1 h as previously described (Lee et al., 2001; Nimmagadda et al., 2015). Noggin proteins were soaked into Affigel blue beads (Bio-Rad Laboratories, Hercules, Canada) of 200 μm diameter for a minimum of 1 h at a concentration of 1 mg/ml (cat. No. 1967-NG, R&D Systems, Minneapolis, USA). Control beads were soaked with DMSO or Tris. Two beads were implanted into the maxillary region on the right side of chicken embryo at stage HH15. For ISH and QPCR, samples were collected 24 h post-bead implantation, embedded into paraffin and processed for ISH.

Immunofluorescence on Slides

Embryos were collected at stage HH24 for MORN5 protein detection. Chicken duodenum was used as a control according to the manufacturer's instruction. Samples were fixed in 4% PFA and processed into paraffin. Following deparaffinization and rehydration, antigen retrieval was carried out using citrate buffer for 1 min at 97°C. Polyclonal antibody to MORN5 (1:50, cat. No. NBP1-91230, Novus Biologicals, USA) was applied overnight at 4°C. The secondary anti-rabbit antibody (1:200, Alexa Fluor 594, cat. No. A-21207) was applied for 30 min at RT. Sections were washed in PBS and coverslipped with Prolong Gold anti-fade reagent containing DAPI (cat. No. P36935, Invitrogen, USA).

Quantitative RT-PCR

Gene expression of *MORN5* was analyzed on tissues isolated from normal chicken prominences at stage 15, 18, 20, and 26. Moreover, Noggin or RA treated maxillary prominences were dissected 24 h following bead implantation at stage 15. Prominences were pooled from at least 15 embryos to produce one sample and 4 biological replicates were analyzed. Total RNA was extracted using the Mini RNeasy Kit (Qiagen, Germany) according to the manufacturer's instructions. The total RNA concentration and purity of each sample were assessed by spectrophotometry using a NanoDrop1000 (Thermo Scientific, Waltham, USA). First-strand cDNA was synthesized using the SuperScript Vilo cDNA synthesis Kit (cat. No. 11754050, Thermo Fisher, USA). The qPCR was performed in 10 μl final reaction volumes containing the one-step master mix (no AmpErase UNG, cat. No. 4324018, Applied Biosystems, Carlsbad, USA) mixed with *MORN5* (TaqMan Assays, Assay ID: AJKAKYV, context sequence: TTCCTGAGAAATGCAGAC GATGAGG, FAM-MGB, Applied Biosystems, Austin, USA) on LightCycler® 96 (Roche, Manheim, Germany) with preheating at 95°C/10 min, followed by 40 cycles of 95°C/15 s and 60°C/1 min. Gene expression levels were calculated using ΔΔCT method with normalization against the *HPRT1* level (TaqMan Assays, Assay ID: Gg033338900_m1, context sequence: TTGAATCATATC

TGTGTGATCAGTG, FAM-MGB, Applied Biosystems, Austin, USA), which was used as the housekeeping gene. Means of 3 technical replicates were generated for each of 3 biological replicates and these values were used for statistical analysis. All procedures were repeated in at least three independent experiments.

Transfection with MORN5 Plasmids in Cell Cultures

The expression vector containing C-terminally FLAG-tagged human MORN5 was obtained from OriGene (Rockville, MD). HEK293T cells were obtained from ATCC (Manassas, VA) and propagated in DMEM media (Sigma-Aldrich, St. Louis, MO) with 10% fetal bovine serum, 1% Pen/Strep and 1% l-glutamin (Invitrogen, Carlsbad, CA). Cells were transfected using FUGENE6 reagent according to manufacturer's protocol (Promega).

HEK293T cells grown on glass coverslips were fixed with 4% PFA (RT/15 min), permeabilized with 0.1%Triton-X100 in PBS (RT/5 min), and incubated with the following antibodies at 4°C overnight: MORN5 (1:100, cat. No. NBP1-91230, Novus Biologicals), FLAG (1:200, cat. No. F1804, Sigma-Aldrich). The secondary antibody AlexaFluor 488 (1:500; cat. No. A21206, Life Technologies) or AlexaFluor 594 (1:500; cat. No. A21203, Life Technologies) were used. Coverslips were mounted into DAPI-containing Mowiol. Images were taken on an LSM700 laser scanning microscope with acquisition done using ZEN Black 2012 software (Zeiss, Jenna, Germany).

siRNA Targeting gMORN5 in Chicken Embryos

Silencer Select custom designed siRNA (gMORN5, cat. No. 4399666, Ambion, Austin, USA) was mixed with FUGENE 6 (Roche, Mannheim, Germany), and then was injected into the maxillary prominence of chicken embryos. Negative siRNA (Silencer select negative control No.1 siRNA, cat. No. 4390843, Ambion, Austin, USA) was used as a control. The first injection of siRNA was performed at stage HH20 and the second one after 24 h about stage HH24. One day later after the second injection, embryos had reached stage HH28 and maxillary prominences were dissected for RNA isolation. Tissues were dissected from 5 embryos to form one sample and three biological samples were used for treated embryos (MORN5 siRNA) as well as for control (Silencer select negative control No.1 siRNA) embryos.

PCR Arrays

Total RNA was extracted from siRNA treated maxillary prominences using the Mini RNeasy Kit (Qiagen, Germany) according to the manufacturer's instructions. First-strand cDNA was synthesized using the SuperScript Vilo cDNA synthesis Kit (cat. No. 11754050, Thermo Fisher, USA). Downregulation of *MORN5* expression after injection was first confirmed using qPCR before further processing for PCR Array analysis.

Custom made Chick-bone plates (KRD, Czech Republic) were used for analysis of BMP pathway genes. The PCR arrays were performed in 12 µl final reaction volumes containing SYBR Premix Ex Taq II (cat. No RR0821A, Takara, Japan) on LightCycler® 96 (Roche, Manheim, Germany) with preheating at 95°C/30 min, followed by 45 cycles of 95°C/5 s, 60°C/20 s and 72°C/15 s. Data were statistically evaluated by $\Delta\Delta$CT method with normalization against *HPRT1* levels. In each PCR array plate, there were three technical replicates for 24 genes, and 2 technical replicates for an additional 13 genes.

Statistical Analysis

All results were expressed as means ± standard deviations (SD) of three samples for each treatment and were compared by unpaired two-tailed Student's t-test for qPCR and PCR Array. Differences were considered to be significant at $p < 0.05$.

RESULTS

Spatiotemporal Gene Expression Pattern of *MORN5* in Facial Prominences

First, we analyzed spatiotemporal expression pattern of *MORN5* in individual prominences of chicken face. Facial prominences begin to form during early embryonic development. *In situ* hybridization showed no expression in chicken face at Hamburger-Hamilton (HH) stage 15 (50–55 h of incubation, **Figures 2A–C**) which is shortly after neural crest cells have entered the face. Later at stage HH17 (52-64 h of incubation, **Figures 2D–F**), *MORN5* expression appeared in the caudal part

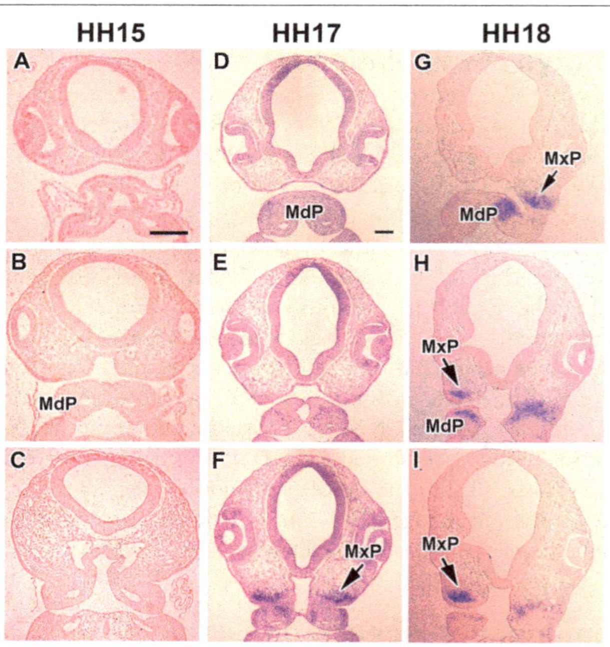

FIGURE 2 | Gene expression of *MORN5* in early chicken face. (A–C) Frontal sections of chicken face at stage HH15. **(D–F)** Frontal sections of chicken face at stage 17. **(D,E)** In the ventral part of maxillary and mandibular prominences, there was no expression. **(F)** *MORN5* expression gradually appeared dorsally in caudal part of maxillary region. **(G–I)** Frontal sections of chicken face at stage HH18. *MORN5* expression was strong in maxilla and also in central part of each mandibular prominence **(G)**. MdP, mandibular prominence; MxP, maxillary prominence. Scale bars = 100 µm.

of the presumptive maxillary mesenchyme close to the maxillo-mandibular cleft. At stage HH18, the bulge of the maxillary prominence contained high levels of *MORN5* transcripts (65–69 h of incubation, **Figures 2G–I**). Expression was also detected in the dorsal (oral side) part of the mandibular prominences close to the maxillo-mandibular cleft (**Figures 2G,H**). At stage HH20 (70–72 h of incubation), there continued to be restricted expression in caudal and medial domains within the maxillary prominences (**Figures 3A–C**). In the mandibular prominences, there was expression in the cranial mesenchyme on either side of the midline groove (**Figures 3A–O**) with the exceptions of mesenchymal condensations of Meckel's cartilage (**Figures 3B,C**). At stage HH24 (4 days of incubation), maxillary prominence enlarged and strong *MORN5* expression was present throughout the mesenchyme (**Figures 3E–G**). Mandibular expression was similar to stage HH20 (**Figures 2E–G**). Thus,

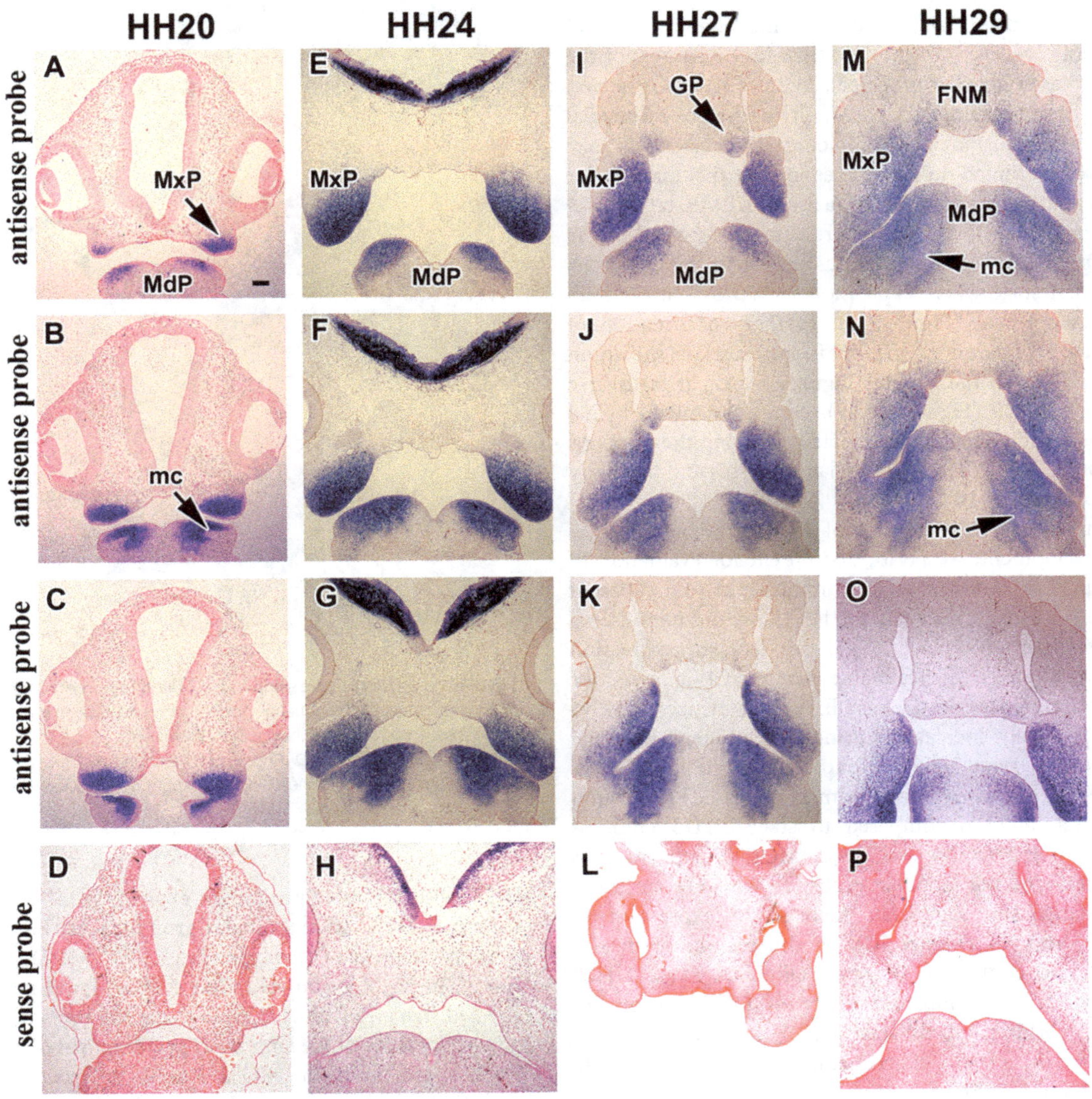

FIGURE 3 | Gene expression of *MORN5* in later stages of chicken embryo. (A–C) ISH analysis in frontal sections of chicken head at stage HH20. There was strong expression in the maxillary prominence. The expression appeared in the cranial part in each mandibular prominence and it continued in dorsal direction. **(B)** No expression was observed in mesenchymal condensations and close to the fusion region of mandibular prominences. **(E–G)** *MORN5* expression in frontal section of chicken head at stage HH24. *MORN5* expression was strong in the mesenchyme of maxillary prominences. *MORN5* expression was localized in the dorsal part of mandibular prominence, but not in mesenchymal condensation and close to the midline. **(I–K)** Frontal sections of chicken head at stage HH27 showed prominent expression in the maxillary prominence. There was weak expression in the globular process. Prominent expression was observed in rostral part of maxillary prominence and also in the mandibular prominence with the exception of midline. **(M–O)** Frontal sections of chicken head at stage 29 where beak is evident. *MORN5* expression was localized in rostral part of maxilla and in fusion region. In the mandibular prominence, there was strong expression but not in the midline. **(D,H,L,P)** ISH analysis using sense probe. FNM, frontonasal mass; GP, globular process; mc, mesenchymal condensation; MdP, mandibular prominence; MxP, maxillary prominence. Scale bars = 100 μm.

MORN5 is expressed in a restricted pattern in neural crest-derived mesenchyme but not in epithelium. Sense probe did not show signal in the maxillary prominence (**Figures 3D,H,L,P**).

MORN5 Expression in the Lip Fusion Zone at Later Stages

The next critical phase of facial morphogenesis is the fusion of the lip. Between stage HH27–29, the cranial-medial edges of the maxillary prominences meet the lateral corners of medial nasal prominences (globular processes) and fuse (Abramyan et al., 2015). At stage HH27 (5 days of incubation), *MORN5* expression was observed for the first time in the corners of the frontonasal mass (globular processes, **Figures 3I,J**). Expression in the maxillary prominences was high in the rostral-medial corner just where fusion with the globular processes will take place. There continued to be expression in the mandibular prominences similar to stage 24 (**Figures 3I–K**). At stage HH29 (6 days of incubation), *MORN5* expression was located in the region of lip fusion (**Figures 3M,N**) as well as in the mandible. This is the first stage where expression of *MORN5* in Meckel's cartilage was detected (**Figure 3M**). Further confirmation of the restricted expression in the lip fusion zone is shown in other embryos cut in the frontal (**Figures 4A–C**) or transverse plane at stage HH29 (**Figures 4A–F**). Note that mesenchymal bridging has taken place by stage HH29, unifying the domains of expression of *MORN5* in the globular processes and maxillary prominences (**Figures 4B,C**).

To quantify the relative levels of expression between the stages of development, we performed QPCR for evaluation of *MORN5* expression level in each prominence at four different stages (HH15, 18, 20, 26). Since stage HH15, we did not observe any expression of *MORN5* by ISH, this level of expression was chosen as the reference value for $\Delta\Delta$Ct analysis for individual prominences. In the maxillary prominence, *MORN5* expression gradually increased during development with the peak level seen at stage HH20 (**Figure 5A**). In the mandibular prominence, we observed significantly increased expression at stage HH20 and 26 compared to stage HH15 embryos (**Figure 5B**). In the frontonasal mass, *MORN5* expression is very low except of the globular processes we were surprised to see a statistically significant increase in expression of stage HH20 embryos (**Figure 5C**). In the section of *in situ* experiments, we could not detect *MORN5* at stage HH20 (data not shown) therefore sensitivity of QPCR is greater than *in situ* hybridization. By stage HH27, there is expression of *MORN5* in the *in situ* experiments; however, QPCR data did not pick up a significant expression level in stage HH26 embryos (**Figure 5C**). Some of the variability may be due to the dissection process and whether the globular process was included in all the samples. We did not compare expression levels between the facial prominences due to the experimental design.

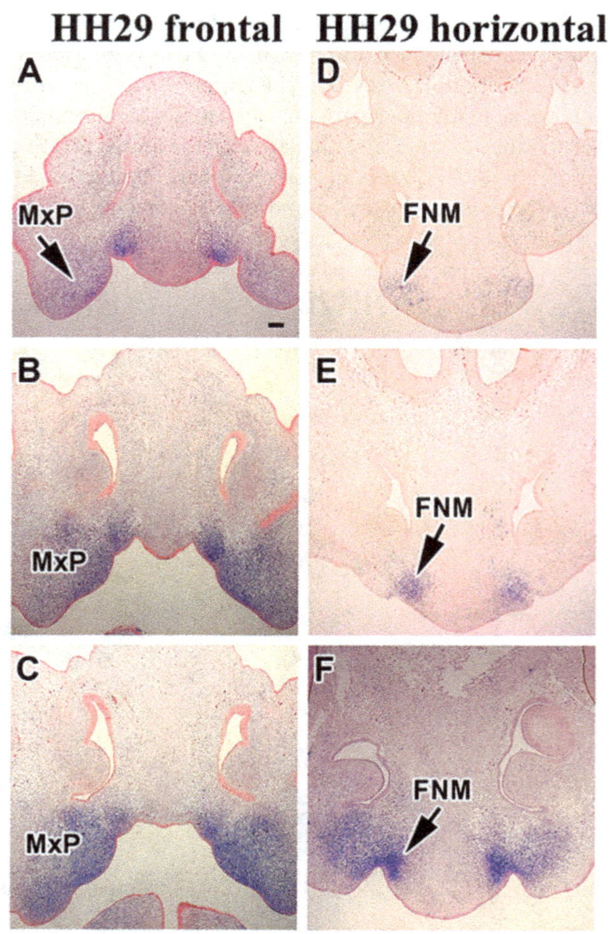

FIGURE 4 | *MORN5* expression in the fusion region at stage 29. (A–C) Frontal sections of chicken head showed strong expression in the maxilla and in the area where edges of the maxillary prominences grow together with medial nasal prominence. **(D–F)** Horizontal sections of chicken head. **(E)** Region of fusion had prominent *MORN5* expression. **(F)** More caudal section (other sample). Scale bars = 100 μm.

MORN5 Protein Expression in the Face

To correlate MORN5 protein distribution with *MORN5* gene expression, we performed immunofluorescence staining. MORN5 protein was localized in developing chicken face at stage HH24, with the most prominent expression in individual cells in the maxillary and mandibular prominences (**Figures 6A–H**). Thus, only a subset of cells expressing *MORN5* RNA expresses the protein. In positive control (adult chicken intestine), there was expected signal in Goblet cells, in the apical parts of enterocytes and in fibroblasts of the lamina propria (**Figures 6I–L**).

The specificity of the MORN5 antibody was also confirmed in HEK293T cells transfected with a MORN5-FLAG plasmid (**Figures 7A–C**). The staining of MORN5 and FLAG antibodies overlapped (**Figures 7A–C**). Similar to tissue section data, exogenous MORN5 protein was found in the cytoplasm in a punctate pattern (**Figures 7D,E**).

Downregulation of *MORN5* after Noggin a Retinoic Acid Treatment

Our study uncovered high levels of *MORN5* expression in normal chicken embryos, however a previous study from

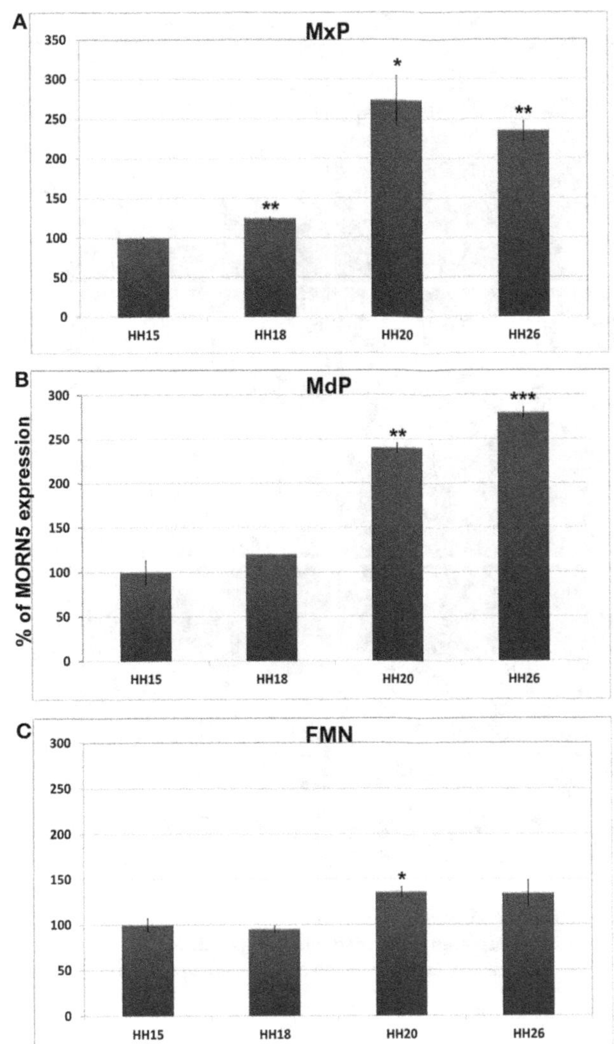

FIGURE 5 | QPCR analysis of *MORN5* expression during face development. (A) In the maxillary prominence, there was most prominent expression at stage HH20. All analyzed stages showed statistically significant overexpression in comparison to stage HH15. **(B)** In the mandibular prominence, we observed significant expression at stage HH20 and 26. **(C)** Very low *MORN5* expression was detected in the frontonasal mass at stage HH15 and 18, but at stage HH20 was *MORN5* expression significantly increased. FNM, frontonasal mass; MdP, mandibular prominence; MxP, maxillary prominence. *t*-test; $^{***}p < 0.001$, $^{**}0.001 < p < 0.01$, $^{*}p < 0.05$.

our group discovered that *MORN5* was downregulated in an experimental paradigm involving beads implanted into the chicken face (Nimmagadda et al., 2015). Beads soaked in the bone morphogenetic protein antagonist, Noggin and retinoic acid (RA) synergistically induced transformation of the maxillary prominence into the frontonasal mass (Lee et al., 2001). The tissues from embryos induced to form this duplicated beak were profiled using microarrays. A significant downregulation of *MORN5* expression was observed in all the treatment groups compared to controls treated with DMSO-Tris beads (-3.77-fold Noggin-DMSO treatment, -3.68-fold Noggin-RA, -2-fold after RA-Tris treatment) (Nimmagadda et al., 2015). We wanted to follow up this findings since it appeared that the RA and BMP pathways were upstream regulators of *MORN5* and that possibly *MORN5* was one of a set of genes mediating the beak duplication phenotype. First, we validated the array results using QPCR on maxillary tissues collected from treated and control embryos. We found a significant downregulation of *MORN5* after Nogin-RA and Noggin-DMSO treatment compared to Tris-DMSO controls (**Figure 8A**). Next, we asked whether there were any spatial differences in *MORN5* expression induced by the bead implants using *in situ* hybridization. Control embryos implanted with beads soaked in DMSO-Tris showed strong expression in the maxillary region and maxillo-mandibular cleft (**Figure 8B**). In contrast, no expression was observed in the maxillary prominence of Noggin-RA or Noggin-DMSO treated embryos. Interestingly, there was residual expression of *MORN5* observed in embryos treated with RA-Tris located just under the epithelium of maxilla-mandibular cleft (**Figure 8B**).

Downregulation of *MORN5* by siRNA Altered Gene Expression of BMP and TGFβ Pathways Members

We had discovered that BMP activity was required for *MORN5* expression but next wanted to investigate the genes that might be downstream of *MORN5*. As the first group of potential targets, we studied genes that are known to be in the BMP pathway. *MORN5* expression in the maxillary prominence was downregulated to 75% of control levels following transfection with siRNA (2 rounds of transfection: at stage 20 and 24; **Figure 9A**). We used a PCR array that included 34 genes specific for the BMP pathway with *HPRT1* acting as the reference control gene (Table S1).

Eight genes showed a statistically significant increase in their expression caused by partial *MORN5* silencing (**Figure 9B**). These included *ENG* (Endoglin), *Gdf2* (Growth differentiation factor 2, also BMP9), *PLAU* (plasminogen activator, urokinase), *FST* (Follistatin), *Runx1* (Runt-related transcription factor 1), *ID1* (Inhibitor of DNA binding 1), *TGFβR2* (Transforming growth factor beta receptor 2) and *TGFβ3* (**Figure 9B**). The most striking increase was seen with *GDF2* (increased 3.5-fold). Statistically significant downregulation was observed only in the case of *BMP5* (**Figure 9B**). It is interesting that *MORN5* normally represses *ID1*, a transcription factor that positively regulates BMP signaling. Although levels of *ID1* were increased, which should imply higher BMP signaling, there is also decreased expression of the *BMP5* ligand. It is likely that cytoplasmic *MORN5* indirectly regulates the expression of these genes and that further work is needed to determine the intermediate mediators of BMP and TGFβ signaling affected by *MORN5*.

DISCUSSION

Here, we found spatially and temporally restricted expression of *MORN5* in the face area during embryonic development suggesting its role in patterning of the maxillary prominences. Moreover, there was expression in the globular processes of frontonasal mass just before their fusion with the maxillary

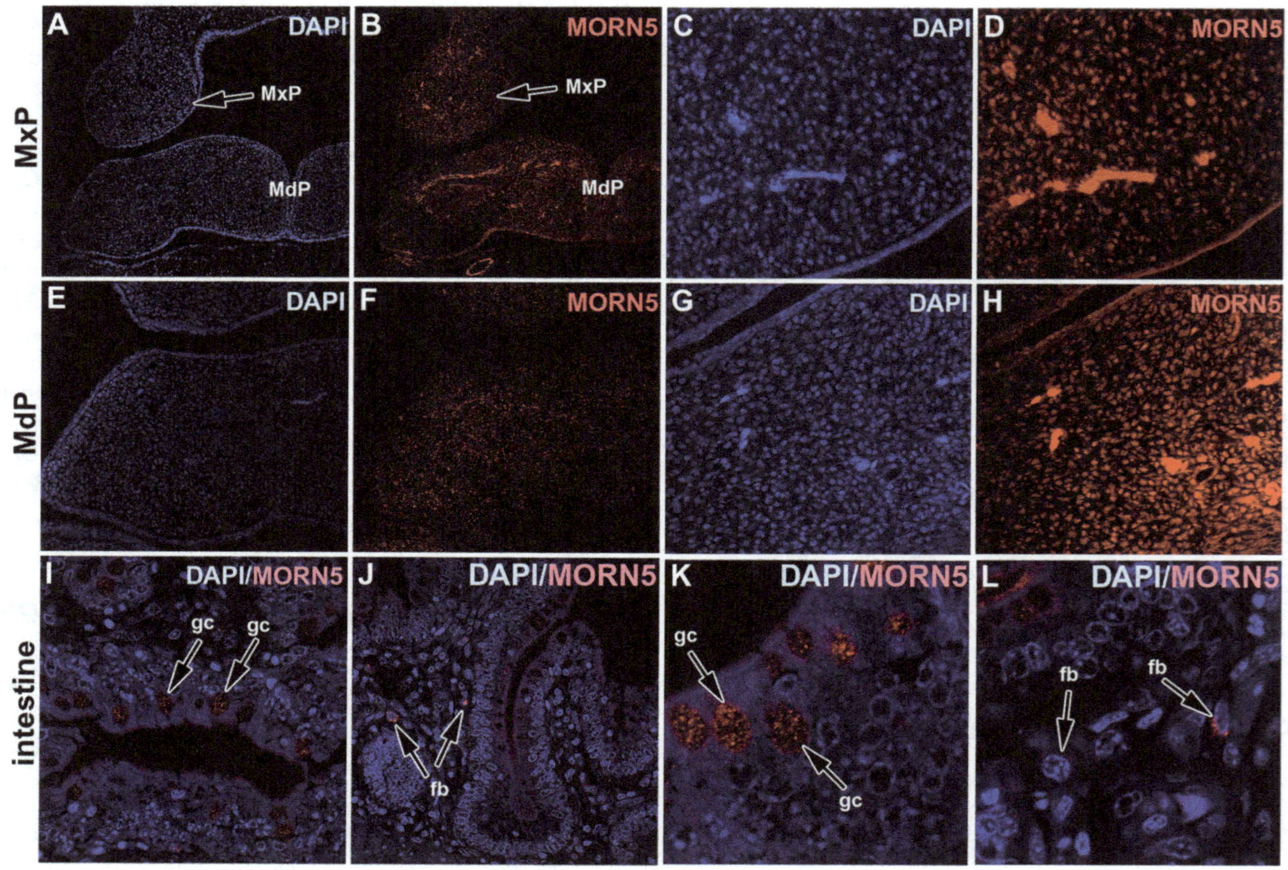

FIGURE 6 | MORN5 protein detected by immunofluorescent labeling. (B,D) MORN5 protein was localized in the maxillary prominences at stage HH24. **(F,H)** In the mandibular prominence, there is very low signal in the mesenchyme. MORN5 expression showed dispersed pattern of distribution. **(A,C,E,G)** DAPI staining. **(I–L)** Chicken intestine was used as a positive control with strong positivity in Goblet cells (gc), in the apical parts of enterocytes and also spotted expression in fibroblasts (fb). MdP, mandibular prominence; MxP, maxillary prominence.

prominences. Previously, a human genetics study found that *MORN5* was associated with non-syndromic cleft lip with or without cleft palate (NSCLP) (Letra et al., 2010). We are the first to document expression of *MORN5* in the relevant parts of the face undergoing lip fusion. In addition, there is strong expression on the medial sides of the maxillary prominences, the sites where palatal shelves will arise. While the chicken has a naturally cleft palate, it is interesting that *MORN5* is expressed in the intermediate stages of palatal shelf formation. Based on previous microarray studies carried out on the chicken face, *MORN5* came up twice, once as a maxillary enriched gene (Buchtová et al., 2010) and second as a differentially expressed gene following Noggin and RA bead implants (Nimmagadda et al., 2015). Taken together, the human genetic and chicken data suggest that *MORN5* is an important maxillary patterning and possibly lip fusion gene. Thus, it would be worthwhile targeting *MORN5* using mouse models and to include this gene in human NSLCP studies.

Complex signaling interactions coordinate the outgrowth of facial prominences to form the adult face. Some of factors have been previously identified by whole genome expression screens or by candidate gene mapping. The BMP signaling pathway regulates many cellular processes of craniofacial development and it is necessary for mesenchymal outgrowth of facial prominences. The expression of BMPs in chicken face was found at the time prior and during lip fusion (Ashique et al., 2002). *BMP4* transcripts were previously detected in the epithelium of the globular processes of frontonasal mass and *MORN5* expression underlays the same area however entirely in the mesenchyme. Also in the maxillary and mandibular prominences, epithelial *BMP4* expression was described in parallel areas to mesenchymal *MORN5*. Furthermore, *BMP2* and *BMP7* were previously detected in the mesenchyme of both facial prominences. Maxillary and mandibular prominences express also several downstream target of BMP signaling. *MSX1* is strongly expressed in the maxillary prominence but in slightly different pattern than *MORN5* in the mandible (Shigetani et al., 2000; Fuchs et al., 2010). There are additional transcription factors that appear to overlap with *MORN5* specifically in the frontonasal mass globular processes and maxillary prominences, *TBX22*, *DLX5*, and *MSX2* (Higashihori et al., 2010). These transcription factors may regulate expression

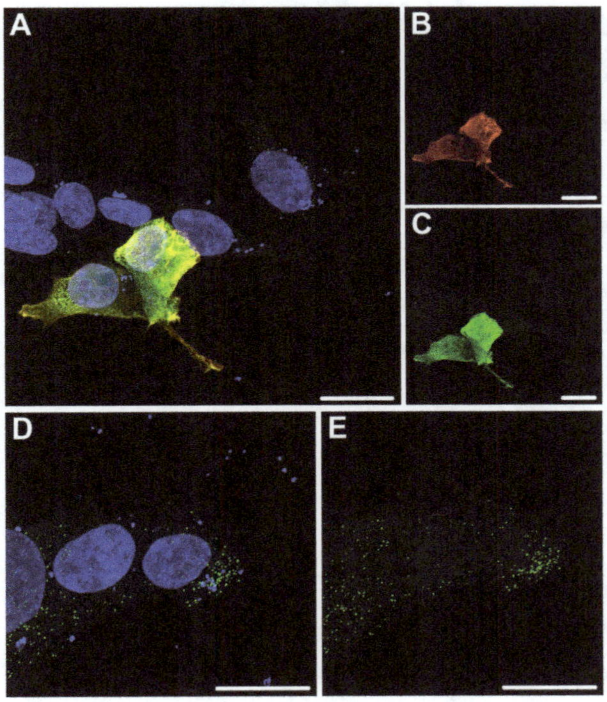

FIGURE 7 | Cytosolic spotted pattern of MORN5 expression in HEK293T cells. (A–C) HEK293T cells were transfected with FLAG-tagged MORN5-expressing vector and immunostained using both FLAG and MORN5 antibodies. Cells expressing transgenic MORN5 were also MORN5-positive pointing to the specificity of the antibody. **(D,E)** In addition, a cytosolic spotted pattern of MORN5 expression was present in non-transfected cells. Scale bars = 100 μm.

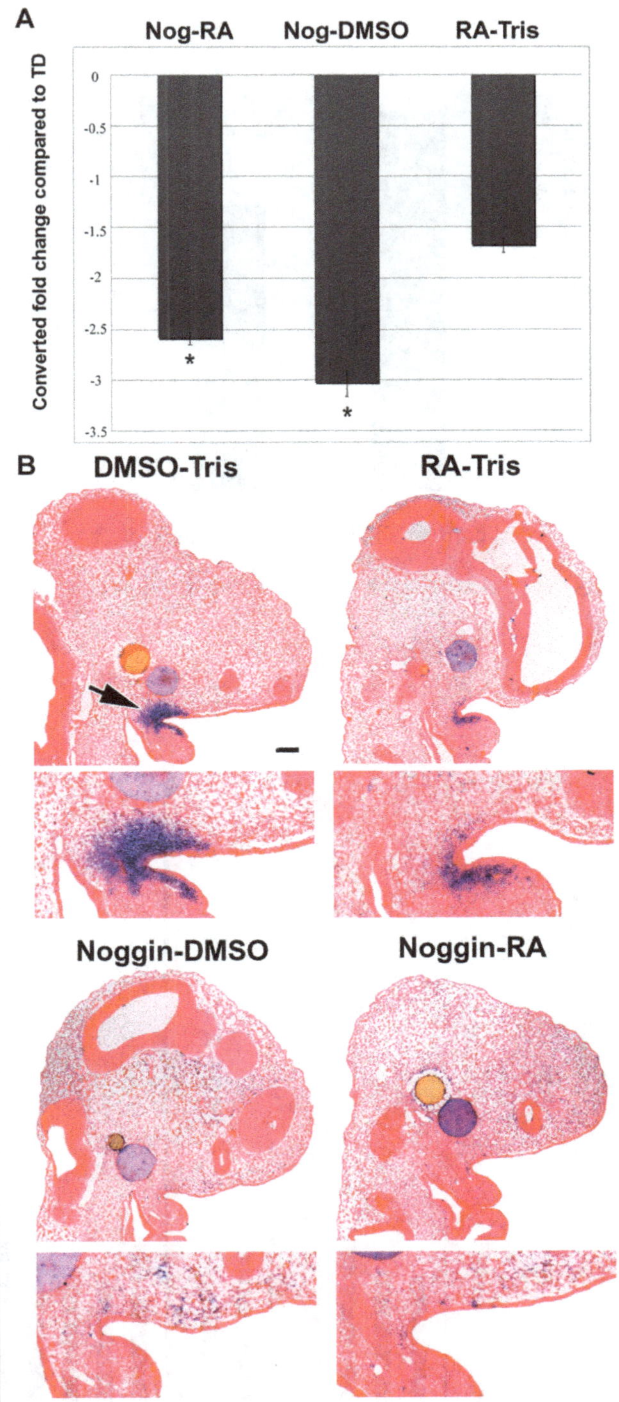

FIGURE 8 | QPCR analysis and ISH of *MORN5* expression after bead implantation. (A) QPCR analysis showed 1.68 times downregulation after RA-Tris, 3.03 after Noggin-DMSO and 2.59 after Noggin-RA treatment in comparison to control DMSO-Tris. **(B)** Control embryos implanted with beads soaked in DMSO-Tris had strong expression in maxillary region and maxilla-mandibular cleft. In RA-Tris treated embryos was very weak *MORN5* expression. After Noggin-DMSO treatment, expression was rapidly decreased. No expression of MORN5 was observed after Noggin-RA treatment. Nog, Noggin; RA, Retinoic acid; TD, Tris-DMSO. Scale bars = 100 μm. *t*-test; $^{*}p < 0.05$.

of *MORN5*. Interestingly, in the microarray study on beak duplicated embryos, *TBX22* was upregulated following Noggin-RA treatment and *TBX22* acts as a transcriptional repressor. It will be necessary to analyze whether *MORN5* is a target of *TBX22* which is a known clefting gene in humans (Kantaputra et al., 2011). It is interesting to note that the gene *LHX6* which is located 3′ to *MORN5* on the opposite strand was reported to be highly expressed in the chicken face (Washbourne and Cox, 2006). Expression of *LHX6* begins in the maxillo-mandibular cleft at stage 18 similar to *MORN5* (Washbourne and Cox, 2006). There is also striking similarity of expression of *LHX6* in the globular processes and medial maxillary prominences at stage 27. This suggests that the two genes may share some common enhancers that drive expression in particular regions of the face.

MORN5 knockdown revealed indirect roles for this gene in controlling the expression of BMP and TGFB signaling pathways. Since we have shown MORN5 is a cytoplasmic protein it is unlikely that it is directly involved in regulating gene transcription. Further biochemical studies are needed to determine the exact function of MORN5 in the cell. Nevertheless, the RNA changes we observed suggest a subset of genes are dependent on *MORN5* for their expression. We did not study the TGFB pathway in our bead implantation studies; therefore, the PCR array data extended our original findings on *MORN5*

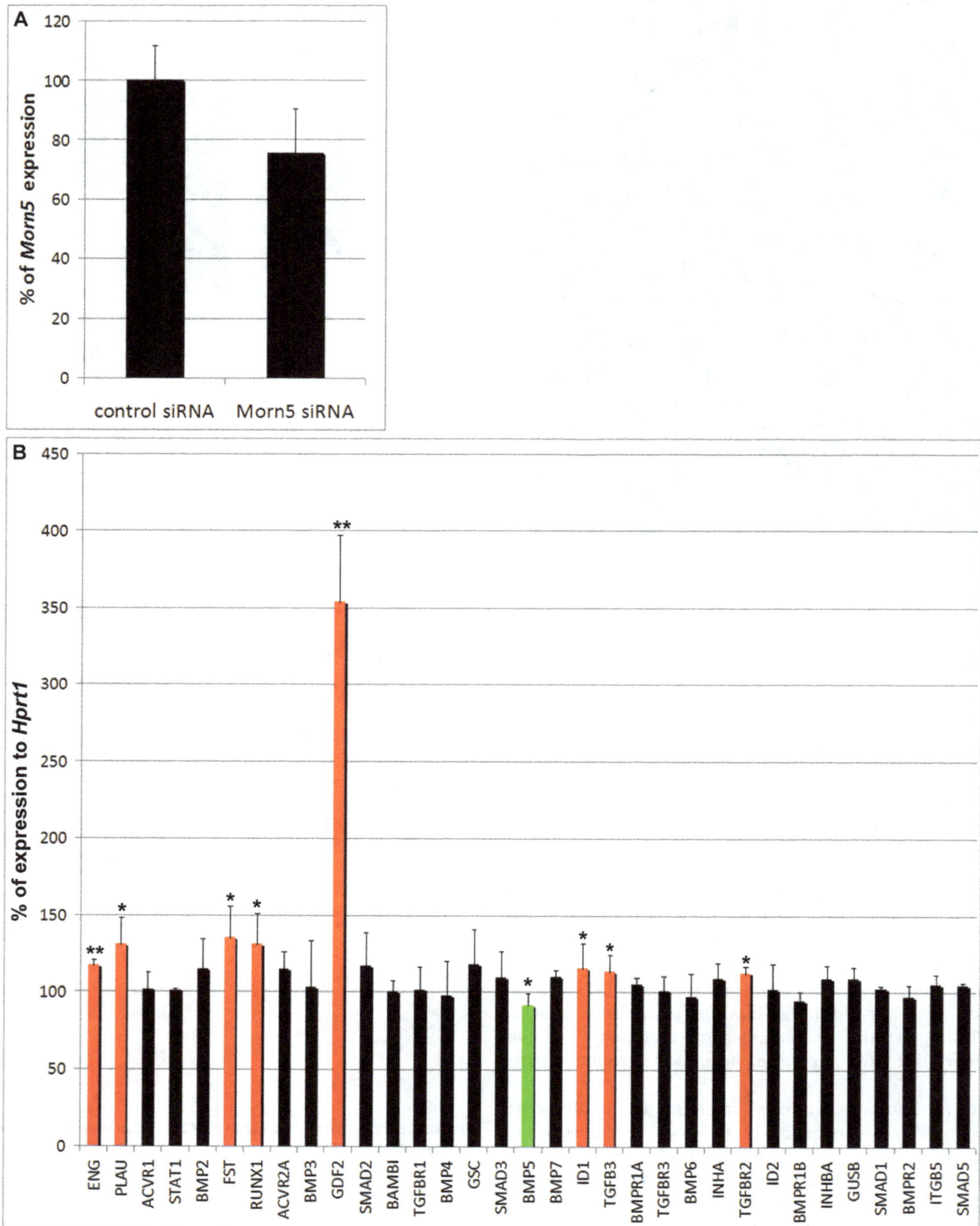

FIGURE 9 | BMP pathway gene expression after *MORN5* downregulation. (A) Downregulation of *MORN5* expression after siRNA treatment. **(B)** *MORN5* downregulation caused significant increase in *GDF2, ENG, TGFBR2, TGFB3, PLAU, FST, RUNX1,* and *ID1* expression. Statistically significant downregulation was observed only in case of *BMP5*. *t*-test; $^{**}0.001 < p < 0.01$, $^{*}p < 0.05$.

function. The most highly upregulated gene, *GDF2,* is known to associate with Endoglin (Castonguay et al., 2011) a glycoprotein located on cell surfaces that serves as a co-receptor for members of the Transforming growth factor-β superfamily (Cheifetz et al., 1992). This suggests that activity of TGFβ family is normally repressed by MORN5. Other changes such as the increase in the antagonist *FST (Follistatin)* may indicate that MORN5 operates in another way to regulate TGF signaling. MORN5 may normally repress this antagonist, which binds members of the TGFβ superfamily with a particular focus on activin (Lambert-Messerlian et al., 2007). We have shown that *FST* does not induce skeletal changes in the palate as compared to Noggin (Celá et al., 2016) therefore *FST* regulation by *MORN5* may serve different functions outside of facial morphogenesis. Several other genes known to be in the TGFB pathway and essential for mouse palate development were upregulated including *RUNX1* (Yamashiro et al., 2002), TGFβ3 (Cui et al., 1998) and *ID1* (Rice et al., 2005). In summary, we discovered that *MORN5* is involved in TGFB signaling at all levels. In conclusion, BMP signaling is required for *MORN5* expression and reduction of *MORN5* derepresses several genes in the BMP and TGFβ signaling pathways. Furthermore, *MORN5* has two potential roles in facial patterning, to specify maxillary identity and to regulate lip fusion that warrant further study in animal models.

AUTHOR CONTRIBUTIONS

MB, JR, and PC conceived the study. PC, MH, KF, MK conducted the experiments. PK provided intellectual contribution. PC, JR, and MB wrote the manuscript. All authors reviewed and approved the final manuscript.

ACKNOWLEDGMENTS

This study was supported by the Grant Agency of the Czech Republic (14-37368G to MB lab), Agency for Healthcare Research of the Czech Republic (15-33232A to PK lab) and institutional support (RVO:67985904).

REFERENCES

Abnave, P., Mottola, G., Gimenez, G., Boucherit, N., Trouplin, V., Torre, C., et al. (2014). Screening in planarians identifies MORN2 as a key component in LC3-associated phagocytosis and resistance to bacterial infection. *Cell Host Microbe.* 16, 338–350. doi: 10.1016/j.chom.2014.08.002

Abramyan, J., Thivichon-Prince, B., and Richman, J. M. (2015). Diversity in primary palate ontogeny of amniotes revealed with 3D imaging. *J. Anat.* 226, 420–433. doi: 10.1111/joa.12291

Ashique, A. M., Fu, K., and Richman, J. M. (2002). Endogenous bone morphogenetic proteins regulate outgrowth and epithelial survival during avian lip fusion. *Development* 129, 4647–4660.

Bhattacharya, M. R., Gerdts, J., Naylor, S. A., Royse, E. X., Ebstein, S. Y., Sasaki, Y., et al. (2012). A model of toxic neuropathy in Drosophila reveals a role for MORN4 in promoting axonal degeneration. *J. Neurosci.* 32, 5054–5061. doi: 10.1523/JNEUROSCI.4951-11.2012

Brunskill, E. W., Potter, A. S., Distasio, A., Dexheimer, P., Plassard, A., Aronow, B. J., et al. (2014). A gene expression atlas of early craniofacial development. *Dev. Biol.* 391, 133–146. doi: 10.1016/j.ydbio.2014.04.016

Buchtová, M., Kuo, W. P., Nimmagadda, S., Benson, S. L., Geetha-Loganathan, P., Logan, C., et al. (2010). Whole genome microarray analysis of chicken embryo facial prominences. *Dev. Dyn.* 239, 574–591. doi: 10.1002/dvdy.22135

Castonguay, R., Werner, E. D., Matthews, R. G., Presman, E., Mulivor, A. W., Solban, N., et al. (2011). Soluble endoglin specifically binds bone morphogenetic proteins 9 and 10 via its orphan domain, inhibits blood vessel formation, and suppresses tumor growth. *J. Biol. Chem.* 286, 30034–30046. doi: 10.1074/jbc.M111.260133

Celá, P., Buchtová, M., Veselá, I., Fu, K., Bogardi, J. P., Song, Y., et al. (2016). BMP signaling regulates the fate of chondro-osteoprogenitor cells in facial mesenchyme in a stage-specific manner. *Dev. Dyn.* 245, 947–962. doi: 10.1002/dvdy.24422

Chai, Y., and Maxson, R. E. Jr. (2006). Recent advances in craniofacial morphogenesis. *Dev. Dyn.* 235, 2353–2375. doi: 10.1002/dvdy.20833

Cheifetz, S., Bellón, T., Calés, C., Vera, S., Bernabeu, C., Massagué, J., et al. (1992). Endoglin is a component of the transforming growth factor-beta receptor system in human endothelial cells. *J. Biol. Chem.* 267, 19027–19030.

Cui, X. M., Warburton, D., Zhao, J., Crowe, D. L., and Shuler, C. F. (1998). Immunohistochemical localization of TGF-beta type II receptor and TGF-beta3 during palatogenesis *in vivo* and *in vitro*. *Int. J. Dev. Biol.* 42, 817–820.

Dixon, M. J., Marazita, M. L., Beaty, T. H., and Murray, J. C. (2011). Cleft lip and palate: understanding genetic and environmental influences. *Nat. Rev.* 12, 167–178. doi: 10.1038/nrg2933

Ferguson, D. J., Sahoo, N., Pinches, R. A., Bumstead, J. M., Tomley, F. M., and Gubbels, M. J. (2008). MORN1 has a conserved role in asexual and sexual development across the apicomplexa. *Eukaryot. Cell* 7, 698–711. doi: 10.1128/EC.00021-08

Fuchs, A., Inthal, A., Herrmann, D., Cheng, S., Nakatomi, M., Peters, H., et al. (2010). Regulation of Tbx22 during facial and palatal development. *Dev. Dyn.* 239, 2860–2874. doi: 10.1002/dvdy.22421

Geetha-Loganathan, P., Nimmagadda, S., Fu, K., and Richman, J. M. (2014). Avian facial morphogenesis is regulated by c-Jun N-terminal kinase/planar cell polarity (JNK/PCP) wingless-related (WNT) signaling. *J. Biol. Chem.* 289, 24153–24167. doi: 10.1074/jbc.M113.522003

Hamburger, V., and Hamilton, H. L. (1951). A series of normal stages in the development of the chick embryo. *J. Morphol.* 88, 49–92.

Higashihori, N., Buchtová, M., and Richman, J. M. (2010). The function and regulation of TBX22 in avian frontonasal morphogenesis. *Dev. Dyn.* 239, 458–473. doi: 10.1002/dvdy.22182

Holland, L. Z., Holland, P. W. H., Holland, N. D. (1996). "Revealing homologies between body parts of distantly related animals by in situ hybridization to developmental genes: amphioxus vs. vertebrates," in *Molecular Zoology: Advances, Strategies, and Protocols*, eds J. D. P. Ferraris (New York, NY: Wiley), 267–282.

Hu, D., Young, N. M., Li, X., Xu, Y., Hallgrímsson, B., and Marcucio, R. S. (2015). A dynamic Shh expression pattern, regulated by SHH and BMP signaling, coordinates fusion of primordia in the amniote face. *Development* 142, 567–574. doi: 10.1242/dev.114835

Jiang, R., Bush, J. O., and Lidral, A. C. (2006). Development of the upper lip: morphogenetic and molecular mechanisms. *Dev. Dyn.* 235, 1152–1166. doi: 10.1002/dvdy.20646

Kantaputra, P. N., Paramee, M., Kaewkhampa, A., Hoshino, A., Lees, M., McEntagart, M., et al. (2011). Cleft lip with cleft palate, ankyloglossia, and hypodontia are associated with TBX22 mutations. *J. Dent. Res.* 90, 450–455. doi: 10.1177/0022034510391052

Kurosaka, H. (2015). The roles of hedgehog signaling in upper lip formation. *Biomed Res. Int.* 2015:901041. doi: 10.1155/2015/901041

Lambert-Messerlian, G., Eklund, E., Pinar, H., Tantravahi, U., and Schneyer, A. L. (2007). Activin subunit and receptor expression in normal and cleft human fetal palate tissues. *Pediatr. Dev. Pathol.* 10, 436–445. doi: 10.2350/06-05-0087.1

Lee, S. H., Fu, K. K., Hui, J. N., and Richman, J. M. (2001). Noggin and retinoic acid transform the identity of avian facial prominences. *Nature* 414, 909–912. doi: 10.1038/414909a

Leslie, E. J., and Marazita, M. L. (2013). Genetics of cleft lip and cleft palate. *Am. J. Med. Genet.* 163C, 246–258. doi: 10.1002/ajmg.c.31381

Letra, A., Menezes, R., Govil, M., Fonseca, R. F., McHenry, T., Granjeiro, J. M., et al. (2010). Follow-up association studies of chromosome region 9q and nonsyndromic cleft lip/palate. *Am. J. Med. Genet.* 152A, 1701–1710. doi: 10.1002/ajmg.a.33482

Lorestani, A., Sheiner, L., Yang, K., Robertson, S. D., Sahoo, N., Brooks, C. F., et al. (2010). A Toxoplasma MORN1 null mutant undergoes repeated divisions but is defective in basal assembly, apicoplast division and cytokinesis. *PLoS ONE* 5:e12302. doi: 10.1371/journal.pone.0012302

Marcucio, R., Hallgrimsson, B., and Young, N. M. (2015). Facial morphogenesis: physical and molecular interactions between the brain and the face. *Curr. Top. Dev. Biol.* 115, 299–320. doi: 10.1016/bs.ctdb.2015.09.001

Murray, J. C., and Schutte, B. C. (2004). Cleft palate: players, pathways, and pursuits. *J. Clin. Invest.* 113, 1676–1678. doi: 10.1172/JCI200422154

Nimmagadda, S., Buchtová, M., Fu, K., Geetha-Loganathan, P., Hosseini-Farahabadi, S., Trachtenberg, A. J., et al. (2015). Identification and functional analysis of novel facial patterning genes in the duplicated beak chicken embryo. *Dev. Biol.* 407, 275–288. doi: 10.1016/j.ydbio.2015.09.007

Rice, R., Thesleff, I., and Rice, D. P. (2005). Regulation of twist, snail, and Id1 is conserved between the developing murine palate and tooth. *Dev. Dyn.* 234, 28–35. doi: 10.1002/dvdy.20501

Richman, J. M., and Lee, S. H. (2003). About face: signals and genes controlling jaw patterning and identity in vertebrates. *Bioessays* 25, 554–568. doi: 10.1002/bies.10288

Schutte, B. C., and Murray, J. C. (1999). The many faces and factors of orofacial clefts. *Hum. Mol. Genet.* 8, 1853–1859. doi: 10.1093/hmg/8.10.1853

Setó-Salvia, N., and Stanier, P. (2014). Genetics of cleft lip and/or cleft palate: association with other common anomalies. *Eur. J. Med. Genet.* 57, 381–393. doi: 10.1016/j.ejmg.2014.04.003

Shigetani, Y., Nobusada, Y., and Kuratani, S. (2000). Ectodermally derived FGF8 defines the maxillomandibular region in the early chick embryo: epithelial-mesenchymal interactions in the specification of the craniofacial ectomesenchyme. *Dev. Biol.* 228, 73–85. doi: 10.1006/dbio.2000.9932

Szabo-Rogers, H. L., Geetha-Loganathan, P., Nimmagadda, S., Fu, K. K., and Richman, J. M. (2008). FGF signals from the nasal pit are necessary for normal facial morphogenesis. *Dev. Biol.* 318, 289–302. doi: 10.1016/j.ydbio.2008.03.027

Washbourne, B. J., and Cox, T. C. (2006). Expression profiles of cIRF6, cLHX6 and cLHX7 in the facial primordia suggest specific roles during primary palatogenesis. *BMC Dev. Biol.* 6:18. doi: 10.1186/1471-213X-6-18

Watkins, S. E., Meyer, R. E., Strauss, R. P., and Aylsworth, A. S. (2014). Classification, epidemiology, and genetics of orofacial clefts. *Clin. Plast. Surg.* 41, 149–163. doi: 10.1016/j.cps.2013.12.003

Yamashiro, T., Aberg, T., Levanon, D., Groner, Y., and Thesleff, I. (2002). Expression of Runx1, -2 and -3 during tooth, palate and craniofacial bone development. *Gene Expr. Patterns* 2, 109–112. doi: 10.1016/S0925-4773(02)00298-8

Zhang, L., Shang, X. J., Li, H. F., Shi, Y. Q., Li, W., Teves, M. E., et al. (2015). Characterization of membrane occupation and recognition nexus repeat containing 3, meiosis expressed gene 1 binding partner, in mouse male germ cells. *Asian J. Androl.* 17, 86–93. doi: 10.4103/1008-682X.138186

Permissions

All chapters in this book were first published by Frontiers; hereby published with permission under the Creative Commons Attribution License or equivalent. Every chapter published in this book has been scrutinized by our experts. Their significance has been extensively debated. The topics covered herein carry significant findings which will fuel the growth of the discipline. They may even be implemented as practical applications or may be referred to as a beginning point for another development.

The contributors of this book come from diverse backgrounds, making this book a truly international effort. This book will bring forth new frontiers with its revolutionizing research information and detailed analysis of the nascent developments around the world.

We would like to thank all the contributing authors for lending their expertise to make the book truly unique. They have played a crucial role in the development of this book. Without their invaluable contributions this book wouldn't have been possible. They have made vital efforts to compile up to date information on the varied aspects of this subject to make this book a valuable addition to the collection of many professionals and students.

This book was conceptualized with the vision of imparting up-to-date information and advanced data in this field. To ensure the same, a matchless editorial board was set up. Every individual on the board went through rigorous rounds of assessment to prove their worth. After which they invested a large part of their time researching and compiling the most relevant data for our readers.

The editorial board has been involved in producing this book since its inception. They have spent rigorous hours researching and exploring the diverse topics which have resulted in the successful publishing of this book. They have passed on their knowledge of decades through this book. To expedite this challenging task, the publisher supported the team at every step. A small team of assistant editors was also appointed to further simplify the editing procedure and attain best results for the readers.

Apart from the editorial board, the designing team has also invested a significant amount of their time in understanding the subject and creating the most relevant covers. They scrutinized every image to scout for the most suitable representation of the subject and create an appropriate cover for the book.

The publishing team has been an ardent support to the editorial, designing and production team. Their endless efforts to recruit the best for this project, has resulted in the accomplishment of this book. They are a veteran in the field of academics and their pool of knowledge is as vast as their experience in printing. Their expertise and guidance has proved useful at every step. Their uncompromising quality standards have made this book an exceptional effort. Their encouragement from time to time has been an inspiration for everyone.

The publisher and the editorial board hope that this book will prove to be a valuable piece of knowledge for researchers, students, practitioners and scholars across the globe.

List of Contributors

Virginie Laugel-Haushalter, Brigitte Schuhbaur and Pascal Dollé
Developmental Biology and Stem Cells Department, Institute of Genetics and Molecular and Cellular Biology (IGBMC), Illkirch, France
Centre National de la Recherche Scientifique, UMR 7104, Illkirch, France
Institut National de la Santé et de la Recherche Médicale, U 964, Illkirch, France
Université de Strasbourg, Illkirch, France

Supawich Morkmued
Developmental Biology and Stem Cells Department, Institute of Genetics and Molecular and Cellular Biology (IGBMC), Illkirch, France
Centre National de la Recherche Scientifique, UMR 7104, Illkirch, France
Institut National de la Santé et de la Recherche Médicale, U 964, Illkirch, France
Université de Strasbourg, Illkirch, France
Pediatrics Department, Faculty of Dentistry, Khon Kaen University, Khon Kaen, Thailand

Eric Mathieu and Joseph Hemmerlé
Université de Strasbourg, INSERM UMR_1121, Biomaterials and Bioengineering, Strasbourg, France

Karen Niederreither
Developmental Biology and Stem Cells Department, Institute of Genetics and Molecular and Cellular Biology (IGBMC), Illkirch, France
Centre National de la Recherche Scientifique, UMR 7104, Illkirch, France
Institut National de la Santé et de la Recherche Médicale, U 964, Illkirch, France
Université de Strasbourg, Illkirch, France
Faculté de Chirurgie Dentaire, Université de Strasbourg, Strasbourg, France

Agnès Bloch-Zupan
Developmental Biology and Stem Cells Department, Institute of Genetics and Molecular and Cellular Biology (IGBMC), Illkirch, France
Centre National de la Recherche Scientifique, UMR 7104, Illkirch, France
Institut National de la Santé et de la Recherche Médicale, U 964, Illkirch, France
Université de Strasbourg, Illkirch, France
Faculté de Chirurgie Dentaire, Université de Strasbourg, Strasbourg, France
Faculté de Médecine, Fédération de Médecine Translationnelle de Strasbourg, Université de Strasbourg, Strasbourg, France
Hôpitaux Universitaires de Strasbourg, Pôle de Médecine et Chirurgie Bucco-Dentaires, Centre de Référence des Manifestations Odontologiques des Maladies Rares, CRMR, Strasbourg, France
Eastman Dental Institute, University College London, London, UK

Matthias C. Schulz, Uwe Eckelt and Ronald Mai
Department of Oral and Maxillofacial Surgery, Medical Faculty "Carl Gustav Carus," Technische Universität Dresden, Dresden, Germany

Jan Kowald
Department of Radiology, Medical Faculty "Carl Gustav Carus," Technische Universität Dresden, Dresden, Germany
Division of Nephrology, Department of Internal Medicine III, Medical Faculty "Carl Gustav Carus," Technische Universität Dresden, Dresden, Germany

Sven Estenfelder
Department of Radiology, Medical Faculty "Carl Gustav Carus," Technische Universität Dresden, Dresden, Germany
Department of Internal Medicine III, University of Ulm, Ulm, Germany

Roland Jung
Experimental Center, Medical Faculty "Carl Gustav Carus," Technische Universität Dresden, Dresden, Germany

Eberhard Kuhlisch
Institute for Medical Informatics and Biometry, Medical Faculty "Carl Gustav Carus," Technische Universität Dresden, Dresden, Germany

Lorenz C. Hofbauer
Division of Endocrinology, Diabetes and Bone Diseases, Department of Medicine III, Medical Faculty "Carl Gustav Carus," Technische Universität Dresden, Dresden, Germany

Christian Stroszczynski
Department of Radiology, University Hospital Regensburg, Regensburg, Germany

Bernd Stadlinger
Clinic of Cranio-Maxillofacial and Oral Surgery, University of Zurich, University Hospital Zurich, Zurich, Switzerland

Paul P. R. Iyyanar and Adil J. Nazarali
Laboratory of Molecular Cell Biology, College of Pharmacy and Nutrition and Neuroscience Research Cluster, University of Saskatchewan, Saskatoon, SK, Canada

Thimios A. Mitsiadis, Pierfrancesco Pagella and Lucia Jimenez-Rojo
Orofacial Development and Regeneration, Institute of Oral Biology, Centre for Dental Medicine, Medical Faculty, University of Zurich, Zurich, Switzerland

Javier Catón
Department of Medical Basic Sciences, Faculty of Medicine, University CEU-San Pablo, Madrid, Spain

Giovanna Orsini
Department of Clinical Sciences and Stomatology, Polytechnic University of Marche, Ancona, Italy

Praneet Chaturvedi
Division of Developmental Biology, Department of Pediatrics, Cincinnati Children's Hospital Medical Center, Cincinnati, OH, USA

Ya-Ting Chang, Elizabeth N. Schock and Samantha A. Brugmann
Division of Plastic Surgery, Department of Surgery, Cincinnati Children's Hospital Medical Center, Cincinnati, OH, USA
Division of Developmental Biology, Department of Pediatrics, Cincinnati Children's Hospital Medical Center, Cincinnati, OH, USA

Isabelle Miletich
Department of Craniofacial Development and Stem Cell Biology, King's College London Dental Institute, Guy's Hospital, London, UK

Guilherme M. Xavier and Martyn T. Cobourne
Department of Craniofacial Development and Stem Cell Biology, King's College London Dental Institute, Guy's Hospital, London, UK
Department of Orthodontics, King's College London Dental Institute, Guy's Hospital, London, UK

Shuji Oishi, Yasuhiro Shimizu, Jun Hosomichi, Yoichiro Kuma, Risa Usumi-Fujita, Sawa Kaneko, Naoki Shibutani and Takashi Ono
Department of Orthodontic Science, Graduate School of Medical and Dental Sciences, Tokyo Medical and Dental University, Tokyo, Japan

Hideyuki Maeda and Ken-ichi Yoshida
Department of Forensic Medicine, Graduate School of Medicine, Tokyo Medical University, Tokyo, Japan

Hisashi Nagai
Department of Legal Medicine (Forensic Medicine), Keio University School of Medicine, Tokyo, Japan

Jun-ichi Suzuki
Department of Advanced Clinical Science and Therapeutics, The University of Tokyo, Tokyo, Japan

Hai-Lei Ding, Kristin B. Artinger and David E. Clouthier
Department of Craniofacial Biology, School of Dental Medicine, University of Colorado Anschutz Medical Campus, Aurora, CO, USA

Peter Batzel and John H. Postlethwait
Department of Neuroscience, University of Oregon, Eugene, OR, USA

B. Frank Eames
Department of Neuroscience, University of Oregon, Eugene, OR, USA
Department of Anatomy and Cell Biology, University of Saskatchewan, Saskatoon, SK, Canada

Joan E. Hooper
Department of Cell and Developmental Biology, School of Medicine, University of Colorado Anschutz Medical Campus, Aurora, CO, USA

Lotta K. Veistinen, Md. Rakibul Hasan and Maarit Takatalo
Orthodontics, Oral and Maxillofacial Diseases, University of Helsinki, Helsinki, Finland

Tuija Mustonen
Orthodontics, Oral and Maxillofacial Diseases, University of Helsinki, Helsinki, Finland Minerva Research Institute, Helsinki, Finland

Yukiho Kobayashi
Orthodontics, Oral and Maxillofacial Diseases, University of Helsinki, Helsinki, Finland
Orthodontics, Tokyo Medical and Dental University, Tokyo, Japan

Dörthe A. Kesper and Andrea Vortkamp
Center of Medical Biotechnology, University of Duisburg-Essen, Essen, Germany

David P. Rice
Orthodontics, Oral and Maxillofacial Diseases, University of Helsinki, Helsinki, Finland
Orthodontics, Oral and Maxillofacial Diseases, Helsinki University Hospital, Helsinki, Finland

Claudio Cantù
Institute of Molecular Life Sciences, University of Zurich, Zurich, Switzerland

Behrouz Zandieh-Doulabi, Antonius Bronckers and Rozita Jalali
Department of Oral Cell Biology, Academic Centre for Dentistry Amsterdam (ACTA), Amsterdam Movement Sciences, University of Amsterdam, VU University Amsterdam, Amsterdam, Netherlands

Johannes C. Lodder and Huibert D. Mansvelder
Department Integrative Neurophysiology, Center for Neurogenomics and Cognitive Research, VU University, Amsterdam, Netherlands

Dimitra Micha
Department of Clinical Genetics, VU University Medical Center, Amsterdam Movement Sciences, Netherlands

James E. Melvin
Secretory Mechanisms and Dysfunction Section, NIDCR/NIH, Bethesda, MD, United States

Marcelo A. Catalan
Secretory Mechanisms and Dysfunction Section, NIDCR/NIH, Bethesda, MD, United States
Departamento de Ciencias Químicas y Farmaceúticas, Facultad de Ciencias de la Salud, Universidad Arturo Prat, Iquique, Chile

Pamela DenBesten
Department of Orofacial Sciences, School of Dentistry, University of California, San Francisco, San Francisco, CA, United States

Jordânia M. de Oliveira Freire and Luzia H. T. de Sousa
RENORBIO, Federal University of Ceará, Fortaleza, Brazil

Iracema M. Melo, Igor I. Castro da Silva and Hellíada V. Chaves
Dentistry School, Federal University of Ceará, Sobral, Brazil

Alrieta H. Teixeira
RENORBIO, Federal University of Ceará, Fortaleza, Brazil
Dentistry School, Federal University of Ceará, Sobral, Brazil

Antônia T. Parente, Nayara A. de Sousa, Gerardo Cristino-Filho and Vicente de Paulo T. Pinto
Medical School, Federal University of Ceará, Sobral, Brazil

Mirna M. Bezerra
RENORBIO, Federal University of Ceará, Fortaleza, Brazil
Medical School, Federal University of Ceará, Sobral, Brazil

Angela M. C. Arriaga and Francisca R. Lopes da Silva
Department of Organic and Inorganic Chemistry, Federal University of Ceará, Fortaleza, Brazil

Karuza M. A. Pereira
Department of Morphology, Medical School, Federal University of Ceará, Fortaleza, Brazil

Paula Goes
Department of Pathology and Legal Medicine, Medical School, Federal University of Ceará, Fortaleza, Brazil

José J. do Nascimento Costa
UNINTA University Center, Sobral, Brazil

Tathyane H. N. Teshima and Silvia V. Lourenco
Department of Stomatology, School of Dentistry, University of Sao Paulo, São Paulo, Brazil

Abigail S. Tucker
Department of Craniofacial Development and Stem Cell Biology, King's College London, London, UK

Marie Landová
Laboratory of Molecular Morphogenesis, Institute of Animal Physiology and Genetics, Academy of Sciences, Brno, Czechia

Iveta Putnová and Hana Dosedělová
Laboratory of Molecular Morphogenesis, Institute of Animal Physiology and Genetics, Academy of Sciences, Brno, Czechia
Department of Anatomy, Histology and Embryology, University of Veterinary and Pharmaceutical Sciences, Brno, Czechia

Vitezslav Bryja
Department of Animal Physiology and Immunology, Institute of Experimental Biology, Masaryk University, Brno, Czechia

Marcela Buchtová
Laboratory of Molecular Morphogenesis, Institute of Animal Physiology and Genetics, Academy of Sciences, Brno, Czechia
Department of Animal Physiology and Immunology, Institute of Experimental Biology, Masaryk University, Brno, Czechia

Jan Štembírek
Laboratory of Molecular Morphogenesis, Institute of Animal Physiology and Genetics, Academy of Sciences, Brno, Czechia
Department of Maxillofacial Surgery, University Hospital Ostrava, Ostrava, Czechia

Michael H. Le and Dawud Abduweli
Department of Orofacial Sciences, University of California, San Francisco, San Francisco, CA, USA

Pamela K. Den Besten, Yan Zhang and Yukiko Nakano
Department of Orofacial Sciences, University of California, San Francisco, San Francisco, CA, USA
Center for Children's Oral Health Research, University of California, San Francisco, San Francisco, CA, USA

Sunita P. Ho
Preventive and Restorative Dental Sciences, University of California, San Francisco, San Francisco, CA, USA

Lillia V. Ryazanova, Zhixian Hu and Alexey G. Ryazanov
Department of Pharmacology, Robert Wood Johnson Medical School, Piscataway, NJ, USA

Matthias Chiquet, Susan Blumer, Manuela Angelini and Christos Katsaros
Department of Orthodontics and Dentofacial Orthopedics, Medical Faculty, School of Dental Medicine, University of Bern, Bern, Switzerland

Daniel H. Doro, Agamemnon E. Grigoriadis and Karen J. Liu
Centre for Craniofacial and Regenerative Biology, King's College London, Guy's Hospital, London, United Kingdom

Julia Meyer
Faculté de Chirurgie Dentaire, Université de Strasbourg, Strasbourg, France

Rabisoa W. Razafindrakoto, Saholy N. Ralison, Jean-Claude Randrianaivo, Georgette Ralison, Rija O. Andriamasinoro, Rija H. Ramanampamaharana, Solofomanantsoa E. Randrianazary, Louise H. Ralimanana, Jeanne A. Rasoamananjara and Simone Rakoto Alson
Institut d'Odonto-Stomatologie Tropicale de Madagascar, Université de Mahajanga, Mahajanga, Madagascar

Marie-Cécile Manière
Faculté de Chirurgie Dentaire, Université de Strasbourg, Strasbourg, France
Centre de Référence des Manifestations Odontologiques des Maladies Rares, Hôpitaux Universitaires de Strasbourg, Pôle de Médecine et Chirurgie Buccodentaires Hôpital Civil, Strasbourg, France

Mathilde Huckert
Faculté de Chirurgie Dentaire, Université de Strasbourg, Strasbourg, France
Laboratoire de Génétique Médicale, Faculté de Médecine, Institut National de la Santé et de la Recherche Médicale U 1112, Université de Strasbourg, Strasbourg, France

Corinne Stoetzel, Véronique Geoffroy and Hélène Dollfus
Laboratoire de Génétique Médicale, Faculté de Médecine, Institut National de la Santé et de la Recherche Médicale U 1112, Université de Strasbourg, Strasbourg, France

Béatrice Richard
UFR Odontologie de Lyon, Université Claude Bernard, Lyon, France

Philippe Gorry
Research Unit of Theoretical & Applied Economics, GREThA (UMR Centre National de la Recherche Scientifique 5113), Université de Bordeaux, Pessac, France

Petra Cela, Marek Hampl and Marcela Buchtova
Institute of Animal Physiology and Genetics, v.v.i., Academy of Sciences of the Czech Republic, Brno, Czech Republic
Department of Animal Physiology and Immunology, Institute of Experimental Biology, Masaryk University, Brno, Czech Republic

Katherine K. Fu and Joy M. Richman
Life Sciences Institute, University of British Columbia, Vancouver, BC, Canada

Michaela Kunova Bosakova
Department of Biology, Faculty of Medicine, Masaryk University, Brno, Czech Republic

Pavel Krejci
Department of Biology, Faculty of Medicine, Masaryk University, Brno, Czech Republic
International Clinical Research Center, St. Anne's University Hospital, Brno, Czech

Index